Principles and Practice of Surgery

A. P. M. Forrest

Kt MD ChM FRCS (Ed., Eng., Glas.) FRSE
HonDSc (University of Wales; Chinese University of Hong Kong);
Hon LLD (University of Dundee); HonFACS HonFRACS HonFRCSCan HonFRCR
Professor Emeritus, University of Edinburgh

D. C. Carter

MD FRCS (Ed., Glas.)
Regius Professor of Clinical Surgery, Royal Infirmary of Edinburgh, UK

I. B. Macleod

BSc MB ChB FRCS (Ed.)
Consultant Surgeon, Royal Infirmary of Edinburgh, UK

SECOND EDITION

CHURCHILL LIVINGSTONE
EDINBURGH LONDON MADRID MELBOURNE NEW YORK AND TOKYO 1991

CHURCHILL LIVINGSTONE
Medical Division of Longman Group UK Limited

Distributed in the United States of America by Churchill
Livingstone Inc., 1560 Broadway, New York, N.Y. 10036
and by associated companies, branches and representatives
throughout the world.

First published 1985
Second edition 1991
    Reprinted 1991
    Reprinted 1992

ISBN 0-443-03909-7

British Library Cataloguing in Publication Data
Forest, Sir, Patrick, *1923–*
    Principles and practice of surgery. — 2nd ed.
    1. Medicine. Surgery
    I. Title   II. Carter, David C. (David Craig), *1940–*   III.
    Macleod, I. B. (Ian Buchanan)
    617

Library of Congress Cataloguing-in-Publication Data
Principles and practice of surgery/[edited by]
    A. P. M. Forrest, D. C. Carter, I. B. Macleod. — 2nd ed.
        p.   cm.
    ISBN 0-443-03909-7
    1. Surgery. 2. Surgery, Operative.   I. Forest, A. P. M.
    II. Carter, David C. (David Craig)   III. Macleod,
    I. B. (Ian Buchanan)
    [DNLM: 1. Surgery. 2. Surgery, Operative.
    WO 100 P9565]   RD31.P85   1991
    617 — dc20
    DNLM/DLC
    for Library of Congress   89-20967

Printed in Great Britain by The Bath Press, Avon

Principles and Practice of Surgery

Preface

The first edition of our textbook *Principles and Practice of Surgery* was written at the suggestion of Dr. John McLeod who was at that time the editor of Davidson's *Principles and Practice of Medicine*. The success of our first edition has confirmed that there was indeed a need for a 'surgical companion' to Davidson's classic textbook. We are now pleased to present the second edition of the textbook and intend to continue to update the work so as to keep pace with the rapidly changing developments in surgery.

Once again we make no apology for not following the trend to shorter and shorter textbooks of surgery for undergraduates. We hope that we have again compiled a reasoned and readable textbook. A large amount of outdated material has been deleted in exchange for coverage of new developments. Careful editing has resulted in a textbook of approximately the same length as the first edition. The book is still aimed principally at undergraduates but we hope that it may prove useful for postgraduates preparing to sit the new Part I examination in Surgery which is being introduced as the initial stage of the Fellowship Examination by the Royal Colleges of Surgeons.

As with the first edition most of this book has been written, cross-checked and edited by the three of us. We have once again incorporated contributions dealing with specialist subjects by Professor J. D. Cash (Transfusion of Blood and Blood Products), Professor G. D. Chisholm (Urological Surgery), Professor E. R. Hitchcock (Neurosurgery) and Professor D. J. Wheatley (Cardiac disease) and practical procedures and medico-legal problems by Mr I. M. C. Macintyre. We have incorporated new contributions from other specialists, namely Mr. G. G. Browning (Head, Neck and Salivary Glands/Mouth, Nose, Throat and Ear), Professor J. G. Collee (Infections and Antibiotics), Mr. J. H. Dark (Chest and Mediastinum), Professor M. H. Irving (Multiple Injury), Mr. C. V. Ruckley (Peripheral Vascular Disease), Professor A. A. Spence (Anaesthesia and the Operation), and Mr. A. C. H. Watson (Wounds and Wound Healing/Burns). We are grateful to all of them for allowing us to edit their work stringently so that it conforms to the style of the rest of the book.

A number of illustrations from the first edition have been deleted and replaced with new drawings. Once again we are grateful to our Medical Artist, Mrs. Anne McNeill for her contribution. We have relied greatly on Mrs. Wendy Taylor for secretarial support and wish to acknowledge gratitude to her for her patience and forbearance. Finally we would like to thank Mrs. Ilske Carter for her painstaking care in preparation of the manuscripts for publication.

Edinburgh, 1990

A.P.M.F.
D.C.C.
I.B.M.

Contributors

G. G. Browning MD FRCS (Ed., Glas.)
Professor of Otolaryngology;
Consultant in Administrative Charge of the
Department of Otolaryngology,
University of Glasgow,
Royal Infirmary,
Glasgow, UK

D. C. Carter MD FRCS (Ed., Glas.)
Regius Professor of Clinical Surgery,
University of Edinburgh;
Honorary Consultant Surgeon,
Royal Infirmary,
Edinburgh, UK

J. D. Cash BSc PhD FRCP (Ed.) FRCPath
National Medical Director,
Scottish National Blood Transfusion Service,
Edinburgh, UK

G. D. Chisholm ChM PRCSE FRCS
Professor of Surgery
University of Edinburgh;
Consultant Urological Surgeon,
Western General Hospital;
Director, Nuffield Transplant Unit,
Edinburgh, UK

J. G. Collee CBE MD FRCPath FRCP (Ed.)
Professor of Bacteriology,
University of Edinburgh;
Consultant in Bacteriology,
Lothian Health Board;
Consultant Adviser in Microbiology,
Scottish Home and Health Development,
Edinburgh, UK

J. H. Dark FRCS
Consultant Cardiothoracic Surgeon,
Freeman Hospital,
Newcastle upon Tyne, UK

A. P. M. Forrest Kt MD ChM FRCS (Ed.; Eng.; Glas.)
DSc(Hon) LLD(Hon) FACS(Hon) FRACS(Hon) FRCS Can(Hon)
FRCR(Hon) FRSE
Professor Emeritus,
University of Edinburgh, UK

E. R. Hitchcock MB ChM FRCS(Eng.) FRCS(Ed.)
Professor of Neurosurgery,
University of Birmingham,
UK

M. Irving MD ChM FRCS
Professor of Surgery,
University of Manchester;
Honorary Consultant Surgeon,
Hope Hospital,
Salford, UK

I. M. C. Macintyre FRCS(Ed.)
Consultant Surgeon,
Western General Hospital,
Edinburgh, UK

I. B. Macleod BSc FRCS(Ed.)
Consultant Surgeon,
Royal Infirmary of Edinburgh;
Honorary Senior Lecturer,
Department of Surgery,
University of Edinburgh, UK;
Surgeon to the Queen in Scotland

C. V. Ruckley ChM FRCS(Ed.)
Consultant Surgeon,
Royal Infirmary of Edinburgh;
Reader, Department of Surgery,
University of Edinburgh, UK

A. A. Spence MD FCAnaes FRCPG
Professor of Anaesthetics,
University of Edinburgh,
UK

A. C. H. Watson FRCS(Ed.)
Consultant Plastic Surgeon,
Lothian Health Board;
Part Time Senior Lecturer,
University of Edinburgh, UK

D. J. Wheatley MD ChM FRCS
British Heart Foundation Professor of Cardiac
Surgery,
University of Glasgow;
Honorary Consultant Cardiothoracic Surgeon,
Greater Glasgow Health Board,
Glasgow, UK

Contents

1. The metabolic response to operation and injury

Following accidental or deliberate injury, a series of changes occur both locally and generally which in due course serve to restore the status quo. The local response of inflammation is supported by a generalized response which conserves fluid and provides energy for repair. The generalized response is protean in its manifestations and is termed the 'metabolic response' to trauma.

There is an *ebb* and a *flow* phase following injury. The short ebb phase corresponds to the period of traumatic shock and is associated with general depression of enzymatic activity and oxygen consumption. The flow phase which follows is divided into two parts. The initial *catabolic phase* is characterized by protein and fat mobilization, with associated increased urinary nitrogen excretion and weight loss, and usually lasts 3–8 days. This is followed by an *anabolic phase* lasting for some weeks during which protein and fat stores are restored and weight is regained (the recovery phase).

It is believed that the changes following injury are due to a complex neuroendocrine mechanism designed to conserve body fluid volume, to mobilize amino acids from protein for gluconeogenesis and wound repair, and to mobilize fat for energy production.

The description that follows concentrates on the catabolic period of the flow phase as this is the period of most concern in the management of patients after operation or serious injury.

FACTORS INITIATING THE METABOLIC RESPONSE

The term 'injury' embraces a wide variety of insults, including trauma, haemorrhage and burns. Other factors which may induce or prolong the metabolic response include infection, myocardial infarction and pulmonary embolism.

Volume depletion

Volume depletion is by far the most important single factor initiating the metabolic response to injury. Fluid loss is obvious in haemorrhage or burns. At the site of any injury or infection there is local oedema due to excess fluid transudation from capillaries. This fluid sequestrates locally and is effectively lost from the circulating fluid volume. Changes in volume result in changes in plasma osmolality, which further modify the response (see Ch.2).

Catecholamines play an important role in volume conservation. They have vasoconstrictive effects on the kidney and on the circulation in general. They also affect intermediate metabolism of carbohydrate, fat and protein. The catecholamines have been described as the 'front runner' hormones in the neuroendocrine response to injury.

Afferent nerve impulses

Afferent impulses, notably pain, play a lesser, though significant, role in the response. On reaching the hypothalamus, they stimulate autonomic nerves and provoke the release of pituitary hormones. In some cases the injury may have been anticipated by the patient and, as a result, the hypothalamic response is triggered by impulses from higher centres before injury. In support of the significance of afferent nerve impulses, it has been demonstrated experimentally that the response to a standardized limb injury is much reduced by the section of nerves to that limb. Patients undergoing surgery under spinal anaesthesia show a delayed response.

Toxic factors

The role of toxic factors in initiating the metabolic response is not clearly defined. It is possible that they exert a modifying rather than initiating effect. They may be exogenous or endogenous.

Exogenous factors. Both exotoxins (e.g. from *Clostridium welchii*) and endotoxins (e.g. Gram-negative organisms) may produce shock (see Ch.3) and initiate the metabolic response.

Endogenous factors. Particulate matter such as fat emboli or small platelet aggregates produced after injury may generate afferent vagal stimuli and thus modify the response to injury. It has been suggested that non-particulate factors released from an injured site or hypoxic area (e.g. ATP, kinins, myoglobin) may also initiate the response.

FACTORS MODIFYING THE METABOLIC RESPONSE

There are many factors which modify the magnitude and duration of the metabolic response. The most important ones are listed below.

1. *Severity of injury.* The greater the injury, the greater the response.

2. *Nature of injury.* Burns produce a greater response than other injuries of comparable size, probably because of the greater heat loss from the burn area (see Ch.13).

3. *Infection.* The metabolic response is potentiated by infection; the catabolic phase persists as long as the infection remains.

4. *Other complications.* Deep venous thrombosis and pulmonary embolism, among others, potentiate the response.

5. *Nutritional status.* Patients in a poor nutritional state at the time of injury have a weaker response than well-nourished patients. Starvation frequently occurs after operation or injury and its effects complement those of the metabolic response (see later).

6. *Ambient temperature.* Much of the increased metabolic activity after injury is directed towards maintaining body temperature. This is particularly true in patients with thermal burns who lose energy due to evaporation of water from the burn. If the usual ambient temperature of approximately 20°C in hospitals in temperate climates is raised to 30–32°C, energy expenditure and consequent metabolic demand are much reduced after injury. This knowledge is exploited in specialized burns units.

7. *Corticosteroids.* These have an important permissive role in that a certain minimum level of circulating corticosteroids is necessary to produce the metabolic response. Adrenalectomized animals do not produce a metabolic response to injury unless given maintenance doses of corticosteroids.

8. *Age and sex.* The metabolic response is less pronounced in children and the elderly. However, there is some doubt whether children would still have a smaller response when body weight or lean body mass is taken into account. Premenopausal females appear to produce a smaller response than males of comparable age.

9. *Anaesthesia and drugs.* Pharmacological and anaesthetic agents may modify the response by affecting the vascular system and hormone production. For example, ether stimulates the output of catecholamines and antidiuretic hormone (ADH, i.e. vasopressin), morphine stimulates release of ADH, and spinal anaesthesia reduces the initial response by blocking afferent pathways.

10. *Other factors.* Meticulous and gentle handling of tissues during operation reduces the severity of trauma and thus the postoperative metabolic demand. Prompt and adequate replacement of fluid loss limits liberation of catecholamines, aldosterone and ADH. In some cases the phase of oliguria and sodium retention may be avoided if replacement accurately balances loss. Provision of sufficient calories (energy) and nitrogen during the catabolic phase may keep to a minimum and occasionally prevent weight loss and negative nitrogen balance. However, it is doubtful whether this has a significant effect on wound healing or the duration of hospital stay in previously healthy patients undergoing elective surgery. In undernourished patients or those with

severe trauma or sepsis, the provision of adequate energy and nitrogen considerably influences recovery. In all patients prolonged post-traumatic starvation adversely affects convalescence.

CHANGES OCCURRING DURING THE METABOLIC RESPONSE

Pulse and temperature changes

Following injury the pulse rate rises temporarily due to catecholamine release. Frequently there is a small rise in temperature lasting 24–48 hours, the so-called 'sympathetic fever'. This reflects a general increase in heat production, accompanied by an altered 'setting' of the temperature regulation centre under the influence of catecholamines. This rise in temperature is not due to infection and does not call for the use of antibiotics.

Water and salt retention

Oliguria is common after injury and normally lasts 48–72 hours. It is a consequence of release of antidiuretic hormone and aldosterone.

Antidiuretic hormone. ADH production is increased when *volume receptors* in the atria and hypothalamus are stimulated as a result of a reduction in blood volume. Neural stimuli reaching the supraoptic nucleus from the injured part also result in ADH release. Any increase in osmolality stimulates *osmoreceptors* in the anterior hypothalamus, causing further secretion of ADH. ADH acts principally on the collecting tubules of the kidney and to a lesser extent on the distal tubule to promote reabsorption of water. If excess water is administered to a patient during this phase, hypotonicity and hyponatraemia will result.

Aldosterone. Aldosterone acts on the kidney to conserve sodium and so further reduces urine volume. Aldosterone secretion is increased by the following mechanisms, of which the *renin–angiotensin* mechanism is much the most important.

1. The juxtaglomerular apparatus of the kidney is sensitive to minor alterations in glomerular arteriolar inflow pressure, and secretes renin if inflow pressure falls. Renin acts with angiotensinogen to form angiotensin I. This is converted to angiotensin II, a substance which stimulates production of aldosterone by the adrenal cortex (Fig. 1.1). The macula densa is a specialized area of tubular epithelium immediately adjacent to the juxtaglomerular apparatus which is sensitive to small alterations in the sodium concentration of urine in the proximal tubule. Any reduction in sodium concentration activates renin release.

2. A minor role is played by receptors in the right atrium which are sensitive to changes in circulating blood volume and by receptors in the carotid artery sensitive to changes in arterial pressure. Any decrease in blood volume and/or drop in arterial pressure results in hypothalamic stimulation and release of corticotropin (ACTH).

3. Aldosterone release may also be activated by a decrease in plasma sodium concentration or an increase in plasma potassium concentration reaching the adrenal cortex. Such changes in plasma concentrations occur frequently after injury.

Aldosterone acts principally on the distal renal tubules to promote reabsorption of sodium and bicarbonate, with increased excretion of potassium and hydrogen ions. Aldosterone also affects the exchange of sodium and potassium across all cell membranes, particularly those of cardiac and smooth muscle, possibly by modifying the effect of catecholamines on these cells. Large quantities of intracellular potassium are released into the extracellular fluid, which may cause a significant rise in serum potassium if renal function is impaired.

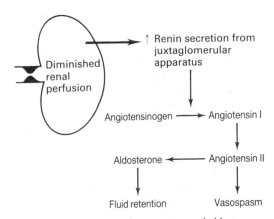

Fig. 1.1 The juxtaglomerular apparatus and aldosterone release

The tendency to retain sodium and bicarbonate after injury may produce metabolic alkalosis with potentially adverse effects on delivery of oxygen to the tissues (see Ch. 3).

In the absence of sweating, the only significant route of excretion of sodium and potassium in healthy individuals is via the kidneys. Approximately 50–80 mmol of each ion are excreted in the urine each 24 hours. Following injury, urinary sodium excretion may fall to 10–20 mmol per 24 hours for 2–3 days, depending on the severity of injury and the degree of fluid and electrolyte replacement. Potassium excretion may rise to 100–200 mmol per 24 hours for a similar period. This should be taken into account when calculating requirements for replacement after injury.

Carbohydrate, protein and fat metabolism

Carbohydrate

In the absence of intake, existing body carbohydrate stores will supply needs for only 8–12 hours. Nevertheless, following injury there is a period of *hyperglycaemia*, the duration of which depends on the severity of injury and the presence of complications such as infection. The hyperglycaemia is produced by a combination of hepatic glycogenolysis and gluconeogenesis, and is initiated largely by catecholamine release and sympathetic overactivity.

Catecholamines increase glycogenolysis directly and also act indirectly by suppressing release of insulin and stimulating that of glucagon. Suppression of insulin release favours the release of amino acids from muscle, which are then available for gluconeogenesis. In addition, the effect of insulin on glucose metabolism is inhibited, possibly as a result of increased growth hormone levels. Glucagon is a potent stimulant of hepatic gluconeogenesis but does not significantly affect the efflux of amino acids from skeletal muscle. Thyroxine can also accelerate gluconeogenesis but its precise role following trauma is not known.

Increased breakdown of muscle protein and gluconeogenesis characterize the catabolic phase following injury, and the resultant hyperglycaemia is sometimes called *the diabetes of injury*. The provision of exogenous glucose and insulin in severely injured patients may lessen this effect. Such therapy has been used in patients whose catabolic demands are excessive, e.g. those with severe burns.

Protein

The average daily intake of protein by a healthy adult is between 80 and 120 g (13–20 g of nitrogen). Of this, 2–4 g of nitrogen are lost daily in the stool and 10–16 g in the urine. After injury the loss of urinary nitrogen increases. Following severe trauma or major burns it may reach three to four times the normal amount. Nitrogen is lost in the form of urea, and the concentration of blood urea rises rapidly if renal function is impaired.

The rise in nitrogen excretion appears soon after injury. Following routine elective surgery, it reaches a peak during the first week, returning to normal after 5–8 days. In major trauma, severe burns or severe infection, the increase in nitrogen excretion may continue for many weeks. Such patients are usually not capable of eating sufficient protein to match this loss, either because of intestinal ileus or the anorexia associated with injury. This is the phase of *negative nitrogen balance*. Provision of adequate energy (calories) and protein by the parenteral (intravenous) route may modify or even prevent this phase, and parenteral feeding is indicated if negative nitrogen balance is likely to last for more than a few days (see Ch.5).

Negative nitrogen balance is associated with weight loss due to loss of muscle mass. The extent can be calculated as follows:

1 g nitrogen = 6 g muscle protein = 30 g wet muscle mass.

A patient with a negative nitrogen balance of 15 g nitrogen a day thus loses approximately 450 g of muscle mass daily. The provision of adequate carbohydrate calories has a protein-sparing effect, reducing the degree of negative nitrogen balance by preventing the need for gluconeogenesis.

Fat

Though energy derived from protein is important,

the principal source of energy following trauma and during starvation is adipose tissue with its large triglyceride store. Catecholamines and glucagon activate adenyl cyclase in the fat cells and produce cyclic adenosine monophosphate (cyclic AMP). This in turn leads to activation of triglyceride lipase and the breakdown of triglycerides to fatty acids and glycerol. Growth hormone and cortisol have a similar, though less important effect. Glycerol provides substrate for gluconeogenesis, while free fatty acids provide energy for all tissues and for hepatic gluconeogenesis. The decreased level of insulin following injury encourages lipolysis. A total of 200–500 g of fat may be broken down daily after severe trauma.

Anabolic phase

Following the catabolic phase of metabolism the patient goes into an anabolic phase characterized by positive nitrogen balance, a regaining of weight, and restoration of fat deposits. The turning point is often obvious clinically in that the patient feels much better and his appetite returns, often quite suddenly. The hormones which contribute to anabolism are growth hormone, androgens and 17-ketosteroids.

The effects of the various hormones affecting energy metabolism during the metabolic response to injury are summarized in Table 1.1.

Changes in blood coagulation

After injury or infection, the blood may be hypercoagulable or hypocoagulable. *Hypercoagulation* appears first and may contribute to the increased incidence of deep venous thrombosis and pulmonary embolism after operation or trauma. It is most marked in the first 12 hours after injury; increased secretion of ACTH and cortisol may be responsible by increasing the number of platelets and their adhesiveness. Noradrenaline also tends to increase coagulability.

Serum fibrinogen levels rise after injury. In patients with severe sepsis this rise is often long

Table 1.1 Effects of hormones on metabolism after injury

Catecholamines — the stress hormones

Hyperglycaemia
1. by action on liver — glycogenolysis
2. by action on muscle glycogen → lactic acid → glucose in liver (Cori cycle)
3. by action on pancreas — suppression of insulin (mainly alpha-stimulation); stimulation of glucagon (beta-stimulation)

Increase in metabolic rate (beta-stimulation)

Mobilization of free fatty acids
direct action on fat cells, which is potentiated by low insulin levels

Insulin — the storage hormone
In non-stress states, insulin secretion in response to increasing blood glucose concentration facilitates the entry of glucose into many tissues with increased glycogenesis and lipogenesis. Low insulin concentrations after injury lead to:
1. accelerated triglyceride breakdown
2. increased release of amino acids from muscle
3. impaired entry of potassium and phosphate ions into cells.

Glucocorticoids, glucagon and growth hormone — the permissive hormones

Glucocorticoids are released in response to elevated ACTH levels after injury or stress and have a permissive role, augmenting specific metabolic responses to stress.
1. Hepatic gluconeogenesis is augmented by stimulating enzymes which increase direct conversion of 3-carbon fragments into glucose.
2. Mobilization of amino acids from the periphery is facilitated.
3. Lipolysis is augmented.

Glucagon has actions on the liver opposed to those of insulin. Its major role after injury is strong stimulation of hepatic gluconeogenesis. It does not contribute to increased efflux of amino acids from muscle, but acts with catecholamines to stimulate lipolysis.

Growth hormone has effects in both the catabolic and the anabolic phase.
1. The insulin response to altered blood glucose levels is 're-set'.
2. Free fatty acid release is augmented.
3. Nitrogen retention is augmented provided there is sufficient supply of non-protein calories.

sustained and followed by a gradual fall. A rapid fall is associated with a poor prognosis.

Hypocoagulation follows hypercoagulation and is associated with increased fibrinolysis and a reduction in serum fibrinogen. This can lead to

FASTING MAN
(24-hour basal requirement 1800 kcal)

ORIGIN AND TYPE
OF FUEL

FUEL CONSUMPTION

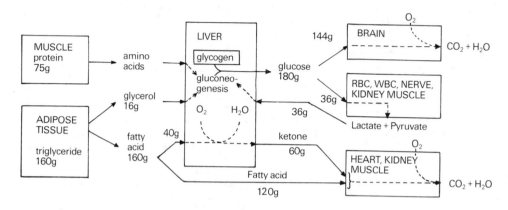

TRAUMATIZED MAN
(24-hour requirement 2400 kcal)

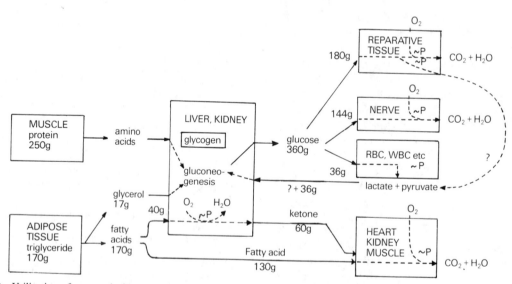

Fig. 1.2 Utilization of energy during starvation. (From Cahill G. F., N. Eng. J. Med. 282: 668, 1970)

generalized bleeding and, though not common, is seen most frequently after severe shock (particularly bacteraemic shock with disseminated intravascular coagulation), after operation on patients with disseminated carcinoma or extensive liver disease, or following cardiopulmonary bypass.

STARVATION AND ITS CONTRIBUTION TO THE METABOLIC RESPONSE

All patients who undergo surgery or suffer severe injury will be starved for a period. It is customary to starve patients for about 12 hours before elective surgery and most are unlikely to take any food on the day of operation itself. Patients undergoing operation on the alimentary tract may not be able to take food for 2–3 days after the operation. Those who develop complications may have to forego food for days or even weeks. Patients with intra-abdominal disease, e.g. carcinoma of the alimentary tract, may have had an inadequate intake for weeks or months before operation.

If the trauma of surgery is relatively minor and followed by only a short period of starvation, as with cholecystectomy, and vagotomy and drainage for example, the changes in metabolism are similar to those caused by starvation alone; after major trauma there are marked differences.

In acute starvation, intermediate metabolism of protein, carbohydrate and fat is altered to preserve the supply of energy to the brain from 6-carbon compounds such as glucose by increasing hepatic glycogenolysis and gluconeogenesis.

Body energy is stored in the form of glycogen, protein and triglycerides. *Glycogen* is stored in the liver and in muscle in combination with water and electrolytes. In this state each gram provides only 2 kcal of energy compared to 4 kcal/g when it is dry. *Triglycerides* are not stored in combination with water, and 1 g of body fat provides just over 9 kcal of energy. *Protein* is stored mainly in muscle and is combined with water, so that muscle contains approximately 20% of its weight as protein. Each gram of dry protein provides 4 kcal. Protein is not used primarily as an energy source but as a source of antibodies and enzymes, and to produce structural and plasma proteins. Ingested protein in excess of that needed to replenish body stores is metabolized; any unused energy is stored as fat. In the absence of intake of food, protein provides energy through gluconeogenesis.

The total energy stores of a healthy 70 kg male are shown in Table 1.2. The plasma proteins (210 g) potentially contribute 840 kcal to the stores. In short-term fasting the body can replenish plasma proteins at a rate equal to utilization. However, in marked catabolism the rate of utilization of plasma proteins exceeds that of liver synthesis. Unless exogenous proteins are provided, hypoproteinaemia results.

In early starvation the basal energy requirement of a 70 kg adult is approximately 1800 kcal per 24 hours. The manner in which the body provides

Table 1.2 Source of energy in a 70 kg male. Assuming a basal expenditure of 1800 kcal, the fasting survival time would be approximately 3 months

Source	Type of fuel	Weight of fuel	Energy produced (kcal)
Fat (adipose tissue)	Triglycerols	15 kg	141 000
Muscle	Protein	6 kg	24 000
Liver and muscle	Glygogen	225 g	900
Circulating	Glucose, fatty acids, triglycerols, etc.	23 g	100
			166 000

and utilizes this energy is shown in Figure 1.2. The brain uses most of the available glucose, but some is broken down anaerobically in kidney and muscle to provide pyruvate and lactate, which are recycled to provide further glucose by gluconeogenesis. The majority of body tissues use fatty acids and ketones as an energy source.

If starvation is prolonged beyond a few hours, the glycogen stores in the liver and muscle become depleted. Muscle protein converted to glucose by gluconeogenesis maintains the brain's energy supply. This process cannot be continued indefinitely, and after 2–3 weeks the brain gradually reduces its glucose consumption and utilizes ketones as an energy source. The amount of muscle protein used falls to about 20 g per day while fat consumption increases. The total energy requirement decreases from 1800 kcal to about 1500 kcal per day.

Differences between effects of trauma and starvation

As can be seen from the above, the general trend of the metabolic changes occurring in starvation is similar to that after trauma, but the combination of trauma and starvation *accelerates* utilization of body stores of protein and fat. However, important differences exist between the two states.

Protein metabolism

In simple starvation the peak nitrogen loss is around 0.1 g/kg body weight per day. The losses are greater in post-traumatic catabolism and in severe injury, and in sepsis may reach 0.4 g/kg body weight per day. The blood urea level normally falls in simple starvation, whereas following major injury the level is normal or elevated. The increases in urinary creatinine excretion which occur after injury are not seen in simple starvation, and reflect differences in protein catabolism.

Blood sugar

During simple starvation, blood sugar levels fall and remain low, despite increased glucagon levels. Following trauma, blood sugar levels are elevated. In simple starvation, administration of glucose produces a rise in insulin secretion. This does not occur after trauma as long as the catecholamine level is increased.

Hormonal response

The increased output of ADH, aldosterone, catecholamines and glucocorticoids seen after trauma does not occur in simple starvation.

Ratio of non-protein to protein calories for tissue synthesis

In simple starvation, the optimal ratio of non-protein to protein calories to ensure that amino acids are used for synthesis rather than as a source of energy is 100 kcal/g nitrogen. After trauma, this ratio is increased to at least 200 kcal/g nitrogen.

Reversibility of metabolic changes

The metabolic changes of simple starvation are rapidly reversed by feeding, either orally or parenterally, and positive nitrogen balance is easily achieved. After major injury, the changes are not reversed until increased hormone secretion reverts to normal and feeding by any route results in a marked wastage of nitrogenous products in the urine. However, it may be possible to achieve a positive balance by giving large amounts of nitrogen rapidly.

2. Principles of fluid and electrolyte balance in surgical patients

The majority of surgical patients with fluid and electrolyte problems cannot take in fluid by mouth so that it has to be administered intravenously. The effect of trauma on the secretion of anti-diuretic hormone (ADH) and aldosterone necessitates careful control of fluid administration in the early postoperative period. Adequate amounts of water, sodium and potassium with anions (supplied as chloride) are routine requirements. In a few individuals, particularly those with chronic gastrointestinal tract loss, deficiencies of calcium and magnesium require correction.

Normal water and electrolyte balance

In calculating fluid and electrolyte requirements it is essential to know how much the patient has lost so that accurate replacement maintains balance. The healthy individual loses fluid by three routes: the kidneys, the gastrointestinal tract, and the skin and respiratory passages. In a 70 kg adult approximately 1500–2000 ml of urine is passed in 24 hours, 200–300 ml of fluid is lost in faeces, and 800–1000 ml is lost as water vapour from the skin and respiratory tract (*insensible water loss*). The onset of sweating (*sensible water loss*) greatly increases water loss from the skin. Water is taken in as fluids and in solid food; an additional 100–200 ml per 24 hours is provided endogenously by oxidation of fat.

In the absence of sweating, almost all the sodium lost is in the urine (50–80 mmol/24 hours). Under the influence of aldosterone the kidney can reduce sodium loss to about 10–20 mmol/24 hours. The principal route of potassium excretion is also via the kidney, some 60–100 mmol being lost in the urine each day. The kidney cannot conserve

Table 2.1 Normal daily losses and requirements

	Volume (ml)	Na$^+$ (mmol)	K$^+$ (mmol)
Urine	2000	80	60
Insensible loss	800	—	—
Faeces	300	—	—
Minus endogenous water	−100	—	—
Requirement	3000	80	60

potassium as efficiently as sodium, but in severe potassium deficiency can reduce losses to 40 mmol per day. The normal daily losses and the requirements to maintain fluid and electrolyte balance are summarized in Table 2.1.

Intravenous administration of normal requirements

When fulfilling these requirements by the intravenous route, sodium is normally provided as 0.9% sodium chloride, which contains 154 mmol sodium and 154 mmol chloride per litre. As it is isotonic with plasma, it is traditionally called *normal* or *physiological* saline. For practical purposes, 500 ml of normal saline supplies the daily requirement of sodium. The remaining volume requirement (2.5 litres) is given as an isotonic non-electrolyte solution such as 5% dextrose. Potassium can be added either to saline or to dextrose from ampoules containing 1.5 g potassium chloride (i.e. 20 mmol of potassium and 20 mmol of chloride). Three ampoules supply a patient's daily need. Increasingly, such additives to intravenous solution bags are added in the hospital pharmacy prior to despatch to the wards, or are added by the manufacturer.

Table 2.2 Provision of the normal 24-hour fluid and electrolyte requirement (4 hours per bottle)

1. 500 ml 0.9% NaCl + 1.5 g KCl
2. 500 ml 5% Dextrose
3. 500 ml 5% Dextrose + 1.5 g KCl
4. 500 ml 5% Dextrose
5. 500 ml 5% Dextrose + 1.5 g KCl
6. 500 ml 5% Dextrose

Instructions for the provision of the *normal* 24-hour fluid and electrolyte requirements are given in Table 2.2.

It is advisable that potassium is not administered in concentrations greater than 80 mmol/l except in severe potassium deficiency (continuous ECG monitoring is then essential). Potassium should *never* be given as an intravenous bolus, as cardiac arrest will occur.

Effect of sweating on requirements

Hyperventilation increases insensible water loss, and pyrexia also raises the water loss from the skin by approximately 200 ml per day for each 1°C rise in temperature. The onset of sweating considerably increases fluid loss, which may reach a rate of 1 l/hour. Calculation of the amount of fluid lost by sweating is difficult and repeated weighing of the patient may be necessary. Sweat contains significant amounts of sodium (20–70 mmol/l) and potassium (10 mmol/l), and these losses must be taken into account when calculating requirements.

Effect of operation on fluid and electrolyte balance

Following operation, release of antidiuretic hormone conserves water by its action on the distal convoluted and collecting tubules. Oliguria results so that the urine volume is reduced to 1000–1500 ml for 2–3 days. Attempts to produce a diuresis by administration of water in the form of 5% dextrose are unsuccessful and only produce hyponatraemia and possibly water intoxication.

Aldosterone secretion conserves sodium and further contributes to oliguria. In the first 2 days after operation the urinary excretion of sodium is reduced to approximately 30 mmol/24 hours.

Potassium excretion is increased during this period to approximately 120 mmol per day, due partly to the influence of aldosterone on the kidney and partly to the liberation of potassium from body cells generally. This liberation is enhanced by cellular damage and further free potassium provided by the infusion of stored blood, so that serum potassium levels tend to rise in the early postoperative period, particularly if the glomerular filtration rate is reduced. For this reason intravenous potassium should not be given in the first 48 hours after operation unless the patient is hypokalaemic or was potassium-deficient preoperatively.

Sequestration of extracellular fluid at the site of operation produces local oedema and temporary loss of fluid from the circulation. Sequestration persists for approximately 48 hours and may involve up to 4 litres of fluid, depending on the severity of the operation or injury. After partial gastrectomy 500 ml per 24 hours is the likely sequestration loss. Sequestration must be taken into account when calculating fluid and electrolyte requirements.

Not all patients require intravenous support following an operation. The majority tolerate 48 hours of fluid deprivation with only thirst and a possible increase in the risk of deep venous thrombosis. However, patients are more comfortable if fluid losses are replaced. If in doubt or if there is evidence of impaired renal or cardiac function, it is better to err on the side of underhydration rather than risk overhydration with the induction of hyponatraemia and/or pulmonary oedema.

Causes of fluid and electrolyte loss from the alimentary tract

The majority of surgical patients requiring intravenous fluid and electrolyte therapy for sustained periods have continuing fluid loss from the gut. This may be due to any of the following circumstances.

Intestinal obstruction

In general terms, the higher the obstruction in the intestine the greater the fluid loss. This is due to failure of fluids secreted by the upper alimentary tract to reach the absorptive areas of the distal jejunum and ileum. Thus a patient with a high small bowel obstruction loses fluid more rapidly than one with a low small bowel obstruction. Major fluid loss from vomiting is not a feature of large bowel obstruction until very late in its course.

Adynamic ileus

This condition, in which the small intestine ceases to function propulsively, may result from infection, electrolyte imbalance (particularly potassium, calcium and magnesium deficiency), hypoproteinaemia, retroperitoneal trauma or haemorrhage, hypoxia, head injury or neurosurgical operations, and often accompanies shock from different causes. Distension of the gut from swallowed air results in an increase in intestinal secretions and reduction of absorptive capacity. Unless the intestinal fluid is removed by nasogastric aspiration, vomiting is persistent.

Intestinal fistula

Fluid loss from an intestinal fistula may be considerable. As with obstruction, the higher the fistula the greater the fluid loss. Fluid loss is not often a major problem with fistulas of the large bowel.

Diarrhoea

Fluid and electrolyte loss from diarrhoea may also be considerable. For example, in cholera and similar superinfections of the gut, some 6–10 litres may be lost each day, resulting in fatal contraction of extracellular fluid volume.

Table 2.3 shows approximate concentrations of electrolytes in some gastrointestinal fluids and may be used to calculate losses over short periods. There is considerable variation in their constitution, and if gastrointestinal loss continues for more than 2–3 days, all the fluid and urine should be collected and sent to the laboratory for accurate determination of electrolyte content. Because of this variation in the constitution of intestinal fluids, the use of specially prepared fluids such as 'gastric solutions' is not recommended. An example of how a patient's short-term requirements may be provided is given in Table 2.4.

In patients requiring replacement for more than 3–4 days, calculations such as those shown in Table 2.4 are likely to be inaccurate. The correction of acid-base imbalance and the provision of parenteral nutrition will have to be considered. The need for ions other than sodium and potassium should be considered if intestinal fluid loss continues, particularly magnesium (up to 1 mmol/kg body weight per 24 hours) and calcium (10–60 ml of 10% calcium gluconate, i.e. 4.5–27 mmol, per day).

Patients who have pre-existing fluid and electrolyte deficiency, or who develop deficiencies under treatment, should have these corrected by adding the calculated deficit to the normal requirement, usually spreading this replacement over 2–3 days.

Table 2.3 Approximate electrolyte concentrations in plasma and various gastrointestinal fluids

	Volume (ml/24 hours)	Na^+ (mmol/l)	K^+ (mmol/l)	Cl^- (mmol/l)	HCO_3^- (mmol/l)
Plasma		140	5	100	25
Gastric juice	2500	50	10	80	40
Intestinal fluid (upper)	3000	140	10	100	25
Bile and pancreatic juice	1500	140	5	80	60
Mixed nasogastric aspirate	—	120	10	100	40
Ileostomy fluid: new	700	125	20	110	30
mature	500	50	5	20	25
Diarrhoea (inflammatory)	—	110	40	100	40

Table 2.4 Calculation of short-term fluid and electrolyte requirements in a patient with ileus

Assuming that the patient is in electrolyte balance and is losing 2 litres/24 hours as nasogastric tube aspirate and 1.5 litres as urine, his 24-hour losses can be calculated as follows:

	Vol. (ml)	Na$^+$ (mmol)	K$^+$ (mmol)
Urine	1500	80	60
Nasogastric aspirate	2000	240	20
Insensible loss	800	—	—
Minus endogenous water produced by oxidation	−300	—	—
Net losses/requirements	4000	320	80

Two litres of normal saline would supply 310 mmol of Na$^+$, which for practical purposes would satisfy the sodium needs; the remaining 2 litres of fluid required would be supplied as 5% dextrose. Thus, in short-term practice, provided urinary losses are normal, replacement of the nasogastric fluid volume-for-volume by normal saline gives the required sodium replacement, while the volume of fluid lost in urine (plus 500 ml) is replaced by dextrose. The required 80 mmol of K$^+$ would be supplied by four 1.5 g ampoules of potassium chloride.

WATER IMBALANCE

Water depletion

A reduction of 1–2% (350–700 ml) in total body water produces the sensation of thirst. Clinically obvious dehydration with intense thirst, a dry tongue, and loss of skin elasticity (particularly over the clavicles) signifies a deficiency of at least 1.5–2 litres. Pure water depletion is rare in surgical practice. Water depletion is usually combined with sodium loss, the combination being generally referred to as 'salt depletion'. The combined loss of sodium and water results in contraction of the extracellular fluid (ECF) volume with circulatory changes (vasoconstriction and tachycardia) as well as the clinical features of dehydration. The most frequent cause of salt depletion is loss of gastrointestinal secretions. Rapid infusion of isotonic saline is indicated.

Water excess

In contrast to pure water depletion, water excess is not uncommon in surgical practice, particularly in elderly postoperative patients who receive excess water in the face of persisting ADH activity. There is dilutional hyponatraemia, yet continued renal secretion of sodium despite the low serum levels. This contrasts with the hyponatraemia due to sodium depletion, in which urinary sodium excretion is minimal and the patient exhibits the clinical signs of reduction in blood volume. Patients with water excess look comparatively well.

Acute renal failure may produce a similar picture if the administration of water is continued in the face of oliguria. Chronic starvation can also produce dilutional hyponatraemia, in this case resulting from excess production of water from the metabolism of body fat in the presence of elevated ADH levels. There is also an increase in aldosterone activity, and total body sodium may actually be increased. A similar effect may be produced by chronic liver disease or congestive cardiac failure.

Inappropriate secretion of ADH can occur in a number of conditions, including sepsis, severe pulmonary infection, ectopic secretion by tumours of lung or pancreas, and disease of or trauma to the brain and meninges.

Treatment

If the condition of dilutional hyponatraemia due to water excess is recognized, any administration of water by mouth or intravenously (as 5% dextrose) should cease and the patient be allowed to 'dry out'. Electrolyte replacement should continue. In severe cases in which there is danger of water intoxication, hypertonic saline (3–5%) should be administered cautiously (100–200 ml over 2 hours) and the patient observed for rapid clinical improvement and a diuretic response. This therapy may be repeated after 12 hours.

SODIUM IMBALANCE

Sodium is the principal extracellular cation, and changes in its total amount or its concentration affect the volume and tonicity of the extracellular fluid. The sodium concentration is the main indicator of extracellular fluid tonicity. The concentration of other ions, e.g. Cl$^-$, HCO$_3^-$, K$^+$, is also affected by acid-base changes and renal function, and therefore does not reflect dilutional change in the same way as sodium, which is relatively uninfluenced by these other factors.

In most clinical situations which involve sodium excess or deficit there is a combination of volume and tonicity changes, either simultaneously or in sequence. It is artificial to consider changes in sodium without at the same time taking into account changes in its solvent, i.e. water. In general terms the significance of an elevated or low serum sodium concentration can best be determined from a study of the patient's history.

Sodium depletion

Causes

Acute sodium loss may be due to: (1) haemorrhage or plasma loss; (2) acute gastric dilatation (the patient may lose up to 1 litre of ECF per hour over a period of 3–5 hours); or (3) massive diarrhoea, e.g. cholera, staphylococcal or pseudomembranous enterocolitis.

Chronic sodium loss may occur as a result of chronic diarrhoea, protracted ileus, ileostomy or chronic renal disease.

As indicated above, true *dilutional hyponatraemia* can occur with a normal total body sodium but an excess of water.

Clinical features

As the fluid lost in these conditions is isotonic, there is contraction of ECF volume, along with the features of dehydration, i.e. thirst, oliguria and concentrated urine.

Treatment

It is essential that *isotonic* fluids are used for replacement. If water or hypotonic solutions are administered either orally or by intravenous infusion, ADH will continue to act in its water-preserving role so that excess water is not excreted: the ECF becomes hypotonic and serum sodium concentration falls. If this drops to below 110 mmol/l there is considerable danger of convulsions and water intoxication. Patients with major trauma or sepsis are likely to have persistent excess

ADH activity and are particularly liable to this form of hyponatraemia.

Isotonic fluid replacement is continued while the patient is allowed to 'dry out'. Treatment with hypertonic saline is rarely necessary and should be considered only if the serum sodium has fallen to 110 mmol/l or convulsions have developed. Correction of the sodium levels should be slow; too rapid changes may worsen the situation.

Mild dilutional hyponatraemia is harmless and does not call for the administration of sodium. In malnourished patients it is corrected by an adequate caloric intake.

Excess urinary loss of sodium due to chronic renal disease may require an increased intake of sodium.

Sodium excess

Causes

True sodium excess is usually iatrogenic, and is due to the continued excess administration of sodium in the face of persisting aldosterone activity. This is particularly likely to occur in the postoperative or post-injury period. The volume of ECF is expanded, increasing the risk of circulatory overload and pulmonary oedema.

Hypernatraemia associated with a true excess of sodium is relatively uncommon but may occur in primary (Conn's syndrome) or secondary hyperaldosteronism. Hypernatraemia occurs more frequently as a result of abnormal loss of water or hypotonic fluids.

1. *Pure water loss from skin or lungs*. The classic example is a shipwrecked sailor without access to water who may compound the situation by drinking sea water (which is hypertonic). In clinical practice pure water loss may occur in patients supported on a ventilator without adequate humidification.

2. *Loss of hypotonic fluid*. Sweat is hypotonic, and if excess sweating is not compensated for by taking fluid, hypernatraemia results. Gastrointestinal secretions may sometimes also be hypotonic, particularly in babies. Frequently the loss is replaced with drinking water, which produces

hyponatraemia; if only isotonic saline is given, true sodium overload with hypernatraemia can develop.

Clinical features

The consequences of hypernatraemia are (1) extreme thirst and (2) CNS symptoms, notably confusion proceeding to coma. The severity of the thirst is such that hypernatraemia is rare in the conscious patient who has access to water.

Treatment

Sodium excess is best treated by administration of pure water or hypotonic solutions. The temptation to achieve rapid correction of the abnormal sodium concentration should be resisted, as sudden changes in the tonicity of extracellular fluid can prove dangerous.

POTASSIUM IMBALANCE

Potassium is the principal intracellular cation. Its intracellular concentration is 150 mmol/l. Only 60 mmol of the total body potassium of 3000 mmol is contained in extracellular fluid, where its concentration varies around 4.0 mmol/l. Levels below 2.5 mmol/l and above 6.0 mmol/l are dangerous and may cause cardiac arrest.

Increasing the intake or output of potassium produces only slow changes in serum potassium concentrations. Rapid equilibration of intra- and extracellular potassium and efficient renal excretion guard against sudden changes in circulating concentrations. However, alterations in acid-base balance affect these exchanges and may produce rapid changes in extracellular potassium concentration.

Effect of acid-base changes on potassium balance

Derangement in acid-base balance causes changes in potassium balance within and outside the cell. Conversely, changes in potassium balance have secondary effects on acid-base balance.

Acidosis. Excess of hydrogen ions in the extracellular fluid causes hydrogen ions to move into the cells in exchange for an equivalent amount of potassium ions, which move out into the ECF. The serum potassium concentration rises and there is increased excretion of potassium in the urine. If the acidosis continues, a considerable deficit in total body potassium may result.

If the acidosis is corrected rapidly, without at the same time providing potassium ions, potassium levels in the serum may fall catastrophically as potassium returns to the cells. This dangerous situation can develop within a few hours and applies equally to metabolic and respiratory acidosis.

Alkalosis. In alkalosis the exchange of potassium for hydrogen ions takes place in the opposite direction. Hydrogen ions move out of the cell in exchange for potassium ions, which move in. Further, the kidneys conserve hydrogen ions at the expense of increased urinary loss of potassium. Hypokalaemia follows.

When the deficiency of potassium becomes severe, the kidney will again allow the excretion of hydrogen ions so that potassium is conserved. This paradoxical aciduria results in worsening of the alkalosis. In patients in this state, adequate replacement of potassium ions is again an essential part of treatment.

Effect of potassium imbalance on acid-base balance

Potassium excess and deficiency have secondary effects on the acid-base balance because of the exchange of potassium for sodium and hydrogen ions across the cell membrane. For every three ions of potassium withdrawn from the intracellular compartment two sodium and one hydrogen ion enter the cell. In states of potassium deficiency there is thus a developing intracellular acidosis and extracellular alkalosis. Conversely, when there is potassium excess with an increase in movement of potassium into the cell, sodium and hydrogen ions are kept out, leading to an extracellular acidosis.

Potassium depletion

Causes

Acid-base balance abnormalities apart, potassium depletion results from either inadequate intake or increased loss.

Inadequate intake. The kidney cannot conserve

potassium as efficiently as it does sodium. Even in the absence of all potassium intake, urinary loss of potassium continues at the rate of approximately 40 mmol per day. This loss is borne primarily by the cells; the level of serum potassium is maintained until late in the deficiency state. The cellular source of the potassium in the urine is indicated by the ratio of potassium to nitrogen, which is 3:1.

A special example of inadequate intake occurs in patients who are metabolically in an anabolic state, particularly when they are receiving intravenous nutrition. The formation of normal cellular components requires potassium, which can be supplied only from the extracellular fluid. If the exogenous source of potassium is not increased (up to 200–300 mmol per day), hypokalaemia may rapidly develop.

Increased loss. This may occur through factors affecting the kidney, e.g. administration of diuretics, excess secretion of aldosterone (this includes primary and secondary hyperaldosteronism and the response to stress) or other adrenocortical steroids, or it may be due to chronic loss of gastrointestinal secretions, e.g. from diarrhoea, malfunctioning ileostomy or the discharge of mucus from a villous papilloma.

In these cases the loss of potassium greatly exceeds that of nitrogen, indicating that it comes mainly from the extracellular fluid compartment. The ratio of potassium to nitrogen in the urine may be as high as 10:1. Hypokalaemia develops more rapidly than when due to starvation alone.

Clinical effects

The principal effect of hypokalaemia is impaired muscle contractility. There is generalized muscle weakness and ileus of the intestinal tract. The associated extracellular alkalosis may produce features of tetany with signs of neuromuscular irritability, including a positive Chvostek sign. Sensitivity to digitalis is increased, and this drug must be used with great care.

Electrocardiographic changes include an increased QT interval, depressed ST segment and inverted T waves. Should the serum potassium fall below 2.5 mmol/l cardic arrest may occur.

Treatment

Adequate replacement of potassium ions is essential. In severe deficiency states the recommended maximum rate of intravenous administration of 15 mmol/hour may be exceeded. Cardiac monitoring should then be instituted. Adequate provision of chloride ions (as NaCl) is necessary to correct the alkalosis.

Potassium excess

Causes

Excessive parenteral administration. Potassium is lost from the body mainly through the kidney. Normal daily potassium intake and urinary excretion each approximate 60–100 mmol. In the presence of normal renal function it is almost impossible to raise serum potassium levels by increasing *oral* intake. However, excessive or too rapid *parenteral* administration (in excess of 15 mmol/hour) may overwhelm the renal excretory mechanism and lead to hyperkalaemia.

Renal failure. Impaired renal function leads to a rapid rise in serum potassium concentration even when exogenous intake of potassium is reduced or prevented. Endogenous release of free potassium continues through cell breakdown, a factor enhanced in the postoperative catabolic phase.

The rise of serum potassium which occurs in acute renal failure approximates 0.1–0.5 mmol/l per day.

Clinical features

The clinical picture of hyperkalaemia is surprisingly similar to that of hypokalaemia. There is muscle weakness, loss of tendon reflexes and development of paralyses. Sensitivity to digitalis is impaired. Electrocardiographic changes include peaked T waves, an increase in the P-R interval and widening of the QRS complex.

Cardiac arrhythmias may develop. If the serum potassium exceeds 7.0 mmol/l, these may proceed to ventricular fibrillation.

Treatment

All administration of potassium is stopped.

Hyperkalaemia may be temporarily counter-acted by the administration of other cations. In an emergency, intravenous administration of 50–100 ml 10% calcium gluconate, 100 ml 1-molar sodium bicarbonate or 100 ml 5% sodium chloride will improve the clinical features for an hour or two.

A slower but longer-lasting depression of serum potassium levels may be achieved by slow (over 4 hours) intravenous infusion of 250 ml 25% glucose with 20 units soluble insulin, which 'drives' potassium back into the cells. This treat-ment may be continued for up to 24 hours.

Ion exchange resins, which exchange three sodium ions for each potassium ion, may be administered orally or rectally. The recommended dose is 10 g of resin orally or 30 g rectally 6-hourly.

If the serum potassium approaches 7 mmol/l, haemodialysis is indicated.

ACID-BASE BALANCE

Metabolic acidosis

Metabolic acidosis is common in surgical practice and is usually a consequence of impaired tissue perfusion (e.g. in shock). It is potentiated by renal failure. Metabolic acidosis can be suspected by the onset of deep rapid respirations in a depleted patient. The diagnosis is confirmed by measurement of arterial hydrogen ion concen-tration, blood gases, and standard bicarbonate. Therapy is directed towards restoring tissue per-fusion. Infusion of bicarbonate is only required when the plasma standard bicarbonate level is less than 15 mmol/l (normal value 24–32 mmol/l).

The amount of bicarbonate required to raise the standard bicarbonate level above 15 mmol/l may be calculated on the basis that 2 mmol of bicar-bonate are necessary to raise the standard bicarbonate level of each litre of cellular fluid by 1 mmol/l, and that the ECF constitutes ap-proximately 20% of body weight. For example, the amount of bicarbonate required to raise the plasma standard bicarbonate level from 10 mmol/l to 27 mmol/l in a 70 kg patient is:

$$(27 - 10) \times 70 \times 20/100 \times 2 = 476 \text{ mmol.}$$

In practice only half of this amount is given slowly over 2 hours, and the standard bicarbonate level rechecked after 4 hours before further ad-ministration is considered. As an 8.4% solution of sodium bicarbonate contains 1 mmol of bicar-bonate per ml, the volume required can be calculated easily if an 8.4% or 4.2% solution is used.

Care must be taken not to overload the patient with sodium and to correct the fall in serum pot-assium which tends to occur after bicarbonate therapy. As many such patients are potassium-depleted, potassium replacement is an important consideration.

Acute renal failure and cardiac arrest produce severe metabolic acidosis and are considered else-where in this volume.

Metabolic alkalosis

Transient metabolic alkalosis follows injury and may occur in shock, but the most frequent surgical cause of metabolic alkalosis is pyloric stenosis. The loss of acid from the stomach is compensated initially by renal conservation of hydrogen ion and an associated increase in potassium output. Thus patients with metabolic alkalosis are always pot-assium-deficient, and many are severely hypokalaemic. Conversely, patients with potas-sium depletion from other causes often develop metabolic alkalosis.

The management of pyloric stenosis consists of stopping all oral intake, hourly gastric aspiration, correction of dehydration by normal saline, pot-assium replacement, and then surgical relief of the cause. The use of gastric lavage in the evenings, with intravenous administration of special 'gastric solution' is not recommended. Replacements should be tailored to the needs of the individual patient.

For patients whose standard bicarbonate level exceeds 35 mmol/l, intravenous ammonium chloride has been recommended, but should not be used in the presence of potassium deficiency.

Respiratory acidosis

Respiratory acidosis is common in surgery and may occur as a consequence of oversedation or postoperative chest complications. Management is directed towards relief of the underlying chest condition, supplemented if need be by assisted ventilation. The administration of bicarbonate is not indicated.

Respiratory alkalosis

There are many causes of respiratory alkalosis. Those encountered in surgical practice are listed below.

1. Hyperventilation on a mechanical respirator or under anaesthesia
2. Pain and apprehension (hysteria)
3. Small areas of pulmonary atelectasis
4. Multiple pulmonary emboli
5. Central nervous system injury
6. Septicaemia (particularly Gram-negative septicaemia).

The underlying cause should be sought and treated. Respiratory suppression (e.g. with phenoperidine) is indicated occasionally. Sustained respiratory alkalosis has a poor prognosis, usually because of the severity of the underlying condition.

Table 2.5 Changes associated with mixed patterns of acid-base imbalance

	H^+	Pa_{CO_2}	Standard HCO_3^-
Metabolic acidosis	↑	↓	↓
Respiratory acidosis	↑	↑	normal
Metabolic alkalosis	↓	normal or slightly ↑	↑
Respiratory alkalosis	↓	↓	normal

Mixed patterns of acid-base imbalance

Many patients have a mixture of respiratory and metabolic components in their acid-base imbalance. Measurement of arterial blood gas tension, hydrogen ion and standard bicarbonate concentrations helps to reveal the contribution of the metabolic and respiratory components, and special nomograms are available for this purpose. The patterns of alterations in these parameters are shown in Table 2.5.

MONITORING OF PATIENTS WITH FLUID AND ELECTROLYTE PROBLEMS

The following should be estimated daily.

1. Urine volume
2. Serum sodium, potassium, bicarbonate and urea concentrations
3. Volume of losses from gastrointestinal tract
4. Haemoglobin concentration and haematocrit (packed cell volume).

In patients with complex problems, the following should also be measured daily.

1. Arterial hydrogen ion concentration, standard bicarbonate and partial pressure of carbon dioxide
2. Urinary sodium and potassium excretion
3. Gastrointestinal fluid sodium and potassium
4. Body weight.

Serum protein should be measured twice a week, and in special circumstances losses of magnesium and calcium should also be measured. Determination of serum and urine osmolalities is useful in patients with severe disorders of hydration.

3. Shock

DEFINITION

Shock may be defined as an acute alteration of the circulation leading to *reduced cellular perfusion* with resultant generalized cellular hypoxia and vital organ damage. Reduced cellular perfusion is common to all patients in shock regardless of the cause.

CAUSES

Shock may result from a variety of causes, the majority of which are associated with a reduced cardiac output. The consequent reduction in tissue perfusion is compounded by the action of catecholamines liberated in response to the 'stress' of the initiating cause (see later).

Hypovolaemia

Hypovolaemia is an important cause of shock, a low venous return leading to a reduced cardiac output. Hypovolaemia may result from any of the following.

1. *Haemorrhage*.
2. *Loss of gastrointestinal fluid*, as in intestinal obstruction, small bowel fistula or diarrhoea.
3. *Trauma and infection*. Injury or infection increases capillary permeability and leads to local sequestration of fluid and oedema.
4. *Burns*. Fluid loss results from direct surface loss (weeping or blistering), tissue sequestration and the loss of the normal waterproof action of the skin.
5. *Renal loss*. Excessive water and electrolyte loss from the urinary tract, e.g. in sodium-losing chronic nephritis, tubular necrosis, diabetic ketosis

or Addisonian crisis, is an occasional cause of prostration and shock (see p. 23).

Pump failure

Primary impairment of cardiac action can cause shock by abruptly reducing cardiac output. This may result from myocardial infarction, acute ventricular arrhythmia, acute cardiomyopathy or acute valvular lesions caused by aortic dissection or by trauma producing severe incompetence. Secondary impairment of cardiac action may result from cardiac tamponade producing constriction of the heart, or major pulmonary embolism producing severe obstruction to right ventricular outflow.

In all shock states myocardial performance is affected adversely as a result of reduced coronary arterial perfusion, and in some cases due to the additional depressant effect of circulating peptides released from the site of infection or injury.

Bacteraemia

Bacteraemic shock is most frequently associated with Gram-negative bacillary infection, although Gram-positive organisms or fungi are sometimes responsible. The most frequent sources of infection are the urinary tract, the biliary tract and the large bowel.

Bacteraemic shock is more complex than hypovolaemic or cardiogenic shock. The bacteria concerned produce toxins, most frequently endotoxins, which participate in an antibody-complement reaction from which substances are produced which profoundly affect the heart and peripheral vasculature. In contrast to hypovolaemic or cardiogenic shock, cardiac output is frequently high, but perfusion is reduced as a result of the opening of many peripheral arteriolar-venular shunts.

Anaphylaxis

Anaphylactic shock closely resembles bacteriogenic shock in that an antibody-complement complex is of central importance in the development of the clinical picture.

Neurogenic factors

True neurogenic shock follows spinal transection or brainstem injury with loss of sympathetic outflow below the site of injury and consequent vasodilatation. The rapid increase in size of the vascular bed 'soaks up' the cardiac output so that venous return falls and cardiac output is reduced.

Pain is a potentially important contributory factor to shock in patients with trauma, particularly those with fractures. Pain increases the output of catecholamines, with adverse effects on the microcirculation. Immobilization (not necessarily reduction) of fractures should therefore come early in the management of patients with multiple injuries.

The most frequently cited example of neurogenic shock is the vaso-vagal attack, or faint, in which intense vagal activity produces marked bradycardia and a fall in cardiac output. The circulation rapidly returns to normal with the involuntary assumption of the horizontal position. This condition is of physiological interest but its transient nature removes it from the true spectrum of shock.

Endocrine factors

Although adrenal failure is by itself a potent cause of the shock syndrome (due to the sudden withdrawal of circulating cortisol and aldosterone), the role of the adrenal cortex in the production of shock by other causes is debatable. In Addisonian states due to chronic adrenal insufficiency the loss of salt and water from kidneys and bowel leads to hypovolaemia. Acute adrenal failure may occur as a complication of septicaemia (Waterhouse-Friedrichsen syndrome), but this is usually regarded as a terminal event.

PATHOPHYSIOLOGY OF SHOCK

The factors producing shock initiate the 'metabolic response' discussed fully in Chapter 1. Release of large amounts of catecholamines in the early stages has important effects on both the macrocirculation and the microcirculation. Failure to rectify the initiating factor results in persistence of the normal response with reduced tissue perfusion resulting in generalized cellular hypoxia and consequent metabolic changes. Different organs vary in their susceptibility to impaired perfusion, and individual organ failure may become manifest.

Macrocirculation

Diminished venous return activates baro-reflexes which increase cardiac rate and cause peripheral arteriolar constriction. These reflexes are supplemented by the rising level of blood catecholamines. The increase in cardiac rate improves cardiac output, while increased peripheral resistance raises arterial blood pressure. Thus a normal blood pressure may be maintained for a time, yet tissue perfusion may not improve and may even be reduced further by the peripheral vasoconstriction.

Peripheral vasoconstriction is more marked in the vessels of the skin and extremities than in central organs. This tendency to preserve flow in central organs has been described as the 'sympathetic squeeze'. The characteristic picture of shock is one of cold pale skin due to peripheral vasoconstriction, and the associated sweating is due to sympathetic sudomotor activity.

Patients in bacteraemic shock present a different clinical picture. The circulation is often hyperkinetic, the cardiac output is higher than normal, and the extremities are warm. The explanation of this 'warm shock' presentation is not entirely certain, but it is due in part to arteriovenous (A-V) shunting induced by kinins from the infected area. The low A-V oxygen difference in these patients supports the 'shunting' theory and indicates that the cells are not utilizing (or receiving) oxygen.

Myocardial function or contractility is adversely

affected and the capacity of the heart to deal with an increased load deteriorates as shock continues. Much of the impairment is a consequence of low coronary arterial flow and myocardial cellular hypoxia. Local and generalized metabolic acidosis, together with alterations in plasma electrolyte levels, alter cardiac contractility and cause further deterioration by provoking arrhythmias.

Microcirculation

Peripheral cellular perfusion is further affected by constriction of precapillary 'sphincters' under the influence of catecholamines. As a consequence less blood enters the capillary bed, the 'vis a tergo' is reduced further and capillary flow becomes sluggish.

In normal conditions only about one third of the capillaries are open at one time. Normally capillaries open in response to hypoxia and close when flow through them has restored tissue oxygen tension. In the sluggish flow conditions of shock the capillaries remain open longer than normal and more capillaries open, further expanding the capillary bed. Consequently, flow in individual capillaries becomes even slower and there is a tendency for blood to 'sludge' in the capillaries. Coagulation time is shortened in shock, and the combination of sludging and slow flow encourages endovascular coagulation, leading to further impairment of flow, worsening hypoxia and local metabolic acidosis, and local cell death. Extensive endovascular coagulation depletes coagulation factors in the blood and may lead to haemorrhage, particularly in subcutaneous tissues and mucous membranes. This syndrome is known as disseminated intravascular coagulation (DIC).

The post-capillary capacitance vessels in shock may be either constricted or dilated. Constriction may briefly improve venous return but will ultimately impair capillary flow by causing obstruction. Dilatation of the post-capillary capacitance vessels results in reduced venous return.

Cells

In order to function normally cells require to extract energy from glucose. This process occurs in

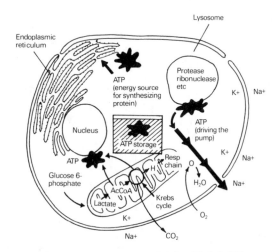

Fig. 3.1 Energy supply in the cell (after Thal & Wilson, in: Current Problems in Surgery, Chicago 1965)

the mitochondria and provides energy for storage in the form of adenosine triphosphate (ATP) and releases free hydrogen. Oxygen is necessary to remove the majority of the freed hydrogen in the form of water (Fig. 3.1). Energy is easily released from ATP and is necessary for cellular protein and enzyme synthesis, for maintenance of the sodium 'pump' and for cell reproduction.

In shock, oxygen is deficient, so that other hydrogen receptors in this chain become saturated. Energy transformation in the Krebs cycle is impaired, and lactic acid cannot be dehydrogenated to pyruvate and thus accumulates. The cell therefore has to rely on anaerobic glycolysis for energy production, which gives a poor yield of ATP compared to aerobic glycolysis (Fig. 3.2). Consequently, vital cellular functions deteriorate: protein and enzyme synthesis fails, sodium leaks into the cell while potassium leaks out, and plasma potassium levels rise. The lysosomal membranes eventually break down, causing intracellular release of proteases, esterases and phosphatases, and cell death occurs (Fig. 3.3). If such changes are widespread, the patient will not recover.

Acid-base balance

Accumulation of lactic acid from anaerobic cellular metabolism leads eventually to generalized metabolic acidosis. This is compensated by buffers and

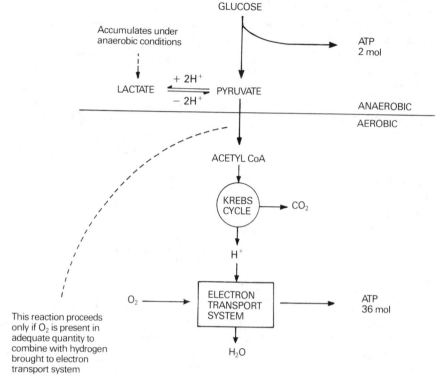

Fig. 3.2 Anaerobic and aerobic metabolism

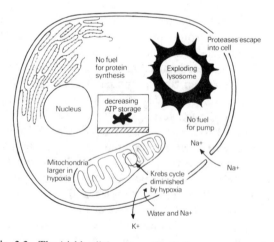

Fig. 3.3 The 'sick' cell (source as Fig. 3.1)

by respiratory and renal mechanisms until the acid load becomes too great. Renal compensation is impaired in shock as a result of reduced renal blood flow, and the development of renal failure greatly increases the tendency to acidosis. Some patients in shock develop alkalosis, which may be respiratory or metabolic or a combination of the two. Respiratory alkalosis due to hyperventilation is more common. Metabolic alkalosis can result from impaired renal handling of bicarbonate and this may be important in patients receiving large transfusions of stored blood (citrate is metabolized to bicarbonate in the body). Alkalosis shifts the haemoglobin oxygen dissociation curve to the left (Fig. 3.4). This, while improving the take-up of oxygen in the lungs, impairs its release in the tissues.

Individual organs

The 'sympathetic squeeze' reduces the effects of shock on vital organs at the expense of the periphery. However, this sparing is relative, and important effects on individual organs are recognizable.

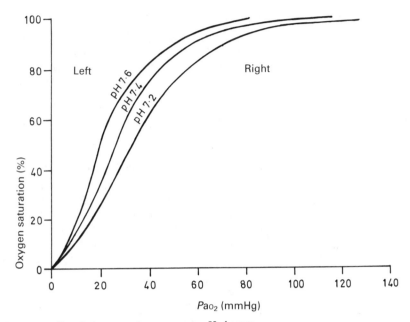

Fig. 3.4 Shifts in the oxygen dissociation curve in response to pH changes

Nervous system

The earliest sign of cerebral hypoxia is restlessness which may give way to stupor and coma. If respiratory alkalosis is present, cerebral blood flow is reduced and this, together with the effect on the haemoglobin oxygen dissociation curve, increases the tendency to anaerobic metabolism. The effects of cerebral hypoxia are usually rapidly reversible in all but the elderly, unless hypoxia has been prolonged.

Kidneys

Renal failure was once a frequent cause of death in shock. Increasing knowledge of the mechanisms of derangement of renal function and more sophisticated management have reduced the incidence of death from this cause.

A fall in urinary output is by far the most frequent effect of shock on the kidneys. Initially this results from reduced glomerular filtration due to reduced renal blood flow, together with the volume-conserving actions of antidiuretic hormone and aldosterone. If the shocked state continues, however, chemical and structural damage to renal tubular cells ensues. *Oliguria* is defined as the production of less than 400 ml of urine in 24 hours, while *anuria* is defined as the production of less than 20 ml of urine in 24 hours. As recovery from the insult occurs, oliguria is followed by a marked diuresis. In some patients, particularly those with sepsis, acute renal failure with rising blood urea occurs in the face of a normal or high urine output without the preceding oliguric phase (high output renal failure).

If oliguria is simply a consequence of attempted volume conservation, the urine has a normal to high specific gravity and low sodium concentration. This situation is managed by increasing fluid administration. Extensive tubular damage is denoted by low urine specific gravity, increasing urinary sodium concentration and a urine osmolality close to that of plasma. A rising blood urea in the presence of adequate hydration and arterial blood pressure indicates acute renal parenchymal damage.

Other factors which contribute to oliguria in shock include tubular necrosis, tubular blockage by debris, intravascular coagulation, jaundice, hyperkalaemia, and nephrotoxic drugs such as the aminoglycoside antibiotics.

Acute renal failure is usually reversible, and fluid restriction and dialysis allow recovery provided the primary cause of shock is controlled.

Lungs

Acute respiratory failure (synonyms: adult respiratory distress syndrome, shock-lung syndrome) is an important cause of death in shock. The development of secondary bronchopneumonia leads to a mortality rate of approximately 50%.

Two principal types are recognized.

1. *Wet lungs*. Pulmonary oedema is the principal component and results from either acute cardiac failure or overhydration, particularly with crystalloid solutions. Pulmonary vein constriction, however, may contribute to the onset of oedema, and pulmonary capillary permeability is increased in shock, possibly as a result of release of histamine or bradykinin. Gas exchange is less impaired than in the second group and the prognosis is better.

2. *Dry lungs*. This situation may be preceded by pulmonary oedema, but gas exchange is severely impaired due to *atelectasis* resulting from plugging of small bronchioles, which is aided by a *reduction in surfactant activity*. Shallow breathing encourages the development of atelectasis. Gas exchange is further impaired by *hyaline membrane* formation. A further problem in these patients is an *increase in pulmonary vascular resistance* which may be more profound and persistent than the rise in peripheral vascular resistance. The cause may include vascular compression from atelectasis, and capillary plugging by platelets, leucocytes, fat embolism or solid particles in blood or plasma infusions. Acidosis and hypoxia also increase pulmonary vascular resistance, and fibrinopeptides (FDPs) released during endovascular coagulation produce further sustained pulmonary hypertension. These changes are usually seen in patients with severe sepsis, and the prognosis is poor.

Heart

Myocardial performance is adversely affected in shock as a result of reduced coronary arterial perfusion. Hypoxia limits aerobic metabolism in the myocardium and acidosis causes problems by depleting myocardial stores of noradrenaline. In addition, contractility and left ventricular function in haemorrhagic and septic shock are further impaired by humoral agents acting directly on the myocardium.

Liver

The liver is the major site for conversion of lactate to pyruvate, and increasing levels of lactate indicate severe impairment of hepatic function, due principally to low liver blood flow and portal venous oxygen desaturation. Routine tests of hepatocellular function show deterioration, and jaundice is a relatively common accompaniment of shock.

Gastrointestinal tract

The splanchnic blood flow is markedly reduced in shock and adynamic ileus is a frequent complication. In patients with atheromatous mesenteric vessels, ischaemic colitis may develop but haemorrhage from the small bowel is not common.

Superficial ulceration of the stomach or duodenum, the so-called *stress ulceration*, may produce major haemorrhage especially in septic shock. Excess corticosteroid secretion or administration and bile reflux have been suggested as possible causes.

Adrenal glands

The adrenal glands play a fundamental role in the response to injury or infection, and in shock the production of corticosteroids and catecholamines is normally well maintained throughout the shocked state (see Ch. 1). Acute pathological changes occurring in the adrenals are rare in shock, although necrosis may occur in meningococcal septicaemia (Waterhouse-Friedrichsen syndrome).

Reticuloendothelial system

The reticuloendothelial system plays a protective role in shock by an undefined but probably non-specific response. For example, exposure of animals to repeated doses of endotoxin protects them against the effects of shock induced subsequently, not only by endotoxin but also by trauma or haemorrhage.

In the shocked patient, however, the impairment of normal reticuloendothelial responses may be demonstrated by depression of detoxification, phagocytosis and antibody formation. The susceptibility of the shocked patient to infection is well recognized clinically. This impairment of reticuloendothelial function may relate to a reduction in blood flow through liver and spleen.

CLINICAL SYNDROME OF SHOCK

The classical appearance of the shocked patient is seen after haemorrhage and is due to intense sympathetic stimulation. The patient is pale and has a rapid thready pulse and cold extremities. The peripheral veins are contracted due to reduced filling and sympathetic venoconstriction. Capillary filling is slow, as judged by the return of colour after pressure on the nail beds or ear lobes. Sweating occurs due to sympathetic sudomotor stimulation. The patient becomes restless as a result of cerebral hypoxia, proceeding to apathy as hypoxia becomes more severe.

Initially the blood pressure is maintained or even raised, particularly in young patients. This is due to increased peripheral vascular resistance. Nonetheless tissue perfusion is markedly reduced with induction of the metabolic changes associated with shock. Arterial hypotension develops sooner or later in all shocked patients and accentuates the impaired perfusion. Central venous pressure falls as return from the capillary bed is reduced. This fall occurs well before the drop in arterial pressure and may precede tachycardia.

The respiratory rate increases as a result of baroceptor stimulation, initially complemented by the development of hypoxia and metabolic acidosis.

Urinary output is low.

The overall picture of haemorrhagic shock is one of low cardiac output. This classic picture is modified in cardiogenic shock, where central venous pressure is elevated due to acute cardiac failure. In bacteraemic shock, the cardiac output may be normal or elevated, the extremities warm and the pulse full. The high flow through inflamed areas is associated with peripheral arteriovenous shunting, but the high metabolic demand in the tissues is not satisfied by this apparent increase in flow.

As the patient responds to treatment, the clinical appearances return towards normal. The value of simple clinical assessment cannot be overemphasized.

PRINCIPLES OF MANAGEMENT

Restoration of adequate perfusion at the cellular level is the essential aim in the treatment of shock. The principles of management are outlined below.

Restoration of tissue perfusion

In the majority of patients this is achieved by adequate *intravenous infusion of fluid*. Patients with clinical evidence of myocardial dysfunction require inotropic drugs to improve function, and certain patients with persisting abnormalities of peripheral vascular tone need vasoactive drugs.

Adequate oxygenation

All shocked patients become hypoxic, and oxygen administration is routine. Patients with respiratory difficulty or a developing acute respiratory distress syndrome require intermittent positive pressure ventilation.

Treatment of the precipitating cause

Haemorrhage is arrested and any infection treated by appropriate antibiotics, drainage of abscesses or removal of the source (e.g. a ruptured appendix).

Monitoring

The response of the patient to therapy is the guide to whether treatment is appropriate or adequate. The response is assessed at frequent intervals following the initial 'baseline' assessment.

General appearance. Note pallor, sweating,

restlessness, venous filling and temperature of extremities.

Cardiovascular parameters. Measure pulse rate, arterial blood pressure and central venous pressure. More sophisticated assessment of parameters such as cardiac output, left ventricular function and pulmonary and peripheral vascular resistance is necessary in some patients. ECG monitoring is required for patients with primary cardiogenic shock or secondary myocardial dysfunction.

Urinary output. Catheterize and measure hourly urine volume and specific gravity. Measurement of urinary osmolality supplements information obtained from determination of the specific gravity.

Haematological and biochemical measurements. Haemoglobin, haematocrit (packed cell volume), urea and electrolyte levels are required for 'baseline' and progress assessment. Arterial blood gas and pH measurements to assess hypoxia and acid/base balance are other essential investigations. Blood lactate levels give a good indication of cellular hypoxia and hepatic function.

In the initial stages of management, clinical and cardiovascular assessments are made every few minutes. The frequency of assessment decreases as the patient responds. Continuous recording of cardiovascular parameters is valuable in some patients in the early stages. Haematological and biochemical indices have to be measured hourly in some patients. In the majority, less frequent determinations are sufficient.

The peripheral circulation in shock has been likened to a marshy swamp in contrast to the normal running stream. The object of treatment is to get the stream running. Early and adequate therapy based on the principles outlined above will achieve this without major cellular damage, and with prompt recovery of organ function. If treatment is delayed or inadequate, it may be possible to restore satisfactory circulation, but at the expense of residual organ dysfunction, e.g. of kidneys, lungs and the liver. Specific management of such organ failure will then be required. More generalized cellular damage resulting in failure of the sodium pump with leakage of potassium from cells (the 'sick cell syndrome') is of serious import. Patients who reach this stage are often refractory to treatment.

MANAGEMENT OF SPECIFIC SITUATIONS

Hypovolaemic shock

Haemorrhage is the most frequent cause of hypovolaemic shock, and the management of haemorrhagic shock exemplifies the approach to all shocked patients.

1. The general condition of the patient is noted, and peripheral perfusion is assessed by noting the temperature of hands and feet, return of colour after blanching the nail bed, and the state of filling of the veins on the dorsum of the hands and feet.

2. An adequate airway is ensured and oxygen given.

3. External injuries and obvious fractures are noted and continuing bleeding is stopped by direct pressure.

4. The pulse rate and arterial blood pressure are recorded.

5. An intravenous infusion is started and blood drawn from the needle or cannula for grouping and cross-matching, and for baseline determination of haemocrit, urea and electrolytes. If haemorrhage is not associated with obvious injury, the platelet count and prothrombin time should be determined. In severely shocked or traumatized patients more than one infusion line should be set up.

The preferred site for initial infusion is the antecubital fossa. If suitable veins are not available here or elsewhere in the arm, the alternatives are to cannulate the subclavian or internal jugular vein or to perform a cut-down to a suitable vein, e.g. the long saphenous. The initial infusion fluid should be crystalloid (either isotonic saline or buffered Ringer lactate solution) and 1 litre should be given as rapidly as possible (over 10–15 minutes). If a blood transfusion centre is nearby, grouped blood can be available for infusion in 10 minutes. The provision of grouped and cross-matched blood requires approximately 1 hour. If a long delay is anticipated, infusion may be continued with albumin 25–50 g per litre of normal saline, or with hepatitis-free plasma. Dextran may cause difficulties with subsequent cross-matching and may give coagulation problems. If haemorrhage continues, group O Rh-positive blood may be used direct from store until adequately cross-matched blood arrives. Once the infusion is running, a central venous line is inserted to allow central venous pressure measurements.

6. The patient is best kept level. The head-down position adversely affects respiration and reduces cardiac output.

7. Pain relief is important to reduce further catecholamine production. Obvious fractures of long bones are immobilized by splinting. Appropriate analgesics are administered intravenously and the dose is noted. Restlessness due to cerebral hypoxia requires restoration of cerebral perfusion, not sedation.

8. The patient is catheterized and hourly urine output and specific gravity are recorded.

9. At this stage a rough assessment of the blood loss associated with obvious injury may be made (see Ch. 14).

The rate and volume of fluid and blood replacement is determined by the patient's response to infusion rather than by any rule of thumb. Individual patients vary greatly in their response to haemorrhage.

The colour and peripheral perfusion of the patient are noted and changes in arterial pressure and pulse rate recorded. The trend in central venous pressure is monitored. As these parameters return to normal, the rate of infusion is slowed. Failure to improve, or deterioration after initial improvement, denotes continuing haemorrhage, and is an indication for urgent operation.

Urinary output should reach a minimum of 50 ml per hour. A lower volume with high specific gravity indicates the need for more infusion, while oliguria with low specific gravity suggests the onset of acute renal failure. If the patient's clinical state suggests that he has been adequately infused, the use of diuretics at this stage may prevent acute renal failure. Frusemide (80–160 mg) is preferred to mannitol. It will initiate a diuresis within 20 minutes unless there is acute renal failure, when specific management is instituted.

Once the circulation is stabilized, the source of haemorrhage is investigated and definitive management undertaken.

Bacteraemic shock

In addition to the principles outlined above for the management of hypovolaemic shock, it is necessary to (1) determine the source of infection; (2) determine the organism(s) responsible and (3) treat the infection.

Serial blood samples are sent for culture, as are specimens of urine and sputum. Swabs are taken for culture from all wounds. Investigations to determine the presence of intrathoracic or intra-abdominal infection or abscesses are initiated.

In the absence of specific bacteriological information, treatment is commenced which will cover both Gram-negative (the more likely) and Gram-positive organisms. A combination of gentamicin (80 mg twice daily) or lincomycin (500 mg 6-hourly) and metronidazole (500 mg 8-hourly) is suitable. Infected wounds and abscesses are drained. Any recognized source of contamination, e.g. perforated appendix, empyema of gall bladder or stones in the common bile duct, is treated by appropriate surgery.

Antibiotic therapy will not be successful in the presence of a continuing source of contamination, and suspected sources of bacteraemia must always be sought and eradicated or drained.

Cardiogenic shock

Fluid infusion in cardiogenic shock requires great caution, and central venous pressure monitoring is mandatory. Attention is directed to three specific areas.

1. *Management of cardiac failure.* Digitalization is usually indicated. Hypokalaemia potentiates the effects of digoxin and care must be taken to avoid induction of arrhythmias. Stimulating drugs such as isoprenaline or dopamine are often used when there is secondary myocardial dysfunction in other types of shock. Again, there is a risk of induction of arrhythmia, particularly in older patients.

Mechanical support using intra-aortic balloon counter-pulsation has been used recently and may be combined with partial left ventricular bypass.

2. *Management of arrhythmia.* Acute arrhythmias are managed by the use of beta-blocking drugs (e.g. propranolol) or quinidine-like drugs, (e.g. lignocaine).

3. *Correction of mechanical factors.* Cardiogenic shock may be precipitated by mechanical factors such as tamponade, valve rupture or massive pul-

monary embolism. Drainage of the tamponade and consideration of valve replacement or embolectomy are necessary.

Neurogenic shock

Neurogenic shock may follow high spinal injury or brainstem injury. Adequate ventilation and fluid replacement is necessary. Vasoconstrictor drugs may be indicated in this type of shock.

Persisting inadequate tissue perfusion

In some patients, despite adequate fluid infusion and management of myocardial and respiratory dysfunction, persisting metabolic acidosis and lactic acidaemia indicate that tissue perfusion remains unsatisfactory. Persisting vasoconstrictor catecholamine activity is usually implicated and is an indication for the use of alpha-blocking vasodilators such as phenoxybenzamine, either alone or in combination with beta-stimulants such as dopamine or isoprenaline.

Drugs of this type result in a large expansion of the peripheral vascular bed, and one must be prepared to infuse large volumes of fluid to ensure adequate venous return. Ideally, when such drugs are being used, the patient should be continuously monitored with frequent determination of cardiac output and peripheral vascular resistance.

Respiratory support in the shocked patient

Hypoxia is invariable in shock. Mild hypoxia is an indication for humidified oxygen by nasal catheter or mask (6 litres/min). Concentrations approaching 100% may be achieved if a tight-fitting mask is used.

If hypoxia is severe, or progressing during oxygen therapy, an endotracheal tube should be inserted and positive pressure ventilation instituted. This may expand atelectatic alveoli while humidification reduces secretion viscosity and allows ventilation of obstructed segments of lung. Secretions are aspirated through the endotracheal tube.

Tracheostomy will be necessary if it is envisaged that ventilation will be required for more than 4–5 days. Ventilation is adjusted to maintain an arterial Po_2 of 70–90 mmHg (9.3–12.0 kPa) and a Pco_2 of 30–40 mmHg (4.0–5.3 kPa). In some patients it will not be possible to maintain adequate oxygenation without significant hypocarbia, and the prognosis is then poor. The use of an extracorporeal membrane oxygenator should be considered at an early stage for such patients. A diuretic such as frusemide should be given to reduce interstitial and pulmonary oedema, and digitalization is indicated if pulmonary oedema is established.

Patients with the acute respiratory distress syndrome frequently develop pulmonary infection, and broad spectrum antibiotics should be given.

Management of acute renal failure

Once acute renal failure is established, it is imperative not to overload the patient with fluid, and input must be carefully equated with fluid loss.

Dialysis. Peritoneal dialysis or haemodialysis is indicated when the blood urea rises at a rate of 7–10 mmol/l per day. It prevents the development of severe metabolic acidosis and potassium intoxication, and the gastrointestinal, cerebral and cardiovascular effects of severe uraemia. Haemodialysis requires heparinization and is best avoided in patients with major soft tissue trauma or a high risk of gastrointestinal bleeding. Peritoneal dialysis is not suitable for patients with intraperitoneal sepsis, recent gastrointestinal resection, or intra-abdominal vascular grafts.

Reduction of potassium levels. Potassium intake must be restricted, and the high levels of potassium in banked blood and crystalline penicillin should be remembered. Emergency measures may have to be instituted to reduce a high serum potassium level.

1. Administration of sodium bicarbonate corrects metabolic acidosis and reduces serum potassium by encouraging transfer into cells.

2. Intravenous administration of 50 g glucose with 20 units soluble insulin also favours transfer of potassium into cells.

3. Intravenous calcium gluconate (2–4 g in 500 ml 5% dextrose) should be given over 4 hours if cardiotoxicity due to hyperkalaemia is present or imminent.

4. Potassium ion-exchange resins may be given orally or as retention enemas, and will extract approximately 1 mmol of potassium per gram of resin. The usual dose is 50–100 g every 24 hours.

Diet. A high-calorie diet is given to ensure protein-sparing. Approximately 40 g protein should be provided each day, and 60–70 kcal/kg body weight should be provided as non-protein calories. Most patients are unable to take this amount orally and parenteral supplementation is necessary.

Acidosis. Metabolic acidosis can occur in shock without evidence of renal failure. Improved tissue perfusion corrects the imbalance and is the primary objective of treatment.

If the standard bicarbonate concentration falls below 15 mmol/l, it is advisable to correct the base deficit. The amount of sodium bicarbonate required is calculated as follows:

Dose (in mmol) = 0.2 × body weight (in kg) × (27 − standard bicarbonate in mmol/l).

Half the calculated dose is given initially, and the subsequent dose is determined by the patient's response.

Non-specific drugs in shock therapy

The role of *steroids* in the management of shock remains debatable. If they are to be effective, they must be given in high dosage (e.g. dexamethasone 2–6 mg/kg body weight 4–6 hourly for 48 hours), but objective clinical evidence of their efficacy remains elusive. Among the advantages claimed for high-dose steroid therapy are improved myocardial function, reduced peripheral vascular tone, stabilization of mitochondrial membranes and reduced intracellular release of lysosomal enzymes, protection against development of severe pulmonary changes, and protection against the action of sensitized antibody-complement complexes in bacteraemic and anaphylactic shock.

The use of *Trasylol* (aprotinin), an antikalli-krein agent, has been advocated in shock. In theory, Trasylol blocks kinin release and avoids the potentially harmful effect of this substance on myocardial and peripheral vascular function. The value of Trasylol has not been confirmed in clinical practice.

Glucagon has actions akin to beta-adrenergic drugs and improves cardiac performance even in fully digitalized patients. Infusion of 3–5 mg per hour has been used in shock, and benefit reported in a few cases. In theory, glucagon would also improve hepatic blood flow.

Disseminated intravascular coagulation (DIC)

In shock, as in other stress states, the blood becomes hypercoaguable and some degree of intravascular coagulation occurs. If this becomes extensive and disseminated, coagulation factors may be consumed to such an extent that a bleeding tendency develops and massive haemorrhage may occur. Platelets, prothrombin, fibrinogen and factors V and VIII become depleted, and, as a result of accompanying fibrinolysis, fibrinopeptides and fibrin degradation products (FDPs) appear in the blood. The laboratory tests to confirm DIC are based on these changes.

The main aim of treatment is correction of the underlying cause, and with successful treatment DIC will resolve. Heparin infusion has been advocated to prevent progression of DIC, and, although clinical results have been disappointing, its use may be justified when DIC progresses rapidly and is associated with severe haemorrhage. In some patients a secondary fibrinolysis becomes the dominant feature, and administration of epsilon-aminocaproic acid (EACA) to inhibit fibrinolysis is advised in addition to heparin. Heparin and EACA must be used with caution and dosage is difficult to control. Direct replacement of platelets and clotting factors is safer and provides some control while the underlying cause is managed.

4. Transfusion of blood and blood products

BLOOD AND PLASMA PRODUCTS

Fifty years ago transfusion was a surgical procedure involving physical connection between donor and patient by tube and cannulas. In the future transfusion therapy may well be supplanted by new synthetic or bioengineered functional substitutes for plasma proteins, red cells and platelets. Currently we are in an intermediate stage. In most developed countries blood and its therapeutic products are readily available, well packaged and relatively straightforward to use. While these materials can be handled like any other pharmaceutical product, one should not lose sight of the fact that blood products are made from people. An individual, whether paid, conscripted or a volunteer, has to part with the raw material. It is therefore a resource which must be used responsibly.

Because of its human source, quality control of the raw material is difficult; it carries the potential for transmission of specific human blood-borne infections. In prescribing blood and blood products, knowledge of the characteristics and side effects of the products, and of the procedures required to ensure safety and compatibility with recipients is necessary.

Source of raw materials

The traditional method of collecting donated blood is to withdraw whole blood into an anticoagulant solution. This is still widely used as the source of red cells, platelets and (in some parts of the world) plasma. The alternative procedure is *apheresis* ('taking away'). *Plasmapheresis* involves withdrawing a donor's blood, separating cells from plasma and returning the cells. As plasma protein levels can be restored much more rapidly than cells, very large volumes of plasma can be withdrawn from one individual over a long period. *Cytapheresis* is the collection of cells (white cells or platelets) by a process which involves blood withdrawal, differential centrifugation, collection of the desired component and return of the remaining constituents to the donor.

In most Western countries whole blood is obtained from unpaid donors. However, a large proportion of the world's supply of plasma is obtained by plasmapheresis of paid donors who may submit to weekly or twice weekly removal of 500–600 ml of plasma. The raw material for most plasma products marketed by pharmaceutical companies (albumin, immunoglobulin, clotting factors etc.) is obtained in this way.

Most blood and plasma collecting organizations apply strict standards to the selection of donors. Priority is given to screening for infection, according to its prevalence in the community concerned. For example, if the hepatitis B carrier state is endemic (as in some Asian populations), the provision of hepatitis-B-negative blood for all recipients may simply not be practicable. In Western countries current priorities are to exclude carriers of hepatitis B and HIV (the human immunodeficiency or AIDS virus). Additional tests to prevent transmission of non-A, non-B hepatitis are also being introduced. It is likely that tests for HIV-related viruses may also have to be introduced.

Blood and plasma processing

Because of the demand for plasma and platelets, most of the blood collected will be processed. The principal stock in the blood bank will be red cell concentrate, not whole blood. Plasma is frozen rapidly to preserve labile coagulation factors. Some of this frozen plasma will be supplied to the hospital blood bank for transfusion as single donor plasma but most will form the starting material for production of plasma fractions. This is a pharmaceutical manufacturing process on a factory scale. Each production batch contains the plasma from many thousands of donations pooled together to provide the raw material for processing. The final product may therefore contain traces of an undetected contaminant, e.g. virus from just *one* of the starting plasma donations. The process must therefore include at least one step to inactivate residual infectivity (e.g. heat treatment). A large number of blood donations is required to produce a single dose of most plasma fractions, emphasizing the human as well as the financial costs of these products.

Blood transfusion can be life-saving and many surgical procedures could not be undertaken safely without good transfusion support. However, transfusion exposes the patient to several types of risk. These depend on the epidemiology of infectious diseases among the donor population, the resources and dedication of the organization which collects, processes and issues blood and blood products for the patient, and the care with which clinical staff order, check and administer them.

Staff who prescribe blood and blood products must be aware of the potential risks of transfusion (see p. 36) and balance these against each patient's need to receive a blood product. Some serious complications such as the development of non-A, non-B hepatitis, hepatitis C or acquired immuno-deficiency syndrome (AIDS) may manifest themselves many months or even years after transfusion and may never be reported to the prescriber.

Blood component therapy

In the past it was difficult to separate the cellular components of blood from the plasma without risk of bacterial contamination. This is still a problem in parts of the world where blood has to be collected in glass containers. As a result, the only product for transfusion was so-called 'whole blood', which is more accurately described as stored blood, diluted with anticoagulant and deficient in platelets and certain coagulation factors. Modern transfusion practice depends on the prescription of separated components of blood. This approach has the advantage of providing specific replacement of a patient's acquired or inherited deficiency of blood cells or plasma proteins. It also permits much more efficient use to be made of donated blood. The range of blood components and plasma fractions, and their use, are described in detail later in this chapter.

COLLECTION AND STORAGE OF BLOOD

Blood is collected from donors who undergo selection intended to exclude those whose blood could be hazardous to the recipient. In many countries there is a legal requirement to test each donation for evidence of hepatitis B, hepatitis C, human immuno-deficiency viruses and syphilis. Such testing is not universal, and in some countries where hepatitis B and/or HIV infection is prevalent, donor testing is incomplete. In these areas transfusion may carry a high risk of transmitting these infections and others, e.g. malaria.

A healthy adult can donate 450 ml of blood without adverse effects. This is collected into a container containing 60–100 ml of a combined anticoagulant–nutrient solution such as CPD-A1. This contains citrate and added nutrients (phosphate, dextrose and adenine) which support red cell metabolism and so permit blood to be stored up to 35 days provided it is kept at 2–6°C.

During refrigerated storage, blood undergoes changes due to continued metabolism and ageing of red cells. Other changes include loss of haemostatic activity of platelets and loss of activity of coagulation factors V and VIII (Table 4.1). Patients who require replacement of platelets or these labile coagulation factors cannot be treated adequately with whole blood and must receive the appropriate blood component.

BLOOD GROUPS AND COMPATIBILITY TESTING

Clinicians who order and administer blood do not usually have to carry out testing for compatibility

Table 4.1 Changes in whole blood stored at 2–6°C in CPD-A1

| | Storage time (days) | | | |
	0	7	28	35
Red cell viability (%)[1]	>90	>90	80	75
Platelet viability (%)[2]	95	0	0	0
Coagulation factors V and VIII (%)[3]	95	30	30	30
Plasma haemoglobin (g/l)	0–0.01	0.1	0.3	0.5
Plasma potassium (mmol/l)	3	12	20	28
pH	7.6			7.0

1. Red cell viability is the proportion of red cells which survive in the circulation 24 hours after transfusion of stored blood.
2. The loss of functional platelets occurs during the first 48 hours of storage at 4°C.
3. Other coagulation factors are stable during storage at 4°C.

with the patient. Nevertheless, essential facts about blood groups and their corresponding antibodies must be understood.

The ABO blood groups

The most important red cell antigens are those of the ABO blood group system (Table 4.2). Blood must be ABO compatible. If ABO incompatible blood is transfused, there is almost certain to be intravascular haemolysis of the transfused red cells. These reactions are rapid and often fatal.

These serious reactions occur because it is normal for the individual's plasma to contain antibodies directed against ABO red cell antigens. These do not arise as a result of previous trans-fusion but are produced in response to the bacteria normally present in the intestine, which have antigens similar to those of blood groups A and B. Patients who are blood group O have antibodies to both A and B antigens. The risk of ABO incompatible transfusion is therefore greatest in these group O patients, who comprise about 50% of most Caucasian populations (see Table 4.2). It is important to remember that the proportion of ABO groups differs considerably among racial groups (Table 4.3).

There are variants of the A and B blood group antigens which occasionally cause difficulties in the initial blood grouping of a patient but do not normally cause problems in supplying compatible blood.

The Rhesus blood groups

The Rhesus blood groups must also be considered when providing compatible blood for all patients. There are five principal Rhesus antigens, usually termed Rh(C), (c), (D), (E) and (e). These may be expressed on the red cells in various combinations depending on the genetic make-up of the individual. The Rh(D) antigen is the most important in transfusion because it is the most immunogenic. If this antigen is present, the patient is Rh(D) positive. About 15% of Caucasians are Rh(D) negative (see Table 4.3). Most to these individuals will develop anti-Rh(D) antibodies in response to a single transfusion of Rh(D) positive blood. In contrast to the ABO system, individuals who are Rh(D) negative do *not* normally have anti-Rh(D)

Table 4.2 The antigens and antibodies of the ABO blood group system in Caucasian populations

Blood group	Approximate frequency in population (%)	Antigens on red cells	Antibodies in plasma	Compatible donor blood group
O	50	None	Anti-A, Anti-B	O
A	35	A	Anti-B	A or O
B	10	B	Anti-A	B or O
AB	5	A or B	None	A, B, AB or O

Note:
1. Blood group frequencies differ with racial group (see Table 4.3).
2. *If the patient's blood group is not known, the only blood which may be transfused is group O. Blood of other groups may kill the patient.*
3. Never transfuse without compatibility testing except in extreme emergency. Incompatibilities other than those due to ABO groups may seriously harm the patient.

Table 4.3 Examples of racial variation in the frequency of blood groups

Racial group	Frequency (%)				
	O	A	B	AB	Rhesus(D) positive
UK (Caucasian)	50	35	10	5	84
Chinese	44	26	25	5	100
West African	52	24	21	3	95
Bengali	22	24	38	16	
South American Indian	100	0	0	0	

in their plasma *unless* they have been immunized either by a previous transfusion or by pregnancy.

The Rhesus system is clinically important for the following reasons.

1. An Rh(D) negative person will usually develop anti-Rh(D) antibodies if Rh(D) positive blood is transfused. Subsequent transfusions of Rh(D) positive blood will lead to haemolysis of the transfused red cells. This may produce a severe haemolytic transfusion reaction and will greatly shorten the survival of the transfused cells, diminishing the effectiveness of the transfusion.

2. Rh(D) antibodies cause haemolytic disease of the newborn. The risk of this serious condition arises when a woman who is Rh(D) negative is carrying a fetus which is Rh(D) positive (due to inheritance of the relevant gene from the father). If the mother's plasma contains anti-Rh(D) antibody, the antibody (IgG) crosses the placenta, enters the fetal circulation and destroys the fetal red cells. This may result in profound anaemia in utero, leading to cardiac failure and oedema, a condition termed 'hydrops fetalis'. After birth, these infants are profoundly jaundiced and may suffer permanent central nervous system damage.

It is therefore essential that Rh(D) negative women of childbearing age are not transfused with Rh(D) positive blood.

A mother may also be exposed to Rh(D) positive fetal cells as a result of small feto-maternal bleeds which may occur during normal pregnancy, delivery or procedures such as amniocentesis or termination. To prevent the development of maternal anti-Rh(D) antibodies, all these Rh(D) negative women should be injected with anti-Rh(D) immunoglobulin immediately after obstetric procedures, termination, abortion, ante-partum haemorrhage or delivery of an Rh(D) positive infant. The administered anti-Rh(D) immunoglobulin removes Rh(D) positive fetal cells from the maternal circulation so that the mother does not produce anti-Rh(D) antibody.

3. There are many patients with Rh(D) antibodies. Sometimes these occur in association with antibodies to other red cell antigens and provision of compatible blood for these patients can be very difficult.

The blood bank must at all times maintain a good stock of Rh(D) negative blood for patients with Rhesus antibodies for use in obstetric emergencies and for emergency transfusion of women of childbearing age.

Other blood group antigens

There are many other red cell antigens. Some of these, in the same way as the Rh(D) antigen, can stimulate production of IgG antibodies when an individual is transfused with red cells, or exposed to fetal antigens during pregnancy. These antibodies are found only in a small proportion of patients but can cause severe transfusion reactions and haemolytic disease of the newborn. The blood bank should always be informed of a history of previous transfusion or pregnancy, and should routinely carry out a screening test to detect red cell antibodies. A patient with IgG antibodies to red cell antigens such as Rh(C), (c), (D) or (E), or to antigens such as those of the Kell, Duffy or Kidd blood group system must only be given red cells which do not express these antigens. This may require extensive testing which can cause long delays in providing compatible blood. Wherever possible, this laboratory work must be done well in advance of the requirement for transfusion.

Leucocyte and platelet antibodies

White cells and platelets have cell surface antigens. Some of these belong to the major histocompatibility system (HLA) and some are cell-type specific. These antigens are not taken into account in routine compatibility testing, but they can cause transfusion problems in those few patients who may develop antibodies to white cells or platelets.

1. In patients who are repeatedly transfused or who have had several pregnancies, leucocyte antibodies can cause unpleasant transfusion reactions. Anti-HLA or anti-platelet antibodies reduce the survival of transfused platelets.

2. Occasionally patients become profoundly thrombocytopenic following transfusion, due to the development of platelet antibodies (post-transfusion purpura).

3. Very occasionally neonates become severely thrombocytopenic or leucopenic due to transferred maternal antibodies.

These problems require expert advice and specialist investigations if transfusion is required.

Plasma protein antibodies

Patients can develop antibodies to transfused human plasma proteins. Usually this does not cause practical transfusion problems. Patients who are profoundly deficient in IgA (frequency approximately 1 in 2500) may make antibodies to IgA. These patients can have severe anaphylactic reactions if transfused with standard blood products, all of which contain at least traces of IgA. This should be remembered as a rare cause of an otherwise unexplained severe transfusion reaction.

BLOOD ORDERING AND PRETRANSFUSION TESTING

Documentation and checking

The object is to ensure that compatible blood is available and identified for the patient when it is required and that the *correct blood* is administered to the patient. The responsibilities for achieving this rest with all those involved in ordering, supplying and administering the blood.

1. *The person who orders the blood.* The patient must be correctly identified, the blood sample for compatibility testing must be placed in a clearly labelled tube, and the request form must be accurately completed and submitted with the correct sample tube.

2. *The blood bank staff.* The labelling of the sample tube and the form must be checked for completeness and consistency, and any available blood bank history should be reviewed. Compatible blood must be selected, documented and delivered.

3. *The person who checks, writes up and administers the blood.* The patient must be positively identified, the labelling of the blood pack shown to correspond to the patient, and the document accompanying the blood must be checked against both patient and blood pack. These checks should be signed for. The instructions for administration should be clearly written on the fluid administration chart and signed for. Instructions for monitoring the patient during transfusion must be given. A record of each unit given must be kept in the patient's case notes.

The most important cause of serious haemolytic transfusion reactions due to incompatible blood is the administration of the wrong blood due to a failure to carry out one of these checks.

For the house surgeon the two greatest risks are (1) placing the blood sample into a tube labelled for the wrong patient and (2) failing to check *in each case* that the details of blood pack and form correspond exactly with those of the patient to be transfused.

'Group and screen' and the blood-ordering schedule

For elective surgical procedures, most clinical units have now developed a blood-ordering schedule which indicates the quantities of blood or red cell units to be ordered routinely. For these procedures, which only rarely require transfusion, it is unnecessary and expensive to have blood cross-matched for the patient, provided the surgeon and anaesthetist are confident that blood can be supplied rapidly in an emergency. The blood bank will determine the patient's ABO and Rh(D) type and also test for the presence of unexpected red cell antibodies (the 'group and screen' procedure). Once this has been done, the blood bank can make compatible blood available for delivery within 10–15 minutes of a request.

In all elective patients who may need transfusion, and especially in those with a history of previous transfusion or pregnancy, this group and screen procedure should be carried out well in advance of planned surgery. This will provide early warning if red cell antibodies are present and allow the blood bank time to select compatible blood.

Ordering blood in an emergency

The house surgeon must know the local arrangements for emergency blood supply: the procedures in a small hospital with no blood bank on site will be different from those in a large hospital with a well-stocked blood bank close to the surgical unit. Transport arrangements may slow the delivery both of the request to the blood bank and of the blood to the patient. Blood banks differ in the speed with which blood can be issued following an urgent request. Whenever blood is needed urgently, the blood bank should be telephoned and the degree of urgency made clear to the doctor or technician responsible. Table 4.4 shows the response times which may be expected.

COMPLICATIONS OF BLOOD TRANSFUSION

The morbidity and mortality of blood transfusion is comparable to that of general anaesthesia. The list of potential complications is formidable.

Febrile reactions

Pyrogens and minor bacterial contamination used to be a common cause of febrile reactions; this is no longer the case. The occasional febrile reaction now seen is more likely to be due to interactions between pre-existing recipient antibodies and transfused leucocytes, platelets or immunoglobulins. These are usually minor but, as some are severe and even fatal, all should be referred to the hospital blood bank for possible investigation. A significant number remain unexplained. They are best managed by stopping the transfusion and administering intravenous antihistamine (chlorpheniramine sulphate 20 mg) and hydrocortisone sodium succinate (100 mg). Further transfusions should be similarly covered. Red cell products with reduced white cells, platelets and plasma protein (see p. 42) may be necessary for patients who require repeated transfusion and who continue to react despite antihistamine cover.

Bacterial contamination

Bacterial contamination of blood donations is rare. However, during donation a small number of skin bacteria can pass into the blood and if it is not stored at 4°C significant growth may occur.

Table 4.4 Time needed to obtain blood for transfusion

Request	Blood bank action	Time required*
Provide blood for a patient who has already been 'group and screen' tested	Check ABO groups Rapid crossmatch	10–15 min
Desperate need — patient exsanguinating, and not previously tested	1. If no patient sample available, issue group O blood (Rhesus D negative if patient is female and of child-bearing age or less) 2. If patient sample available and adequately identified, issue blood of patient's ABO and Rh type	5–10 min
Blood needed within the hour; patient not previously tested	Full compatibility procedure needed, including ABO and Rh (D) type, antibody screen and crossmatch	30–60 min
Blood for elective surgery	Full compatibility procedure as above. Laboratory processes requests in batches so response is slower	3 hours to 1 day (depends on local system)

* Time from request reaching blood bank until blood is ready for issue. *Transport times are additional.*

Heavily contaminated blood is almost black and on transfusion causes sudden and severe endo-toxaemia, which is usually fatal. Treatment is by intravenous infusion of antibiotics to cover both aerobic and anaerobic organisms and other supportive measures for bacteraemic shock (see Ch. 11). The offending blood donation must be returned immediately to the blood bank for investigation.

Circulatory overload

This complication is most likely to occur in anaemic elderly patients with cardiac insufficiency. Such patients should be transfused with red cell concentrates or packed red cells. Unless blood loss and anaemia is acute, only one unit of red cells should be given every 24 hours. Each unit should be accompanied by 20 mg frusemide intra-venously. In some patients exchange transfusion may be required.

Haemolytic reactions

The most serious haemolytic reactions are caused by ABO incompatability. Less than 50 ml of ABO incompatible blood can give rise to sudden and severe pain in the back and at the injection site, marked dyspnoea and profound hypotension. Haemoglobinuria and haemoglobinaemia occur and the patient becomes icteric within 24 hours. Within one hour of transfusion, acute renal failure may have developed. Disseminated intravascular coagulation (DIC), initiated by antigen/antibody complexes formed on the red cell membranes, may cause bleeding. General anaesthesia may mask many of these signs and symptoms. Sudden unex-plained hypotension may warn of a haemolytic reaction.

Most other antibodies do not cause intravascular haemolysis: the antibody-coated red cells are destroyed more slowly by the reticuloendothelial system. Jaundice usually develops, but renal failure and DIC are rare.

Massive haemolysis can follow administration of compatible blood which is heavily contaminated or has accidentally been frozen and thawed, or heated above 40°C.

It must again be emphasized that *the commonest causes of incompatible blood transfusions are mistakes made in the ward or theatre, errors in identification or cross-matching of blood samples, or failure to check blood before administration.*

The investigation and management of major in-travascular haemolytic transfusion reactions are outlined in Table 4.5.

Transmission of disease

Transmission of viral hepatitis remains the most frequent serious complication of the administration of blood and blood products. In the United Kingdom before hepatitis B testing became routine, the morbidity and mortality rates of post-

Table 4.5 Management of intravascular haemolytic transfusion reactions*

Investigations	Therapy
Check for evidence of incompatible blood on pack, bottle or labels. Return suspect donation to blood bank for immediate investigation.	Stop transfusion Hydrocortisone 100 mg i.v. Insert urinary catheter, empty bladder and monitor urine flow
Withdraw 30 ml blood and send for investigation immediately. Inform blood bank medical staff. (10 ml for serological testing at blood bank; 10 ml for blood urea and electrolyte determination; 10 ml for coagulation screen)	100 ml mannitol (20%) and 100 ml 0.9% saline 150 mg frusemide i.v. If 2 hours after mannitol and saline the urine flow is less than 100 ml/hour, assume acute renal failure and treat accordingly.
Electrocardiogram for evidence of hyperkalaemia	If there is clinical, ECG or laboratory evidence of hyperkalaemia, start Resonium/insulin/glucose therapy.
Repeat coagulation and chemical screens 2–4 hourly until stabilized	Patients with evidence of DIC may require blood product support and heparin therapy

* If possible, avoid further blood transfusion until blood bank staff have checked compatibility of blood to be given. In the meantime, manage hypovolaemia with albumin solutions, artificial colloids or crystalloids. DIC = disseminated intravascular coagulopathy.

transfusion hepatitis were 27 and 8 respectively per 10 000 units transfused. Although type B hepatitis virus remains a significant cause of post-transfusion hepatitis, most cases are due to another viral agent, so far unidentified, and are described as non-A, non-B hepatitis. Other viruses rarely cause post-transfusion hepatitis.

In most countries blood donations are routinely tested for hepatitis B virus, using the surface antigen (HBsAg) as a marker. This reduces the overall risk of post-transfusion hepatitis by about 25%. Only two blood products (albumin and immunoglobulin) are without risk. It is likely that some heat-treated coagulation-factor concentrates will also prove not to transmit hepatitis.

All donations are screened for syphilis. As spirochaetes have limited viability, blood stored for more than 4 days at 4°C is safe. Other infectious diseases which can be transmitted by blood transfusion include brucellosis, toxoplasmosis, malaria and trypanosomiasis.

Since 1983 it has become evident that blood and some blood products may transmit the human immunodeficiency virus (HIV), the cause of acquired immunodeficiency syndrome (AIDS). In most countries blood donations are now routinely tested for evidence of this infection, using a test which detects antibody to the virus. This test is combined with other measures designed to exclude donors who are at high risk of exposure to HIV. This programme has ensured that in countries such as the United Kingdom the risk of transmitting HIV by a single blood donation is not likely to be greater than one in a million. Moreover, because HIV is particularly sensitive to thermal damage, it now seems certain that heat-treated plasma fractions (such as coagulation factors VIII and IX, and albumin) do not transmit HIV. Current evidence also suggests that the standard process used to fractionate plasma to produce immunoglobulin preparations also kills HIV. Knowledge about human retroviruses is developing extremely rapidly. It is already evident that there are other retroviruses which can be transmitted by blood transfusion.

Although transfusion-transmitted AIDS is likely to be very rare in countries which take effective preventive measures, it provides a grave reminder of the microbiological risks of transfusion, and the problem of non-A, non-B hepatitis remains unsolved. Recent studies have suggested that a considerable proportion of all transfusions of red cells, platelets and especially of fresh frozen plasma are not clinically justified. The most effective way of reducing transfusion-transmitted infection is to avoid these unnecessary transfusions.

Complications of massive transfusion

If four units of blood are transfused at a rate in excess of 100 ml/min a number of complications may arise.

Citrate toxicity. Patients who are hypotensive or who have liver or renal damage fail to metabolize or excrete the large load of citrate in transfused blood. As a result of the increase in serum citrate levels there is a decrease in ionized calcium (with which it forms a complex), leading to muscle tremor, tetany and cardiac arrhythmias. The citrate load is much smaller if red cell concentrate is given.

Potassium toxicity. Since potassium leaks from red cells during storage, rapid administration of large volumes of stored blood may elevate the serum potassium concentration to cardiotoxic levels. This is particularly likely to occur in patients with renal damage or severe crush injuries with extensive muscle damage. Excessive hydrogen ions in stored blood potentiate this effect.

Platelet deficiency. Stored blood has few viable platelets. Massive transfusions may lead to dilution thrombocytopenia and bleeding.

All these problems can be reduced by taking the following precautions.

1. Warming the blood (25°C) prior to transfusion using a correctly designed blood warmer (blood must not be warmed by placing packs on radiators, in incubators, in sinks of hot water etc.). This helps to avoid hypothermia and the risk of reduced citrate metabolism. If there is evidence of hypocalcaemia after more than 5 units of whole blood have been administered, 10 ml of 10% calcium gluconate should be given for every two further units. Bolus administration of calcium gluconate must be avoided as this can be cardiotoxic. Infusion should take at least 3 minutes.

2. Using red cell concentrate. This reduces the load of citrate transfused.

3. Using the freshest available blood to reduce potassium load.

4. Administering platelet concentrates if there is thrombocytopenia and bleeding, which suggests failure of haemostasis.

Microaggregates of platelets and leucocytes are formed during the storage of blood and it has been suggested that when transfused in large amounts they may contribute to the adult respiratory distress syndrome. The use of microaggregate blood filters has become popular but there is little evidence of their benefit, certainly in patients receiving up to 5 units of blood.

AUTOLOGOUS TRANSFUSION

Because of the risk of immunological and infective complications from receiving donor blood, many hospitals now, wherever possible, use the patient's own blood to provide support during surgery: this is called 'autologous transfusion'. Alarm about transfusion-transmitted AIDS has strengthened this method of reducing a patient's exposure to another person's blood. It also reduces the demand for conventional blood donations. The procedures are described in more detail below.

Preoperative bleeding and haemodilution

This procedure is widely used in cardiothoracic surgery. Immediately before operation, one or two units of blood are withdrawn from the patient and stored in the theatre in standard blood packs. The immediate volume deficit is replaced with a crystalloid solution. During or after surgery, the patient's blood can be reinfused to provide not only red cells but (because the blood is fresh) also platelets and all coagulation factors. An additional benefit is the preoperative reduction of the patient's packed cell volume (PCV), or haematocrit, to give optimal capillary perfusion.

Intraoperative blood salvage

If during surgery there is heavy bleeding into the operative field, it may be possible to collect large volumes of the patient's blood by suction. Equipment is available with which the collected blood can be washed in a sterile solution to produce a suspension of the patient's red cells suitable for reinfusion. This method may be particularly useful for cardiothoracic procedures. Staff and equipment to carry out the additional procedures during the course of the operation are required.

Preoperative bleeding with liquid storage of the patient's blood

Blood can be stored for up to 5 weeks using standard blood bank conditions. Patients who are awaiting planned surgery may therefore donate blood to be stored for use during or after their operation. Careful selection is required to ensure that patients are medically fit for this procedure. Suitable patients can lay down 2–4 units of blood preoperatively.

Frozen storage of autologous donations

Frozen red cells can be stored for long periods. This permits autologous red cell donations to be stored for a planned procedure. This procedure is expensive and the facilities are unavailable in many hospitals.

Of these procedures, immediate preoperative bleeding and haemodilution is the most widely established and is standard practice in many surgical units. The extent to which the other procedures contribute to transfusion practice remains to be evaluated. Autologous blood is a most desirable option for the patient because of its biological compatibility. However it is suitable only for planned procedures. The majority of patients (e.g. trauma victims and patients with major obstetric haemorrhage or gastrointestinal bleeding) still require heterologous transfusions. The development of autologous transfusion can never be a substitute for a safe conventional blood transfusion system linked to a critical approach to the prescription of all blood products.

BLOOD PRODUCTS AND THEIR CLINICAL USES

By separating plasma from blood and fractionating

it into its components, a range of concentrated blood derivatives, e.g. platelet and coagulation factor concentrates, can be produced. These allow specific replacement therapy without the risk of circulatory overload. Table 4.6 lists the range of blood components and plasma fractions generally available.

Blood replacement

Acute haemorrhage

An average healthy adult can lose 500 ml of blood rapidly without ill effect. Provided circulatory volume is maintained (with crystalloids and/or colloids), the loss of 1–2 litres of blood will not lead to irreversible hypotension. Children, the elderly and those with cardiopulmonary disease tolerate haemorrhage less well; they are also more susceptible to volume overload from overtransfusion.

Accurate assessment of blood loss is difficult, particularly after acute haemorrhage. Measurements of blood volume are time-consuming and often inaccurate, particularly in anaemic and/or debilitated patients. Estimations of haemoglobin and PCV (haematocrit) are misleading during haemorrhage since both plasma and red cells are lost. Serial clinical observations showing increasing pulse rate, falling blood pressure and urine output, irritability, sweating, cold extremities, intolerance to exertion and frequent changing of posture are the best indications for blood transfusion in haemorrhage. Blood or red cells should not be transfused on the basis of a single clinical observation of pulse and blood pressure unless there is additional evidence of major bleeding. A systolic pressure of less than 100 mmHg following blood loss suggests a deficit of more than 30% of the circulating volume, and the need for transfusion.

There is no need for specific action to replace coagulation factors unless the patient has a congenital deficiency (e.g. haemophilia) or impaired

Table 4.6 Examples of products which contribute to blood component therapy

Blood product	Shelf-life	Main indication for use
Whole blood	21 days (ACD) 28 days (CPD) 35 days (CPD-A1)	Severe life-threatening haemorrhage; components of a transfusion policy
Red cell concentrate	As whole blood	All routine transfusions and as part of a transfusion policy (see text)
Fresh frozen plasma	1 year	Some bleeding conditions (see text)
Platelet concentrate	5 days	Severe non-immune thrombocytopenia
Albumin 5% 15–20%	4 years 4 years	Acute volume expansion Severe symptomatic hypoproteinaemia
Cryoprecipitate	6 months	Haemophilia A management; von Willebrand's disease; hypofibrinogenaemia
Freeze-dried factor VIII concentrate	1 year	Haemophilia A management
Factor IX II, VII, IX, X II, IX, X	2 years 2 years	Acquired deficiencies (liver disease; oral anticoagulant reversal) Management of haemophilia B and of haemophilia A with inhibitors
Immunoglobulin (i.m.) Normal Hyperimmune anti-Rh(D) anti-tetanus anti-zoster anti-HBV anti-rabies anti-cmv	4 years	Prophylaxis against hepatitis A Prevention of Rh disease of newborn Prevention and treatment of tetanus Prevention of zoster Prevention of hepatitis B virus infection (needle-stick accident) Prevention of rabies following infected bite Management of some cmv infections
Immunoglobulin (i.v.)	2 years	Replacement therapy — immune deficiency states; management of immune thrombocytopenia

liver function, is on oral anticoagulant therapy or there is accompanying disseminated intravascular coagulation. Coagulation factor levels may drop by up to 50% in severe haemorrhage, but this is still compatible with normal haemostasis. Movements from the extravascular space together with release and synthesis of coagulation factors from a normal liver readily compensate for the losses associated with even severe bleeding.

The balance between oxygen-carrying capacity and capillary flow must be considered. In patients *without* cardiopulmonary disease an ideal balance between capillary flow and tissue oxygenation is achieved by a haematocrit of 30%. A haematocrit below 30% is compatible with normal tissue metabolism, provided oxygen is also administered. Because of the absence of fibrinogen, fluid replacement with crystalloids or synthetic colloids reduces blood viscosity more effectively than plasma.

In planning blood replacement for a patient, it is not appropriate simply to replace blood loss millilitre for millilitre. If there is clinical evidence of hypovolaemia then up to 2 litres of crystalloid and colloid solutions should be infused initially. Solutions which do not transmit hepatitis viruses should be used. Reconstituted freeze-dried plasma is not a desirable alternative, since (1) it contains fibrinogen, which may increase blood viscosity and reduce capillary flow, (2) it transmits viruses and (3) its potassium content is high. Administration of red cell concentrates and whole blood can follow. The first two units should be red cell concentrates; thereafter red cell concentrates or whole blood may be used. Guidelines for transfusion requirements are given below:

1. Previously healthy adults:
   Begin with 1000 ml crystalloid;
   followed by 1000 ml colloid;
   followed by two units of red cell concentrates;
   followed by whole blood or red cell concentrate as required.
2. Elderly patients and those with significant cardiopulmonary disease:
   Begin with 500 ml crystalloid;
   followed by 500 ml colloid;
   followed by red cell concentrate;
   followed by whole blood or red cell concentrate as required.

By using these regimens the majority of patients transfused for blood loss associated with elective surgery will not require red cell transfusion.

Dextrans and gelatin solutions are the colloid preparations of choice. They are contraindicated in patients with haemostatic failure, in whom plasma or albuminoid should be used.

Patients with severe liver disease or those on full doses of oral anticoagulants should receive 500 ml fresh frozen plasma (FFP) along with the two red cell concentrates. Further doses of FFP may be required.

Chronic anaemia

Transfusion is usually not appropriate for patients with anaemia due to a chronic disorder, as the rise in haemoglobin is only temporary. In haematinic disorders such as severe pernicious anaemia, transfusion is usually contraindicated because of the risk of cardiac failure.

Blood transfusion should only be considered when haematinics have failed. Acute haemorrhage in a severely anaemic patient is hazardous and every effort must be made to maintain the haemoglobin level above 7 g/dl by transfusion. In some patients it may be acceptable to avoid transfusion by delaying surgery, to permit a response to haematinics. This decision must be based on an assessment of the relative risks and benefits for each patient.

If transfusion is essential, concentrated red cells should be given slowly together with diuretics, and serum electrolytes should be monitored closely. Frequent transfusion is valuable in α-thalassaemia major but should be avoided in α-thalassaemia minor or in haemoglobinopathies such as the sickle-cell diseases. Exchange transfusion is useful in sickle crisis.

Although major surgery can be performed on patients with haemoglobin levels below 5 g/dl without peroperative transfusion, many surgeons and anaesthetists still prefer an initial haemoglobin of 10 g/dl before commencing any elective major operation. Provided pre-existing anaemia is asymptomatic, surgical haemorrhage can be controlled by intraoperative transfusion and a lower figure, e.g. 7 g/dl, can be accepted. The blood product of choice for transfusing anaemic patients is red cell concentrate. Each donation (250 ml of concentrate) should raise the haemoglobin by 1.0 to 1.5 g/dl. To minimize the risk of circulatory overload in the extremely anaemic patient (Hb less than 5 g/dl), the elderly or when significant cardio-pulmonary disease is present, it is wise to cover each unit of red cells with 20 mg frusemide intravenously. Ideally, preoperative transfusions should be completed 24 hours before surgery.

An overall transfusion policy

Over the last 20 years the routine use of whole donor blood for red cell replacement has been recognized as an incorrect and inefficient use of a scarce therapeutic resource. Demand for special blood products which can only be produced from plasma now exceeds the requirement for red cells by a factor of almost two to one.
This imbalance can be resolved if:
  1. red cell concentrates are used for all forms of chronic anaemia requiring transfusion; and
  2. in acute haemorrhage (including intra-operative blood loss) following crystalloid administration, the first two donations of blood are given as red cell concentrates. This may be followed by whole blood or red cell concentrate, as required, over the subsequent 24-hour period.

BLOOD COMPONENTS
Whole blood

As indicated in the transfusion policy above, whole blood should be reserved for patients with severe uncontrolled haemorrhage and clinical signs of hypovolaemia. Fresh whole blood (less than 6 hours old) to ensure haemostasis is no longer in-dicated. It should only be given to a bleeding patient with a haemorrhagic diathesis if an ap-propriate blood component is not available. The results of tests for hepatitis B virus and HIV will not usually be available prior to administration of fresh blood.

Red cell concentrates

Red cell concentrate is prepared by removing plas-ma from a donation of whole blood and resuspending the cells in anticoagulant nutrient solution to give a haematocrit of 70%. This is the product of choice for routine transfusions and should account for 60–70% of all units transfused.

Packed red cell concentrates. This product has a haematocrit in excess of 90%. It is reserved for patients with severe anaemia and cardiac failure.

Leucocyte- and platelet-depleted red cells. Patients who experience non-haemolytic trans-fusion reactions (see p. 36) may require red cells from which white cells, platelets and plasma proteins have been removed. The following preparations may be used.
  1. Buffy coat depleted red cells. Approxi-mately 50% of white cells and platelets are removed by centrifugation.
  2. Filtered red cells. Special filters are used to remove about 90% of white cells and platelets. Red cells are also washed to remove plasma.
  3. Frozen, thawed red cells. Red cells can be preserved for long periods by freezing. This is a useful but costly method.for storing blood of very rare groups. The thawed product is washed and contains minimal residual white cells, platelets and plasma.

Platelet concentrates

Platelet concentrates contain 60–70% of the platelets present in the original donation, suspended in approximately 40 ml plasma. An adult requiring platelet replacement usually needs platelets pooled from five to six donations to achieve haemostasis. Platelet concentrates should be infused rapidly (over 15–30 minutes) and must be administered immediately after receipt from the blood bank. Platelets must not be refrigerated before administration.
    Platelet therapy is indicated in patients with bleeding due to thrombocytopenia (less than $20\,000 \times 10^9/l$) or with clinical evidence of platelet malfunction. Platelet concentrates are also of value in the patient with haemorrhage following massive transfusion of stored blood (see Table 4.6 and p. 38). They are of little value in patients with immune thrombocytopenia or splenomegaly, for they are rapidly removed from the circulation before they can exert their haemostatic effects. Prophylactic platelet therapy may be indicated in patients undergoing intensive chemotherapy, as this can severely deplete the platelet count.

As platelet concentrates contain small amounts of red cells, it is advisable, but not essential, to provide ABO and Rhesus(D) compatible donations. Efficacy is best assessed by clinical observation; post-transfusion platelet counts are unreliable. Repeated platelet transfusions may lead to an immune refractory state. If this arises, platelets from HLA compatible donors may be required to achieve a haemostatic effect.

Fresh frozen plasma

Plasma separated from fresh blood and stored at $-30°C$ contains all coagulation factors. Thawing takes approximately 60 minutes. The thawed plasma should be used within 4 hours, as coagulation factors V and VIII deteriorate rapidly. Fresh frozen plasma should be ABO compatible with the recipient.

Fresh frozen plasma is not a panacea for all bleeding states. Its main indication in surgical practice is in the management of patients on oral anticoagulants or with severe liver disease who are bleeding or require emergency operation. In an adult 800 ml (four donations) should be infused over 60 minutes. In elderly patients, circulatory overload may be prevented by administration of frusemide (40 mg intravenously). Fresh freeze-dried plasma is available in some countries. It has the advantage that it can be stored in a domestic refrigerator.

Outdated (freeze-dried) plasma

This product is no longer available in the UK but is still produced in some countries. It is prepared from a pool of donations; usually different ABO groups are mixed so that the final product can be given to patients of any ABO group. Each bottle is made up with 400 ml distilled pyrogen-free water. As the potassium content is high (up to 30 mmol/l), it should be given with caution in patients with renal impairment. There is a considerable risk of virus transmission.

Outdated freeze-dried plasma once had a major role in the management of hypovolaemia, but with the introduction of safer colloids (dextrans, gelatins) and preparations of human albumin, its use has declined. Its main indication now is in the management of burns, but in most countries it has been replaced by albumin preparations.

As freeze-dried outdated plasma can be stored for up to 5 years, it is still useful as an acute volume expander in countries without facilities for plasma fractionation. In concentrated form (made up in 150 ml distilled water) it provides a useful source of coagulation factors other than the labile factors V and VIII.

Factor VIII

There are two main types of human factor VIII preparation: cryoprecipitate and freeze-dried factor VIII concentrate. When fresh plasma is frozen to $-40°C$ and then allowed to thaw at $4-8°C$, a precipitate forms which contains 40–80% of the factor VIII, fibrinogen and factor XII of the original plasma. It also contains clinically significant quantities of the factors which stimulate synthesis and release of factor VIII and increase platelet adhesion. These are deficient in patients with von Willebrand's disease. The cryoprecipitate from each donation is stored at $-30°C$ in a small volume (20–50 ml) of the plasma supernatant. It dissolves rapidly at $37°C$ and should be infused within 4 hours of reconstitution. Material from several donations is usually pooled prior to administration. Each donation of cryoprecipitate contains 50–150 units of factor VIII. Freeze-dried factor VIII concentrate is produced by plasma fractionation. It has significant advantages over cryoprecipitate: each vial contains a standard and stated dose, it can be stored in a domestic refrigerator, and it is much more convenient to administer. As it is prepared from large plasma pools, it has in the past carried a high risk of transmitting viruses. Current factor VIII preparations are treated by heat or other virus-inactivating processes. These remove HIV infectivity and may also reduce hepatitis virus transmission.

Factor VIII preparations are used in the management of haemophilia A. Minor episodes of joint or muscle pain usually require a single intravenous dose of factor VIII; more serious haematomas need to be treated for 2–4 days. If major surgery is required, factor VIII must be administered 8-hourly for the first 2 days and 12-hourly for the next 10–14 days. Major surgery in an adult haemophiliac may require the factor VIII content of over 1000 donations. As there are trace amounts of anti-A and anti-B in most preparations, large doses occasionally cause mild haemolysis in those of group A, B or AB.

Home therapy is a recent development in the management of haemophilia. The patient or relative administers a small dose (250–500 units) of factor VIII concentrate as soon as pain is felt in a joint or a muscle. This can abort a more serious bleed and avoid hospital admission.

Factor IX

Two types of freeze-dried concentrate are available. One is a mixture of coagulation factors II, IX and X and the other of II, VII, IX and X. Both are used primarily in the management of hereditary coagulation factor deficiencies, particularly factor IX deficiency (Christmas disease or haemophilia B). The principles of replacement therapy in Christmas disease are similar to those in haemophilia A.

Factor IX concentrate can also be used to produce rapid transient reversal of oral anticoagulant therapy and to prepare patients for liver biopsy.

Factor IX concentrates have in the past carried the same risk of transmitting hepatitis as concentrates of factor VIII. Similar virus inactivation processes are now applied to most currently available factor IX products. Some preparations may be thrombogenic, particularly in patients with severe liver disease. Thrombogenic activity increases if the concentrates are left standing after reconstitution with distilled water. They should therefore be infused immediately after reconstitution.

Factor IX concentrates can be used in the management of haemophilia A patients with inhibitors to factor VIII. Their use in this context requires expert advice.

Fibrinogen

Fibrinogen concentrate fractionated from large plasma pools is still available, but cryoprecipitate, available as a single donation containing 0.1–0.3 g of fibrinogen per pack has considerably less risk of transmitting hepatitis. Fibrinogen is occasionally indicated in surgical patients with disseminated intravascular coagulation.

Albumin solutions

Preparations of human albumin are available in two forms: a 4.5–5.0% solution (salt content approximately 140 mmol/l) used for acute volume expansion, and a 15% or 25% solution poor in salt (salt-poor albumin; SPA) used to correct hypoproteinaemia. Human albumin preparations are heated to destroy contaminating viruses. Some have a significant kinin content which may produce transient hypotension. Such reactions are rare and invariably benign.

Human albumin is very expensive. The 5% preparation costs about 10 times more than colloid volume expanders such as dextrans. Albumin infusions should be reserved for hypovolaemic patients who are likely to develop significant hypoproteinaemia (i.e. those with crush injuries, septic peritonitis, severe acute pancreatitis, prolonged intestinal obstruction and mesenteric vascular occlusion) and those with failure of haemostasis in whom artificial colloids are contraindicated. The 5% preparation can be used in the management of hypovolaemia associated with burns.

Albumin infusions are quite unsuitable as a nutritional source. Albumin must be broken down to amino acids before it is incorporated into body proteins, and this process is slow (half-life 18 days). Moreover, the content of essential amino acids (particularly tryptophan) is poor. Infused albumin increases the catabolic rate. Its main value in hypoproteinaemia is as an oncotic agent.

Patients are at risk from low oncotic pressure when the total plasma protein level falls below 52 g/l (albumin less than 25 g/l). Albumin solutions (25%) should be administered in amounts calculated as:

$$2 \times (\text{desired} - \text{actual albumin level}) \times \text{plasma volume},$$

assuming a plasma volume of 40 ml/kg. This calculation allows for the extravascular deficit which will consume approximately half the administered dose.

Immunoglobulin preparations

Immunoglobulin preparations consist of IgG with only trace amounts of IgM and IgA. Immunoglobulin preparations are usually administered intramuscularly, do not transmit viruses, and only rarely cause untoward reactions. The concentration of protein is usually 15 g/100 ml, but antibody content is variable and depends on the donors used. There are two types.

1. *Human normal immunoglobulin* (HNI) is prepared by fractionation of large pools of plasma from over 2000 ordinary donations. It is used as replacement therapy in hypogammaglobulinaemia and for passive protection against hepatitis A infection and measles.

2. *Human specific immunoglobulin* (HSI) is produced by fractionation of donations known to have particularly high titres of a specific antibody. They include anti-Rh(D), anti-tetanus, anti-zoster, anti-rabies and anti-hepatitis B.

Anti-Rh(D) immunoglobulin has proved outstandingly successful in preventing immunization against the Rhesus D antigen during pregnancy. It is also indicated if Rh(D) positive blood is transferred accidentally to a Rh(D) negative recipient. The dose is 50 i.u. per millilitre of red cells administered.

Anti-tetanus immunoglobulin is available as a 250 i.u. dose for prophylactic therapy. It should be given to patients who have not had appropriate active immunization (full initial course or a booster) within the last 5 years and who present with a dirty (soil-contaminated) wound or one which has not received medical attention for over 72 hours. A more concentrated preparation (3000 i.u.) is available for use in established tetanus.

Anti-hepatitis B immunoglobulin can be used prophylactically to diminish the severity of hepatitis B viral infections. The recommended adult dose is one vial given within 5 days of exposure. The material is in short supply and most frequently used for health service staff and emergency workers who accidentally inoculate themselves with the body fluids of a patient known to be HBsAg positive. This occurs from needle pricks or from splashes onto cuts or mucous membranes. Hepatitis B vaccine should normally be administered in addition to immunoglobulin in these cases.

Anti-rabies immunoglobulin is used together with rabies vaccine for post-exposure prophylaxis of rabies. Both must be used to give maximum protection to patients bitten by potentially infected animals.

Immunoglobulin preparations are now available which can safely be administered intravenously allowing large doses of IgG to be given rapidly. These offer the best replacement therapy for patients with hypogammaglobulinaemia but the value of this treatment in surgical infections remains to be established. High doses of IgG can elevate the platelet count in some patients with immune thrombocytopenia. This treatment, in conjunction with high-dose corticosteroids, may be useful in preparing such patients for splenectomy.

5. Nutritional support in surgical patients

Many patients coming to surgery have associated nutritional disorders. This is particularly true of patients with gastrointestinal disease, those with serious infections and those who have suffered major injuries. Some are admitted with a disease which has caused the nutritional disorder, for example carcinoma of the oesophagus, while others may develop it during treatment of a disease not normally associated with malnutrition. It is a disturbing fact that the risk of developing a nutritional disorder increases the longer a patient stays in hospital.

Although minor degrees of protein and calorie malnutrition do not appear to affect the outcome of surgical operations, there is no doubt that major nutritional disorders jeopardize recovery by impairing wound healing, lowering the body's resistance to infection and prolonging the recovery period.

Nutritional disorders in surgical practice have two principal components. Firstly there is starvation, caused either by the effects of the disease or restriction of oral intake, or both. Secondly there are the metabolic effects of inflammation, namely increased catabolism and reduced anabolism. These cause a kwashiorkor-like effect with a low serum albumin concentration, muscle wasting and water retention. While in some patients malnutrition may be purely the result of starvation, in most surgical patients it results from a combination of the two components.

Assessment of nutritional status

Although most patients undergoing surgery, including those with a minor degree of nutritional disorder, can withstand 3–4 days of starvation without obvious detriment, early detection and correction of progressing malnutrition is vital if recovery is not to be jeopardized or delayed.

There are many ways to detect protein-calorie malnutrition, ranging from simple anthropometry to sophisticated isotopic investigations. Happily, valuable information can be obtained from such simple measurements as changes in body weight, arm muscle circumference and serum albumin concentration. However, it has to be stressed that these changes can be difficult to interpret, especially in the short term, because of complicating factors such as water retention. Simple criteria of nutritional disorder in surgical patients include the following.

1. Recent unintentional weight loss of 10% or more
2. Body weight less than 80% of ideal for height
3. Serum albumin less than 30 g/litre
4. Total lymphocyte count below 1.2×10^9/litre
5. Mid-arm muscle circumference less than 80% of value in comparable population

Normal nutritional requirements

The recommended daily basal requirements for adults are shown in Table 5.1. Even after quite major surgical procedures these requirements change very little. However, if complications occur, such as intestinal ileus or abdominal sepsis, catabolism increases and energy requirements rise. In some patients, e.g. those with burns or major injuries, the metabolic requirements increase dramatically from the moment of injury (Table 5.2).

Nutritional requirements are usually estimated

Table 5.1 Recommended daily basal requirements

	Per kg body weight	Per 70 kg patient
Water (ml)	35	2450
Non-protein calories	30	2100
Carbohydrate (g)	2.0	140
Fat (g)	3.0	210
Protein (g)	0.7	50
Nitrogen (g)	0.1	7
Sodium (mmol)	1.0	70
Potassium (mmol)	1.0	70
Vitamin B (mg)	0.5	35
Vitamin C (mg)	1.0	70

Table 5.2 Average daily nitrogen and energy requirements in different metabolic states

Metabolic state	Nitrogen (g/70 kg)	Energy (kcal/70 kg)
Normal	7–9	2000
Starvation	9	2000
Moderate injury	12	2200
Hypercatabolic (e.g. multiple injury, major burns, sepsis)	up to 30	up to 3000

on the basis of the patient's clinical condition, but for a more accurate estimate his metabolic state can be assessed by measurement of urinary nitrogen excretion and indirect calorimetry.

Causes of inadequate intake

The ideal way for a surgical patient to take in adequate nutrients is to eat and drink palatable food. However, this may not be possible for a variety of reasons. The patient may be too weak and anorexic, or have a mechanical problem such as obstruction of the gastrointestinal tract. Patients with increased metabolic demands may have difficulty in taking in sufficient food to meet these demands. Some patients suffer from what is best described as 'intestinal failure'. This may be defined as a state in which the amount of functioning gastrointestinal tract is reduced to below a level where it can digest and absorb sufficient food to nourish the patient. The four principal causes of intestinal failure are:

1. the *short bowel syndrome* caused by massive resection of ileum and jejunum;

2. *fistula formation* in which the bowel content is lost externally or is short-circuited (internal fistula) before it can be adequately digested and absorbed;

3. *motility disorders* of the small bowel such as paralytic ileus and chronic intestinal pseudo-obstruction; and

4. extensive *small bowel disease* such as Crohn's disease.

In these difficult cases specialized nutritional treatment is required if the patient is to remain normally nourished. As a general rule, nutritional treatment is not effective in the presence of active sepsis. The priority in such patients is to eliminate the sepsis.

Methods of providing nutritional support

Nutrients can be given via the gastrointestinal tract, i.e. by enteral nutrition, or directly into the blood stream, i.e. by parenteral nutrition, otherwise known as intravenous feeding. Parenteral nutrition is indicated only when enteral feeding is not feasible. Very few patients are not suitable for some form of enteral feeding. Certainly all those who have a normal length of functioning gastrointestinal tract and most of those who have a reduced amount can be fed by this route.

ENTERAL NUTRITION

The first approach to enteral nutrition must be to try and encourage the patient to take in an adequate normal diet by mouth. If he cannot do this because of difficulty in swallowing, the food can be liquidized. If this approach is not successful, or not feasible, enteral nutrition using chemically prepared liquid feeds should be instituted. Such preparations can be used either for supplemental feeding or total feeding. In *supplemental feeding* the liquid diet is drunk or infused into the stomach or proximal jejunum at regular intervals to complement an otherwise inadequate food intake. *Total enteral nutrition* is indicated in patients who cannot eat or drink normally because of conditions that prevent them from doing so. These include:

- unconsciousness
- neurological dysphagia
- inflammatory bowel disease
- short bowel syndrome
- post-traumatic weakness
- postoperative weakness
- post-irradiation weakness
- head and neck surgery
- chemotherapy
- burns
- old age

Composition of liquid enteral feeds

A wide range of enteral feeding preparations are available, the main difference between them being the way in which the energy and protein content are presented. Liquid whole-protein feeds are cheaper and more palatable than those based on oligopeptides and amino acids, the so-called elemental diets. Although oligopeptides and amino acids are said to be better absorbed, especially in patients with shortened or diseased bowel, there is no firm evidence for this.

The energy content of most liquid diets is provided in the form of glucose, oligosaccharides, maltodextrin, corn syrup, medium chain triglycerides, sunflower seed oil, etc. Other essential nutrients such as electrolytes, minerals, trace metals and vitamins may be added in varying quantities, depending on the product. Several of the liquid feeds and supplements do not contain lactose and can thus be used in patients with lactose intolerance. An ideal nutritionally complete enteral regimen should supply 2000–3000 kcal (8.4–12.6 megajoules) of energy and 10–15 g of nitrogen per day in 2–3 litres of fluid. The proportion of energy provided by fat should be 30–40%, and the mixture should contain minerals, trace metals and vitamins.

Methods of administration

Nasogastric tube. If the patient is unable to drink or sip the liquid feed for mechanical reasons, or if he is unconscious or on a ventilator, the preparation can be given via a fine tube passed through the nose into the stomach or proximal small bowel. The position of the tip of the tube should be checked by X-ray before nutrients are infused. Modern feeding tubes are of fine bore and made of polyurethane or Silastic. They are well tolerated and can remain in position for long periods without the risk of oesophageal ulceration or chest complications such as those associated with large nasogastric tubes. Some patients who need prolonged enteral feeding can learn to pass a fine-bore tube into the stomach each evening and feed themselves overnight. This technique when carried out in the patient's own home is called 'ambulatory home enteral nutrition'.

Gastrostomy and jejunostomy. If nasogastric feeding is not possible because of disease or obstruction in the upper alimentary tract, nutrients may be given through a tube placed into the gastrointestinal tract below the lesion. Thus a patient with pharyngobulbar palsy or an oesophageal fistula can be fed through a gastrostomy, while a patient with a gastric or duodenal fistula may be fed through a jejunostomy.

Although these methods may be adequate in the short term, they tend to be less satisfactory in the long term because of local complications such as leakage around the tube and an increased incidence of problems such as diarrhoea.

Complications of enteral nutrition

Simply because liquid feeds are administered directly into the gastrointestinal tract, it cannot be assumed that enteral nutrition is free from complications. Patients being fed by this route are at risk from aspiration, vomiting and diarrhoea, and disturbances of metabolism and water balance. In addition, careless handling of the preparation can result in it becoming infected and causing gastroenteritis. The commonest complications of enteral nutrition are listed below.

- Gastric retention
- Aspiration
- Nausea and vomiting
- Abdominal cramps
- Diarrhoea
- Dehydration
- Hyperosmolar coma
- Hyperglycaemia
- Tube misplacement

- Oesophageal erosion
- Infection

PARENTERAL NUTRITION

Intravenous administration of nutrients is indicated when patients cannot be fed adequately by mouth, nasogastric tube or enterostomy, or when they are in a state of complete or partial intestinal failure. This situation may be permanent, as in the short bowel syndrome, or it may be reversible, as in paralytic ileus, when a fistula closes or when residual small bowel adapts.

Parenteral nutrition can provide a patient's total requirements of protein, energy, electrolytes, trace metals and vitamins. Because of the need to restrict volume, concentrated solutions of amino acids, carbohydrate and fat have to be used. As most such solutions are irritant and therefore intensely thrombogenic, they have to be administered through catheters with their tips positioned in large veins such as the superior vena cava.

As with enteral feeds, many different intravenous preparations are commercially available but all have the same principal components.

Carbohydrate solutions

Although many different types of carbohydrate have been used to provide energy, glucose is now considered to be the best source. Solutions used for intravenous feeding vary in concentration between 29% and 50%. The greater the concentration of glucose the more likely it is to precipitate diuresis and hyperosmolar problems. In some patients, especially those with infections, simultaneous administration of insulin may be required to avoid hyperglycaemia and ensure glucose utilization.

Other sources of energy such as xylitol, fructose, sorbitol and ethyl alcohol, although having theoretical advantages, are no longer used in the United Kingdom.

Fat emulsions

Preparations used in the United Kingdom are usually prepared from soya bean oil and are available in concentrations of either 10% or 20%. They are non-thrombogenic and not osmotically active. They are particularly valuable as a source of energy, providing 9 kcal/g. Thus, one litre of 20% fat emulsion together with its emulsifier will provide 2000 kcal. The amount of fat required for parenteral nutrition depends on the patient's condition. Patients with infections who find it difficult to metabolize glucose may need up to 50% of their energy requirement as fat, whereas those without infection may only need a weekly infusion of 500 ml of 10% fat emulsion to provide essential free fatty acids.

Amino acid solutions

In the past, amino acid solutions were prepared by hydrolysis of proteins such as casein, while modern solutions are a mixture of synthetic L-amino acids in crystalline form. These amino acids are delivered into the body's amino acid pool whence they are removed to form the 'building blocks' for the body's proteins. There is no agreed ideal formulation for intravenous administration but most solutions contain a mixture of essential and non-essential amino acids similar in composition to that of high quality protein such as egg white. A choice of amino acid mixtures is available, most providing between 7 and 17 g of nitrogen per litre.

Mixed solutions for total parenteral nutrition

Although total parenteral nutrition can be provided by either sequential or simultaneous infusion of glucose, fat and amino acids from separate bottles, it is now more common to mix the day's requirements into one 3-litre bag (this should be done in the pharmacy to avoid accidental contamination) and administer the mixture over 12–24 hours, depending on the patient's clinical condition. To prevent wasteful use of glucogenic amino acids as a source of fuel (energy), non-protein calories must be administered at the same time in sufficient quantity to prevent this happening. The recommended ratio is 150–200 kcal of non-protein energy for every gram of nitrogen administered.

In addition to adequate provision of energy and nitrogen, the patient's fluid and electrolyte requirements must be met. Many patients on parenteral nutrition need additional water, sodium and potassium because of excess fluid loss from, for example, a high-output fistula. Trace elements and vitamins must also be incorporated into the daily feeding regimen, often in increased quantities because of the demands created by infection and excessive loss. Special preparations of vitamins and trace elements are available for intravenous feeding.

Example. A 70 kg man with a high-output fistula from the duodenum is referred for intravenous feeding. The daily loss from the fistula is 800 ml of enteric contents. He needs an intravenous feeding regimen providing approximately:

2500 ml of water (normal daily requirements);
500 ml of water (to partially replace fistula losses);
80 mmol of Na^+ (normal daily requirements);
80 mmol of Na^+ (to replace fistula losses);
60 mmol of K^+ (normal daily requirements);
40 mmol of K^+ (to replace fistula losses);
16 g of nitrogen; and
2100 kcal of energy.

The above can be provided (within acceptable clinical limits) by:

1 litre of amino acid solution containing 14 g of nitrogen, 70 mmol of sodium and 60 mmol of potassium;
1 litre of 40% glucose solution providing 1600 kcal of energy;
0.5 litres of 10% lipid emulsion providing 500 kcal of energy; and
0.5 litres of 0.9% saline containing 75 mmol of sodium; to which are added 40 mmol of potassium, trace metals and vitamins.

All the above can be incorporated under sterile conditions by a skilled pharmacist into one 3-litre bag and infused into the patient using a simple pump.

Central venous administration

Sites for insertion of cannula for parenteral feeding

As the solution is hypertonic and has to be infused into a vein with a high blood flow, such as the superior vena cava, access has to be gained by cannulating tributaries of the chosen vein. Although veins in the lower limb can, and occasionally have to be used, this approach is best avoided because of the higher risk of thrombosis and infection.

The best veins to use are the internal jugular, the subclavian and the cephalic veins. The internal jugular vein is approached by direct puncture of the skin between the two heads of the sternocleidomastoid muscle, and the subclavian vein by direct puncture either above or below the clavicle. The cephalic vein is approached directly by cut-down into the deltopectoral groove. To allow patients greater mobility, the external portion of the cannula inserted via the jugular and subclavian veins is usually run through a subcutaneous tunnel which emerges through the skin over the middle of the sternum. The veins in the elbow, although easily accessible, should be avoided.

Modern cannulae are made of Silastic rubber and are of fine bore. Before use the position of the tip should be checked by chest X-ray. With good care a correctly positioned cannula can remain in position for several months.

Indications for parenteral nutrition

The chief indications for parenteral nutrition are those already mentioned under 'intestinal failure'. Although many surgeons have advocated preoperative parenteral nutrition as a means of improving the condition of a patient prior to operation, there is no good evidence that the outcome is affected. It is, however, sensible to commence parenteral nutrition in any patient with intestinal failure as soon as the condition is recognized. In such patients, operative removal of the lesion causing the nutritional disorder will be followed by more rapid recovery if nutritional support continues uninterrupted.

In contrast to preoperative parenteral nutrition, postoperative parenteral nutrition, when required, is effective and often life-saving. The vast majority of patients undergoing elective surgery have an uneventful postoperative course and do not require parenteral nutrition. However, when complications do occur, especially when these prevent enteral administration of nutrients and when accompanied by infection, parenteral nutrition becomes mandatory. Examples are paralytic ileus lasting more than three days, small bowel fistula and gross intra-abdominal sepsis. Intravenous feeding may also be necessary in patients with increased metabolic demands, e.g. after multiple injury or major burns.

Parenteral nutrition should continue until intestinal function has recovered sufficiently to allow the patient to maintain nutrition by the oral or enteral route. In cases of intestinal fistula, parenteral feeding should be continued until the fistula has either closed spontaneously or is closed surgically. Patients in whom enteral nutrition cannot be resumed may be taught the necessary techniques of parenteral administration and allowed to return home and to work. This is called 'ambulatory or home parenteral nutrition.'

Complications of parenteral nutrition

Catheter problems. Catheters can be wrongly positioned, with the tip lying in a vein other than the chosen one (usually the superior vena cava). It is essential not to start infusion of nutrients until the position of the cannula has been checked by X-ray. Sometimes the tip of the cannula penetrates the vessel wall so that it comes to lie outside the venous system. This should be suspected when blood cannot be freely aspirated from the cannula.

Careless handling of a cannula inserted through a needle can result in the cannula fracturing, with consequent embolization of the tip. In the event of such a mishap, the fragment can usually be recovered by interventional radiological techniques.

Thrombophlebitis. Thrombosis of the vein through which the cannula passes or in which its tip lies is a frequent complication, especially if a long line is used, if the tip is not in an area of high blood flow, or if extremely hypertonic carbohydrate solutions are used. The tell-tale signs are redness and tenderness over the vein carrying the cannula, together with oedema and swelling of the whole limb if the thrombosis is more proximal. Occasionally a superior mediastinal syndrome develops in patients with superior vena caval thrombosis.

The diagnosis should be confirmed by venography and anticoagulant therapy started with heparin. An attempt should be made to lyse the clot with urokinase. If this fails, the cannula must be removed and repositioned in an unoccluded vein.

Infection. Infection and septicaemia are the most serious complications of parenteral nutrition. The usual offending organisms are coliforms or staphylococci, but the incidence of fungal infections is increasing, possibly because many of the patients requiring parenteral nutrition are also taking broad spectrum antibiotics.

However, most catheter infections are the result of poor care of the intravenous feeding lines. The catheter insertion site should be dressed on alternate days using an antiseptic cream. Drip tubing should be changed daily and the line used *only* for infusion of nutrients and never for taking or giving blood or for drugs. Great care should be taken to avoid contamination when changing bottles or the 3-litre bag.

If the patient develops an unexplained pyrexia, the catheter insertion site should be examined for redness or purulent discharge. Blood should be taken from a peripheral vein and through the line and sent for culture. If this shows any evidence of infection, the catheter can be flushed out with heparin containing an antibiotic solution. If this fails to relieve the infection, the catheter is removed and its tip sent for culture. After 48 hours, provided the patient has recovered, a new cannula can be inserted.

Metabolic complications. Metabolic complications can arise especially if the solution is given too rapidly or if feeding continues for a long time.

An osmotic diuresis may occur as a result of renal overspill of hyperosmolar solutions, especially if they are given too rapidly. The problem can be minimized by increasing the time over which the infusion is given. The urine should be checked regularly for sugar. If glycosuria persists, the infusion rate should be further slowed.

Occasionally over-rapid infusion of hypertonic glucose causes an acute hyperosmolar syndrome. This is managed by slowing the rate of infusion and by the administration of insulin. Too rapid cessation of glucose infusion may result in rebound hypoglycaemia.

Long-term parenteral nutrition may lead to deficiencies in essential trace substances. Zinc deficiency may present as a skin rash, while folate deficiency can cause thrombocytopenia as well as the more commonly recognized anaemia. Hypophosphataemia may occur in patients receiving only glucose as an energy source.

Some patients develop sensitivity reactions to individual components of the nutritional regimen while others may react adversely to overprovision of a particular nutrient. Hepatomegaly and disordered liver function may occur as a result of excessive glucose provision.

Peripheral vein nutrition

Because of the undoubted risks associated with conventional parenteral nutrition, solutions have been developed which can be administered through peripheral veins. These contain isotonic amino acids and lipid emulsions which are less irritating to veins. While there is no doubt that they can be used over short periods, their value has not been substantiated. In patients who need long-term intravenous feeding conventional techniques should still be used.

6. Investigation and diagnosis of surgical problems

The general approach to a patient with a 'surgical condition' differs little from that used in other branches of medicine. However, there are matters of detail and sometimes of timing which are influenced by the particular nature of a surgical disease. Establishment of a clear diagnosis and assessment of the severity and extent of disease are the foundations for rational therapy, which need not necessarily include operation.

The approach may have to be modified if the rate of progress of disease does not allow time to confirm the suspected diagnosis before treatment becomes mandatory. The surgeon must then use his experience and judgement to decide the course to be followed. For example, approximately 20% of appendices removed on a clinical diagnosis of 'appendicitis' are normal. This figure can be reduced if patients are observed until the diagnosis is 'certain', but this must not result in an increased incidence of perforated appendicitis, peritonitis and even death.

Fundamental to the selection of appropriate investigative procedures is a clear definition of the patient's problems based on a detailed history and meticulous clinical examination. Neglect of this principle leads to unnecessary and indiscriminate investigation with inherent risks, discomfort and expense.

Investigations are required not only to confirm the diagnosis but also to monitor the course of the disease and the response to therapy. For example, radiology and endoscopy are used to monitor the response of a gastric ulcer to treatment, while serial liver function tests are needed to monitor the progress of a patient with obstructive jaundice.

EXAMINATION OF THE URINE

Routine analysis

Analysis of the urine is mandatory on admission to hospital. Diabetes may come to light in this way by detecting glycosuria, and this may have important implications for the conduct of anaesthesia. Microscopic examination of the urine may help to define the cause of acute abdominal pain, e.g. pyelonephritis (pus cells), renal colic (red cells, abnormal crystals) or appendicitis (usually, but not always, clear).

Microscopic examination of the urine may also be used to monitor progress. For example, the number of red cells reflects recovery after renal injury, while counts of casts can be used to monitor rejection of a kidney transplant.

Specific gravity (osmolality)

Measurement of the specific gravity of urine is all too often neglected. In the shocked patient who develops oliguria, it will help to differentiate acute renal tubular failure from inadequate renal perfusion due to hypovolaemia. The treatment of these two conditions is quite different. Only one drop of urine is needed for measurement of urinary specific gravity in a portable 'refractometer', which measures total solids. Measurement of urine osmolality by freezing-point depression is a more sophisticated technique for estimating the total concentration of solids in the urine of patients with complicated fluid and electrolyte problems.

24-hour collection

In some instances, 24-hour urine collections are

required to determine the excretion of particular substances. These include:

1. *creatinine* to determine creatinine clearance as a test of renal function;

2. *11-hydroxycorticosteroids, 17-oxosteroids* and *oestrogens* in the diagnosis of adrenocortical hyperactivity;

3. *3-methoxy-4-hydroxymandelic acid (VMA)* in the diagnosis of phaeochromocytoma;

4. *5-hydroxyindoleacetic acid (5-HIAA)* in the diagnosis and monitoring of the carcinoid syndrome;

5. *calcium* in suspected hyperparathyroidism or to monitor the progress of metastatic disease of bone;

6. *porphyrins* so that porphyria may be excluded as a cause of abdominal pain;

7. *amylase* to estimate amylase clearance relative to that of creatinine in the diagnosis of acute pancreatitis;

8. *electrolytes* (Na, K, Cl) when complicated problems of fluid balance require estimation of losses from all sources; and

9. *hydroxyproline* (OHP) to monitor progress of metastatic disease in bone.

EXAMINATION OF THE BLOOD

Venous blood should be sampled routinely for haematological and biochemical measurement. The indications for specific investigations are discussed elsewhere with reference to individual clinical situations. In most, if not all, cases it is necessary to know the haemoglobin concentration and white cell count, the blood urea, and the serum sodium, potassium and bicarbonate concentrations.

The haemoglobin concentration does not reflect the magnitude of acute haemorrhage, as compensatory haemodilution may not be complete for 48 hours. A patient admitted with acute haemorrhage who has a low haemoglobin concentration has probably suffered chronic blood loss as well.

As a general rule, a patient should not be submitted to surgery unless the haemoglobin concentration is 10 g/dl or more. Patients who are anaemic because of blood loss may benefit from a blood transfusion before operation. Except in an emergency, anaemia of unknown origin should be investigated before attempting surgery.

For all but minor operations, the patient's blood group should be determined. For more major procedures, each surgical service will have its own rules about the number of units of cross-matched blood that will be kept in readiness on the day of operation.

In patients treated by intravenous infusion and nasogastric aspiration, it is essential that the urea, sodium, potassium and bicarbonate concentrations are estimated daily.

Patients with a history of jaundice should be screened for hepatitis B surface antigen (HBsAg). A positive test indicates potential infectivity and the necessity of taking special precautions against spillage of or contamination with the patient's body fluids. Screening of patients suspected of being infected with human immunodeficiency virus (HIV) for HIV-antibodies is not yet routine.

Bio-assays employing bacteria, e.g. determination of serum cyanocobalamin (B_{12}) and folate, are affected by antibiotics and should therefore *not* be performed while the patient is receiving antibiotic therapy.

EXAMINATION OF THE STOOL

Examination of the abdomen is incomplete without digital examination of the rectum (Fig. 6.1). Rectal examination is in turn incomplete without inspection of any faeces on the examining finger and testing for the presence of faecal occult blood. Every rectal tray should carry the appropriate reagents (e.g. Haemoccult test cards).

Simple inspection of the stool is helpful in patients with diarrhoea. Slime and obvious blood may point to an inflammatory process, clay-coloured stools to obstructive jaundice; and bulky or frothy stools to malabsorption.

Microscopic examination of a fresh specimen of faeces is indicated in patients with diarrhoea. Pus cells, trophozoites, cysts of *Entamoeba histolytica*, and worms such as *Giardia lamblia* may be found. The presence of undigested meat fibres points to malabsorption. A preponderance of coccal organisms occurs in certain superinfections of the intestine. Bacteriological culture of the stool is es-

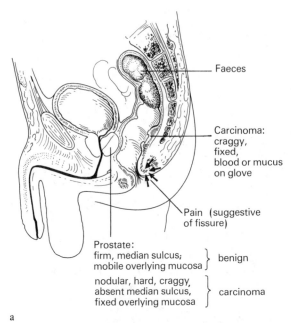

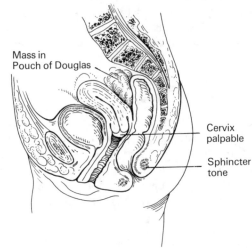

Fig. 6.1 Possible findings on digital examination of the rectum. (a) Male. (b) Female

1. Direct smears and culture of body fluids, tissues, exudates and excreta may provide evidence of infection. The swab is an inefficient sampling device. If it is used, it should be well loaded with material and sent to the laboratory without delay. Fragments of excised necrotic or devitalized tissue and specimens of frank pus in small bottles or capped syringes may yield much useful information. Special transport media may be used in some circumstances.

2. Determination of the type and sensitivity of an infecting organism is necessary for rational antibiotic therapy. Ideally, the administration of antibiotics should be delayed until sensitivities are known. If delay is dangerous, the bacteriologist and clinician together select 'blindly' the therapy which will deal best with the organism(s) believed most likely to be causing the infection.

3. From time to time, surgical wards develop a 'run' of infection in patients who have undergone operation. The bacteriologist can define precisely the type of organism and its sensitivity to antibiotics, and may then trace the source by bacteriological examination of nursing and medical staff, and of the ward and theatre environment. The source may prove to be an asymptomatic carrier, a faulty sterilizer or a patient with sepsis. It is important to keep a daily ward record of the state of all surgical wounds, preferably in a special 'wound book'.

4. Bacteraemia should always be considered as a possible cause of unexplained shock in a surgical patient. Serial blood samples are taken for culture. The ideal time for taking these samples relative to temperature elevations is still under debate. A good rule is to take one or two sets of blood cultures before starting antibiotic therapy. The responsible organism is often a Gram-negative bacillus and arises most frequently from the urinary tract, biliary tract or large bowel. Persistent pyrexia after an operation suggests an infection associated with the surgical procedure.

ENDOSCOPY

Endoscopy is defined as the viewing of the interior of hollow viscera and body cavities by instruments introduced through natural or created orifices. The development of flexible fibreoptic instruments in

sential in the investigation of patients with diarrhoea.

BACTERIOLOGICAL INVESTIGATIONS

Bacteriological investigations are important in surgical practice for several reasons.

which the light image is transmitted through thousands of tiny glass fibres, each coated with an opaque medium, has extended the scope, range and diagnostic accuracy of endoscopy. Most endoscopes have facilities for irrigation and suction, tissue biopsy and photography.

Upper gastrointestinal tract

The first oesophagoscopes and gastroscopes were rigid. Their passage was uncomfortable and general anaesthesia was usually required. Perforation of the oesophagus in the neck or at the entrance to the stomach was a well-recognized risk. This has been reduced by the introduction of fibreoptic endoscopes. These modern instruments are flexible, have controllable tips and can be swallowed relatively easily under mild sedation and local anaesthesia. However, rigid endoscopes are still used for sigmoidoscopy and cystoscopy, and in some clinics for bronchoscopy and oesophagoscopy.

The following flexible instruments are available.

Oesophagoscopes are end-viewing instruments which are rather shorter and thicker than the gastroscope.

Gastroscopes are available in end-viewing or side-viewing forms. The end-viewing instrument is better for all-purpose use, whereas the side-viewing gastroscope allows better inspection of the lesser curvature, particularly in its upper part.

Gastroduodenoscopes are longer versions of the gastroscope which can be negotiated through the pylorus to inspect the duodenum. Using the side-viewing instrument, the ampulla of Vater can be cannulated and radio-opaque contrast injected to visualize the common bile duct and pancreatic duct (Fig. 6.2) This is called endoscopic retrograde choledochopancreatography (ERCP). The investigation may be used to define the lower part of the bile duct in patients with jaundice or with a history suggesting gallstones in the bile duct and is of great value in the investigation of patients with suspected pancreatic disease. Cytological examination of pancreatic secretions may help in the diagnosis of pancreatic disorders.

Choledochoscopes are used primarily to inspect the interior of the bile ducts during operation and to detect residual calculi. Modern instruments

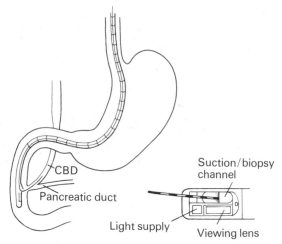

Fig. 6.2 Endoscopic retrograde cannulation of the pancreatic and biliary ducts (ERCP). CBD=common bile duct

have a wider channel which permits passage of a 'stone catcher' for the removal of retained stones. The instrument can also be inserted postoperatively along the drainage track following choledochotomy.

Lower gastrointestinal tract

The *proctoscope* is a short instrument (10 cm) which is introduced per anum to inspect the anal canal and lower rectum (Fig. 6.3). Haemorrhoids and other lesions of the anal canal, e.g. fissure and carcinoma, can be detected. Haemorrhoids can be injected and tumours biopsied. Proctoscopy is nor-

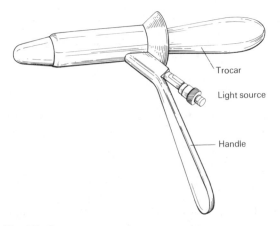

Fig. 6.3 *Proctoscope*

mally undertaken with the patient lying in the left lateral position, with the knees drawn up to the chest. It is always preceded by careful inspection of the perianal area and digital rectal examination. The instrument is well lubricated with KY jelly and introduced gently so that it passes upwards and forwards in the direction of the anal canal. Painful conditions such as acute fissure-in-ano are associated with marked anal spasm, so that proctoscopy is usually impracticable. In these circumstances the examination should be abandoned and the patient examined later under general anaesthesia. If the patient adopts the knee-elbow position, up to 10 cm of rectum can be visualized through the protoscope. However, this position is embarrassing for the patient and is therefore seldom used.

The standard *sigmoidoscope* is a rigid steel or plastic instrument, 25–30 cm in length, which is used to inspect the interior of the rectum and lower sigmoid colon. In modern instruments the lighting system is fibreoptic. During inspection of the rectum, the bowel is *gently* distended with air to allow better visualization of the mucosa.

Sigmoidoscopy is best carried out with the patient in the left lateral position and without special preparation. Before introducing the instrument, the rectum is examined digitally.

This relaxes the anal sphincter and determines whether the rectum is empty. If the rectum is full of faeces, examination is deferred pending bowel preparation.

The lubricated instrument, with its obturator in place, is then passed gently through the sphincter, following the direction of the anal canal for a few centimetres. It is then directed more posteriorly and the obturator is removed. The eyepiece and insufflator are attached and the instrument is now passed upwards under vision for its full length or until further progress is prevented by a pathological process or an anatomical feature. Negotiation of the pelvic-rectal junction (12–15 cm from the anal verge) can be difficult if there is an acute bend in the bowel and may give rise to considerable patient discomfort. One should not persist if this is the case.

The bowel wall is carefully inspected while the instrument is slowly withdrawn, and specially designed forceps can be used to take punch biopsies from obvious lesions or from the rectal mucosa.

Two sizes of rigid sigmoidoscope are available, and flexible fibreoptic instruments are now also in use and are preferred if the examination is to be carried beyond the pelvic-rectal junction. If a biopsy has been taken during sigmoidoscopy, the patient must not have any form of enema, *including barium examination*, for five days. Otherwise there is a definite risk that the forcible distension of the rectum by the enema will perforate the bowel at the biopsy site or result in air or barium embolization. In some radiological departments barium enemas are delayed for a week after any sigmoidoscopy, even when no biopsy has been taken.

The following are noted during examination.
1. General appearance of the mucosa (colour, consistency, signs of inflammation).
2. Presence of contact bleeding. In contrast to normal mucosa, inflamed mucosa bleeds if stroked lightly with forceps, a swab or the edge of the sigmoidoscope.
3. Any abnormalities, such as ulcerating neoplasia.
4. The nature of the bowel content (e.g abnormal faeces, the presence of mucus, fresh or altered blood, pus). These findings may signify pathology beyond the reach of the instrument. If faeces are encountered, a specimen is tested for occult blood.

Biopsies are taken of obvious abnormalities or, in some instances, of apparently normal mucosa.

Some lesions such as small polyps may be removed completely at sigmoidoscopy. Larger polyps are normally removed under anaesthesia using an *operating sigmoidoscope*. This is a shorter and broader version of the instrument. Diathermy can be used to fulgurate small mucosal lesions.

The *colonoscope* is a fibreoptic instrument which can be used to inspect the whole of the interior of the large bowel. It is particularly useful in the investigation of patients with colonic polyps, as these tend to be multiple and are frequently difficult to demonstrate radiologically. Any abnormal areas may be biopsied and polyps can be removed for histological examination with a diathermy snare. The procedure requires considerable patience on the part of both the operator and the patient, and meticulous bowel preparation is essential to its success.

The peritoneal cavity

The interior of the peritoneal cavity can be inspected through a *laparoscope*. General anaesthesia is preferred so that the abdominal wall can be relaxed for induction of a pneumoperitoneum. A needle is inserted through the abdominal wall just below the umbilicus and carbon dioxide is delivered through a water seal which acts as a safety valve to prevent excessive intra-abdominal pressure. The laparoscope is inserted through a small subumbilical incision and, by appropriate elevation of the head or foot of the operating table, different parts of the peritoneal cavity are inspected. Structures lying posteriorly cannot be visualized. Laparoscopy is particularly useful for:

1. examination of pelvic organs in the female and sterilization by tubal diathermy;

2. inspection of the liver in jaundiced patients (the detection of multiple hepatic metastases may obviate the need for laparotomy); and

3. biopsy of organs under direct vision. This is particularly useful for liver biopsy as the biopsy needle can be directed to areas of obvious pathology (Fig. 6.4).

The procedure is well tolerated even by frail patients, and is followed by little discomfort. Considerable care is needed in patients who have previously undergone laparotomy. Adhesions limit the view and bowel adherent to the anterior abdominal wall may be perforated during introduction of the instrument. Laparoscopy is being used increasingly as an aid to the differential diagnosis of acute abdominal disease, particularly when of pelvic origin.

The respiratory system

The *laryngoscope* may have a curved or straight blade and is used to inspect the pharynx and laryngeal inlet. It is usually inserted before a tracheal tube is passed or may be used for sucking out the pharynx under direct vision in the unconscious patient.

The *bronchoscope* is used to inspect the trachea and main bronchi under either local or general anaesthesia. A rigid instrument is still preferred by some. Large biopsies can be taken through this instrument and pus can be aspirated from the bronchial tree in patients with postoperative pulmonary collapse or severe chest infection. The flexible fibreoptic bronchoscopes now available are smaller than the rigid instruments and allow inspection of smaller bronchi. They may detect more peripheral lesions, but substantial biopsies cannot be obtained (Fig. 6.5).

The *mediastinoscope* is a rigid instrument which is introduced into the mediastinum through a short transverse incision in the suprasternal notch. Mediastinal tissues can be biopsied. The finding of involved mediastinal nodes in a patient with bronchogenic carcinoma may prevent fruitless operation.

The *thoracoscope* is an instrument similar to the laparoscope which is used to visualize the pleural space. Pleural or peripheral lung lesions may be biopsied without recourse to formal thoracotomy.

The urinary system

The interior of the bladder may be inspected through a *cystoscope*, a rigid instrument which is introduced via the urethra (Fig. 6.6). The bladder is subsequently distended with distilled water so that its entire interior can be viewed clearly. Modern cystoscopes have fibreoptric lighting systems which provide excellent illumination without

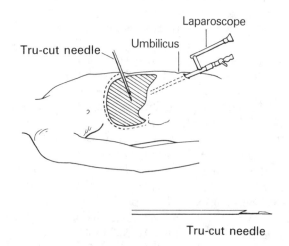

Fig. 6.4 Laparoscopy and liver biopsy

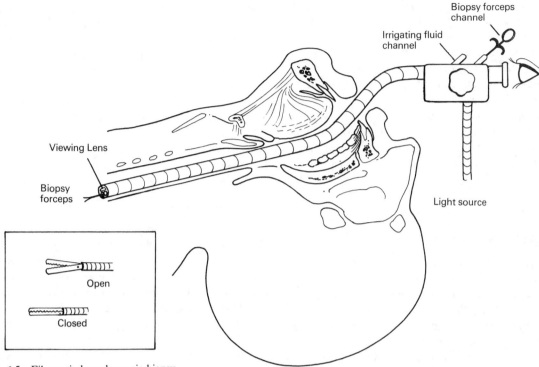

Fig. 6.5 Fibreoptic bronchoscopic biopsy

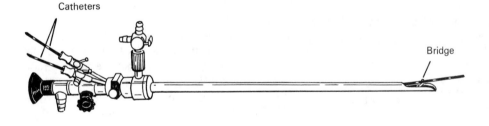

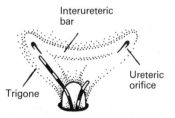

Fig. 6.6 Cystoscope and ureteric catheterization

heat. Forceps or diathermy leads can be introduced through the instrument for biopsy or fulguration.

The ureteric orifices are visible at cystoscopy and can be cannulated by fine catheters. Radio-opaque contrast medium introduced through these catheters allows visualization of the renal pelvis and ureter (retrograde pyelography).

Flexible fibreoptic *ureteroscopes* have been developed recently which can be introduced into the ureter to allow direct inspection of small lesions of the ureter or renal pelvis.

The urethra can be examined with a *urethroscope* in patients with urethral trauma, urethral stricture or prostatic disease.

A *nephroscope* is an instrument which, when inserted percutaneously through the renal substance, allows visualization of the renal pelvis. Stones in the pelvis or upper ureter may be extracted.

DIAGNOSTIC IMAGING

Principles of radiology

X-rays are produced by bombarding a tungsten target with an electron beam (Fig. 6.7). An image can be produced on a fluoroscopic screen which is activated by X-rays to produce light, or a silver precipitate can be made on a photographic plate or film coated with an emulsion sensitive to both light and X-rays. An X-ray film is normally enclosed in a cassette containing a fluorescent screen. This screen is activated by X-rays and produces light rays which reinforce the action of X-rays on the film.

The intensity of the image produced by target substances depends on their ability to absorb X-

rays. Metal absorbs them completely and is absolutely radio-opaque; fat and air are non-absorbent and are therefore completely radiolucent.

Passages of X-rays through solid objects depends not only on the radiation density of the object, but on electromagnetic properties of the X-rays, their quantity and time of exposure. By varying the kilovoltage of the machine (which determines the amount of radiation in the beam) and the time of exposure, the radiologist can visualize tissues of varying densities.

Three-dimensional and moving images

An X-ray plate gives a two-dimensional reproduction of a three-dimensional target so that radiologists frequently take additional films at 90° to the original plane. Anteroposterior and lateral films are routine when X-raying bones and chest. Various obliquities of projection help to demonstrate tissues at varying depths from the X-ray tube.

By moving the X-ray tube and film in opposite directions around a fulcrum in the plane of the object to be studied, the shadow of structures outwith that plane can be intentionally blurred. Only the plane under study is left in focus. Each film represents a 'slice' or section of the body or tissue and is called a *tomogram*. This technique has been brought to its ultimate sophistication by computerized transverse axial tomography (CT), as described below.

Stereoscopic techniques are also used in radiology. Two pictures are taken, the second after shifting the X-ray tube by a distance equal to that between our eyes. When viewed through a stereoscopic projector, the image appears three-dimensional. In the past this technique was most commonly used to detect small linear fractures of the skull but it is now being applied to the examination of soft tissues.

Moving organs or the flow of contrast material can be studied by observing sequential changes either on serial radiographs taken on rapid-change cassettes or by continuous viewing of the image on a fluorescent or television screen (Fig. 6.8). These techniques have proved of particular value in such dynamic investigations as coronary angiography or the study of deglutition.

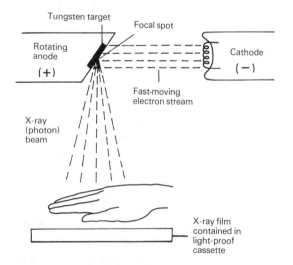

Fig. 6.7 Principles of radiology

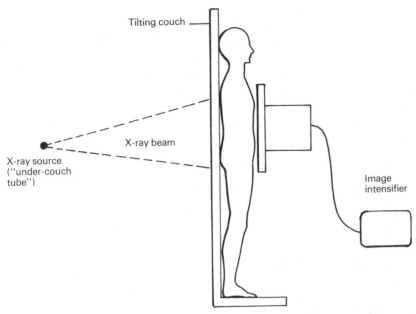

Fig. 6.8 Principles of television screening

Precautions

Radiological investigations expose the patient, radiologist and radiographer to potentially harmful irradiation. Radiation received by staff is monitored constantly by a small badge containing an X-ray film. Protective lead clothing is worn whenever staff are in an exposed situation. The hands of the radiologists are particularly vulnerable and lead gloves are worn when appropriate. The first sign of excessive radiation is vertical ridging and brittleness of the nails, followed by atrophy of the skin, excess keratinization and fisures.

Protection of the patient is also the responsibility of the radiological staff. They must know which levels of irradiation are safe and how much radiation is involved in routine investigations. In addition, it is now recommended that elective radiological investigations in women of childbearing age are carried out only in the first 10 days following menstruation so that irradiation of an unsuspected recently conceived fetus is avoided. This is the '10-day rule'.

Because of the radiation risk, requests for unnecessary radiological investigations must be avoided.

Special techniques

Contrast studies

In plain films the different densities of the body tissues, liquids and contained air provide contrast between adjoining structures and produce shades of grey on photographic film. Natural contrasts can be augmented by introducing air, barium sulphate or media containing iodine into body cavities and hollow viscera, and by oral or parenteral administration of radio-opaque materials which are secreted or excreted in body fluids.

An emulsion of barium is used to examine the alimentary tract. It may be swallowed to outline the oesophagus, stomach and small intestine or introduced by enema to outline the rectum and colon. Relatively small amounts of barium are used. Accuracy is improved if air is insufflated to distend the organ and spread the barium thinly on the mucosa. These 'air contrast' or 'double contrast' studies allow detection of fine mucosal abnormalities. At some sites distension is possible only if a relaxing agent is administered. For example, air distension of the duodenum requires injection of an anticholinergic agent such as propantheline or hyoscine butylbromide (Buscopan) and may reveal abnormalities not shown by routine barium studies. If there is clinical evidence of obstruction or perforation of the bowel is suspected, barium must not be used. It may provoke complete obstruction or cause dense adhesions in the peritoneal cavity. In these circumstances the water-soluble iodine-containing 'Gastrografin' is preferred.

A variety of other iodine-containing organic chemicals are available for contrast radiology of hollow viscera, ducts and other conduits. Water-soluble compounds specifically filtered and excreted by the kidneys are used for excretion urography, but can also be injected to outline arteries, veins, sinus tracts or ducts.

Compounds prepared in an oily base are used to visualize lymphatics and those sinus tracts in which only a more viscous medium will remain long enough to be radiographed. Oily media are particularly suitable for lymphangiography, as they are trapped by phagocytes in lymph nodes and allow serial X-rays to be taken over a period of months. Iodine-containing fluids of varying solubility are available which mix freely with particular body fluids and can thus be used to outline joints (arthrography), the spinal canal (myelography) or the ventricles of the brain (ventriculography).

Some compounds containing iodine have been developed specifically to be excreted by the liver. Some are fat-soluble and used to visualize the gallbladder. Others, such as Biligrafin, are water-soluble and following intravenous injection are excreted directly by the liver and outline the bile ducts (intravenous cholangiography).

Xeroradiography

Xeroradiography uses a plate consisting of an aluminium sheet coated with a thin layer of positively charged selenium. The charge is retained until the plate is exposed to light or X-rays, when it leaks out from the exposed areas. The pattern of the charge which remains is determined by the amount of X-radiation which has passed through the part examined and therefore by the radiation-absorbing properties of the tissues. The pattern of the remaining charged particles is made visible by blowing a blue plastic powder containing negatively charged particles onto the plate.

This adheres to the positively charged ions to produce an image which is impressed on plastic-coated paper by heat (Fig. 6.9).

A special feature of this technique is the 'edge enhancement' due to heaping-up of powder at lines of differing electrical charge. This makes it particularly suitable for the study of soft tissues, such as the breast, and for the detection of foreign bodies.

Thermography

Every object at a temperature above absolute zero emits infrared radiation which can be recorded by an infrared camera as a thermogram (Fig. 6.10). Thermograms must not be confused with conventional infrared photographs which are taken with an ordinary camera equipped with filters to remove visible light, and with film sensitive to long-wave light. In infrared photography the object must be illuminated by an external source, whereas a thermogram may be taken in total darkness. An infrared camera for thermography contains mirrors which focus the infrared rays onto a detector. Differences in temperature induce electrical activity which can be displayed on an oscilloscope and photographed. Areas of increased metabolic activity or vascularity are 'warmer' than surrounding areas.

Thermography is non-invasive and records natural body emissions. It has the drawback that the patient must be cooled in a constant ambient temperature for 15 minutes. It has been used for a variety of purposes, including detection of breast tumours, determination of tissue viability following trauma or burns, definition of inflammatory lesions and recognition of incompetent communicating veins in patients with varicose veins.

Computerized axial tomography (CT scanning)

Computerized axial tomography uses a slit beam of X-rays which are directed at points on the circumference of a narrow section of the body in the transverse axis. These rays fall sequentially on multiple scintillation crystal detectors with photomultipliers, each of which feeds impulses into a computer to build up a picture of the section

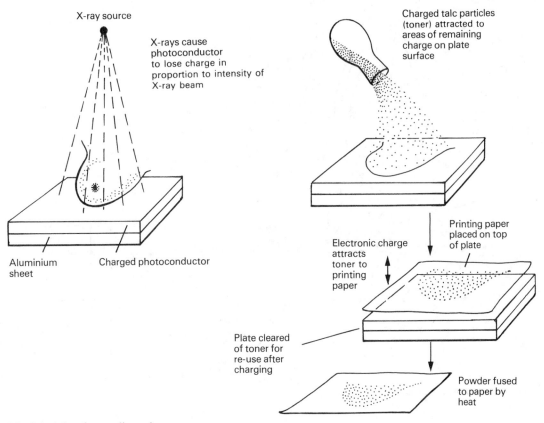

Fig. 6.9 Principles of xeroradiography

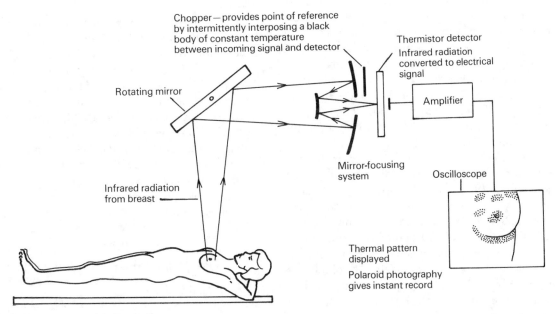

Fig. 6.10 Principles of thermography

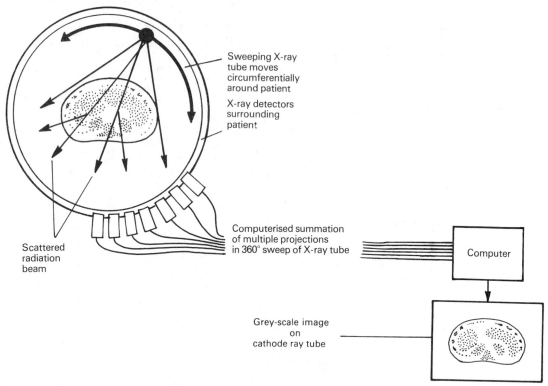

Sweeping X-ray tube moves circumferentially around patient

X-ray detectors surrounding patient

Scattered radiation beam

Computerised summation of multiple projections in 360° sweep of X-ray tube

Computer

Grey-scale image on cathode ray tube

Fig. 6.11   Principles of CT scanning

being examined (Fig. 6.11). The picture can be displayed on a console, printed out, or stored on tape or disc. The patient is gradually moved through a ring of tubes and detectors so that the whole body can be examined in a series of transverse sections. The dose of radiation to the skin is similar to that received in routine radiology.

CT scans can detect minor differences in tissue density. Resolution is extremely fine, one point on the matrix representing an area of tissue 0.75 mm × 0.75 mm.

CT scanning is already widely used in the investigation of intracranial disease, and for examination of the thorax and abdomen. Owing to respiratory and cardiac movement, intrathoracic and intra-abdominal structures are shown in less detail than intracranial structures but techniques of 'gating' images synchronously with respiration or heart beat are now available. Resolution is improved by the simultaneous injection of iodine-containing media which enhance contrast of abnormal tissues.

Radioactive isotopes and scintiscans

Trace studies

Isotopes emitting beta- or gamma-rays may be used as 'trace' substances to measure their non-radioactive counterparts in the body. For example, the size of body fluid compartments may be determined by injecting small amounts of radioactive substances, allowing time for equilibration, counting the isotope concentration and then calculating the total volume in which they are dissolved according to the 'dilution principle'. Assuming that the substance is equally distributed and not excreted or metabolized, the amount of substance injected (Q) equals the product of [S] and V, where [S] is the concentration of the dissolved substance and V the volume in which it is dissolved:

$$Q = [S]V$$

Since both Q and [S] are known, the volume is given by:

$$V = \frac{Q}{[S]}$$

The turnover of radio-isotopically labelled proteins and other substances can give valuable information on metabolism and organ function.

Scintiscans

As gamma-rays penetrate several centimetres of tissue, they can be detected by an external counting device. The counter usually consists of a detector which emits scintillations of light when exposed to gamma-radiation. These scintillations are magnified by photomultiplier circuits and counted or displayed visually. A mobile detector can be used to scan the patient (as in a rectilinear scanner) or multiple detectors can be used in a fixed device (as in the gamma-camera). The pattern of isotopic emissions can be printed out on paper or displayed on an oscilloscope screen.

Scintiscans can be used to study the circulation by estimating the flow of an isotopically labelled substance through an organ or part of the body. However, they are used most widely to visualize organs which selectively concentrate specific isotopes after oral or intravenous administration. The organ is scanned or photographed by the gamma-camera and its position and size assessed. Areas of abnormally high or low uptake may point to contained disease. Scintiscanning does not disturb patients to any extent.

To prevent radiation damage, isotopes suitable for scintiscanning should be excreted rapidly and have a short half-life. Thorium (Thorotrast), which was used at one time to outline the cerebral circulation, had a half-life of millions of years, accumulated in the liver and induced cancer formation.

Liver scans. The liver can be visualized by injecting dyes such as ^{131}I-labelled Rose Bengal which are concentrated by parenchymal cells (hepatocytes), or by injecting colloidal particles such as ^{99m}Tc-labelled sodium pertechnitate which are removed by reticuloendothelial (Kupffer) cells. In normal liver these isotopes are distributed uniformly. Lesions within the liver appear as areas of diminished uptake but must be at least 2 cm in size to be demonstrated. Liver scintiscans have a false negative rate of 25%.

Simultaneous liver and lung scans may be used to demonstrate a subphrenic abscess by revealing a gap between the upper margin of liver and lower margin of lung.

Pancreatic scans. Methionine labelled with selenium-75 is taken up by acinar cells and has been used for pancreatic scintiscanning. Its accuracy is too low and it is seldom used.

Lung scans. Two types of lung scan are used. In 'perfusion scans', microaggregates of serum albumin labelled with ^{131}I or ^{99m}Tc are injected intravenously to outline the pulmonary circulation. In 'ventilation scans' radioactive xenon (^{133}Xe) is inhaled to outline the bronchi and alveoli. An area of diminished uptake on the perfusion scan may indicate pulmonary embolus. Postoperative atelectasis diminishes both perfusion and ventilation and produces an abnormality on both scans. A ventilation scan should be performed whenever interpretation of a perfusion scan is in doubt.

Thyroid scans. Radioactive isotopes of iodine (^{131}I and ^{125}I) are trapped selectively by thyroid acinar cells. The determination of uptake by the gland relative to its concentration in the blood and excretion in the urine was once the basis of thyroid function tests. This approach has been replaced by biochemical estimation of circulating thyroid hormone levels in peripheral blood.

Thyroid scanning is still used to detect localized increased or decreased uptake in patients with palpable thyroid nodules. However, radioiodine has now been superseded by ^{99m}Tc sodium pertechnicate, which is also taken up by the iodine-trapping mechanism but is easier to prepare and exposes the patient to a lower dose of irradiation. The nodules are described as 'hot' if the isotopes are taken up to a greater degree than in the surrounding gland, 'cool' if the concentration is the same, and 'cold' if less. The function of a palpable nodule is a valuable pointer to its pathology. A hot nodule is most likely to be a benign adenoma, whereas a cold nodule is likely to be a cyst, degenerate benign nodule or cancer.

Total body scans after the injection of ^{131}I are used to detect metastatic lesions in patients with thyroid cancer.

Brain scans. ^{131}I-labelled human serum albumin, [^{99m}Tc] sodium pertechnicate and [^{113m}In] indium chelate are used to investigate patients with suspected intracranial lesions. The increased vascularity of brain tumours results in higher uptake than in normal brain. Non-malignant cystic lesions appear as areas of diminished uptake. Haematomas may also show increased uptake but, as the isotope has to diffuse into the haematoma, activity appears more slowly than in tumours. Serial scans may differentiate between the two. Brain scintiscans have now been superseded by CT scans.

Skeletal scintiscans. Increased turnover of bone minerals in areas of osteoblastic activity can be demonstrated by scintiscans following intravenous injection of bone-seeking isotopes. Fluorine-18, strontium-85 and calcium-47 were initially used but ^{99m}Tc-labelled diphosphonates and polyphosphates are now preferred.

Bone scanning is used mainly to detect bone metastases when typically multiple 'hot spots' are seen. The osteoblastic activity surrounding these metastases may be detected several months before radiological change. Areas of increased uptake may also be seen in Paget's disease, in arthritis and other degenerative conditions and at fracture sites.

Venous thrombosis. The early detection of deep venous thrombosis is facilitated by scintiscanning of the legs after intravenous injection of ^{125}I-labelled fibrinogen. This is administered before operation and the legs are scanned daily for 7–10 days. As a venous thrombosis forms, it incorporates labelled fibrinogen and produces a localized hot spot. Prevention of deep venous thrombosis is more important than early detection and this technique has proved particularly useful in assessing the value of prophylactic regimens.

Ultrasonography

The tissues of the body vary in their capacity not only to absorb radiation but also to absorb sound. When an ultrasonic wave strikes the interface between two media of different acoustic impedance, some of the energy is reflected into the first medium as an ultrasonic echo whose amplitude depends on the relative impedance of the two media and is greatest at the interface between solids and liquids (Fig. 6.12). The echo is recorded by a detector in line with the generating ultrasonic beam and can be displayed on an oscilloscope as an unidimensional wave (a scan). If a sweeping beam is used, a two-dimensional black

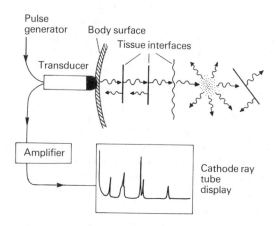

Fig. 6.12   Principles of ultrasonography

and white picture can be constructed (B scan). In modern machines the intensity of the image can be modulated according to the amplitude of the reflected wave, and a picture of varying shades of grey can be produced. This is called *grey-scale ultrasound.*

Multiple generators and detectors in different planes can be used to construct an ultrasonic tomogram. Three-dimensional images are also possible; in some sites, e.g. the pancreas, the quality of the image rivals that of CT scanning. 'Gated' images synchronous with the heart beat allow good resolution of intracardiac structures.

Ultrasound is non-invasive, carries no radiation risk and has high resolution. In surgical practice it is used most commonly to determine whether a mass is solid or cystic. The progress of pancreatic cysts, deep-seated abscesses or an aortic aneurysm can be followed by serial examinations. Ultrasonography is also used to detect displacement of the falx cerebri by space-occupying intracranial lesions. Other uses include scanning of the liver for metastases, monitoring the fetus in utero and defining intracardiac anatomy.

Ultrasonic flow meters have been developed which function on the Doppler principle. Movement of red blood cells causes a shift in the frequency of the signal reflected from their interface with fluid blood. Transcutaneous flow meters consist of an ultrasonic transmitter, a receiver, an audio-amplifier and loudspeakers. When the transducer (which contains transmitter and receiver) is placed over a vein, venous flow is audible. In obstruction there is silence. In the normal limb, squeezing the leg distal to the transducer augments the venous flow and causes a roar from the loudspeaker, indicating patency of the vein. A similar system is used to study flow in peripheral arteries.

A sophisticated form of ultrasonography is echocardiography which is used to obtain a time-based tracing of movements within the heart. The reflection of the moving valves and chamber walls can be printed out in grey-scale fashion, and intra-cardiac lesions can be defined. Similarly, arterial lesions can be defined by sophisticated imaging of red cell movements.

BIOPSIES

In many situations a sample of tissue must be obtained for histopathological or biochemical examination before a definitive diagnosis can be made. This is particularly important in the differentiation between benign and malignant disease, and in the liver or kidney, where diseases of different aetiology can produce similar changes in form or function.

Cytology

Cytology is the examination of the architecture of cells, while histopathology is the examination of the architecture of tissue and its cellular components.

Two main methods are used to obtain cells for examination.

Exfoliative cytology. Cells shed by epithelial linings of hollow viscera or ducts can be separated from secretions or excretions and examined for abnormalities. As the cells are suspended individually or in clumps, the recognition of abnormalities rests on examining cellular as opposed to tissue morphology, and considerable skill and experience are required. Exfoliative cytology is readily applied to diseases of the upper gastrointestinal, respiratory, urinary and female genital tracts.

Needle aspiration cytology. A 1.5 mm needle is attached to a syringe and inserted into the tissue to be sampled. Suction is applied and the needle advanced several times through the tissue so that a small drop of cellular material is drawn into the needle shaft. The needle and syringe are then withdrawn and the contents of the needle are smeared onto a slide (Fig. 6.13).

Apart from obtaining material for cytological ex-

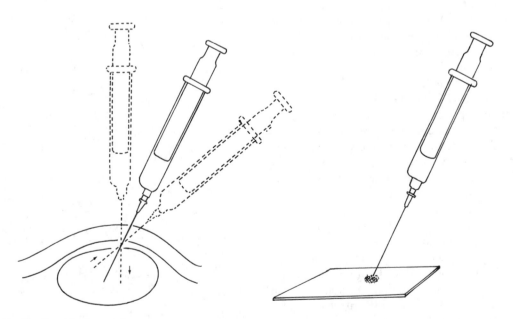

Fig. 6.13 Needle aspiration cytology

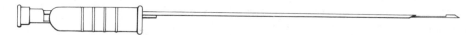

Fig. 6.14 Tru-cut biopsy needle

amination, needle aspiration can be used to differentiate cystic from solid swellings. Cysts of the thyroid, breast and kidney can be readily distinguished from solid tumours and operation avoided. Radiological screening with X-rays or ultrasonic scanning can aid accurate direction of the needle into a deep-seated lesion. For example, a lesion detected on mammography, even if not palpable, can be sampled and a diagnosis reached without, or prior to, its surgical removal.

Histopathology

Needle biopsy. Various types of hollow needle have been used for 50 years to obtain small cores of tissue. Most have a trocar, cutting tip and a mechanism to retrieve the tissue sample. The Vim-Silverman and Menghini needles have been largely superseded by the Tru-cut needle (Fig. 6.14), which is used to obtain biopsies of liver, kidney and muscle. Specially designed cannulae with cutting edges are used for bone and marrow biopsies.

Drill biopsy. Modern drill biopsy apparatus consists of a small sharp cannula attached to a high-speed compressed air drill which rotates at 15–20 000 r/min. The technique is cumbersome, noisy and seldom used.

Punch biopsy. Punch biopsy forceps are used for removing pieces of tissue from skin tumours and from lesions within the mouth or nose. Small punch biopsy forceps can be passed through endoscopes and have been used to obtain tissue samples from the gastrointestinal tract, the urinary system and the bronchi. However, the recent introduction of miniature forceps which can be passed through fibreoptic endoscopes now allows biopsies to be obtained from any part of the gastrointestinal tract, from within the bile ducts and from the lungs (see Fig. 6.5). As these biopsies are small, multiple samples should always be taken, otherwise the true nature of a lesion may be missed.

Crosby capsule biopsy. This technique is used to obtain samples of small bowel mucosa and is particularly valuable in the investigation of malabsorption. The Crosby capsule is a small metal cylinder containing a biopsy channel and a guillotine. It is attached to fine tubing through which suction can be applied (Fig. 6.15). It is swallowed by the patient and its position monitored radiologically. When the capsule is in the desired position, suction is applied to the tube. This draws a portion of mucosa into the capsule which is snipped off and retained by the guillotine. The capsule is withdrawn slowly by traction on the suction tube. Alternatively, the tubing is cut and the capsule recovered from the faeces.

Modifications of this capsule allow biopsy specimens to be sucked up the tube so that multiple biopsies from different sites can be obtained.

Open biopsy. Open operation may be necessary if the site is otherwise inaccessible, if closed methods are thought dangerous, or if a large piece of tumour is required. The biopsy may be ob-

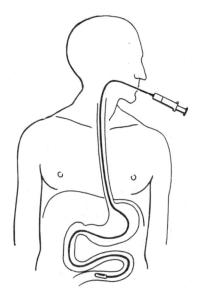

Fig. 6.15 Crosby capsule used to biopsy small bowel mucosa

tained by incision (cutting into the tissue to obtain a sample) or excision (removing the whole of the abnormal tissue). Immediate histological examination by frozen section technique is indicated when diagnosis is required urgently, e.g. so that the surgeon may proceed with definitive operative treatment.

Surgical exploration

In some patients it is necessary to resort to formal exploratory operation to establish the presence, extent and nature of disease. This is not an admission of diagnostic failure, and when used appropriately may save the patient numerous expensive and painful investigations. Further, the operative findings and immediate histological diagnosis may allow the exploratory procedure to be converted into a therapeutic one.

POPULATION SCREENING

Screening of normal populations of men and women for early signs of disease has been used in this country to detect malignant disease of the uterine cervix, the lung and the breast. In Japan, where cancer of the stomach is common, screening of normal persons by radiology and endoscopy has resulted in early detection of this cancer and may have reduced mortality.

As screening is expensive, the condition sought must be sufficiently serious to pose an important health problem and its natural history must be well understood. There must be a recognizable early stage and evidence that treatment at that stage confers more benefit than treatment later. The method chosen should be acceptable to the patient, highly sensitive (i.e. it should detect over 90% of established lesions) and preferably non-invasive and of high specificity, i.e. the false positive rate must be low. The availability of simple tests to identify individuals at risk from the disease is an advantage in that it allows screening to be concentrated on those most likely to require it. The cost of introducing a screening programme must be balanced against the benefit it provides.

Before launching any large-scale screening programme, it is essential to demonstrate conclusively that early detection will reduce the mortality caused by the disease in question. Such evidence usually requires a controlled trial in which the mortality of the disease in the population offered screening is compared with that in randomly allocated controls.

TESTS OF FUNCTION

The techniques described above are concerned mainly with the detection of anatomical abnormalities. Many disease processes, however, do not produce anatomical change but are the result of aberrations of function. These can be detected by tests of organ and tissue function.

Simplest are the range of biochemical tests commonly used in the initial investigation of a patient — 'the biochemical profile'. For example, plasma urea and creatinine concentrations reflect renal function, while those of albumin, bilirubin and liver enzymes reflect hepatic function. Serum electrolytes give an indication of general metabolic functions. Some abnormalities may reflect impaired function of one of several tissues. For example, a raised alkaline phosphatase may be caused by disease of the liver, bone or intestinal tract.

A whole range of complex biochemical investigations are now available to study the synthetic, secretory, absorptive and excretory functions of organs. It is important to remember that many organs and tissues have other than biochemical functions. For example, the gastrointestinal tract displays motor activity, a nerve conducts impulses, a muscle contracts. Measurements of intraluminal pressure, of electrical impulses and of the effects of stimuli are all used to study disease processes. Many of these sophisticated techniques have originated in physiological and clinical research laboratories and should be applied clinically only when proven to be safe and to give valid information.

Details of the use of these and other investigations in specific diseases are given elsewhere.

7. Preoperative assessment and preparation

Preoperative assessment and preparation are an essential part of any surgical procedure. Elective operations should be carried out under optimal conditions with full physical and psychological preparation of the patient, who should be adequately informed of the reason for the operation, its nature and its implications. In an emergency this may not be possible and an operation may have to be performed in less than ideal circumstances (see Ch. 10).

OUTPATIENT VISIT

Assessment and preparation begin at the first outpatient consultation. A good referral letter from the general practitioner is invaluable, providing an assessment based on a long professional relationship between family doctor and patient. The first responsibility of the consulting surgeon is to reach the most probable diagnosis based on a careful history, detailed physical examination and the results of investigations. Many of these can be carried out during outpatient visits but some require admission to hospital.

A decision to recommend operation is made once the cause of the patient's problem has been diagnosed and it is known to be amenable to surgical treatment. The patient must be fully informed of the nature of his illness and, if he wishes, given an accurate prognosis. He should understand the reason for the operation and its implications in terms of mortality, complications and long-term morbidity. Thus, the likelihood of residual deformity and disability, e.g. from an amputation or artificial stoma, should be discussed frankly from the outset. The surgeon should indicate the likely duration of stay in hospital, the period of convalescence and the time of absence from work or household duties.

By the end of his outpatient visits the patient should be fully aware of what lies ahead. He will appreciate an estimate of the date of admission so that he can make appropriate arrangements.

The surgeon should write to the general practitioner after every outpatient visit to keep him informed of progress.

Assessment of fitness for operation

The pre-admission clinic

In most hospitals the house surgeon is primarily responsible for recording a full history and clinical findings in the patient's case notes. This serves as a data base and defines secondary problems which may merit consideration. In addition, fitness for anaesthesia and operation must be carefully assessed.

Ideally all patients awaiting elective surgery should be seen at a 'pre-admission' outpatient clinic some days before the admission date. This ensures that undiagnosed medical conditions such as diabetes or hypertension are identified before admission and appropriate therapy is instituted. Current medication can be modified or stopped according to need. The patient can then be admitted to the ward on the night before operation with all necessary investigations completed.

The following should be ascertained routinely.

Fitness for anaesthesia. Any disease which increases the risk of anaesthesia and surgery should come to light during the systematic enquiry. The use of drugs should be noted, particularly of steroids, insulin, drugs given to treat cardiac failure or arterial hypertension, anticoagulants, bronchodilators, antibiotics and psychotropic agents. Women of child-bearing age should be asked whether they are taking the contraceptive pill. Because of the risk of miscarriage or exposure to drugs which may be teratogenic, elective non-urgent operations are not performed on pregnant women. Particular attention is paid to a history of past cardiovascular, respiratory or renal disorders.

Allergies and hypersensitivity. Any previous adverse or idiosyncratic response to a drug or other substance should be recorded clearly. Sensitivity to Elastoplast and penicillin are common. Knowledge of sensitivity to iodine-containing compounds is essential, as deaths have been reported from X-ray departments following the injection of contrast media containing iodine in sensitive patients. A similar risk is attached to some preoperative radiological investigations, such as cholangiography carried out before cholecystectomy.

Previous operations and anaesthetics. Any complications, particularly chest, cardiac or renal complications, jaundice or infection, following a previous operation or anaesthetic should be noted. A history of unexplained jaundice after halothane administration or prolonged apnoea following the use of suxamethonium chloride may influence the conduct of anaesthesia. The case notes from previous admissions must be read in their entirety. It is recommended that halothane is not given twice to a patient within a 3-month period unless there is a specific indication for its further use.

Alcohol and drug abuse. Possible abuse of alcohol and psychotropic drugs must be recorded. These can affect the tolerance to anaesthetic agents and lead to difficulty in inducing and maintaining anaesthesia. If chronic intake of these agents has led to drug dependence, withdrawal symptoms can be anticipated in the postoperative period.

Smoking. Cigarette smoking is associated with a major increase in postoperative chest complications. All patients should be encouraged to stop smoking once the decision to operate has been made. The longer the interval between stopping smoking and operation, the lower the risk of postoperative problems.

Physical examination

General metabolic status

The patient's weight and height should be recorded. The dose of some drugs is determined by body surface area rather than weight. Emaciated malnourished patients withstand surgery poorly. The serum albumin and total protein levels are measured and, if necessary, nutritional status is improved by preoperative dietary supplements, nasogastric tube feeding or parenteral nutrition (see Ch. 5).

Obese patients present many problems: venepuncture and intravenous infusions are more difficult; landmarks are obscured; surgical exposure is tedious; postoperative respiratory problems are common; and the risks of thrombo-embolism, wound infection and wound dehiscence are increased. Unless operation is urgent, it should be postponed until a substantial weight reduction has been achieved. The basic requirements regarding haematological and biochemical measurements have been mentioned in Chapter 6. A coagulation screen is performed if:

1. there is a history of a previous bleeding disorder or of undue bleeding at a previous operation;
2. the patient has received cytotoxic chemotherapy or drugs affecting coagulation;
3. there is acute or chronic liver disease; or
4. there is evidence of purpura or spontaneous bruising.

Specific disease states can significantly influence the risk of anaesthesia and operation. Of equal importance to knowing the diagnosis is an understanding of the associated functional disturbance and its implications for the perioperative period.

Respiratory system

The chest should be examined clinically and a chest X-ray obtained if there are any respiratory symptoms or signs. In many hospitals it is considered appropriate to obtain a chest X-ray routinely in any patient over the age of 45 years and all those undergoing abdominal surgery. An added advantage of this policy is that it serves not only as a screening procedure for lung tumours but also establishes a preoperative record for comparison should postoperative respiratory difficulties occur. If there is a productive cough, a specimen of sputum is sent for bacteriological examination.

Chronic bronchitis and emphysema are associated with an increase in intrapulmonary shunting presenting as arterial hypoxaemia. The arterial Po_2 should be considered in the light of the fact that, without special precautions, abdominal or thoracic surgery causes additional short-term hypoxaemia which could be life-threatening. Patients with the severest form of chronic bronchitis (type 2 respiratory failure), in which hypoxaemia is accompanied by carbon dioxide retention, are a high-risk group and likely to need artificial ventilatory support in the postoperative period. In view of their short life expectancy, in any case, they should not be considered for anything other than the most urgent operations.

Patients with asthma and other diseases causing reversible airway narrowing may develop postoperative respiratory failure because of the excessive work of breathing. It is important, therefore, to assess the severity of airway constriction and, if necessary, to take steps to lessen the work of breathing by administering appropriate bronchodilators such as salbutamol.

The best index of the state of the airways is the ratio of the forced expiratory volume in 1 second (FEV_1) to the forced vital capacity (FVC) expressed as a percentage, i.e. 100 FEV_1/FVC. A value less than 50% which cannot be improved by appropriate therapy is likely to be associated with the need for artificial ventilatory support in the postoperative period. Values above 75% are normal. A crude but useful test of normality is to ask the patient to extinguish a lighted match held 25 cm (10 inches) from the mouth by blowing with the mouth open, not with pursed lips as for birthday candles. 'Normal' people can achieve a high enough airflow to extinguish the flame.

Patients with chronic pus production in the bronchial tree, as in bronchiectasis, need a good cough effort to dispose of secretions and prevent them from descending further into the bronchial tree with absorption collapse. Antibiotic therapy and inducement to cough and drain the lungs, supervised by a competent physiotherapist, may lessen the problem. If such patients undergo abdominal or thoracic surgery, the pain in the postoperative period may prove a major impediment to coughing. Special attempts are then made, perhaps with local anaesthetic nerve blocks, to render these patients pain-free.

Healthy patients in the acute phase of the common cold should not be submitted to elective anaesthesia and surgery. The drugs that they are likely to receive will inhibit ciliary activity and encourage the spread of infection into the distal bronchial tree with consequent risk of bronchopneumonia.

Cardiovascular system

The cardiovascular system should be examined carefully, taking special note of the arterial pressure, pulse rate and rhythm, and any signs of right or left heart failure.

The fundamental requirement is adequacy of oxygenated blood flow to the vital organs: brain, liver, kidney and myocardium (see below). Factors which compromise perfusion are a reduction in cardiac output as a result of heart muscle disease or ineffective cardiac rhythm, and obstruction to flow in major blood vessels as a result of disease such as neoplasia. Of course, these processes may be interrelated: generalized vascular disease may cause hypertension leading to left ventricular strain and eventually failure, while coronary artery disease can cause areas of ischaemia with consequent arrhythmia.

Patients with clinical signs of cardiac failure should be assessed with a view to introducing new treatment or altering existing drug treatment so that their cardiovascular system is in an optimal state before the operation begins. Drugs to control cardiac failure or treat cardiac arrhythmias should usually be continued over the period of operation, but with additional precautions, if necessary (see below). The same is true of most types of antihypertensives.

If a raised arterial pressure is found on

preoperative examination in a patient not previously known to be hypertensive, the first step is
to give a reassuring explanation and then repeat
the measurement 4-hourly over 24 hours. Often,
after one or two measurements the pressure falls
to within the normal range. Persistent hypertension is an indication to postpone the operation
until the cause of hypertension is known and appropriate treatment established. In very urgent
cases the advice of an experienced physician
should be sought with a view to rapid control of
pressure with various combinations of diuretics,
beta-blockers, vasodilators and calcium channel-
blockers, according to the severity of the
condition. The goal is a diastolic pressure of
105 mmHg or less.

There is good evidence that surgery in untreated
hypertensive patients is associated with an increased risk of cerebrovascular accident and
myocardial infarction.

Whenever possible, anaesthesia and surgery
should be avoided in the first year after a myocardial infarct (except for operations on the heart
which are designed to improve the vascular supply). The risk of operation causing re-infarction is
very high (1 in 2 or worse) in the first 4–6 weeks
after infarction, falling markedly over the next 6–
12 months (see Fig. 10.1).

Patients with evidence of myocardial ischaemia
are likely to suffer myocardial infarction if the
effects of anaesthesia increase myocardial oxygen
demand, decrease coronary blood flow, or both.
Drugs or techniques which increase heart rate and
consequently alter filling time for diseased
coronary arteries, or which raise ventricular and
diastolic pressure and alter perfusion gradients,
must be used with great care. Many anaesthetic
drugs have this potential.

Great care is needed in the surgical and anaesthetic management of patients who have a 'fixed'
cardiac output, e.g. those with severe aortic
stenosis or cardiac tamponade. Even very small
haemodynamic changes induced by anaesthetic
agents or modest degrees of blood loss can lead to
sudden acute cardiac failure or myocardial infarction if the coronary perfusion is compromised.

Cardiac arrhythmias occurring in the
preoperative period should be discussed with a
cardiologist. While the underlying problem may

be relatively benign (e.g. runs of ventricular extra-
systoles can be a feature of sudden withdrawal
of nicotine in a person who normally smokes
heavily), it can also be of serious import. For
example, arrhythmias may signal an area of
ischaemia or a metabolic or drug problem causing
disturbance of the potassium ratio across the cell
membrane. Atrial fibrillation, a common arrhythmia, has a wide variety of causes, ranging from
myocardial ischaemia to thyrotoxicosis. In many
cases the fibrillation cannot be altered but its effect
on ventricular rate may need to be controlled.
Patients with a heart block may require a temporary pacemaker.

Patients with valve disease, typically after
rheumatic fever, should be given prophylactic
antibiotics before any surgical operation to prevent subacute bacterial endocarditis.

The concept of available oxygen. The carriage
of oxygen to the tissues is governed by three
factors:

1. the arterial *oxygen tension*, which in turn
depends on the adequacy of lung alveolar Po_2 and
the proper matching of alveolar gas and pulmonary capillary blood — the ventilation/per-
fusion relationship (V/Q ratio);

2. the *oxygen-carrying capacity* of blood, which
depends on the concentration (measured in g/dl)
of effective haemoglobin (carboxyhaemoglobin and
methaemoglobin are ineffective); and

3. the *cardiac output* and *regional blood flow*.

The available oxygen is calculated by multiply-
ing the total oxygen content by the flow. At a Po_2
of 12 kPa (90 mmHg), 100 ml blood with an
effective haemoglobin concentration of 13 g/dl
contains approximately: 0.27 ml O_2 in simple
solution and 17.42 ml combined with
haemoglobin, i.e. a total of 17.69 ml of oxygen.

If the cardiac output is 5 litres/min, the tissue
availability of oxygen is 884.5 ml. The resting
metabolic demand is usually about 200 ml/min so
that there is an apparently impressive safety
margin. However, the venous Po_2, a useful index
of tissue Po_2, should not fall below 5.3 kPa
(40 mmHg), which approximates to an oxygen
content of 12.31 ml/dl.

Thus, halving either the cardiac output or the
haemoglobin concentration, with maintenance of

oxygen consumption, will reduce venous $P\text{O}_2$ to an unacceptably low value.

A combination of low-flow, uncompensated anaemia and increased tissue oxygen demand (fever) is obviously undesirable.

Hypovolaemia. Loss of intravascular volume, either as a result of haemorrhage or from fluid and electrolyte losses by other means, causes a reduction in cardiac output. In some instances there may be dilutional anaemia. By the time such patients are obviously hypotensive there will be a reduction in pulmonary perfusion with worsening of the ventilation-perfusion relationship in the lung and consequent risk of arterial hypoxaemia. An adequate blood volume should be restored, with appropriate monitoring of arterial and central venous pressure, before anaesthesia commences. That advice is modified in the case of operations to stop persistent haemorrhage. For further details see Chapters 2 and 3.

Hepatic function

All jaundiced patients and those with a previous history of liver disease, hepatomegaly, splenomegaly or high alcohol intake require tests of liver function, testing for circulating hepatitis-B associated antigen, and a coagulation screen (including prothrombin time).

Urinary system

Postoperative urinary retention can be anticipated in male patients with prostatic hyperplasia. In all elderly males prostatic size is checked by rectal examination and bladder distension excluded by abdominal palpation and percussion. Suspected chronic retention of urine (i.e. incomplete empty-ing of the bladder) should be investigated preoperatively.

Plasma urea and creatinine concentrations are useful but insensitive indicators of renal function. Suspicion of renal disease demands more sensitive tests, e.g. creatinine clearance. A sample of urine must always be tested by 'dipstick' before oper-ation for sugar, ketones, bilirubin, urobilinogen and blood. Microscopic examination and culture of urine are indicated if there is any suspicion of urinary tract infection or haematuria.

ADMISSION TO HOSPITAL

Many hospitals now have admission departments where basic information such as the patient's name, address, date of birth, religion, occupation, next of kin, and the general practitioner's name and address are recorded in the patient's case folder. The patient should have received a booklet explaining hospital procedure. Once the documen-tation is complete, the patient is admitted to the ward.

On arrival, the house surgeon checks that the patient's notes are complete and that the results of preoperative investigations have been received. He should explain again to the patient the nature of the operation and the risks and problems involved, and see that the consent form is completed and signed.

Some procedures (e.g. for breast and colorectal disease) require extensive counselling which may be best achieved by specialist personnel. Where possible, patients should be permitted to become familiar with any appliances they may require in the postoperative period. For example, patients who will need crutches should practise before surgery. Of particular importance is the adequate counselling of patients likely to require an intes-tinal stoma; they should be given the opportunity to wear a stoma bag for 24 hours to ensure that its position is correct lying, standing or sitting.

Arrangements are made to inform the relatives about the diagnosis, the operation to be performed and its likely outcome. This is mandatory in all serious diseases.

Finally, the house surgeon ensures that all is ready for the final check in the preoperative pro-cedure — the preoperative ward round (see below). In some wards a preoperative check list is used.

Special preparation of the patient may be re-quired, depending on the procedure proposed. For example, for large bowel surgery the bowel must be empty. This may be achieved by whole gut lavage with either 4 litres of polyethelene glycol or 1 litre of 10% mannitol, by the use of a strong aperient such as magnesium citrate (200 ml) or by large bowel enemas. These can be administered on the day preceding surgery. Patients undergoing minor anorectal procedures should be given two glycerine suppositories inserted rectally at 06:00 hours on the morning of surgery.

THE PREOPERATIVE WARD ROUND

On the day before surgery the surgeon, his medical staff, and a member of the ward nursing staff visit the patient. The anaesthetist will also visit the patient, usually the evening before the operation.

Final examination of the patient. The surgeon re-examines the patient to confirm previous findings and to ensure that the proposed operative procedure is correct. In the case of unilateral conditions, e.g. hernia, breast lumps or varicose veins, the operation side is marked with an indelible marker. The patient's records are checked to make certain that all essential investigations have been completed and that, if appropriate, blood is available for transfusion.

Instructions to medical staff. The need for preoperative intravenous infusion is discussed. In many cases, an infusion is not established until the patient arrives in theatre. Urethral catheterization may be required, e.g. in pelvic operations. If possible, this should be delayed until the patient has been anaesthetized.

When peroperative radiology is required (e.g. operative cholangiography during gallbladder surgery), the radiology department should be informed so that facilities are available at the desired time. If an immediate pathological report on a specimen is likely to be required, the requisite pathology form should be completed and the pathologist informed.

Discussion of procedures. At the preoperative round the surgeon will discuss the plan of the operation and particular points in postoperative care. Patients are always greatly reassured by a brief outline of the procedures leading up to the start of anaesthesia, and to be told where they will be (e.g. in the recovery room), how they will feel and what will be attached to them in the way of monitoring and infusion equipment when they recover from the anaesthetic. In all of these matters good planning and clear communication between members of the operating team and the theatre and ward staff has top priority. The house surgeon has a key role in this.

Instructions to nursing staff. The nursing staff are responsible for several standard preoperative procedures. For example, they remove dentures, rings and other jewellery, administer the premedication and fix a plastic wrist band around the patient's wrist indicating name, religion, dose and time of administering premedication. An orderly is usually responsible for washing and shaving the operation site if required (see below). These duties may require modification in the light of particular problems brought to light at the preoperative round.

To minimize the risk of regurgitation and aspiration of vomitus during anaesthesia patients usually receive no food or fluids after 23:00 hours on the day before operation unless the operation is planned for the afternoon, in which case a light breakfast can be allowed.

A depilating cream is less likely to give rise to wound infection than shaving but, as it has to be applied for several days, it is not usually a practical alternative. Shaving is best performed as soon before surgery as convenient, i.e. immediately before the call to theatre or even after anaesthesia has been induced. If shaving is carried out on the previous evening there is a greater risk of wound infection. Patients who are to receive an implant of foreign material should not be shaved until the last possible moment. It is not necessary to shave a patient requiring an abdominal operation radically from 'nipple to knee'. A full pubic shave is rarely required even for procedures of the perineum.

Early on the morning of surgery patients should shower with a 10% povidone-iodine or 0.05% chlorhexidine solution, directing particular attention to groin and axilla.

Patients undergoing gastrointestinal surgery will need a nasogastric tube. This may be passed 2 hours before operation unless there is a history of gastric retention, when it may be inserted several days before operation. In some cases it may be possible, and kinder, to insert the tube after anaesthesia has been induced.

If the operation involves the large bowel, the surgeon should confirm that this has been prepared properly.

The patient's drug chart is checked and essential medication prescribed. Problems such as diabetes and impaired coagulation require special attention.

A fluid balance chart is commenced before all major operations and in all patients with abnormalities of fluid and electrolyte balance.

When all preparations have been checked, the surgeon has a final word with the patient to reassure him or her and allay anxieties. He makes certain that the operation consent form has been correctly completed, that relatives have been informed and that arrangements have been made for him or a member of his staff to meet them postoperatively.

Premedication. The anaesthetist should be alerted as early as possible to any physical or disease problems which are likely to pose difficulties with anaesthesia. If there is any doubt, he should be asked to see the patient in consultation before the timing of the operation is planned.

The aim of premedication is to sedate the patient and relieve anxiety, and to reduce pain if this is present before operation. It should be remembered that drugs are no substitute for explanation and reassurance.

The commonest premedicants are the benzodiazepines and opiates, the former having the advantage that they can be given by mouth. In some cases, for example when stimulation of the mouth or pharynx is anticipated, an anticholinergic agent (usually atropine) is given by intramuscular injection. (The main objection to the administration of anticholinergics before operation is that the patient may suffer from a very dry mouth.) Atropine has the added advantage of helping to block vagal influences of the heart, thus preventing profound bradycardia. It is for this reason that atropine is sometimes injected at the time of induction of anaesthesia in those who have not received it as part of the premedication.

Many patients receiving drugs for longstanding medical conditions can take these as normal early on the morning of operation subject to discussion with the anaesthetist.

Prophylaxis against deep venous thrombosis should be instituted according to the agreed protocol of the surgical unit. If indicated, prophylactic antibiotics can be administered intravenously immediately after induction of anaesthesia.

8. Anaesthesia and the operation

The patient's name and identifying number should be clearly marked on all records and samples, and on a tag affixed to the patient, usually to a wrist bracelet which cannot be removed casually. At all stages during the patient's stay in hospital the staff should be satisfied that they are dealing with the correct individual. These precautions are particularly important if the patient is sedated, confused or unconscious for any reason. Where there is any possible doubt about the site of operation (e.g. right or left side), a mark should be made on the skin with a felt pen or similar marker to indicate the site of the lesion (e.g. in a breast) or proposed incision.

GENERAL ANAESTHESIA

The basic aims of general anaesthesia are a reversible loss of awareness and temporary blocking of gross response to stimulation, i.e. skeletal muscle movement and autonomic effects (tachycardia, hypertension, sweating etc.). At deeper levels of general anaesthesia with inhalation agents, profound muscle relaxation may occur and thus facilitate access for the surgeon, for example in abdominal surgery.

When anaesthesia was introduced in 1846–47 these aims were achieved with a single drug, ether or chloroform. Inhalation proved an effective route to the blood and thence to the central nervous system. The trouble with single-agent anaesthesia is that a relatively high concentration has to be given to achieve the desired effect. If the agent is very soluble in body tissues other than the central nervous system (CNS), as is the case with ether, recovery is very slow because of the large mass of drug to be eliminated. Chloroform, which is less soluble but toxic to the heart and vomiting centre in high dose, caused much morbidity when used as a single agent.

The ED_{50} of an inhalation anaesthetic is called the *minimum alveolar concentration* (MAC). This is the concentration (in vol %) or, more precisely, the tension (measured in kPa) which prevents half the population given that agent from moving in response to a painful stimulus. As there is no synergism between anaesthetics, fractions of MAC can be added to each other.

Nitrous oxide has hardly any unwanted side effects, but is poorly soluble and has a very high MAC (105 kPa) so that it cannot be given as the sole anaesthetic. If 66% nitrous oxide in oxygen is used as the carrier gas to vaporize chloroform or ether (or any other volatile agent), the concentration or tension of these volatiles required becomes less. Two-thirds of the anaesthetic effect is due to the nitrous oxide. As the unwanted effects of chloroform or ether are greatly minimized, recovery is more rapid than with ether alone, and cardiac and emetic effects are less common than with chloroform alone.

Although chloroform and ether have been taken as examples because they are historically important, neither drug is much used in Britain today. Ether is still widely used in less advanced countries because it is the safest anaesthetic for non-professionals to use. Many volatile anaesthetics have been introduced over the years (Table 8.1) but those currently used in British hospitals are halothane, enflurane and isoflurane.

Thus, probably the simplest anaesthetic given today is nitrous oxide with oxygen and one of the modern volatiles, with the patient breathing spontaneously.

Table 8.1 Some important features of volatile anaesthetics

Drug	MAC(kPa)	Main advantages	Main disadvantages
Diethylether ('ether')	1.7	Inexpensive; wide availability of apparatus for safe use in developing countries	Flammable in air, explosive with oxygen-rich gas; slow uptake/recovery; vomiting
Chloroform	0.8	None	Cardiac arrhythmia; vomiting
Trichlorethylene		Good analgesic effect which lingers postoperatively; used in obstetrics	Cardiac arrhythmia; tachypnoea; difficult to control depth of anaesthesia
Methoxyflurane	Not known	Good analgesic effect; used in obstetrics	Very slow uptake and recovery; high-output renal failure with high dosage
Halothane	0.8	Huge successful international experience over 30 years	Cardiac arrhythmia (nodal rhythm); bradycardia; very rare hepatic necrosis alleged, especially if drug is repeated within 3 months (thought to be due to metabolite)
Enflurane	1.7	Less metabolized than halothane	Half potency of halothane; contraindicated in epilepsy or renal failure
Isoflurane	1.2	Least metabolized of modern volatiles	Very high cost; hypotension; possible problems in myocardial ischaemia

MAC = Minimum alveolar concentration

The anaesthetic machine

This is commonly referred to as Boyle's machine, after H.E.G. Boyle, a London anaesthetist who introduced trolleys for mounting gas cylinders and the means of vaporizing ether and chloroform. It is not called after the eminent scientist Sir Robert Boyle, although his well-known law relating pressure and volume is obeyed in the filling and emptying of gas cylinders. The anaesthetic machine has facilities for delivering and metering gases which the patient needs or may need (oxygen, nitrous oxide, carbon dioxide and sometimes medical air and cyclopropane) and carries accurately functioning vaporizers for the volatile anaesthetics.

The patient's breathing system (sometimes called the circuit) is connected to the main outlet from the anaesthetic machine. There are many designs of circuit but all must meet the following minimum criteria.

1. A reservoir of gas sufficient to supply the largest tidal volume and to enable the means of intermittent positive pressure ventilation of the lungs must be available.

2. Resistance to breathing must be low.

3. The inspired gas concentrations must be known with accuracy.

Thus, exhaled gas can only be rebreathed safely if carbon dioxide has been absorbed and 'consumed' gases, notably oxygen, have been replaced. This is the basic reason for designing circular systems with CO_2 absorbers (soda lime). Alternatively, the exhaled gas may be discharged from the system by suitable placement of valves. This will result in higher gas and vapour consumption than is strictly necessary. In addition there must be an arrangement for scavenging — directly discharging gases safely to the outside of the hospital building — to avoid pollution of the theatre atmosphere.

It is convenient to use the anaesthetic machine as a trolley for monitors, an automatic lung ventilator, and a work surface for the record chart and for dispensing drugs. Monitors include the ECG, a blood pressure measuring device, a neuromuscular block monitor, meters for measuring gas concentrations and a spirometer. The design and complexity of these arrangements varies from place to place, and as with modern cars often reflects the needs and practices of the user and to some extent his personality. Prototype systems are increasingly directed to automation of record keeping, rather like the 'black box' in an aircraft (and with a similar purpose in mind).

Induction of anaesthesia

A normal person who has received no anaesthetic or CNS depressant is deemed to be fully conscious; someone who receives an increasing overdose will eventually die. It is thus important to recognize the clinical signs at various depths of anaesthesia. Arthur Guedal, an American, proposed the following division of anaesthesia into four stages.

Stage 1 spans full consciousness to loss of consciousness.

Stage 2 is a very unpleasant stage characterized by reflex hyperexcitability, breath-holding, the risk of regurgitation, bladder emptying etc. As the concentration of anaesthetic in the brain increases, however, the patient reaches the third stage of anaesthesia.

Stage 3 is characterized by the return of a regular breathing pattern. As anaesthesia deepens through the third stage, the respiratory muscles fail increasingly, starting with the accessories, and finally the diaphragm.

Stage 4 is respiratory arrest and will soon lead to cardiac arrest unless oxygenation can be maintained.

Thus, stage 3 is the depth of anaesthesia for surgical operations. It is further divided into four planes; plane 2 is referred to as the 'surgical plane'.

Plane 2 or surgical anaesthesia can be achieved by commencing directly with inhalation of an anaesthetic mixture but, depending on the speed of uptake, patients will be aware of the unpleasant effects of stage 2. Moreover, many patients do not like having a face mask applied when they are conscious, even if premedicated. The intravenous induction agents allow a rapid, pleasant onset of unconsciousness to the point at which the patient will tolerate application of a face mask and inhalation of the anaesthetic mixture without the unpleasant features of the second stage. Sodium thiopentone (Pentothal) is a thiobarbiturate

classified among the barbiturates as an ultrashort-acting agent. It has enjoyed pride of place for intravenous induction of anaesthesia for 50 years in spite of its apparently appalling pharmacokinetic profile. It has a long half-life of about 18 hours which renders it quite unsuitable for repeat administration or infusion, and a hangover effect which extends well into the postoperative period. Attempts to replace it have been unavailing in spite of the regular emergence of new compounds. The problems with these alternatives range from severe pain on injection to an unacceptable incidence of idiosyncratic reactions.

Propofol (Diprivan) is a new intravenous induction agent which appears to be showing some promise. It is difficult to dissolve in water and is presented as an emulsion. It has a short half-life and may be suitable not only for repeat administration during anaesthesia but possibly for continuous sedation over long periods in intensive care (see later).

Ketamine (Ketalar) produces a state of dissociative anaesthesia. In smaller doses than are required for induction of anaesthesia it can be used as an analgesic. Unlike the other two intravenous anaesthetics, it has minimum effects on the cardiovascular system. On the other hand, it can cause bizarre psychomimetic effects (it is chemically related to phencyclidine).

The concept of 'balanced anaesthesia': the muscle relaxants

In the 1940s anaesthetists began to use small doses of tubocurarine ('curare') injected intravenously. This produces partial neuromuscular blockade causing muscle relaxation at lighter levels of anaesthesia so that dose requirements and unwanted effects can accordingly be reduced. Unfortunately, sensitivity to neuromuscular blockers varies enormously. In susceptible individuals, difficulty with breathing can result in the need for assisted ventilation. With experience it became clear that the best course was to increase the dose of tubocurarine, accept a greater degree of neuromuscular block in all patients, and ventilate the lungs with 'lighter' anaesthetic mixtures. This move was one of the more important developments in modern surgery for the following reasons.

1. By reducing anaesthetic toxicity it opened the way for operations in patients who would have been regarded as unsuitable for anaesthesia previously.

2. It allowed safer and more extensive surgery of the heart, lungs and brain.

3. It changed the practice of anaesthesia from an empirical art to a discipline based on scientific principles and requiring specialist practitioners.

Expertise in artificial ventilatory support was the springboard for developing surgical intensive care units where ventilatory support is still the principal and most successful therapeutic mode. A wide range of neuromuscular blocking agents are used in modern anaesthetic practice. Suxamethonium has a short duration of action (5–10 min) unless the patient has a deficiency or inherited abnormality of cholinesterase (pseudocholinesterase), when blocking will be prolonged from 30 min to 8 hours. Suxamethonium is the only *depolarizing* blocker used, and usually muscle fasciculations can be seen shortly after the drug has been injected.

Among the non-depolarizing neuromuscular blockers (sometimes called competitive blockers), tubocurarine, pancuronium and alcuronium have a longer duration of action than the recently introduced atracurium and vecuronium. The two new drugs have a shorter onset and offset of effect, accumulate less and have fewer unpredictable side effects such as changes in heart rate and blood pressure.

All of the non-depolarizing blockers can be antagonized with neostigmine, an anticholinesterase. This must be given with atropine to block the muscarinic effects of acetylcholine (bradycardia, bronchospasm, increased gut motility, salivation etc.), leaving the nicotine effect on the neuromuscular junction as the desired action, and restoring normal neuromuscular conduction with (as the first sign) return of spontaneous breathing.

The airway in anaesthesia

One of the major challenges in general anaesthesia is the protection of the laryngeal inlet from foreign material, including regurgitation of stomach contents, and the maintenance of a clear airway through the mouth or nose.

Protection of the larynx and trachea

The best guarantee against aspiration of gastric material is an empty stomach. Preparation of the patient by starvation helps greatly but is not necessarily totally effective. Gastric emptying rates differ and there is always the possibility that the starvation regimen may not have been adhered to rigorously. In emergencies there may not be time to ensure that gastric emptying has taken place. In any case, severe injury may delay emptying; opioids given for pain relief also cause delay.

Less common, but equally sinister, are the risks of tracheal soiling from haemorrhage in the upper airway or cerebrospinal fluid (CSF) leakage following skull fracture.

The airway through the nose is less likely to become obstructed than that through the mouth but in some patients the nasal airway is not very effective in the first place. The difficulty with the oral airway is that the muscle relaxation induced by general anaesthesia causes a loss of normal tone in the muscle groups related to the hyoid bone. The support which keeps the tongue in the normal position is thus lost and the tongue tends to fall back towards the posterior pharyngeal wall. In some patients this can very easily cause total airway obstruction and sudden death from asphyxia is a recognized danger. Such airway obstruction can be lessened by turning the patient on his side (rather than leaving him supine). Insertion of an oropharyngeal airway may help greatly. However, the best guarantee of maintaining an airway under anaesthesia is to insert a tracheal tube. The orotracheal route is commonest but nasotracheal intubation is a more suitable alternative if the operation is to take place within the mouth.

The commonest design of tracheal tube has an inflatable cuff which provides a seal between the outer surface of the tube and the tracheal lining. This helps to prevent contamination of the trachea by the ingress of material which may have found its way to the pharynx. The cuff also ensures that the airway is through the tube rather than round the tube so that, once the anaesthetic breathing system is connected to the tube, only the planned anaesthetic mixture is inhaled, without contamination by air inhaled around the outside of the tube.

Insertion of a tracheal tube is easier if the

patient has received a neuromuscular blocking drug. If there is no great hurry before the tube has to be placed and the cuff inflated, a competitive drug may be given. In other circumstances the very rapid onset of block from suxamethonium is an advantage: intubation can be performed immediately after the fasciculations have ended.

There are many circumstances in which it is not necessary to maintain neuromuscular blockade throughout the operation. The patient may then breathe the anaesthetic mixture via a face mask after an oropharyngeal airway has been inserted. Alternatively a tracheal tube may be inserted after suxamethonium has been given. After 4–5 min, or whatever time is necessary for the recovery from suxamethonium, the patient breathes spontaneously although the tracheal tube remains in place.

LOCAL ANAESTHESIA

A local 'anaesthetic' blocks transmission of impulses along nerve fibres by altering membrane permeability. Used to block sensory nerves, it prevents appreciation of painful stimuli so that operative procedures can be carried out within the area subserved by the blocked nerve. The anaesthetic agent may be injected into the operation site or proximally around the main trunks of the appropriate nerves. At higher concentration the local anaesthetic may also block motor nerves. This can be a considerable advantage, for example in spinal anaesthesia, where the profound relaxation of muscles may be useful in aiding surgical access.

Local anaesthesia is also of value in the control of postoperative pain.

For clinical use a local anaesthetic must be non-irritating, rapid in action, completely reversible and readily sterilized. If absorbed systemically, there is stimulation of the central nervous system and depression of the myocardium. Lignocaine and bupivacaine are the local anaesthetics used most frequently. The total doses of local anaesthetics that are safe to administer depend on the age and weight of the patient, the site of injection, the concentration of the drug in solution and whether or not adrenaline has been added to the solution. Local anaesthetics should never be administered without consulting the data sheet and being thoroughly familiar with the constraints of their use.

Topical anaesthesia

As anaesthetic agents are absorbed through the surface of mucous membranes, solutions and creams containing 0.5%–4.0% lignocaine are used to anaesthetize the conjunctiva, mucosa of the mouth, nasopharynx and larynx, the urethra and the urinary bladder. They are applied as sprays, gargles, soaked pledgets of cotton wool, or gels. Anaesthesia develops rapidly and lasts for 30–60 min. As local anaesthetics can be absorbed very rapidly into the systemic circulation from topical administration, the general guidance given on maximum doses applies here also.

Local infiltration

Solutions of lignocaine are available for local infiltration through a fine needle inserted into or through the skin. Because of the dangers of rapid absorption, local anaesthetics must not be injected into inflamed tissues. The altered pH of the tissues also affects the action of the anaesthetic agent.

The addition of adrenaline to local anaesthetic solutions causes vasoconstriction at the site of injection and may prolong the duration or action of the drug. It is important that the amount of adrenaline is kept to a minimum and a concentration of 1:200 000 should not be exceeded. Because of the risk of intense vasoconstriction leading to cessation or inadequacy of flow through the affected blood vessel, adrenaline should not be injected close to arteries which constitute the sole supply to the part(s) in question. Examples are the digits and the penis.

Sometimes it is expedient to use local anaesthetic infiltration in combination with general anaesthesia. In that event the solution should never contain adrenaline if the patient is receiving halothane, as adrenaline is likely to increase myocardial irritability in its presence.

Nerve block

Nerve block is performed by injecting small amounts of local anaesthetic around the main nerve trunk. Lignocaine or bupivacaine can be used with or without adrenaline. The anaesthetist or surgeon carrying out the injection must be aware of the anatomical course of the nerve, its surface relationships and the type of surrounding tissues. As with all injections, aspiration must precede injection so that intravascular injection is avoided. Common sites for nerve block are the brachial plexus in the axilla or root of neck; the ulnar nerve at the elbow; the anterior or posterior tibial nerve at the ankle; the digital nerve at the roots of the fingers or toes; and the intercostal nerve below the ribs (Fig 8.1).

When multiple sensory nerves supply a part,

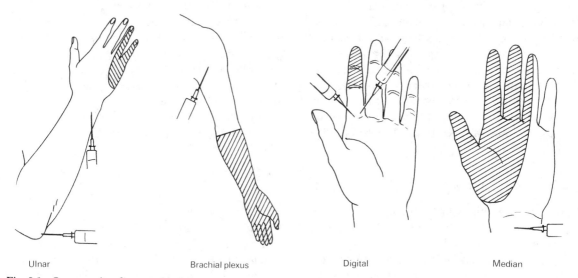

| Ulnar | Brachial plexus | Digital | Median |

Fig. 8.1 Common sites for nerve blocks

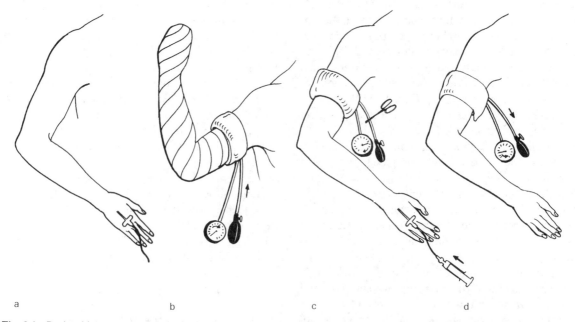

a   b   c   d

Fig. 8.2 Regional intravenous anaesthesia. (a) Insertion of cannula. (b) Limb elevated and exsanguinated using an elastic bandage. The cuff is then inflated. (c) Injection of local anaesthetic. (d) The cuff is deflated at the end of the procedure

e.g. the groin or scalp, a 'field block' can be carried out by using a series of injections to block all the nerves.

Regional intravenous anaesthesia

Reduction of closed fractures and other simple surgical procedures on extremities can be performed under regional anaesthesia induced by injection of a dilute solution of local anaesthetic into a vein while the limb is kept ischaemic by a tourniquet (Fig. 8.2). The principle of the method is that the venous compartment of the isolated limb is filled with dilute local anaesthetic solution which tracks in the vasa nervorum to the nerve tissue where it produces a block.

A blood pressure cuff is first applied to the upper arm or thigh and an indwelling cannula inserted into a distal vein. The limb is elevated and an elastic bandage applied to empty it of blood. The cuff is then inflated to above arterial systolic pressure (usually to 250 mmHg) and 40 ml of 0.5% prilocaine injected. Bupivacaine should not be used.

If the limb is painful, as with a Colles' fracture, when application of an elastic bandage is unacceptable, it is adequate to elevate the arm for a period of 5 min before occluding the limb. Emptying of

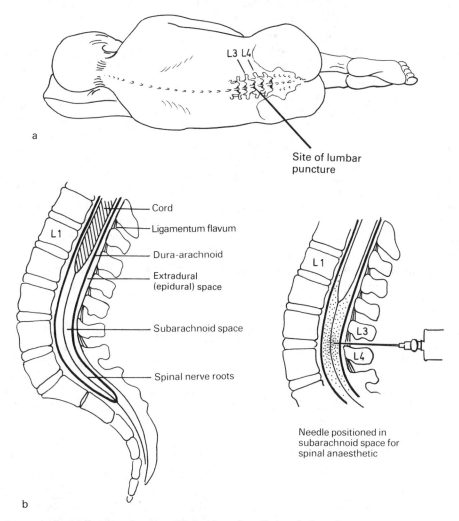

Site of lumbar puncture

Cord
Ligamentum flavum
Dura-arachnoid
Extradural (epidural) space
Subarachnoid space
Spinal nerve roots

Needle positioned in subarachnoid space for spinal anaesthetic

Fig. 8.3 Spinal anaesthesia. (a) Position of patient. (b) Position of needle in spinal canal

the veins will be less effective than if the bandage were applied, but the method usually works reasonably well.

Anaesthesia lasts 30–60 min but the pressure of the cuff becomes intolerable after 30 min. The cuff must *not* be released before 15 min have elapsed or there is a danger of release of the agent into the general circulation with induction of cardiac arrhythmia.

Spinal and epidural anaesthesia

Local anaesthetic agents can be injected into the subarachnoid or epidural spaces to block spinal nerve roots as they course from the spinal cord to intervertebral foramina. Spinal anaesthesia is performed by injecting the agent through a lumbar puncture needle inserted between L3 and L4 (Fig. 8.3). Solutions of lignocaine or bupivacaine are used. Some anaesthetists prefer 'heavy' solutions which, by virtue of the addition of 6% dextrose, are heavier than cerebrospinal fluid. Thus the whole solution moves under the influence of gravity, giving some control over the spread of the block when injection has been made into the subarachnoid space. Leakage of CSF may cause headache and the patient should lie flat in bed for at least 12 hours after a spinal anaesthetic.

For epidural anaesthesia the needle is inserted into the epidural space which lies between the ligamentum flavum and the dura-arachnoid membrane (Fig. 8.4). The injection can be made at any level of the spinal column, including the caudal canal. The solution spreads upwards and downwards from the site of injection so that a band of anaesthesia can be created depending on the segments involved. Additionally, it is possible to insert a fine catheter through the needle before the needle is withdrawn. The catheter allows repeated injections of a local anaesthetic to maintain anaesthesia for hours or even days if necessary. Thus epidural anaesthesia can be of value in the control of postoperative pain. It is also well known as an effective means of relieving the pain of labour.

The sympathetic outflow along anterior nerve roots is also blocked by spinal and epidural anaesthetics. Vasomotor paralysis can cause hypotension and bradycardia. These effects are particularly dangerous in hypertensive arteriosclerotic patients.

Complications

The main complication of local anaesthesia is overdose. Excitement, apprehension, muscle irritability and convulsions result from stimulation of the nervous system. This is followed by depression and a shock-like state. Cardiovascular and respiratory depression occur and death from hypoxia may follow. The most important steps in treatment are to oxygenate and if necessary ventilate the patient. Control of convulsions by injection of diazepam is occasionally necessary. Sodium thiopentone or muscle relaxants have also been used to control convulsions but these are very likely to induce apnoea. The administrator should be prepared to maintain the airway by tracheal intubation and positive pressure ventilation of the lungs.

THE OPERATION

Surgery exposes the patient to three main risks: infection, the effects of trauma, and postoperative thromboembolic disease. Great care is taken to reduce these hazards to a minimum.

Infection

Infection of the operation wound can arise from four sources: (1) the theatre air; (2) instruments and materials used in the operation; (3) surgical and nursing staff in the operating theatre; and (4) the patient himself.

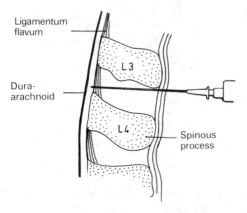

Ligamentum flavum

Dura-arachnoid

L3

L4

Spinous process

Fig. 8.4 Epidural anaesthesia

Theatre air

The ventilation systems of modern theatres ensure that there are frequent changes of air so that the density of organisms is kept low. Fresh filtered air is blown into the theatre at pressure so that old air is expelled outwards into surrounding areas. The theatre atmosphere cannot be completely sterilized and there is always a 'fall-out' of organisms onto the operation site, the drapes used to surround the wound, and the floor. Laminar flow systems which blow a current of filtered air over the operating table will reduce, but not abolish, this fall-out.

As an operation 'list' proceeds, the bacterial count in the atmosphere increases and infection is more common in patients at the end of a list. If more than four major operations are to be performed in the same theatre, there should be a break of one hour after the fourth case to allow the bacterial count to fall.

Infection rates increase when 'clean' and 'infected' cases are treated in the same theatre. Ideally, infected cases should undergo surgery in a separate theatre. If this is not possible, they should be treated at the end of the list after all 'clean' cases have been dealt with.

Occasionally, a patient undergoing a 'clean' operation is found unexpectedly to have an abscess or other infective condition. After completion of such an operation, the list should be suspended for one hour while the theatre is cleaned.

The longer an operation, the greater the risk of infection. Longer procedures inevitably involve greater tissue manipulation and damage, and longer exposure to the atmosphere.

Excessive movements of staff in theatre cause currents of air. These may carry organisms from the floor or from crevices in the furniture to contaminate wounds or instruments. Movements of theatre staff should be orderly. Excess numbers of staff should not be allowed 'on the floor'. Cross-infection is further considered in Chapter 11.

Instruments and materials

In well-run theatres, the risk of infection from instruments and other materials is slight. Routine checks of sterilization procedures and equipment (autoclaves etc.) are the responsibility of a bacteriologist (see Ch. 11). At the end of each operation, all contaminated materials are removed from the theatre for re-sterilization or disposal.

If an instrument or swab is inadvertently left in a wound at the end of the operation, infection is the rule. This is frequently serious and may be fatal. Standardized counting procedures are used to keep a tally of swabs, instruments and needles. The surgeon is responsible for ensuring that the count is correct and expects that the nurse in charge of the case will account for all instruments and materials before completion of an operation.

Surgical and nursing staff

Humans harbour millions of organisms in and on their bodies. Organisms are numerous on the hands and perineal skin, and in the axillae, groins and other skin-fold areas. Bacteria shed from the hands include those of the resident commensal flora and those transiently acquired by contact with other potentially infective sites.

There is an abundant commensal flora in the oropharynx, the terminal ileum, the colon and the genitourinary tract. The commensal flora is not usually virulent; the exceptions are *Staphylococcus aureus*, which may be carried in the anterior nares and the perineum, and *Streptococcus pyogenes*, which is sometimes present in the throat of an asymptomatic person ('healthy carrier'). If a healthy carrier of *Strep. pyogenes* is detected, or if a member of theatre staff has a septic focus such as a wound, pimple or boil (usually staphylococcal infections), he or she is banned from theatre until the lesion has healed completely. As nasal carriage of *Staph. aureus* is very common, it is not practicable to regard this as ground for permanent exclusion from theatre duty. Scrupulous attention to detail in theatre practice must take account of this. However, a nasal carrier of a staphylococcus traced as the likely source of an infection should be removed from the theatre team and treated with a nasal antibiotic cream to eliminate the organism. As the recognition of carriers is important, routine nasal swabs should be taken from all theatre staff.

The hands. The 'scrub-up' technique is designed to remove surface organisms from hands and forearms. It cannot remove organisms from sweat glands and hair follicles. After routine cleansing the skin surface is recolonized in approximately 20 min. Excess scrubbing should be avoided and many scrub-up rooms are equipped with a stop-clock.

The problem of recolonization is overcome in two ways: (1) the use of sterile rubber gloves and gowns worn over a fresh laundered 'scrubsuit'; and (2) modern washing agents which combine a detergent with an antiseptic and remain active on the skin surface for a long time. Organisms arriving at the skin surface are killed for up to 2 hours after scrubbing with povidone-iodine (Betadine) or chlorhexidine (Hibitane). Gloves are frequently punctured during operations. After a 3-hour operation, 70% of gloves usually contain puncture holes. If a puncture is recognized, gloves should be changed. If the sleeve or any other part of the gown becomes wet, thus creating a channel for the transfer of organisms, the gown should be changed.

The upper respiratory tract. A mask to cover the nose and mouth is worn routinely in theatre. This reduces the number of bacteria and bacteria-laden droplets expelled from the mouth and nose during respiration and conversation. The source of infection in surgical patients is occasionally traced to a member of the surgical or theatre staff who is a nasal 'carrier' of a pathogenic organism.

The general body surface. Showers of bacteria and skin flakes are continually being shed from the body surface. Organisms from the perineum are particularly likely to be pathogenic. Shedding of flakes and bacteria increases for a period of about 2 hours after a shower, which should not be taken immediately before an operation. Shedding is reduced by wearing a 'theatre cap' to cover the hair, and trousers gathered in at the ankle to prevent dispersion from the perineum.

The patient

The most potent source of organisms causing wound infection is the patient. Such 'endogenous' infections are common and may occur in four ways.

1. The patient may be an asymptomatic 'carrier' of pathogens. This is more likely if he has been exposed to the hospital environment for some time. Some surgeons insist that in such patients nose, throat and perineal swabs are taken preoperatively, followed by appropriate antibiotic treatment if necessary.

2. The patient may have an intercurrent infection unrelated to his surgical problem. This may be an infected skin lesion, a bad tooth or an infection of the respiratory or urinary tract and should be treated before elective surgery. If operation cannot be postponed, the intercurrent infection should be treated with appropriate antibiotics during and after surgery.

3. The disorder for which the patient is undergoing operation may have produced local sepsis, e.g. an appendix abscess. When it is not possible to avoid entering the 'contaminated' area, steps must be taken to protect the wound from infection, e.g. by delay in its suture or administration of antibiotics.

4. The operation may have involved entry into a contaminated viscus such as the small or large intestine. In elective procedures this hazard is reduced by preparation of the intestinal tract (see Ch. 32).

Effects of trauma

Tissue damage is inevitable with any operation. Its degree affects:

1. the *metabolic demands* on the patient;
2. the risk of *infection* (dead or injured tissue is more liable to colonization by bacteria);
3. the extent of postoperative *oedema* (the sequestration of circulating fluid reduces effective circulating blood volume which, if severe, may lead to circulatory shock); and
4. the amount of operative *blood loss*.

A good surgeon handles tissues and instruments gently and protects all tissues which lie outside the immediate operative field.

Thromboembolic disease

It is now recognized that in the majority of patients in whom deep venous thrombosis develops, the process starts during the operation itself. Measures taken in the postoperative period are therefore unlikely to affect the incidence of thrombosis, and emphasis is now placed on prophylactic measures before and during surgery.

These include low-dose subcutaneous heparin, the wearing of supportive stockings and prevention of calf pressure while muscles are relaxed (see Ch. 9).

THE RECOVERY PERIOD

Towards the end of the operation the level of anaesthesia is lightened and, where applicable, the neuromuscular block is antagonized. If an opioid has been given in large dosage (to reduce or avoid the need for a volatile anaesthetic) it too may be antagonized (with naloxone). The aim of these manoeuvres is to render the patient capable of breathing spontaneously with adequate alveolar ventilation and competent laryngeal reflexes so that soiling of the trachea is avoided. When the conditions are judged to be right, the cuff on the tracheal tube is deflated after careful suction of the mouth and pharynx, and the tube is withdrawn.

If a nasogastric tube is in position, it should be allowed to drain freely to a suitable bag. It is dangerous to close a tube with a spigot since this increases the risk of regurgitation around the outside of the tube.

Unless there is a surgical contraindication (a limb in traction, for example) the patient is safest in the prone position to promote free drainage of any pharyngeal contaminants which accumulate.

Recovery room

The recovery room is an area where specially trained nurses look after the surgical patient in the first 1–2 hours after the operation. This includes the following.

1. Careful monitoring of vital signs (heart rate, blood pressure, respiratory rate) and special attention to the integrity of the airway. The nurses are competent to give first aid in case of airway obstruction.

2. Institution and development of a satisfactory analgesic regimen.

3. Improvement of oxygenation. In the first hour all patients will need enrichment of the inspired oxygen concentration. A controlled oxygen mask delivering 28% oxygen is appropriate except in patients with type 2 respiratory failure.

4. Early detection of haemorrhage should this occur.

5. Establishing a fluid balance regimen.
6. Instituting the postoperative chart.

The recovery room is regarded as having continuity with the operating room, so that the anaesthetist and surgeon remain aware of the condition of the patient and can move there quickly in the event of a problem. When the surgical team are happy that the patient is awake, stable and comfortable, return to the ward can be arranged.

INTENSIVE CARE

There are many types of intensive care unit in larger hospitals (e.g. renal, oncological, neonatal, coronary). The principal area is usually called the general intensive care unit and deals with, among others, the problems of surgical patients and those who have sustained trauma. The unit has continuity of experienced medical staff, a high nurse-to-patient ratio, a concentration of the equipment necessary for the care of the acutely ill, and effective links with the many departments of the hospital whose assistance is needed around the clock — and often urgently (e.g. ex-directory biochemistry, haematology, bacteriology, renal dialysis). The unit is in the charge of a coordinator (anaesthetist, physician or surgeon) who has undergone special training for the purpose. He acts as a common point of reference because many different specialists may be involved in patient care. For example, a patient who has been severely injured in a road traffic accident may need the attention of a general surgeon, an orthopaedic surgeon, neurosurgeon, ophthalmologist, faciomaxillary surgeon and a nephrologist.

In general the most effective method of arranging continuous patient monitoring is also the simplest. An ECG cardiac monitor is relatively cheap and easy to use and allows continuous monitoring of pulse rate. Blood pressure is measured readily by sphygmomanometry, and central venous pressure by a simple saline manometer through a central venous line. Urinary output is measured by a calibrated reservoir and catheter; electrolytes and blood gases by automated laboratory equipment.

Sophisticated methods of monitoring are required in some cases, but the equipment is

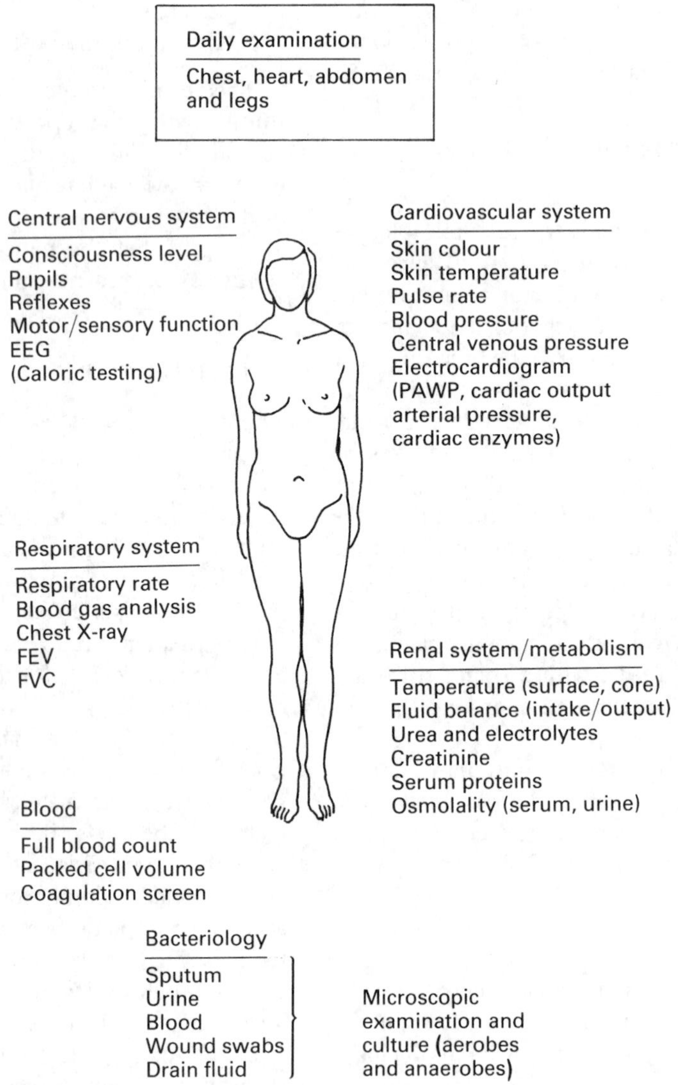

Daily examination

Chest, heart, abdomen
and legs

Central nervous system

Consciousness level
Pupils
Reflexes
Motor/sensory function
EEG
(Caloric testing)

Cardiovascular system

Skin colour
Skin temperature
Pulse rate
Blood pressure
Central venous pressure
Electrocardiogram
(PAWP, cardiac output
arterial pressure,
cardiac enzymes)

Respiratory system

Respiratory rate
Blood gas analysis
Chest X-ray
FEV
FVC

Renal system/metabolism

Temperature (surface, core)
Fluid balance (intake/output)
Urea and electrolytes
Creatinine
Serum proteins
Osmolality (serum, urine)

Blood

Full blood count
Packed cell volume
Coagulation screen

Bacteriology

Sputum
Urine
Blood
Wound swabs
Drain fluid

Microscopic
examination and
culture (aerobes
and anaerobes)

Fig. 8.5   Monitoring of patient following major operation. FEV = forced expiratory volume; FVC = forced vital capacity;
PAWP = pulmonary arterial wedge pressure

expensive and techniques are often invasive. Continuous monitoring of arterial blood pressure requires an arterial line; monitoring of pulmonary wedge pressure requires an indwelling Swann-Ganz catheter, which also allows the estimation of pulmonary venous blood gas concentration or cardiac output. Some sophisticated measurements can be obtained without invasive techniques; e.g. deep body or core temperatures can be measured by sensitive surface thermometers and aortic blood flow by an ultrasonic flow meter placed over the chest. Equipment apart, the main value of an intensive care unit is that it allows continuous care of a patient by trained personnel. Changes in skin colour, the level of consciousness, the quality of the pulse and peripheral circulation are still important guides to progress (Fig. 8.5). Recognition of 'pattern' changes is still of the greatest significance and good nursing care remains the basis of intensive therapy. Intensive care units are not without their danger, e.g. in relation to spread of infection. This is discussed in Chapter 11.

9. Postoperative care and complications

POSTOPERATIVE CARE

Following an operation, there are three phases of patient care.

1. *Immediate (recovery room) care.* As indicated in Chapter 8, the patient is returned from the operating theatre to a recovery area where he remains until fully conscious. During this period any of the following problems may arise: myocardial ischaemia, cardiac arrest, respiratory failure, or airway obstruction. These will be discussed in more detail later in this chapter.

2. *Care on return to the surgical ward.* Regular observation by medical and nursing staff continues on return to the ward. There is a continuing need for skill in the diagnosis of myocardial infarction, respiratory failure, deep venous thrombosis and other medical conditions which may complicate recovery. Complications during this phase, except for haemorrhage or cardiopulmonary catastrophe, rarely pose an immediate threat to life and are usually specifically related to the operation performed. However, all staff in surgical wards (as in recovery areas) must still be skilled in the first aid management of cardiac arrest.

After a major operation, this period of care generally lasts for a week.

Some patients may have to be transferred to intensive care before returning to the ward, usually because of a need to ventilate the lungs artificially. Many modern hospitals now also have an intermediate critical care area between recovery room and ward, called a *high dependency unit*. This is intended for a stay of about 24 hours, usually without the need for artificial ventilation but with intensive monitoring and careful attention to pain relief and maintenance of oxygenation. The philosophy is to prevent the development of conditions that would require later admission to intensive care.

3. *Rehabilitation and convalescent care.* Although by now the patient is well on his way to full recovery, he may still require a period of professional care before he is able to return home and resume domestic and other duties. This is provided in a convalescent hospital or, if there is need for a programme of graded activity, in a rehabilitation centre.

Immediate postoperative care

Myocardial ischaemia

Postoperative cardiac failure is most likely to occur in the immediate recovery period. While in most cases there is a history of preceding cardiac disease, myocardial ischaemia or cardiac arrest can occur in an otherwise fit patient. Patients with myocardial ischaemia may complain of gripping chest pain, but this is not invariable (particularly in the postoperative period) and hypotension may be the only sign. If ischaemia is suspected, electrocardiography is performed urgently and arrangements are made for cardiac monitoring. A sample of blood is withdrawn for estimating concentrations of cardiac enzymes.

Cardiac arrest

Cardiac arrest results in an absence of pulse, unconsciousness and apnoea. External cardiac massage is started immediately, a cuffed tracheal tube is inserted and the lungs are ventilated artificially. Sodium bicarbonate (100 mmol) is administered intravenously during the first 10 minutes to combat acidosis and this may be repeated as long as the circulation remains inadequate. Care should be taken to avoid rendering the patient grossly alkalotic. An ECG is obtained. If this reveals asystole, the heart can be stimulated by calcium solutions or adrenaline. Ventricular fibrillation can be corrected by electrical defibrillation. The extent of recovery depends on the degree of cerebral damage and is related to the duration of arrest. Persistent fixed dilatation of the pupils denotes irreversible cerebral damage.

Respiratory failure

Respiratory failure is defined as an inability to maintain normal partial pressures of oxygen and carbon dioxide (Pao_2 and $Paco_2$) in the arterial blood. Blood gas estimations are essential for its early recognition and should be repeated frequently in patients with previous respiratory problems. The normal Pao_2 is over 13 kPa at the age of 20 years, falling to around 11.6 kPa at 60. For practical purposes respiratory failure is denoted by a value below 6.7 kPa. Severe hypoxaemia may result in visible central cyanosis.

Airway obstruction

The airway must be kept clear at all times. The main causes of obstruction are summarized below.

1. *Obstruction by the tongue.* This can occur during unconsciousness (loss of muscle tone causes the tongue to fall against the posterior pharyngeal wall) and may be aggravated by masseter spasm during the emergence from unconsciousness. It may also be due to haemorrhage into the tongue or soft tissue of the mouth or pharynx after operation in these areas.

2. *Obstruction by foreign bodies* (e.g. secretions, blood). Dentures should be removed before operation.

3. *Laryngeal spasm.* This occurs at light levels of unconsciousness and is aggravated by stimulation.

4. *Laryngeal oedema.* This occurs in small children after traumatic attempts at intubation and with infection (epiglottis).

5. *Tracheal compression* (e.g. from haemorrhage after thyroidectomy).

6. *Bronchospasm or blockage.* This may be due to inhalation of a foreign body or aspiration of irritant material. It may also be an idiosyncratic reaction to drugs and can of course occur in asthmatic patients.

If the airway is clear, *hypoxia* is likely to be due to underventilation of areas of the lungs with discrepancies between ventilation and perfusion. Blood gases are measured and oxygen is administered by a mask such as the Ventimask which delivers 28% oxygen or some other known concentration depending on the oxygen flow rate and the design of the mask. The delivered concentration is marked on the mask itself. Mechanical ventilation via a cuffed endotracheal tube may still be required if an adequate Pao_2 or $Paco_2$ cannot be maintained.

Special problems

More complex methods of monitoring are required for certain groups of patients. For example, patients undergoing adrenalectomy will require steroid replacement therapy and thus careful monitoring of steroid levels. Patients having neck surgery must be observed for accumulation of blood in the wound which can cause rapid asphyxia; and those undergoing open heart surgery will require intensive cardiovascular monitoring. These problems are dealt with in other chapters.

Care on return to the surgical ward

General care

On return to the ward, observation continues with regular hourly or two-hourly checks on pulse, blood pressure, respiratory rate and wound drains. In some patients hourly monitoring of urine volume is indicated. The surgeon gradually relaxes these measures as recovery continues and the patient stabilizes. Thereafter the patient is visited by medical staff morning and evening to ensure that there is steady progress towards recovery without complication.

Awareness of the normal postoperative course for a particular operation and of its common complications is important. Anxiety, disorientation and minor changes in personality, behaviour or appearance are often the earliest manifestation of impending complications. Sleeplessness can be troublesome and depressing and it is important to recognize patients in need of quiet and rest. The general circulatory state and adequacy of oxygenation are noted, and the pulse, blood pressure and respiratory rates checked from the nurses' chart. The surgeon should also enquire about the patient's urinary and bowel function and whether he is coughing freely and expanding his chest.

The chest is examined physically and any sputum inspected. The legs are examined for any swelling, discoloration and calf tenderness. Fluid balance must be carefully controlled in all patients recovering from a major operation. If an intravenous infusion has been established, the nature and amount of intravenous fluids and the urinary volume are checked at least twice daily by the medical staff. Serum electrolyte concentrations are measured daily in all patients receiving intravenous fluids (see Ch. 2).

Once intravenous fluid therapy has been discontinued, oral fluid intake is monitored until it is clear that the patient can drink freely. Nutritional requirements must also be borne in mind. A short period of starvation (i.e. a few days) causes little harm but if this is prolonged, nutritional support by parenteral or enteral means is required (see Ch. 5).

Care after abdominal surgery

In patients recovering from abdominal operations, the abdomen must be examined carefully each day for evidence of excessive distension, tenderness or drainage either from drain sites or wounds. The main abdominal complications are the slow recovery of intestinal motor function, anastomotic leakage and occult bleeding or abscess formation. Return of bowel sounds and the free passage of flatus reflect recovery of peristaltic activity.

If a nasogastric tube has been passed, it should be kept open at all times and allowed to drain freely into a small plastic bag. The tube serves as an air vent, but free drainage is usually combined with continuous or intermittent suction. Many surgeons do not allow patients to drink while a nasogastric tube is in place. Others permit the patient to drink measured small amounts of fluid at regular intervals. The time at which a tube is removed also varies; many surgeons prefer to retain the tube until the volume of hourly aspirate suggests that gastric stasis has resolved.

Soft tissue and wound care

Surgery involving soft tissue only is generally associated with few complications, and care of the wound and its underlying tissues is the main concern.

Bulky dressings are not normally used for incised wounds and the area is inspected daily for signs of wound infection. Drains prevent accumulation of blood or fluid. Mild suction is usually applied and the amount of drainage measured daily. Once this falls to a few millilitres, the drain is removed unless the surgeon has indicated that it should be retained for longer.

Traditionally, skin sutures remained in place until the wound had soundly healed, but many surgeons now prefer early removal to prevent unsightly 'cross hatching'. Replacement of sutures with adhesive strips (e.g. Steristrips) avoids tension and improves healing. At many sites subcuticular sutures of non-absorbable synthetic material are now preferred, as these may be left in until the skin has healed without producing a mark.

If the wound becomes infected, it may be necessary to remove one or two sutures prematurely to allow egress of infected material.

COMPLICATIONS OF ANAESTHESIA

Nausea and vomiting can be caused by anaesthesia or operation or both. If the condition is troublesome, an antiemetic of the phenothiazine group should be given.

Headache

Spinal anaesthesia may cause headache due to leakage of cerebrospinal fluid, and it is advisable that the patient remains flat on his back for 12 hours following this form of anaesthesia. If headache persists, it may be necessary to seal the injection site in the arachnoid by a 'blood patch', i.e. an injection of the patient's blood which will clot and close the leak.

Sore throat

Passage of an endotracheal or nasogastric tube can cause trauma to the mucous membrane and a sore throat. Dryness of the mouth contributes to this. Symptoms are usually of short duration, although ulceration of the larynx with granuloma formation can cause persistent hoarseness.

Vascular complications and nerve injuries

Intravenous administration of irritant drugs or infusions can cause bruising, haematomas, phlebitis or even venous thrombosis. Venous catheters can break, with carriage of the tip to great vessels, heart or lungs. Arterial cannulas and needle punctures are now the commonest cause of arterial injury, and may lead to arterial occlusion, impaired circulation and gangrene. Nerve palsies can be caused by stretching or compression of nerve trunks and by extravascular injection of irritant solutions. The nerves most commonly affected are the ulnar nerve at the elbow joint, the radial nerve in the upper arm and the brachial plexus at the shoulder. Care must also be taken to guard against nerve palsies when positioning the patient on the operating table.

Muscle pain

Myalgia affecting the chest, abdomen and neck may begin 24 hours after the operation and last for 1–7 days. This is a specific complication of the administration of suxamethonium.

Damage to teeth

Patients whose teeth are loose, or who have crown and bridge work may suffer dental damage during intubation. They should be warned of this possibility before operation. Aspiration of a loose tooth into a bronchus is a possible risk.

Damage to eyes

Patients whose eyes do not close during anaesthesia may develop corneal damage. In severe cases, this will lead to ulceration. This complication is usually prevented by the anaesthetist taping the eyelids during anaesthesia.

COMPLICATIONS OF SURGERY

Respiratory problems

Respiratory failure in the immediate postoperative period due to hypoxia and airway obstruction has already been discussed. Once the patient has fully recovered from anaesthesia, the main respiratory problems are caused by incomplete expansion of the lungs and accumulation of secretions. This leads to pulmonary collapse and may progress to pulmonary infection. Pulmonary embolism is a complication of deep venous thrombosis and is considered separately.

Pulmonary collapse

Inability to breathe deeply and to cough up bronchial secretions after surgery is the primary cause of pulmonary collapse. This may be due to various factors, including paralysis of the cilia by anaesthetic agents, impairment of diaphragmatic movement and pain in the wound. As a result of the accumulation of secretions, the patient does not aerate his lungs fully and collapse may follow.

With complete obstruction of a major bronchus, air in the lung, a lobe or a segment which it supplies is absorbed, the alveolar space closes (atelectasis) and the affected portion of the lung contracts and becomes solid.

Pulmonary collapse after surgery thus varies from closure of a small segment to massive collapse of a lobe or, if a main bronchus is obstructed, the whole lung. In most instances, this occurs within 24 hours of operation.

The clinical signs of a lobar collapse include rapid respiration, slight cyanosis and tachycardia. Breath sounds are diminished and there is dullness over the affected lobe. Blood gas estimations reveal a low PaO_2 and on an X-ray of the chest there are areas of increased opacity. With massive collapse there is severe dyspnoea and the affected side of the chest is uniformly dull with absent breath sounds. The mediastinum is drawn over to the affected side and there is compensatory hyperinflation of the unaffected lung, which is hyperresonant on percussion.

Management. For the prevention of pulmonary collapse it is essential that the patient is encouraged to move around, to breathe deeply and to cough during the postoperative period. Regular visits by a physiotherapist should be arranged. Coughing and deep breathing are best encouraged after a small dose of analgesic or narcotic while the abdominal wound is supported with the hands or a temporary binder. Intermittent injection of local anaesthetic through an indwelling catheter in the epidural space of the midthoracic region may also help to relieve pain. Inhalation of salbutamol relieves bronchospasm. Oxygen should be administered by nasal probes or a mask if there is hypoxia.

In more severe cases, stimulation of the trachea with a catheter or instillation of 1–2 ml of sterile saline will encourage the patient to cough up secretions. Bronchoscopy may be required to suck out a plug of inspissated secretions. If hypoxia is severe, endotracheal intubation, artificial respiration and repeated bronchial aspiration may be required. Prophylactic antibiotic therapy is advised after sputum specimens have been sent for bacteriological culture and sensitivity determination.

Posture is important. If collapse is extensive, the patient should initially be placed on the unaffected side so that he is forced to expand the affected lung. Thereafter, frequent changes of posture and intensive physiotherapy are essential to aid re-expansion.

Pulmonary infection

Pulmonary infection commonly follows pulmonary collapse. Aspiration of gastric secretions is a potent and not uncommon cause of pulmonary infection. Pyrexia and a viscid green sputum are typical features. Pulmonary signs are those of collapse and consolidation with absent or diminished breath sounds. Bronchial breathing and coarse crepitations from surrounding areas of partial bronchial occlusion may be present. Chest X-ray usually demonstrates patchy, fluffy opacities.

The patient must be encouraged to cough and antibiotics are indicated. The choice of antibiotic depends on the sensitivity of the likely infecting organism but ampicillin benzylpenicillin or Augmentin are the agents which are generally preferred. Oxygen administration is indicated if there is hypoxaemia, and more intensive respiratory support, including bronchoscopy and assisted ventilation, may be deemed necessary if respiratory function continues to deteriorate.

Cardiac failure

As indicated above, acute cardiac failure is most likely to occur in the immediate postoperative period. However, patients suffering from ischaemic or valvular heart disease, arrhythmias or severe trauma are liable to develop cardiac failure in the subsequent recovery period. Excessive administration of fluid in the early postoperative period is a common predisposing cause which can be prevented by monitoring central venous pressure. Treatment with digitalis and diuretics is indicated.

Hypovolaemia and the complications of sepsis are major sources of cardiac insufficiency in patients during the recovery phase. Treatment is directed at the primary cause. Therapeutic measures include restoration of circulating blood volume, elimination of hypoxaemia, correction of acid-base balance and administration of inotropic agents to increase cardiac output.

Renal failure

Acute renal failure after surgery results from protracted periods of inadequate perfusion of the kidneys. This may be due to hypovolaemia, sepsis or anaphylaxis (e.g. as a result of mismatched blood transfusion). Patients with pre-existing renal disease and those who are jaundiced are more susceptible to the effects of poor perfusion and more likely to develop acute renal failure after a less severe insult.

Acute renal failure can largely be prevented by adequate fluid replacement before, during and after the operation so that urine volume is maintained at 40 ml/h or more. Monitoring the hourly urine volume after catheterization is a necessary precaution in all patients recovering from major surgery and in those considered at risk from renal complications. Early recognition and effective treatment of bacterial and fungal infections is also important.

The cardinal feature of acute renal failure is oliguria associated with a dilute urine (specific gravity less than 1010; urea concentration less than 300 mmol/l). Oliguria with a concentrated urine indicates that the kidney is functioning but is inadequately perfused. This is an indication to give more fluid, and rapid infusion of 1 litre of normal (isotonic) saline should increase urine output. In such patients a careful check must be made for continued bleeding as a cause of hypovolaemia.

If oliguria is associated with a dilute urine (and the patient is well hydrated and has a stable circulation) or if it does not respond to a saline infusion, 20–40 mg frusemide should be administered intravenously. If there is no response, acute tubular necrosis has probably occurred and treatment for renal failure is instituted.

Ischaemic renal lesions are usually reversible and the mainstays of treatment are replacement of observed fluid loss with a supplement of 600–1000 ml/24 h for obligatory insensible loss; restriction of dietary protein to a maximum of 20 g/24 h; avoidance of hyperkalaemia and acidosis; and haemodialysis if conservative measures fail to prevent rapid rises in the concentrations of urea and potassium in the venous blood.

Thromboembolic phenomena

These are described in detail in Chapter 21. Management is summarized here for convenience.

Deep vein thrombosis

Prophylaxis against deep vein thrombosis usually includes care to avoid compression of the leg veins during operation and in the postoperative period, the wearing of tapered support stockings and, in high-risk patients, low-dose subcutaneous heparin (calcium heparin 5000 units 12-hourly). Many surgeons now use low-dose heparin in all patients requiring a general anaesthetic who are over 40 years of age.

Thrombosis is suspected clinically by the development of tenderness over the calf veins, by swelling of the foot or leg, or by areas of increased uptake of ^{125}I-fibrinogen (injected as a marker of forming clot) on serial scintiscans. In such patients bilateral ascending phlebography is essential to confirm thrombosis and to determine whether the clot occludes the vein lumen and whether it is located in the iliofemoral segment or in more distal veins. Some surgeons also perform a ventilation-perfusion (VQ) lung scan to establish a baseline for future reference should pulmonary embolism develop.

Treatment of venous thrombosis confirmed on phlebography depends on the location of the clot.

1. Thrombosis confined to the calf vein carries a low risk of embolism and in a mobile patient is treated by support stockings and encouragement to move around. If the patient is immobile and confined to bed, heparinization may be considered.

2. Thrombosis in the iliofemoral segment carries a significant risk of embolism, particularly when the clot is non-occlusive. The patient is heparinized and confined to bed for 48 hours with the foot of the bed elevated. Thereafter, support stockings are fitted and the patient is mobilized. If phlebography shows a tail of non-occlusive thrombus, consideration should be given to insertion of a filter in the inferior vena cava.

Heparinization is commenced with an intravenous bolus of 5000–10 000 units followed by 1000 units/h by continuous intravenous infusion. The whole blood clotting time is estimated at 6 hours and the dose adjusted to maintain a clotting time of two to three times the control values. Heparinization is usually continued for 7–10 days and then replaced by long-term oral anticoagulant therapy. This is introduced during heparin administration, using an initial dose of 10 mg of warfarin a day. Further dosage depends on the prothrombin time, which should be maintained at a ratio to normal of around 3 : 1.

Pulmonary embolus

Massive pulmonary embolus with severe chest pain, pallor and shock demands immediate cardiopulmonary resuscitation, heparinization (10–15 000 units intravenously as a bolus dose) and urgent pulmonary angiography. If the diagnosis is confirmed, the catheter may be left in the pulmonary artery so that pulmonary arterial pressure can be monitored. Arterial and central venous pressure (CVP) lines are also inserted to monitor pressures. If the patient's condition improves, heparinization is continued. If it deteriorates, the embolus must be removed either by the administration of a thrombolytic agent such as streptokinase to dissolve the clot or by pulmonary embolectomy under cardiopulmonary bypass.

If a small pulmonary embolus is suspected because of the occurrence of chest pain and haemoptysis, particularly when accompanied by tachypnoea and/or a pleural effusion, it is necessary first to confirm or refute the diagnosis. A chest X-ray and ECG are obtained to rule out alternative causes and, if normal or compatible with a pulmonary embolus, perfusion and ventilation lung scans are ordered. If one or more lobar or segmental defects are seen, the patient should be fully heparinized and carefully observed.

In all such cases, it is important to investigate the patient for the source of embolus by bilateral phlebography. If this shows thrombosis with propagated clot lying loose in the vessel, a filter is inserted into the vena cava.

10. Special problems in surgical care

The previous chapters dealt with the care of patients before, during and after operation who are generally fit for anaesthesia and operation. However special problems may arise in particular groups of patients; these are considered in this chapter.

THE EMERGENCY CASE

Time for detailed preparation (as outlined in Ch. 7) may not be available when a patient admitted as a surgical emergency requires urgent operation. Priority must then be given to correction of a life-threatening condition and relief of pain. However, the following must not be disregarded.

1. A detailed enquiry must always be made regarding conditions likely to affect anaesthesia, particularly cardiac, respiratory, metabolic and endocrine disease. The course of previous anaesthetics should be ascertained and a note made of any drugs taken over the past 3 months. In elderly men urinary problems are of particular importance, as chronic retention and uraemia may be unsuspected hazards during the postoperative phase.

2. The cardiovascular and respiratory systems are always examined fully. Pulse rate and blood pressure are recorded, haemoglobin concentration is estimated, and a chest X-ray is obtained. An ECG is necessary if there is any suspicion of cardiac disease and is advisable in all patients over 55 years of age. Arterial blood gas and pH determinations may be useful in patients who are shocked or who have respiratory disease.

3. The state of nutrition and hydration is assessed, and blood urea and electrolyte concentrations are estimated in all patients. For all major procedures, a sample of venous blood is taken preoperatively for blood grouping and cross-matching.

4. Obvious deficiencies or illness are treated as far as possible before operation. Anaemia or blood loss should be corrected by transfusion; congestive cardiac failure by digitalization and diuretics; and dehydration by fluid and electrolyte replacement.

5. A nasogastric tube is passed before anaesthesia in all patients who have vomited or who may have intestinal obstruction, peritonitis or a perforated ulcer. A 4–6 hour fast is desirable before operation. If this is not feasible, a nasogastric tube should be passed, the stomach emptied and the anaesthetist informed. In shocked patients a urinary catheter is passed to monitor urine volume. If large quantities of fluid or blood are being infused, a central venous line is inserted and pressure monitored.

6. Consent forms must be signed (children under 16 years require parental consent). The side of the operation is marked, and the nursing staff should carry out their normal preparations. The type and dose of analgesic is determined only after discussion with the anaesthetist.

THE NEONATE

As the body of a newborn infant has a higher water content than that of an adult (700 mg/kg compared to 600 mg/kg), little fluid is normally required in the first few days of life. However, abnormal losses from the gastrointestinal tract can produce *dehydration* and *electrolyte depletion* within a few hours and an intravenous infusion is essential for all infants undergoing surgery. The neonate has a blood volume of 88 ml/kg, compared to 70 ml/kg in adults, and is very susceptible to *blood loss*. One unit of fresh blood should be cross-matched so that operative blood loss can be replaced rapidly, and 1 mg of vitamin K_1 (phytomenadione) is injected before operation to compensate for possible deficiencies in clotting factors.

Hypothermia can develop rapidly, particularly in premature or dehydrated infants. This is due to the relatively large surface area of the newborn and his lack of subcutaneous fat. Hypothermia must be corrected rapidly or acidosis, hypoglycaemia and hyperkalaemia can occur. Heat loss is reduced by placing the infant on a warming pad during operation, and in an incubator set at 32°C postoperatively. Oxygen may be added to the air inflow, and humidity is maintained at 90–100% to reduce insensible water loss from the skin and to prevent crusting of bronchial secretions.

Hyperthermia may complicate anaesthesia in febrile infants with insufficient preoperative fluid replacement. Rapid cooling is achieved by placing the patient in an ice-cooled alcohol bath.

Overhydration is readily produced postoperatively in premature babies. Provided operative blood losses are made good, postoperative intravenous infusion is unnecessary unless there are gastrointestinal losses.

Hypoglycaemia may complicate neonatal surgery and is treated by infusion of 10% glucose for several days. Every effort should be made to recommence oral feeding soon after surgery; otherwise parenteral feeding is required.

THE ELDERLY

Any surgical operation in the elderly carries a greater risk than in younger patients. Although the increased mortality is associated primarily with major operations, even the simplest procedure, e.g. hernia repair, may be hazardous. Because of structural and functional changes in the respiratory, cardiovascular and renal systems, and their altered metabolism, old people are less able to withstand the effects of operation than those who are young or middle-aged.

Respiratory system

With age, structural changes occur in the lungs and chest wall which reduce air space and restrict ventilation. Lung capacity, forced respiratory volume and compliance are reduced; gas exchange is less efficient and Pao_2 falls. Rigidity of the pulmonary blood vessels produces an imbalance between ventilation and perfusion. Relatively unoxygenated blood 'shunts' from pulmonary artery to vein, further adding to hypoxia.

In elderly patients requiring elective surgery in whom respiratory impairment is suspected, a full investigation of the respiratory system should be carried out before operation. This includes estimation of forced vital capacity (FVC) and forced expiratory volume (FEV), and blood gas analysis. The sputum should be cultured and, if positive, an appropriate antibiotic given. Full oxygenation during and after operation is critical. Factors causing postoperative respiratory distress, such as pain and nasogastric intubation, are avoided. Intensive pre- and postoperative physiotherapy to the chest should be arranged.

Cardiovascular system

Atherosclerotic disease is common and thrombotic episodes are frequent. Many old people have ischaemic heart disease, and postoperative acute myocardial infarction may occur. A preoperative ECG is essential in all patients over 55 years of age. Fatal postoperative myocardial infarction is more common in those with previous infarcts, and pre- and postoperative cardiac monitoring is instituted in those with ischaemic changes. An elective operation should normally not be performed within 6 months of a proven infarct.

As vasomotor reflexes are defective, the elderly are intolerant to changes in blood volume. Hypovolaemia is avoided by monitoring blood pressure and ensuring good control of fluid and electrolyte balance.

The risks of postoperative deep venous thrombosis and pulmonary embolism increase with age. Prophylactic measures should be taken (see Ch. 21).

Renal system

The elderly are likely to have impaired renal function and are prone to develop acute tubular necrosis. Hypotension must be avoided. Urinary volume is monitored postoperatively so that oliguria can be recognized and treated promptly.

Metabolic effects

Body composition changes with age. Loss of cells, poor dietary intake, reduced caloric (energy) demands and endocrine hypofunction result in a chronic wasting state. Serum proteins must be estimated preoperatively and any specific deficiencies treated.

Drug metabolism is altered in the elderly and dosage must therefore be carefully controlled. Oversedation should be avoided as it may cause disorientation and unnecessary immobilization.

THE PSYCHIATRIC PATIENT

All patients are anxious before operation. A calm and reassuring approach by ward staff and a truthful explanation of what lies ahead can do much to allay fear. Tranquillizers are rarely necessary. If preoperative anxiety is excessive, operation should be postponed until a full psychiatric assessment has been made.

It must be remembered that psychiatric patients develop the same surgical diseases as 'normal' people. On the other hand, some hysterical patients produce a bewildering variety of symptoms in the hope of persuading a surgeon to operate. If careful investigation fails to elicit organic disease, a psychiatric opinion should be sought.

Patients with abnormal psychiatric behaviour or a history of psychiatric disorder need careful assessment by a psychiatrist during the pre- and postoperative periods. This should be undertaken together with the surgeon. Drug therapy should be interrupted as little as possible during operation. Patients with suicidal and aggressive tendencies may require special supervision during their stay in a general hospital.

The management of postoperative mental disturbance requires recognition and treatment of precipitating factors, a sympathetic, calm and orderly approach to the patient, and if necessary sedation with diazepam (Valium) 15–30 mg daily in divided doses or 10 mg intramuscularly repeated in 4 hours, or with chlorpromazine (Largactil), starting with 25 mg orally three times a day, or 100 mg by suppository or 25–50 mg intramuscularly. Antidepressant therapy should not be given without psychiatric advice.

When treating mentally disturbed patients the following factors should be kept in mind.

1. Old patients in a strange environment often become disorientated, particularly at night. Adequate light and a sympathetic approach may be all that is necessary to settle them.

2. Disorientation may, however, reflect hypoxia and may then be resolved with oxygen and respiratory care.

3. Acute retention of urine in the elderly may cause abnormal behaviour. Catheterization of a distended bladder will give relief.

4. Mental changes ('toxic psychosis') occur in septicaemia and may be the first sign of septicaemic shock. Patients who become confused must be examined for evidence of chest, wound or urinary tract infection. If an intestinal anastamosis has been performed, leakage should be suspected.

5. Postoperative disorientation can occur from withdrawal of alcohol. Excessive alcohol intake may not have been suspected preoperatively or may be denied by the patient. If in doubt, his relatives should be consulted and treatment instituted.

THE JAUNDICED PATIENT

Operation in the presence of jaundice carries specific risks which are described in detail below.

Impaired coagulation

Bile salts in the intestine are necessary for the absorption of fat-soluble vitamins (A, D, E and K). In jaundice, bile salts are absent or present only in reduced amounts and absorption of vitamin K is impaired. Hepatic insufficiency leads to diminished hepatic synthesis of factors II, VII, IX and X.

The prothrombin ratio (PTR) can be used to monitor levels of these factors. If the prothrombin time is prolonged, synthetic vitamin K_1 (phytomenadione) 10 mg/24 h is given intravenously or intramuscularly for several days before operation. If there is evidence of hepatocellular dysfunction, a full coagulation screen is required. Replacement of coagulation components may be necessary.

Acute renal failure ('hepatorenal syndrome')

The risk of renal failure in jaundiced patients is increased for several reasons.

1. Dehydration is common and compounded by anorexia or vomiting.

2. Patients with obstructive jaundice excrete conjugated bilirubin in the urine which is believed to reduce glomerular perfusion and to be toxic to tubular cells.

3. Disordered coagulation increases the risk of heamorrhage and hypotension during operation, leading to reduced renal perfusion.

4. Infection of the biliary tree (cholangitis) commonly complicates biliary obstruction. Surgical manipulation of infected bile ducts can cause bacteraemia with toxic effects on the kidney.

Assuming that coagulation defects have been corrected, the most important prophylactic measures are to ensure full hydration of the patient before operation and to monitor urine volume. The patient is catheterized, and sufficient intravenous fluids are given to ensure a urinary output of at least 40 ml/h during operation and for 48 hours thereafter. Some surgeons administer diuretic agents such as frusemide or mannitol (100 ml of a 20% solution commencing 1 hour before operation and given over 30 min) routinely during surgery but this is only necessary if adequate hydration fails to achieve adequate urine volumes. In patients with obstructive jaundice, the operation should be carried out under antibiotic cover to avoid bacteraemia. Cotrimoxazole (trimethoprim 80 mg and sulphamethoxazole 400 mg in 5 ml diluted to 125 ml, given 8-hourly) or a cephalosporin are preferred.

Hepatotoxicity due to anaesthetic agents

Many drugs given in the perioperative period are potentially hepatotoxic and care should be exercised when these are given to patients with liver damage. The anaesthetist will probably wish to avoid the use of halothane.

Hepatocellular injury is associated with delay in metabolism of drugs normally dependent on the liver for excretion.

Hepatitis virus

Jaundiced patients with serum hepatitis constitute a potential danger to medical and nursing staff. All jaundiced patients undergoing surgery must therefore have their serum tested for hepatitis B surface antigen so that adequate precautions can be taken should this prove positive.

THE MALNOURISHED PATIENT

Malnourishment presents special surgical hazards.

1. As blood volume is reduced, any further reduction by haemorrhage is not well tolerated.

2. Hypoproteinaemia leads to increased sequestration of fluid at the operation site and further reduces blood volume. The risk of pulmonary oedema following intravenous infusion of crystalloids is increased. If an intestinal anastomosis has been performed, local oedema may impair patency and delay return of normal intestinal function.

3. Protein and vitamin deficiencies impair synthesis of collagen and delay wound healing. Wound dehiscence and anastomotic disruption are more common in patients who are malnourished.

4. Resistance to infection is reduced by impaired production of antibodies.

5. Protein reserves may be further depleted by the catabolic phase of the metabolic response.

The general nutritional state of these patients should be improved before operation if at all possible. If surgery cannot be delayed, full nutritional support must be given postoperatively. Elemental minimal residue diets (Vivonex, Triosorbon and Flexical) are mixtures of synthetic carbohydrates, amino acids, fats (usually medium-chain triglycerides) and all essential vitamins and trace elements. They can be used as dietary supplements or to provide a complete daily intake of all necessary foods in milky drinks of varying palatability. Alternatively, various commercially available high-calorie low-residue food extracts can be used.

Alimentary feeding

Preoperative nutrition is best provided by the alimentary route using normal food. A daily intake of 3000–3500 kcal/100–120 g protein with added vitamins should be continued until body weight is within 15% of ideal.

If oral feeding is impracticable, e.g. in patients who cannot eat or who have an oesophageal or gastric obstruction, enteral feeding may be required. This can be given through a fine nasogastric tube or by gastrostomy or jejunostomy. The delivery of foodstuffs directly into the small intestine may cause diarrhoea, and hyperosmolar solutions should be avoided.

Intravenous feeding (parenteral nutrition)

If oral or enteral intake is not possible or inadequate, parenteral feeding (see Ch. 5) is the best method of supporting those who are malnourished. Solutions of synthetic amino acids and emulsified fats are available which can be administered intravenously to provide a nutritionally balanced diet. Parenteral nutrition is particularly valuable in patients with excessive losses, e.g. from intestinal fistulas.

IMPAIRED HAEMOSTASIS

Haemostasis may be impaired by defective coagulation, disorders of the capillary endothelium, or platelet deficiency. The following are of surgical relevance.

Anticoagulant therapy

Heparin. Heparin interferes with platelet aggregation and has antithrombin and antithromboplastin action. A single intravenous dose of 5000–15 000 units prolongs clotting time to two to three times the normal value for 2–5 hours. Rapid reversion to normal follows when therapy is discontinued.

Protamine sulphate combines with heparin to form a stable complex without anticoagulant activity and is used to counteract heparin if urgent operation is required. A dose of 1.0–1.5 mg antagonizes each 100 units of heparin. Protamine is given by *slow* intravenous injection. The quantity required decreases rapidly with the time elapsed after heparin injection: after 30 min only about 0.5 mg is required to antagonize each 100 units injected. As low-dose heparin therapy has been shown to prevent postoperative deep venous thrombosis, heparinized patients requiring surgery are best treated by subcutaneous injection of low doses (5000 units prior to operation followed by 5000 units thereafter).

Oral anticoagulants. Anticoagulants of the coumarin and indanedione class act as substrate competitors with vitamin K and depress manufacture of vitamin K-dependent clotting factors II, VII, IX and X. As they take 36–48 hours to exert their full effect, heparin is used concomitantly when instituting therapy. The dose depends on the prothrombin time, now expressed as an international normalized ratio (INR). Currently recommended ratios are 2–2.5:1 for prophylaxis of deep vein thrombosis; 2–3:1 for treatment of deep vein thrombosis; and 3–4.5:1 for arterial grafts and prosthetic heart valves. Provided that the prothrombin ratio is not greater than 2.0:1, major surgery can be performed without excessive bleeding.

As these drugs are bound to albumin and there is negligible renal excretion, the duration of action is long. If liver function is adequate, 10–30 mg of synthetic vitamin K_1 (phytomenadione) given by intravenous or intramuscular injection will restore the prothrombin ratio to normal within 24–48 hours. More rapid restitution can be achieved by natural vitamin K_1 (pylloquinone) or by transfusion of factor concentrates, plasma or blood.

In patients on long-term treatment with warfarin who are to undergo elective surgery, oral anticoagulants should be stopped 48 hours before operation and the prothrombin ratio estimated daily. Heparin may be substituted if this falls to less than 2.0:1. In an emergency situation where oral anticoagulants may predispose to haemorrhage, e.g. in acute pancreatitis, a similar regimen should be instituted on admission.

Haemophilia

Operations are potentially disastrous in haemophiliacs and close cooperation with a haematologist is essential. The level of anti-haemophilic globulin (factor VIII) must be maintained between 30 and 40% of normal by transfusion of concentrates of human anti-haemophilic globulin or, alternatively, fresh blood or plasma. The adequacy of transfusion is monitored by sequential estimates of factor VIII (see Ch. 4); the prothrombin time is normal in haemophilia. Infection with human immuno-deficiency virus (HIV), which has had disastrous effects in haemophiliacs, should no longer be a risk in view of the routine testing of donors for HIV-antibodies and heat-treatment of factor VIII.

The allied condition of Christmas disease (factor IX deficiency) is less common and usually less severe. Operation can be covered by transfusion of fresh frozen plasma or factor concentrate.

Thrombocytopenia

Thrombocytopenia may be 'idiopathic' or secondary to problems such as drug reactions, hyper-splenism, disseminated intravascular coagulation, or marrow destruction by radiotherapy or tumour. Patients receiving multiple transfusions of stored blood may also develop thrombocytopenia, as such blood does not replace platelet losses.

A platelet count of $40–50 \times 10^9/l$ is normally adequate for haemostasis, and platelet transfusions should be used to attain this level in thrombocytopenic patients requiring surgery. This can be given by a 'bolus' infusion preoperatively.

Disseminated intravascular coagulation (DIC)

The causes of this rare syndrome include major trauma, septicaemia, hypoxia, transfusion reaction, metastatic carcinoma and amniotic fluid embolism. An unusual cause is transfer of peritoneal fluid to the systemic venous system by an artificial shunt, as used in treatment of ascites. Coagulation systems are activated and platelet aggregation occurs within the vascular system, leading to thrombocytopenia, deficiencies of clotting factors and secondary activation of the fibrinolytic system. The level of fibrin degradation products (FDP) is raised.

In surgical patients, DIC is encountered most frequently in the postoperative period. Treatment is complex and may include steroids, heparin and epsilon-aminocaproic acid. A haematologist should be consulted.

Fibrinolysis

Primary fibrinolysis is occasionally seen in patients with liver disease and metastatic carcinoma and is quite distinct from the secondary fibrinolysis of the DIC syndrome. The plasma fibrinogen level is diminished, platelet count is normal, thrombin time is normal or only slightly prolonged, and there is an early increase in plasma levels of fibrin degradation products. Heparin is contraindicated; epsilon-aminocaproic acid acts as a fibrin substitute and is the treatment of choice. Its administration must be controlled by a haematologist.

CARDIAC DISEASE

As already stated, a preoperative ECG is obtained in all patients over 55 years and in those with cardiac symptoms to detect any arrhythmias and ischaemic changes, and to serve as a base for postoperative comparison. If cardiac disease is present, a cardiologist should be consulted preoperatively.

Recent myocardial infarction seriously affects the response to surgery, and only emergency procedures are performed within 6 months of a proven infarct. Only after that time does the risk of a further infarct become acceptably low (Fig. 10.1).

Patients with angina should be fully investigated before any operation. In mild cases of angina of effort, operation is safe provided anaemia is corrected, and full and continued oxygenation of the blood is achieved during and after operation.

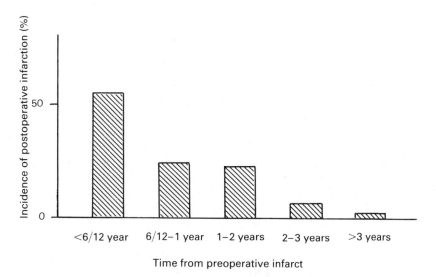

Fig. 10.1 Risk of postoperative myocardial infarction in patients with preoperative infarct

Respiratory depression must be avoided at all costs.

Wherever possible, operation is postponed in patients with severe angina, particularly when it is of the 'crescendo type'. In such patients coronary angiography and, if considered necessary, coronary artery revascularization has priority.

Cardiac arrhythmias are corrected before surgery if possible. Preoperative digitalization may be required to control rapid atrial fibrillation, and lignocaine may be given to suppress multiple ventricular ectopic beats. Antiarrhythmic therapy with amiodarone is becoming more popular in this country.

Cardiac failure is an obvious risk factor, and in patients with acute congestive failure, operation should be delayed if possible until failure has been corrected by digitalization and diuretics. Elderly hypertensive patients must be examined carefully for evidence of congestive failure; this again should be treated preoperatively if possible.

In patients with congestive failure particular care is taken with fluid replacement. Saline infusion is limited to 500 ml daily, urine volume is monitored, and diuretics are given as required. If large volumes of fluid or blood are required for resuscitation or correction of electrolyte deficiencies, monitoring of central venous pressure is essential.

Patients with valvular heart disease present a particular problem. Not only are they liable to arrhythmias and cardiac failure, they may also be taking drugs which can complicate the course of operation. Some of these patients may require replacement of the affected valve before any other surgery can be considered.

Patients with some types of artificial heart valve are likely to be receiving oral anticoagulants (e.g. warfarin). This should be stopped preoperatively and heparin substituted when the prothrombin ratio falls below 2.0:1. A low-dose heparin regimen is normally used. Vitamin K_1 should not be given to patients with a prosthetic heart valve as it may make them resistant to anticoagulant therapy for several days. Fresh frozen plasma is preferred. The patient's normal anticoagulant regimen is reinstituted as soon as the risk of acute bleeding has passed. Postoperative arterial emboli indicate the presence of intracardiac thrombus, and emergency cardiac surgery may be required to avert a fatal embolic episode.

Drugs used to control hypertension are not normally withdrawn except on the day of operation. Beta-adrenergic blockers are commonly used for antihypertensive therapy. As they impair normal cardiac responses, cardiac function must be monitored carefully during anaesthesia and in the postoperative period.

CHEST DISEASE

Preoperative assessment and management

All patients requiring general anaesthesia are screened for chest disease. This demands a careful history, physical examination and chest X-ray. Particular note is made of the patient's occupation and smoking habits, dyspnoea on exertion, and any history of previous chest infection.

When impaired pulmonary function is suspected, forced expiratory volume over a standard period of 1 second (FEV_1) and forced vital capacity (FVC) are measured by spirometry. In obstructive airway disease the FEV_1 may be less than 1 litre and the ratio of FEV_1 to FVC below the normal 80–65%. Arterial oxygen and carbon dioxide tension (Pao_2 and $Paco_2$), bicarbonate and hydrogen ion concentration are determined to provide a baseline for future comparison. Normal values are: $[H^+]$ 36–44 nmol/l; Pao_2 12–15 kPa; $Paco_2$ 4.4–6.1 kPa; and plasma bicarbonate 21–27.5 mmol/l.

If the patient has a productive cough, a specimen of sputum is sent for bacteriological examination. If the sputum is green and purulent, preoperative antibiotic therapy is required; the choice of antibiotic depends on the results of culture and sensitivity determination.

Preoperative physiotherapy helps clear the chest and is valuable training for deep breathing and coughing in the postoperative period. Smoking should be forbidden. If possible, the patient should stop smoking for at least 2 weeks before elective surgery. Bronchodilation with salbutamol by mouth or inhalation is useful in obstructive airway disease, and regular postural drainage should be instituted in patients with bronchiectasis or excess sputum.

Only life-saving operations should be undertaken in patients who are unable to maintain satisfactory ventilation and gaseous exchange at rest. Local or epidural anaesthesia should be considered as an alternative to general anaesthesia.

Postoperative care

Inhalation anaesthetics irritate the bronchial mucosa, inhibit ciliary action, increase bronchial secretions and reduce lung compliance. Wound pain impairs ventilation after thoracic and abdominal surgery. Sedation diminishes ventilation, and prolonged deep sedation is contraindicated in patients with chest disease. Frequent small doses of narcotics are preferred to infrequent large doses.

The patient should expand his lungs fully by deep breathing every 30–60 min and clear accumulated secretions by coughing. This is made easier if the abdominal wound is supported by a physiotherapist or nurse placing her hands around the lower chest. Regular physiotherapy is essential to encourage the patient to clear his chest of secretions. He must not be allowed to lie passively in bed taking shallow breaths. These fail to maintain lung expansion and allow accumulation of secretions, resulting in increasing atelectasis and bronchopneumonia. The chest is examined clinically twice daily and, in patients with chronic chest disease, radiologically once daily. Respiratory efficiency is monitored by blood gas estimations.

If the patient is not able to cooperate, tracheal suction is used to clear the airway and stimulate coughing. Bronchoscopy may be required if significant airway obstruction persists.

Oxygen therapy is indicated for arterial hypoxaemia; it should be given at a known concentration and its effect monitored by regular blood gas estimations. In patients with ventilatory failure necessitating artificial ventilation, the inspired oxygen is set to achieve the desired Pao_2. This should be at least 8–9 kPa. Individuals with chronic respiratory disease may live normally with a lower Pao_2, and in such patients only small increases in inspired oxygen (using a Ventimask or similar *controlled* oxygen therapy device) should be attempted.

Antibiotic therapy is continued postoperatively. Bronchodilators are continued in patients with obstructive airway disease. Intravenous fluid administration is monitored carefully, as even slight overload may precipitate pulmonary oedema.

Assisted ventilation

Patients with severe chest disease may require assisted ventilation for hours or days after general anaesthesia. The anaesthetist will not remove the endotracheal tube until spontaneous ventilation is adequate. Assisted ventilation is required if a steady increase in Paco$_2$ is accompanied by clinical deterioration and/or a rise in hydrogen ion concentration to above 44 nmol/l. Other indications for ventilatory support are a Paco$_2$ of less than 8 kPa in a patient breathing 100% oxygen; failure to remove copious bronchial secretions; and a respiratory rate faster than 35/min.

There are two main types of ventilator: volume-limited and pressure-limited. In the volume-limited type a preset tidal volume is delivered. Pressure-limited ventilators cycle when the peak pressure in the trachea reaches a preset value.

A volume-limited respirator is preferred in patients with acute respiratory failure. Its high peak velocities compensate adequately for increased airway resistance and decreased pulmonary compliance. Oxygenation can be improved further by the use of positive end-expiratory pressure (PEEP), i.e. by adjusting the ventilator to deliver the desired air/oxygen mixture under positive pressure (5–10 cmH$_2$0) throughout the expiratory phase. This modification prevents alveolar collapse, decreases the diffusion distance for oxygen by thinning the alveolar wall, and encourages movements of fluids out of the alveoli and their adjoining interstitial space.

DIABETES

In the days before insulin, diabetic patients undergoing surgery were at considerable risk of developing fatal ketoacidosis. This risk is now reduced by meticulous attention to insulin and carbohydrate requirements and by regular testing of blood and urine. As a general rule, it is imperative to *avoid hypoglycaemia*; a degree of hyperglycaemia is acceptable provided that ketoacidosis does not occur.

Elective operations in diabetic patients

All diabetics must be admitted 2–3 days before operation to ensure that control is adequate. General anaesthesia can induce ketosis, and infection, starvation and trauma all increase the risk. Elective operations in diabetics are best carried out

early in the day, with the patient placed first on the operating list. Specific management depends on the type of control of the patient's diabetes.

Patients controlled by diet alone require no particular action other than 4-hourly finger-prick blood glucose estimations and regular testing of urine for sugar and ketones. Insulin may be needed temporarily if the blood glucose rises and ketosis develops.

Patients whose diabetes is controlled by an oral hypoglycaemic agent should omit their tablets on the morning of the operation and restart as soon as oral feeding recommences. Otherwise management is as for patients controlled by diet alone.

Patients whose diabetes is controlled normally by insulin are easier to manage if soluble insulin rather than long-acting preparations are used. On the day before surgery the dose of depot insulin is halved and supplemented by soluble insulin later in the day. Hypoglycaemia is the major danger on the day of operation and *no* insulin is given prior to surgery.

Blood glucose concentration is estimated preoperatively. If it is less than 6.7 mmol/l, intraoperative hypoglycaemia is avoided by giving 25–50 g of glucose intravenously as a 10% solution. If it exceeds 11 mmol/l (and this is unusual) one-third of the daily insulin requirement is given as soluble insulin *once operation has been completed*.

Following minor surgery, the patient should be able to take carbohydrate orally. Drinks of 25 g glucose are given every 3–4 hours, each covered by 12 units of insulin.

After major operations, it may be some days before oral feeding is possible. Caloric (energy) requirements are supplied by intravenous infusion of glucose (100 g/l) covered by soluble insulin (0.5 units/g) and monitored by twice-daily estimates of blood glucose. Postoperative complications increase the tendency to ketosis. Each specimen of urine must be tested for glucose and ketones; ketonuria indicates the need to increase insulin dosage. Arterial blood gases and hydrogen ion concentration are estimated to establish whether significant acidosis has developed. Electrolytes must be checked daily.

Once the patient is eating normally, he can revert to his usual insulin regimen. A temporary increase in insulin requirements is common after major surgery.

Emergency operations in diabetic patients

An intravenous infusion is established and blood glucose, arterial gases and hydrogen ion concentration are determined. The urine is tested for sugar and ketones. Glycosuria can usually be ignored *provided there is no ketosis.*

Ketoacidosis is an indication to defer surgery until acidosis and fluid and electrolyte abnormalities have been corrected by soluble insulin and intravenous fluids. Complete correction may not be possible until the precipitating surgical cause has been dealt with. Timely incision and drainage of an abscess may lead to marked improvement in the metabolic state. Considerable clinical judgement is required for optimal timing of surgical intervention. The operation is usually performed under cover of an infusion of 10% glucose to avoid hypoglycaemia. Postoperative carbohydrate and insulin requirements are determined by frequent testing of the blood and urine.

ALCOHOL ABUSE

Alcoholics are prone to malnourishment with hypoproteinaemia, chronic vitamin deficiency and poor liver function. Plasma proteins and liver function should be checked. Preoperatively, the patient's nutritional state should be improved by ensuring an adequate caloric (energy) intake, and daily injections of a multivitamin preparation (e.g. Parentrovite, which supplies vitamins B and C). If liver function tests are abnormal, the prothrombin time should be estimated. If prolonged, 20 mg of synthetic vitamin K_1 is given daily by mouth or by intravenous or intramuscular injection.

Induction and maintenance of anaesthesia may require larger doses of anaesthetic than usual. The anaesthetist must be informed that the patient has a history of alcohol abuse.

Withdrawal symptoms can pose problems particularly in the postoperative period. These may take the form of autonomic disturbances, hallucinations, sleep disturbance, tremor and various affective states. Possible fatal complications include epileptiform fits, hypovolaemia, circulatory collapse and hyperthermia.

Management

The patient is nursed in quiet surroundings, isolated from the main ward. As alcoholic patients tend to be dehydrated and liable to hypoglycaemia and hypomagnesaemia, intravenous infusions of saline, glucose, vitamin and magnesium are recommended.

Sedation is required. *Chlormethiazole* (Heminevrin) is still sometimes used. As the duration of the effects of alcohol withdrawal are not shortened by treatment, a full 9-day course must be given. The preparation is available in the form of capsules (each containing 192 mg chlormethiazole base) or as a syrup. Recommended doses are: 9–12 capsules on day 1, 6–8 capsules on day 2, and 4–6 capsules on day 3, given in divided doses three or four times daily. The dose is then reduced to the minimum amount which will control symptoms. In view of the risk of dependence, treatment with the drug should not be prolonged beyond 9 days. 5 ml of Heminevrin syrup can be substituted for each capsule, if desired.

If the patient will not swallow the capsules or syrup, or oral administration is impractical for other reasons, an 0.8% solution of chlormethiazole edisylate can be administered by slow intravenous infusion. The solution is administered at a rate of 60 drops/min (i.e. 4 ml/min) until the patient is drowsy and then at 10–15 drops/min (1 ml/min) to maintain sedation. Constant close supervision is necessary, and the infusion should be replaced by oral therapy with chlormethiazole capsules as soon as possible.

As chlormethiazole is metabolized by the liver, its action may be prolonged in patients with liver decompensation.

Diazepam (Valium) is now generally preferred to chlormethiazole. It is given initially by slow intravenous injection as an 0.5% solution, in a dose of 150–250 μg/kg body weight and at a rate not exceeding 5 mg/min. This is repeated if necessary after an interval of 4 hours or followed by an intravenous infusion to a maximum of 3 mg/kg over 24 hours. Treatment may be continued by oral medication (15–30 mg daily).

Facilities for reversing respiratory depression must be available when using either regimen.

THE CONTRACEPTIVE PILL

Thromboembolic episodes are increased in women taking oral contraceptives, particularly those which contain oestrogen. Current thinking favours continuing taking the pill, as it is now believed that the risks of subsequent venous thrombotic disease, should pregnancy occur, far outweigh those of an operation performed during administration of the pill. If the pill is continued, full prophylaxis against deep vein thrombosis should be given (see Ch. 21).

PREGNANCY

Pregnancy may influence surgical diseases in several ways.

1. Certain intra-abdominal conditions occur more frequently during pregnancy. Those of surgical importance are urinary tract infection, cholecystitis and intraperitoneal haemorrhage.

2. While acute abdominal inflammatory disease (e.g. appendicitis) is not more common in pregnancy, its course may be altered. The gravid uterus interferes with the normal walling-off of infective lesions by bowel or omentum, thus facilitating the spread of infection.

3. The altered position of the viscera and laxity of the abdominal wall can modify the signs of acute abdominal disease and lead to delays in diagnosis. Although removal of a normal appendix during pregnancy should be avoided, it is equally important not to allow appendicitis to proceed to the point of perforation.

4. The need to avoid abdominal X-rays during the early months of pregnancy can increase diagnostic difficulties.

5. The altered hormonal balance during pregnancy may influence the course of disease outside the abdomen. For example, breast cancer occurring during the second half of pregnancy can be particularly fulminating.

Elective surgery

Elective surgery should be avoided during pregnancy. Operation is particularly dangerous during the first trimester, when hypoxia, hypotension and drugs may cause developmental malformations in the fetus.

Essential surgery

If operation during pregnancy is mandatory, the anaesthetist must be forewarned. Drugs with teratogenic properties must not be given. As ovarian function is necessary for preservation of the fetus to the 16th week, ovaries should only be removed when there is no alternative.

Postoperatively the patient should be nursed in quiet surroundings. For most procedures the postoperative course is uneventful. If uterine pain, vaginal bleeding or vaginal discharge occur, an obstetrician must immediately be summoned.

ENDOCRINE DYSFUNCTION

The endocrine system consists of glands which by virtue of their secretion of steroid, polypeptide or protein hormones influence the function of a wide variety of 'target' tissues. Removal of a normal endocrine gland may have profound effects, and in the case of certain glands can prove fatal. Essential hormones must be replaced following ablative endocrine surgery.

Further illness, particularly if necessitating operation, can bring additional problems to patients with endocrine dysfunction.

Pituitary-adrenal system

A particular problem is posed by patients with pituitary or adrenal disorders in whom any additional stress may impose demands which cannot be met by secretion of glucocorticoid or mineralocorticoid hormones. This is particularly important in patients whose pituitary and adrenal glands have been removed, or when therapy with steroid hormones has resulted in suppression of normal endogenous secretion. Any operation or acute illness places such patients in danger of acute adrenal failure.

Normally patients are aware of this problem and have been warned to increase the dose of maintenance steroids in such circumstances. In patients requiring a general anaesthetic, steroid cover is best provided by intravenous injection of 100 mg hydrocortisone (cortisol) sodium succinate at the start of the operation. This dose may be repeated during the operation and further doses given by intravenous infusion (100 mg/500 ml saline every 4–6 hours). Thereafter, intramuscular or oral administration of hydrocortisone in decreasing daily amounts will provide adequate steroid support.

Any surgical procedure is hazardous in patients with a catecholamine-secreting phaeochromo-cytoma of the adrenal medulla or paragangli-onic tissue. Such patients have an extremely labile circulation and are prone to attacks of acute hypertension, hypotension and circulatory col-lapse. A history of paroxysmal adrenergic over-activity (hypertension, sweating, pallor, headache) or the discovery of hypertension in a young person should arouse suspicion. If there is no opportunity for a full preoperative investigation, adrenergic blocking drugs and intravenous hydrocortisone sodium succinate should be available, and the blood pressure carefully monitored during induc-tion and maintenance of anaesthesia.

Thyroid

It is also important to assess thyroid status in patients requiring surgery. Thyrotoxicosis is likely to precipitate serious cardiac and metabolic crises and must be controlled before any operation. Anti-thyroid drugs such as carbimazole are not suitable for this purpose, as it takes up to 10 days before they exert their full inhibitory effect. The beta-adrenergic blocking agents rapidly antagonize the peripheral effects of thyroid hormone, and propanolol 10–30 mg three times a day should be given to any thyrotoxic patient requiring emer-gency surgery. Postoperatively, the patient is sedated and antithyroid medication instituted.

Equally important is the recognition of hypothyroidism. Such patients may develop car-diac arrythmias and arrest during anaesthesia, and hypothermia and electrolyte deficiences may occur postoperatively. Careful administration of small doses of tri-iodothyronine, supplemented by hydrocortisone, is accepted treatment but must be carefully regulated. These problems are further discussed in Chapter 23.

11. Infections and antibiotics

Wound infection

An open wound is invariably contaminated with organisms which may be derived endogenously from the patient's skin or exogenously from an external source such as the soil or air, or the hand of an attendant. The outcome of the microbial challenge depends on many factors, including the circumstances of contamination.

If contamination is minimal, as in an elective surgical incision performed under good conditions on a patient in good general health, the defences of the host cope completely. If contamination is severe, and particularly when other adverse factors operate, the challenge may rapidly result in a fulminating and overwhelming infection unless prompt and adequate action is taken to counter it.

Such conditions arise for example with a lacerated wound following a road accident in an elderly person or a perforated lesion of the colon in a debilitated patient.

Contamination usually denotes the passive presence of a relatively small number of various species of bacteria. When one or more contaminants have a survival advantage over the others and replicate in the wound, *infection* is initiated and microbial pathogenicity is expressed (Fig. 11.1). There may be bacterial invasion, toxin production or a combination of these. Less commonly there may be viral or fungal infection.

Thus a wound infection implies the implantation of a potentially infective inoculum under conditions that allow the organisms to evade or overcome host defences; it is a function of the

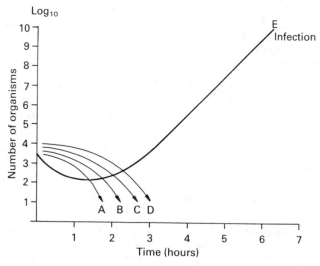

Fig. 11.1 In contamination a number of different species (A,B,C,D,E) may be present in small to moderate numbers. In infection one (or more) species expresses a survival advantage and multiplies to produce a significant challenge (E).

number of organisms in the inoculum, their quality or nature, and the efficacy of local and general host defence mechanisms.

Predisposing factors

Factors that predispose to or promote infection include:

contamination with potential pathogens;
foreign material in the wound;
virulence-enhancing effect of some materials such as soil,
calcium salts and iron salts;
delay in primary attention;
pathogenic synergy (see later);
devitalized tissue;
oedema/pressure/constriction;
impaired blood supply;
extravasation of tissue fluids and blood; and
host factors lowering resistance, e.g. age, debility, obesity, immunocompromised states, diabetes, alcoholism.

Several of these factors are more likely to be present in accidental wounds, and prompt and adequate surgical treatment should be given before the stage of bacterial contamination has led to bacterial proliferation and passed into that of active infection. Ideally this should be within 1–2 hours of injury and must include thorough cleansing of the wound with removal of all debris (surgical toilet) followed by excision of all devitalized tissue (debridement). If primary surgical care is not given within 6 hours, infection must be presumed.

Factors concerned with healing, and problems of wound management are considered in Chapter 12.

Tissue oxygenation

Primary host defences against wound infection include phagocytosis and intraleucocytic microbicidal systems. Effective phagocytosis, good tissue perfusion and oxygenation are requirements for optimal operation of these defences. All wounded tissue is less aerobic than normal tissue; impaired oxygenation persists for

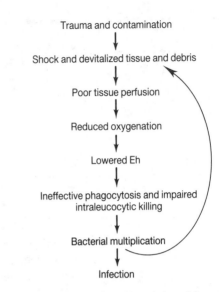

Fig. 11.2 The 'vicious circle'. Association of factors that may be involved in the change from contamination to infection in a wound. Eh = oxidation-reduction potential

some days until healing is established. If the patient is initially shocked, tissue perfusion is further constrained and a vicious circle may result (Fig. 11.2).

Signs of infection

It is important to detect infection in a wound early. Cardinal local signs include erythema, warmth, oedema, tenderness and possibly serous or seropurulent exudate. The patient's temperature may rise and local tenderness may increase to pain and muscle guarding in the affected part.

Pyogenic organisms provoke a polymorphonuclear leucocytosis. The erythrocyte sedimentation rate (ESR) increases and the level of C-reactive protein rises. If the infection is severe, with early progression to bacteraemia and septicaemia, the patient may quickly and insidiously develop bacteriogenic or 'septic' shock (see below) with facial pallor giving way to an ominous, slightly cyanotic flush. As the blood pressure falls and perfusion of vital organs is reduced, the patient's mental state changes from one of anxious malaise to clouded consciousness and then coma. Multiple organ failure and death ensue. The time course of these events may be as short as a few hours.

When an operation involves an unavoidable and significant microbial challenge to the tissues, as in colonic surgery, it is standard practice to protect the patient by giving antimicrobial prophylaxis to cover the period of challenge (see p. 128). It is important that this should be for as short a time as possible. For example, a suitable antibiotic may be given just before operation and continued for 1–2 days postoperatively, but not for longer.

Septic shock

A range of shock syndromes are associated with a considerable spectrum of microbial challenges. These are variously described as *bacteraemic, septicaemic,* or *septic shock.* Other synonyms such as *Gram-negative shock* and *endotoxic shock* reflect the fact that Gram-negative bacteria are often (but not invariably) responsible and that bacterial lipopolysaccharide endotoxin is thought to be a significant mediator or at least significantly involved in a final common pathway.

While Gram-negative sepsis is more commonly associated with septic shock, Gram-positive sepsis may be. The possibility of septic shock should be considered whenever cardiovascular instability is evident in a patient with major infection, or in a postoperative or injured patient in whom a major infection may be developing. The condition may present suddenly, but some patients become progressively shocked over a period of time. Clinical awareness and prompt action are essential.

Two phases are recognized although in a fulminating case the patient's condition may deteriorate so rapidly that the dramatic features of the second phase may be all that is noted.

Phase 1. This is the *hyperdynamic* phase which is characterized by tachycardia, hyperventilation, warm dry extremities, but an ominous degree of hypotension. The patient may be anxious and restless, and then confused, lethargic, drowsy and weak.

Phase 2. The patient's colour may progress to a curious facial flush with a slightly mauve cyanotic tinge heralding the transition to the *hypodynamic* phase. Here there is cyanosis, marked hypo-

tension, vasoconstriction, oliguria and mental confusion, followed by multiple organ failure, coma and then death.

The pulmonary component of multiple organ failure is the adult respiratory distress syndrome (ARDS) with acute dyspnoea and hypoxaemia, widespread infiltrates in the lungs with increased permeability and inflammatory changes, and pulmonary oedema. ARDS may be associated with a range of causes. In at least 50% of patients the cause is septicaemia and the mortality rate in this group is very high. ARDS as a complication of septicaemia is sometimes loosely called 'septic lung'. The term denotes acute respiratory failure in a patient with sepsis or septic shock, but the lung is not primarily involved in the bacterial infection and is reacting as one of the components of multiple organ failure.

In septic shock, the organs that fail include the heart, the lungs, the brain, the kidneys and the liver.

Tumour necrosis factor (TNF)

TNF is a macrophage factor (synonym: cachectin) with several known activities. It inhibits lipid uptake by adipose tissue and is involved in the wasting (cachexia) typical of chronic diseases. It is a pyrogen, like bacterial endotoxin, and it induces the synthesis of interleukin 1.

Bacterial endotoxin is a potent inducer of TNF. Thus a cascade of mediators of the components of the septic shock syndrome includes TNF as a key factor.

Hospital infections

Patients who remain in hospital for some time acquire hospital organisms on the skin, in the nose and mouth and in the gut. Such hospital strains of bacteria may have evolved a special facility for colonization and infection. A patient who is unwell and old has both reduced tissue and reduced general resistance, and is more susceptible to colonization and infection. The length of stay of such a patient in an acute hospital must be kept to a minimum.

After any prolonged series of inpatient investigations it is wise to allow the patient to return home before surgical treatment so that his normal flora can be restored away from the hospital environment.

Sites of colonization

It is possible to monitor the acquisition of flora and this may be of clinical value, e.g. in the preparation of a patient for intestinal surgery or before treatment with cytotoxic agents. Hospital practice often fails to recognize the significance of a patient's endogenous flora in relation to both potential protective and potential pathogenic effects. For example, long-stay patients, particularly when old, should not be treated in an acute surgical ward, as dispersal of acquired skin flora, e.g. from an infected bedsore into the ward environment and onto surfaces in toilet areas, poses dangers to other patients.

The 'colonization resistance' of the gut is markedly reduced by some forms of antibiotic therapy, so that the opportunities for exchange of antibiotic resistance between strains and species of gut bacteria are increased.

Hospital microbial challenges

Hand-borne or surface-mediated challenges

The hands of patients and staff are of great importance in conveying microbial challenges. Related hazards and possible control measures are summarized in Table 11.1. Some sophisticated

measures, such as special containment facilities, are costly but simple methods of control are not, yet they are often neglected.

Air-borne challenges

Potential microbial challenges from air and effective measures to control them are listed in Table 11.2. Some basic control measures are not unduly expensive and if applied conscientiously reduce the advantages of more sophisticated measures, such as unidirectional filtered air-systems, to marginal proportions.

Ingested challenges

Significant microbial challenges may be delivered to the gastrointestinal tract in hospital (Table 11.3). Food hygiene is of paramount importance and hospital catering systems must be of a high standard. The numbers of organisms delivered to our patients in hospital food may be unacceptably high. Resistant organisms may reach the gut of patients as a result of the multiplication of animal strains that contaminate some foods.

Inoculated challenges

Infection with hepatitis B virus is an important

Table 11.1 Hand-borne challenges and contact hazards, and possible control measures

Hazard	Control measures
Hand contact (Direct and mediated contact)	Hand-washing Antiseptics and disinfectants Gloves No-touch techniques
Trolley surfaces, etc. Contaminated instruments Contaminated solutions	Disposable or 'dedicated' instruments Adequate staff adequately trained Adequate facilities
Shared facilities e.g. shared toilets, basins, towels	Separate facilities Special containment facilities

Table 11.2 Air-borne hazards, associated problems and possible control measures

Hazard	Control measures
Contamination of ward and theatre air	Ventilation in theatre and ward Adequate interspace in ward
Wound dressing	Avoidance of contamination by restriction of action in ward
Bedmaking Floor polishing Toilet flushing, etc.	Avoidance of generation of air-borne particles Avoidance of use of aerosols Treatment of fabrics Control of dangerous dispersers
Hot-air blowers	Filtration and laminar-flow systems Special containment facilities
Transmissible respiratory infections	Attention to anaesthetic equipment, respirators, etc.

example of the serious potential hazard of skin-penetrating injuries in all clinical staff. This arises from cross-contamination with blood or other body fluids from a patient with a recognized infection or one who may be a known or unknown carrier. Many other pathogenic agents can be transmitted by accidental inoculation of blood or blood products. In surgical staff, punctures of surgical gloves occur in up to 30% of operations, and skin-penetrating injuries with needles and knives are common events demanding constant caution. Currently attention is focused on the viruses of hepatitis B, non-A non-B hepatitis, and AIDS as infecting agents. The carrier rate for hepatitis B in the UK is around 0.1%, while in some countries in Africa and Asia it is as high as 5–15%. In high-risk groups in the UK and USA (some immigrants, drug addicts, patients with Down's syndrome, male homosexuals) the carrier rate is 5–10%. Surgeons, obstetricians, dentists, haematologists and their staff, laboratory workers and workers in transfusion services are particularly at risk and should take care to avoid skin-penetrating injuries in circumstances in which contamination with blood or blood products or other body fluids is likely. Active immunization with three injections of hepatitis B vaccine is recommended for all those at risk.

The infective state of a patient or carrier in relation to hepatitis B is demonstrated by the detection of hepatitis B surface antigen (HBsAg), and in particular hepatitis B 'e' antigen (HBeAg) in the serum.

If a non-immunized person has a skin-penetrating injury with likely hepatitis B con-tamination, emergency (post-exposure) passive protection can be given by intramuscular injection of hyperimmune hepatitis B immunoglobulin (HBIG) within 48 hours.

Hazards associated with intensive care

Special infective hazards may be posed by a variety of procedures performed in an intensive care unit, including the use of ventilators and respirators, nasogastric tubes, suction apparatus, intravenous lines, percutaneous needles, and catheters. It is paradoxical that our most severely compromised patients should be exposed to such inadvertent challenges.

Pathogenic potential of microbes

Exaltation and attenuation

When an organism is serially passaged in vivo, its virulence may be exalted and its capacity to spread from one host to another increased.

The concept of increased pathogenic potential as a result of exaltation in vivo must be linked with the ability of some commensal or opportunist bacteria to acquire and pass on new potentially dangerous genetic information. This may affect an organism's ability to colonize, to infect, to produce toxin or to gain multiple antibiotic resistance. The 'hospital staphylococcus' illustrates some of the alarming possibilities that result when an organism acquires new genetic material in the course of its colonization. Gram-negative bacilli, especially klebsiella organisms, have also demonstrated a potential for dangerous genetic exchange. The extending range of beta-lactamases in such widely different genera as *Haemophilus*, *Neisseria* and *Bacteroides* is a matter for concern. The transmission of organisms from patient to patient must be rigorously avoided. Hand-washing on the ward is critical, as is the wearing of disposable gloves in situations where transfer of flora from one patient to another may occur.

Pathogenic synergy

Two or more organisms may combine forces in a mixed infection and demonstrate enhanced ag-

Table 11.3 Ingested challenges, associated problems and possible control measures

Hazard	Control measures
Contaminated hospital food	Strict food hygiene
Contaminated special diet formulations	Good, easily cleaned equipment Safe kitchen practices
Contaminated drug preparations	Bacteriological monitoring Trained staff
R-factor transmission from animals	Control of antibiotics Care in food preparation

gression and virulence. Examples include acute ulceromembranous gingivitis (Vincent's infection), Meleney's synergistic gangrene and various fusospirochaetal or mixed infections with anaerobic components, all of which may lead to progressive destruction of tissue or a fulminating invasive infection. Mixed infections are common in a wide range of conditions, e.g. cerebral, dental, lung and pelvic abscess and peritonitis. When bacteroides organisms are present in such infections, they interfere with normal phagocytic mechanisms and inhibit intraleucocytic bactericidal systems. This may partly explain the observed synergistic action of coexisting pathogens.

Asepsis

Surgical ritual

In surgical areas, clear and specific instructions must be given on preoperative skin cleansing of the patient and on adequate disinfection of the operation site (see Ch. 8). The relative advantages of masks, gowns and drapes at operation are debated and the limitations of these precautions should be understood. Only suitable materials should be used.

There should be a clear disinfectant policy and an antibiotic policy to ensure that antibacterial agents are used sensibly on the wards and in the operating theatres. Strict adherence to the principles of sterilization and disinfection is essential when cleansing and processing surgical instruments and anaesthetic equipment.

Sterilization

This is an absolute term denoting complete removal or inactivation of viable microorganisms (protozoa, fungi, bacteria and viruses). It can only be achieved by strict attention to detail. Instruments or articles can be classified as sterile if they have been subjected to any of the following.

1. Wet heat in an autoclave at 121°C for 20 minutes or at a higher temperature for a shorter time (HTST) to provide an equivalent exposure (Fig. 11.3).

2. Dry heat in a hot-air oven at 160°C for 1 hour (see Fig. 11.3).

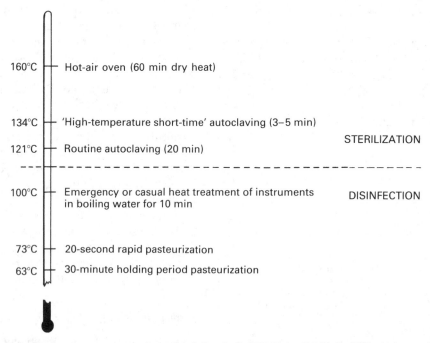

Fig. 11.3 A summary of heat-treatment temperatures (after Collee, J. G. 1981 in *Applied Medical Microbiology*, p. 104. Blackwell, Oxford)

3. Gamma-radiation under strictly controlled conditions.

4. Special sterilizing chemicals, liquids or gases, such as formaldehyde, glutaraldehyde or ethylene oxide, under strictly controlled conditions.

Some transmissible agents are now known to challenge these conventional assumptions, e.g. those responsible for Creutzfeldt-Jakob disease.

Disinfection

This denotes a significant reduction in the numbers of organisms present, particularly those that might cause infection. With few exceptions, chemical disinfectants are not sterilizing agents. *Antiseptics* are relatively mild disinfectants that can be used on living tissues without causing undue harm.

Disinfection and preparation of the skin for surgery. Before a surgical incision is made in intact skin, the transient and resident flora at the operation site can be markedly reduced by thorough cleansing and then largely inactivated by the application of a suitable antibacterial agent. This will inactivate vegetative forms of bacteria only; it cannot be expected to kill bacterial spores. Accessible vegetative bacteria on the skin can be quickly inactivated by applying 70% ethanol, or 70% isopropyl alcohol, in water. Another antiseptic such as chlorhexidine or iodine 1–2% may be incorporated into the application. It is the alcohol at its optimum concentration of 70% in water that achieves a quick kill of vegetative bacteria.

Surgical sepsis

Postoperative wound infection

Bacterial infection of a surgical wound is still a common postoperative complication. The following generalizations reflect current experience in Britain.

Clean wounds in healthy tissue should heal promptly. With adequate facilities, an infection rate of less than 2% should be the aim of a good surgical team. Infections with *Staphylococcus aureus* occur from time to time. A series of such infections in a surgical unit suggests that a member of the team may be a carrier of *S. aureus*. Infec-

tions with coagulase-negative staphylococci are particularly associated with the implantation of heart valves, orthopaedic prostheses, or other artificial materials.

Abdominal wounds. Perioperative antimicrobial prophylaxis has significantly reduced the incidence of infection in abdominal surgery. Operations on the oesophagus, stomach and proximal small bowel are at risk of infection with oropharyngeal flora such as cocci, bacteroides organisms and coliform bacteria. A 10% infection rate is not uncommon, especially if gastric achlorhydria allows bacterial multiplication in the stomach. This has special relevance to patients receiving cimetidine or other secretory inhibitors.

Colorectal surgery and operations on patients with complicated appendicitis are associated with higher postoperative infection rates, ranging from 10% to 35% or more. Coliform bacteria and bacteroides organisms are common pathogens, often acting synergistically. Mixed infections with faecal streptococci and proteus or pseudomonas organisms pose special problems in clinical management.

The hazard of infection can be reduced by careful choice of antimicrobial prophylactic agents and meticulous preoperative preparation of the patient. Acute emergency cases are at special risk.

Antimicrobial prophylaxis is also important in surgery of the biliary tract, where potentially infective organisms include faecal streptococci, coliform bacteria, pseudomonas organisms and *Clostridium perfringens*. Despite antimicrobial measures, infection rates of 5–10% are still recorded in such patients.

Peritonitis

Chemical ('abacterial') peritonitis arises when irritant substances such as pancreatic juice, gastroduodenal contents or blood gain access to the peritoneum. Staphylococcal infection sometimes follows surgical intervention.

Various bacteria may be associated with a primary infection. Peritonitis occurring as a complication of continuous ambulatory peritoneal dialysis (CAPD) is a special problem.

Infections most commonly associated with peritonitis secondary to perforation of an abdominal or pelvic viscus are due to aggressive elements of the commensal flora. These infections are mixed: coliform bacteria, bacteroides organisms and Gram-positive cocci are usually prominent. Clostridia are sometimes involved. Pure anaerobic infections without coliform or facultative bacteria may be encountered, especially in pelvic abscesses.

Pelvic inflammatory disease

This is a cause of much morbidity in female patients, who are especially prone to pelvic infection. It is most commonly acquired from the genital tract with inflammation in the region of the uterus, fallopian tubes and ovaries, giving rise to symptoms and signs of local peritoneal irritation. As in other forms of pelvic sepsis, there may be mixed coliform organisms and anaerobes, usually bacteroides and/or anaerobic cocci. Chlamydial infection is common and must not be missed. Pelvic sepsis in male or female patients may follow peritoneal infection arising from a non-genital source, e.g. a perforated appendix.

Burns

Burned areas of skin are highly vulnerable to bacterial colonization with organisms such as *Streptococcus pyogenes* (group A beta-haemolytic streptococcus), various staphylococci and coliform organisms (including pseudomonas), proteus bacteria and faecal streptococci.

Bacteraemia, septicaemia and septic shock

These may occur postoperatively after abdominal or genitourinary operations, following invasive manipulations, or in patients in intensive care after serious injuries or major surgery. Blood culture can be helpful in identifying the pathogens and guiding therapy, but it is necessary to start active antimicrobial treatment on a 'best-guess' emergency basis.

Urinary tract and respiratory tract infections are discussed elsewhere in this volume.

Pressure sores

Ulceration of the skin over pressure areas in im-

mobilized patients results from ischaemia. There is direct pressure on small blood vessels which causes endothelial damage leading to activation of the clotting system. Predisposing factors include vascular disease, anaemia, obesity, incontinence, malnutrition, loss of cutaneous sensation, chronic debilitating disease, and imposed restriction of movement associated with the control of fractures.

Prevention requires careful teamwork and vigilance. A sheepskin or other special mattress (e.g. a water ripple mattress) may be necessary to avoid uneven distribution of the patient's weight. The skin should be kept dry and clean. Treatment of a pressure sore includes cleansing and the application of water-miscible preparations containing dimethicone (a silicone). Dietary supplements of vitamin C and oral zinc may help to promote good healing.

ANAEROBIC INFECTIONS

Tetanus

Clostridium tetani is an anaerobic spore-forming bacillus that occurs in soil and faeces and may contaminate an accidental wound. Survival of anaerobic bacilli in a wound is favoured by hypoxia, the presence of haematoma, soil and foreign bodies, and devitalized tissue. Failure to cleanse and excise the wound, coupled with ill-judged primary closure, provides favourable conditions for clostridial spores to germinate and for the bacteria to multiply and produce toxins.

When infection is established, the tetanus bacillus contributes little to local wound inflammation. However, it produces an exotoxin (tetanospasmin) which increases muscle tone, resulting in exaggerated responses to trivial stimuli and intermittent muscular spasms. These progress to generalized muscular spasms. In 30% of cases the initial injury may be a minor puncture wound so small as to be ignored by the patient.

The incubation period between injury and development of symptoms varies from a few days to three months. Most cases declare themselves within two weeks. The onset period is that between the first symptom and the onset of generalized muscle spasms. The prognosis is better if the incubation and onset periods are long.

Clinical presentation

The clinical presentation is often insidious. Tingling or ache or stiffness in the wound area is usually the first symptom. Jaw movements become restricted (hence the traditional name 'lockjaw'), facial muscle spasms produce a sardonic grin (risus sardonicus) and the muscles of the neck and back become stiff. Dysphagia, laryngeal spasm and spasm of the chest wall muscles and diaphragm can compromise ventilation and threaten life.

In severe cases, painful muscle spasms become more widespread and increase in frequency and duration. Arching of the back muscles can produce a state known as 'opisthotonos'. Sphincter spasm may cause micturition difficulties.

The patient remains conscious, although consiousness is frequently clouded. Muscle spasms are painful and exhausting and may be triggered by minor stimuli. The temperature is normal or only slightly elevated despite profuse sweating and tachycardia. These features are due to sympathetic overactivity, which may also cause worrying swings in blood pressure.

It is important to appreciate that these are the clinical features of a severe attack. Some cases are milder and do not progress to the full spectrum of generalized muscle spasms.

Diagnosis

Diagnosis is essentially clinical, but is supported by the demonstration of typical slender bacilli with drumstick spores in material from the devitalized wound tissue, and confirmed by the demonstration of tetanus toxin in cultures by toxin-antitoxin neutralization tests in mice.

Prevention

Tetanus is a preventable disease. Its low prevalence in countries with well developed medical services depends on prompt and adequate attention to wounds (Figs. 11.4 and 11.5) and programmes of active immunization.

Active immunization of all children in Britain is achieved by the use of a combined vaccine, the so-called triple vaccine (diphtheria, pertussis, tetanus vaccine), which includes adsorbed tetanus toxoid and is given in three doses within the first year of life. The first and second injections are separated by an interval of 6–8 weeks and the third is given about 4–6 months later. Adults should receive booster injections of adsorbed toxoid at 5 and 15 years and thereafter at 10-year intervals until middle age. In this way they can maintain lifelong immunity.

If possible, the immunization record of all patients with lacerated wounds should be checked. Patients immunized more than 5 years ago are given a booster injection of 0.5 ml of adsorbed toxoid (the need for this is debatable if the period since their last booster is less than 5 years). A full course of active immunization with toxoid is advisable if there is any doubt regarding past immunization, and immediate protection by simultaneous passive immunization is necessary if the patient has not been previously immunized.

Passive immunization with equine immune globulin (anti-tetanus serum; ATS) is associated with the risk of hypersensitivity and should now be abandoned if human immune globulin is available.

Human tetanus immune globulin (HTIG) is available in many countries to give immediate transient protection to non-immune patients. Its use is reserved for those considered to be tetanus-prone and then as an adjunct to active immunization and antibiotic treatment (see below). An intramuscular injection of 250–500 i.u. is given at a site distant from that used for the toxoid and from a different syringe.

Tetanus-prone wounds are those complicated by delay in treatment of more than 6 hours; stab and other puncture wounds; animal or human bites; penetrating wounds; and wounds heavily contaminated with agricultural or horticultural materials or soil. They require particular care in their assessment. Following wound toilet they are carefully excised as necessary. Local antisepsis with an iodophor is advised. The wound should not be sutured but drawn together with Steristrips or lightly packed. Delayed primary closure should be considered in 4–5 days.

The assessment of puncture wounds is difficult, and adequate excision and exploration is not always practical. Such wounds should be regarded as potentially contaminated (see Fig. 11.5).

Antibiotic prophylaxis

A dose of long-acting penicillin should be given just before the wound is cleaned and explored. If the patient is allergic to penicillin or a more prolonged course of antibiotic is considered advisable, erythromycin 500 mg twice daily is given for 5 days, the first tablet being administered just before wound toilet. It must be stressed that antibiotic treatment does not replace the need for basic surgical care of the primary wound, but it may be a necessary adjunct.

Tetanus treatment

Treatment of tetanus is intensive and must begin as soon as the diagnosis is made.

Destruction of the infecting organism and neutralization of the toxin. At least 10 000 units of human tetanus immune globulin is given by slow intravenous infusion diluted in saline. The wound is excised, cleaned and left open. Penicillin 1 mega-unit 6-hourly by intramuscular injection or intravenous infusion, and metro-nidazole 1 g rectally 8-hourly by suppository will kill surviving bacteria and prevent further production of toxin. The first dose of antibiotic and the antitoxin should be given immediately, and before wound excision if possible. The duration of antibiotic therapy depends on the individual response of the patient and bacteriological guidance. A case can be made for giving a further dose of 5000 units of antitoxin after a few days.

Life support. The effects of toxin that has been fixed to receptors in the nervous system must be countered if the patient is to survive. He is nursed well-sedated in a quiet, shaded, intensive care room. Muscle spasms are controlled by tubocurarine or other neuromuscular blocking agents which necessitate intubation and assisted ventilation. Tracheostomy may be required to relieve respiratory embarrassment and is best performed early in the disease. Diazepam and chlorpromazine are given to depress excitability and control spasms and to help the patient to cope with a terrifying experience.

The patient is in a hypercatabolic state and nutrition must be maintained. A nasogastric tube

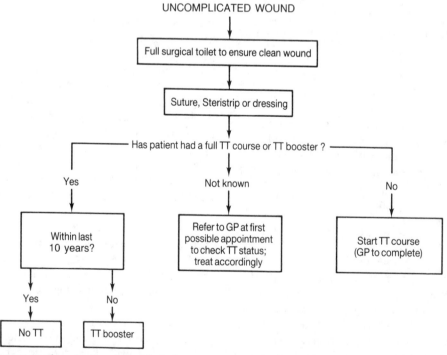

Fig. 11.4 Management of uncomplicated wounds, including tetanus prophylaxis schedule. TT = tetanus toxoid (adsorbed); GP = General practitioner. (Collee, MacLeod and Little, and Lothian Health Board, 1987)

facilitates feeding and lessens the risk of aspiration. Regular turning is necessary to avoid pressure sores and to keep the patient's chest clear.

Intense sympathetic activity can be controlled by beta-adrenergic blockers, which also control arrhythmias and labile blood pressure.

Several weeks of such intensive therapy may be required.

Gas gangrene and other clostridial infections

Clostridium perfringens (previously called *Cl.* *welchii*) is the principal cause of clostridial myonecrosis or gas gangrene. Other clostridial species alone or in combination may be associated with gas gangrene, often in concert with facultative organisms. The organisms form spores which reside in soil and faeces, and contaminate skin and clothing. They are strict anaerobes and their growth is favoured by failure to debride contaminated wounds.

The pathogenic clostridia of the gas-gangrene group produce a number of toxins, including phospholipase (lecithinase), collagenase, proteinases, hyaluronidase, lipase and various

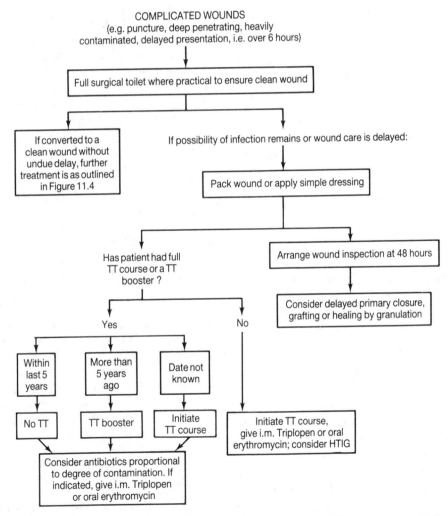

Fig. 11.5 Management of complicated wounds, including tetanus prophylaxis schedule. TT = tetanus toxoid (adsorbed); HTIG = human tetanus immunoglobulin. (Source as Fig. 11.4)

haemolysins. These toxins and aggressins devitalize cells, destroy the local microcirculation and favour dissemination of infection along tissue planes with active destruction of muscle. When the products of the infection gain entry to the systemic circulation, the patient's initial anxiety gives way to a clouding of consciousness and delirium. There is tachycardia, pallor and jaundice, with subsequent circulatory collapse and death.

The spectrum of infection extends from superficial contamination of an open wound, through invasion of subcutaneous tissue, the production of crepitant cellulitis and localized painful myositis, to the full-blown picture of clostridial myonecrosis and gas gangrene. Localized forms of infection need not be associated with signs of systemic upset, or there may be relatively mild upset with fever and tachycardia. Diffuse myositis and gas gangrene produce profound systemic upset and quickly threaten the affected limb and life of the patient.

Infection typically takes 2–3 days to become manifest, sometimes as an unexplained deterioration in the patient's general condition. The wound and surrounding tissues must be inspected, after removal of plaster casts if need be. A brown seropurulent discharge with characteristic odour, oedema, crepitus and pain on examination support the diagnosis, which is confirmed microscopically by the presence of Gram-positive rods. Subsequent culture and special tests determine the species involved. *Clostridium septicum* and *Cl. novyi* (*Cl. oedematiens*) can be detected directly by immunofluorescence microscopy with special stains.

Blood culture sometimes helps to establish the diagnosis and to guide management.

Prevention

As for tetanus, prompt and adequate primary wound care by excision and debridement is essential. Contaminated wounds must not be closed by primary suture. Penicillin remains the prophylactic antibiotic of choice, with erythromycin as a good alternative. Polyvalent gas gangrene antitoxin was once available but its efficacy was in doubt and allergic reactions were common. It is no longer used.

Treatment

An established infection is treated radically. The wound is opened widely, fascial compartments are freely incised and dead tissue is meticulously removed. Devitalized muscle must be excised widely until bleeding viable tissue is encountered. In some cases, amputation is inevitable.

Wounds are loosely packed and left open, to be closed only when they appear healthy. Wide tissue defects may require subsequent tissue reconstruction and skin grafting. Amputation stumps are also left open in the first instance.

The patient is shocked and frightened. Intensive supportive therapy to correct and maintain fluid and electrolyte balance is necessary. Hypovolaemia is common and multiple transfusions may be required. Antibiotic therapy is essential. Penicillin is given in very high dosage together with metronidazole to control anaerobes. Additional antibiotics may be needed to control components of mixed infections that may be encountered. Intensive antibiotic therapy should be started before radical surgery, but not at the expense of losing valuable time.

The use of hyperbaric oxygenation in a pressure chamber has reduced mortality but is not a replacement for adequate surgery and the other measures described above. An increased arterial Pa_{O_2} cannot drive oxygen into dead tissues or eradicate established infection in devitalized tissues. However, it has a favourable effect in critical situations, when it may limit the amount of radical surgery required.

A particular mixed form of clostridial infection follows penetrating injury to the colon or rectum, the source of infecting organisms being the bowel. The mixed infection is likely to include clostridia and bacteroides organisms, anaerobic cocci, faecal streptococci, coliform bacteria and pseudomonas organisms. Wide debridement, free drainage, intensive antibiotic therapy and a proximal colostomy are essential measures.

Progressive bacterial gangrene and necrotizing fasciitis

These form a spectrum of advancing bacterial gangrene which may occur after a seemingly trivial injury or an operation, typically in the lower abdomen or perineum.

Progressive bacterial gangrene (bacterial synergistic gangrene, dermal gangrene, Meleney's gangrene) involves only the skin and advances relatively slowly. A variety of organisms have been incriminated, and synergistic action between a microaerophilic streptococcus and associated organisms is considered important. Predisposing factors include general debility, diabetes and hypoxia.

Necrotizing fasciitis (Fournier's gangrene) affects primarily the subcutaneous fat and deep fascia of the perineum or abdomen. The skin dies as a result of thrombosis of its blood supply. It is a rapidly advancing, frequently fatal disease. The rapidity and extent of tissue destruction are very alarming. The initial cellulitis is associated with the appearance of dusky purple patches in its centre which progress to skin necrosis. There may be crepitus. The patient becomes very ill and develops septic shock.

Treatment. It is important to determine the haemoglobin, blood glucose, blood urea and electrolyte concentration. Shock must be corrected with intravenous infusions. Blood, swabs and excised tissue are sent for culture. Diabetes should be considered and, if present, brought under control.

Intravenous antibiotics are started immediately; a combination of large doses of benzylpenicillin, metronidazole and gentamicin or tobramycin is recommended. These are modified in the light of culture reports as they become available.

As soon as the patient's condition allows it, radical excision of the affected area, including skin, subcutaneous tissue and deep fascia, is performed. The patient returns to theatre daily for inspection and further necessary excision until the infection is under control. The resulting defect in the skin and deep fascia, which frequently is very large, requires skin grafting.

Other anaerobic infections

The Gram-negative non-sporing anaerobic pathogens include bacteroides organisms (*Bacteroides fragilis, Bacteroides melaninogenicus* etc.) and fusobacteria such as *Fusobacterium necrophorum*.

These often occur in association with anaerobic cocci and other facultative organisms in a wide range of mixed putrefactive infections, including cerebral abscess, periodontal disease, ulceromembranous gingivitis and dental abscess, cancrum oris, Ludwig's angina, aspiration pneumonia, lung abscess, infected bite wounds, synergistic gangrene, Fournier's gangrene (necrotizing fasciitis), peritonitis, pelvic abscess, perianal and ischiorectal abscess, balano-posthitis, vaginitis/vaginosis and decubitus ulcers.

The common anaerobic component of many of these infections must be appreciated if the results of treatment are not to be disappointing. In some cases there is alarming pathogenic synergy which overwhelms the patient if effective treatment is delayed.

ANTIMICROBIAL MANAGEMENT OF WOUND INFECTIONS

It is important to know when a wound is being significantly colonized by a potential pathogen. Regular inspection of wounds is essential, and bacteriological assistance should be sought when necessary. The decision to treat a wound infection should be based on clinical judgment and should not be an automatic response to a positive culture report. In some cases, removal of a suture at an inflamed point (minor stitch abscess) may be all that is needed to allow host defences to operate. Similarly, the isolation of coliform bacteria from a mild superficial infection of an abdominal wound need not call for active antimicrobial therapy if the patient's general condition does not indicate any constitutional upset. On the other hand, a positive blood culture obtained from a patient with signs of impending shock, or the isolation of a significant pathogen (e.g. *Streptococcus pyogenes*) from a wound with signs of regional lymphadenitis, calls for immediate and positive antimicrobial treatment.

Inconsistent or incompatible findings must be discussed with senior experts. For example, a report on a secondary plate culture obtained after a specimen of pus has been subjected to enrichment culture in cooked meat broth might yield a profuse, almost pure growth of *Clostridium perfrin-*

gens derived from spores contaminating skin adjacent to the wound. If the wound is giving no clinical cause for alarm and the patient's general condition is satisfactory, a diagnosis of gas gangrene is most unlikely to be justified. Heroic treatment must not be instituted on the basis of such evidence.

Suggestions for specific antibiotic therapy are given in Table 11.4, and initial ('best-guess')

therapy is indicated in Table 11.5. The antibiotic sensitivities of common anaerobic pathogens are outlined in Table 11.6.

PRINCIPLES GOVERNING THE CHOICE AND USE OF ANTIBIOTICS

Antibiotics should be used with care. The clinician should attempt to recognize self-limiting infec-

Table 11.4 Antibiotics in surgery: suggestions for specific therapy 1989

Organism	First choice	Alternatives
Staphylococcus aureus (coagulase-positive staphylococcus)	Flucloxacillin	Erythromycin, cefuroxime, fusidic acid, clindamycin, Augmentin
Coagulase-negative staphylococci including *Staph. albus*	Vancomycin	?Teicoplanin
Streptococcus pneumoniae (the pneumococcus)	Benzylpenicillin	Erythromycin
Streptococcus pyogenes (group A β-haemolytic streptococcus)	Benzylpenicillin	Erythromycin
Streptococcus faecalis (the enterococcus)	Ampicillin (amoxycillin)	Gentamicin with penicillin or ampicillin; trimethoprim
Bacteroides species	Metronidazole	Augmentin, erythromycin, clindamycin
Escherichia coli 1. Sepsis including bacteraemia 2. Urinary tract infection	Gentamicin* or cefuroxime Cefuroxime or trimethoprim	Cefotaxime, ceftazidime Gentamicin*, cefotaxime, ceftazidime, cotrimoxazole, ampicillin
Haemophilus influenzae	Ampicillin (amoxycillin)	Trimethroprim, erythromycin, Augmentin, chloramphenicol (meningitis)
Klebsiella species	Gentamicin* or cefuroxime	Cefotaxime, ceftazidime, ciprofloxacin, imipenem
Proteus species	Gentamicin*	Cefotaxime, ceftazidime
Pseudomonas aeruginosa	Gentamicin*	Azlocillin, ceftazidime, ciprofloxacin
Clostridia	Benzylpenicillin, metronidazole	Erythromycin, clindamycin
Clostridium difficile	Vancomycin (oral)	Metronidazole

* or other aminoglycoside (tobramycin, amikacin, netilmicin).
? = possible

Table 11.5 Initial ('best-guess') therapy for acute infections

Type of infection	Antibiotic
Chest infection	
Probable pathogens:	
Streptococcus pneumoniae (pneumococcus)	Benzylpenicillin
Haemophilus influenzae	Ampicillin (amoxycillin), Augmentin
Staph. aureus	Flucloxacillin
Enterobacteria	Gentamicin*, cefuroxime
Urinary tract infection	
1. Relief of acute, but not dangerous infection	Trimethoprim, ampicillin, Augmentin
2. Emergency treatment of potentially severe pyelonephritis	Gentamicin*, cefuroxime, cefotaxime, ceftazidime
Wound infection	
1. Abdominal and pelvic	Gentamicin* with benzylpenicillin and metronidazole, *or* metronidazole with 2nd or 3rd generation cephalosporin
2. If *Staph. aureus* suspected	Flucloxacillin *or* cefuroxime *or* erythromycin
3. Amputations and ? gas gangrene	Benzylpenicillin, metronidazole
Septicaemia and septic (bacteriogenic) shock	Gentamicin* with benzylpenicillin and metronidazole. Consider ceftazidime, chloramphenicol
Severe pseudomonas infections	Gentamicin* plus azlocillin *or* piperacillin. Ciprofloxacin, ceftazidime

Note: these suggestions are for occasions when immediate treatment is necessary. Therapy must be adjusted as bacteriological investigations proceed.
* or other aminoglycoside (tobramycin, amikacin, netilmicin).

Table 11.6 In-vitro activity of antimicrobial drugs against anaerobic bacteria

Antibiotic	Relative activity* against		
	B. fragilis	Anaerobic cocci	Clostridia
Metronidazole	+ + + +	+ + + +	+ + + +
Penicillin	± (often R)	+ +	+ +
Amoxycillin plus clavulanic acid (Augmentin)	+ + +	+ + +	+ + +
Erythromycin	+	+ +	+ + +
Clindamycin	+ + +	+ + + +	+ +
Chloramphenicol	+ + + +	+ + + +	+ + + +
Tetracycline	+	+	+
Cephradine	+	+ +	+ +
Cefuroxime	+	+ + +	+ +
Cefotaxime	+	+ +	+
Cephamycins	+ + +	+ +	+ + +
Imipenem	+ + +	+ + + +	+ + + +
Gentamicin	R	R	R

* ±, +, + +, + + +, + + + + indicate increasing degrees of activity.
R = resistant.
Data from Dr Brian Watt, Department of Bacteriology, City Hospital, Edinburgh.

sensitivity tests are necessary to guide the clinician in many cases. It is reasonable to initiate therapy on clinical evidence but the drugs selected must be reviewed once the bacteriological report is available. When an antibiotic has been selected, an adequate dose must be given by the recommended route at the correct time intervals. In hospital practice, there is often a disturbing difference between the practical interpretation of '8-hourly' and 'three times a day'.

When an organism acquires resistance to an antibiotic, it has an advantage over others of the same species in the presence of the relevant antibiotic. If the antibiotic is used extensively or carelessly in a ward, resistant organisms may become predominant.

It is important to restrict the use of an antibiotic where possible and to ensure that body fluids from patients receiving antibiotics are disposed of carefully so that residual antibiotic is not irresponsibly distributed into the ward or adjoining rooms, where it may influence the bacterial flora of patients, staff and the environment.

The staphylococcal menace of the last two decades has been largely controlled, but staphylococci with multiple resistance (MRSA) are a threat. Many other bacteria exploit mechanisms

tions while taking account of the potential toxicity and cost of any antibiotic. As antibiotic resistance is increasing, antibiotic abuse carries collective penalties for the individual patient and for the community.

The choice of therapy should be positively determined. Some organisms associated with certain illnesses are almost invariably sensitive to certain antibiotics. For example, the haemolytic streptococcus (*Streptococcus pyogenes*) is always sensitive to benzylpenicillin. On the other hand, hospital staphylococci are frequently resistant to penicillin and a range of other drugs. Antibiotic

of resistance to gain inroads into the patient they invade.

In general, an effort should be made to use a single effective antibacterial agent in the treatment of a particular infection. If a combination of antibiotics is used, the decision should be based on positive evidence that this is rational. In some cases, for example when a patient is seriously ill and a mixed infection is likely (as in acute peritonitis), it may be necessary to give more than one antibiotic to cover a likely combination of pathogens. This blunderbuss strategy should be reserved for such desperate situations and should be rationalized at the earliest opportunity in the light of the patient's progress and available bacteriological guidance.

Antibiotic policy

A policy for the use of antibiotics is desirable. It must be kept under regular review because of continuing changes in the patterns of bacterial resistance to antibiotics. In conjunction with the hospital bacteriologists, the resistance patterns of all pathogens isolated from sputum, urine, bile, pus and blood should be regularly recorded and periodically reviewed, e.g. at 6-monthly intervals. A policy may then be devised which 'rests' those antibiotics to which resistance is developing. Knowledge of resistance permits more appropriate use of antibiotics in circumstances where it is necessary to give 'blind' treatment, for example in life-threatening infections where antibiotics must be prescribed before the results of culture and sensitivity tests are known. The following guidelines should be observed when prescribing antibiotics.

1. Select an antibiotic to which the known or presumed pathogen is likely to be fully sensitive. The spectrum of an antibiotic should be known accurately. A broad spectrum antibiotic is avoided if a suitable narrow spectrum antibiotic is available.

2. Restrict the use of antibiotics to which resistance is developing (or has developed).

3. Antibiotics that are used systemically should not be used topically.

4. Antibiotics should be given in full dose by an appropriate route and at the correct intervals.

5. With only a few rare exceptions (e.g. lung abscesses) antibiotics are not used to treat abscesses without also ensuring that effective surgical drainage is achieved.

6. The side effects of antibiotics should be known and monitored.

7. Expensive antibiotics are not used if equally effective and cheaper alternatives are suitable.

Prophylactic use of antibiotics

The prophylactic use of antibiotics is established in the following situations.

Chronic bronchitis

Patients with chronic bronchitis subject to intermittent exacerbations may be given prophylactic antibiotics before a planned operation. The matter is fiercely debated and opinions are divided. Amoxycillin or cefuroxime are favoured by some workers. The use of epidural anaesthesia has special advantages for these patients. Prophylactic antibiotics are commenced shortly before operation and discontinued soon afterwards.

Tetanus

Patients with tetanus-prone accidental wounds are given prophylaxis as described on page 123, but the wounds must still be treated by meticulous debridement or, if treatment is delayed, by excision.

Gas gangrene

Patients with ischaemic limbs that require major surgery are at considerable risk of developing gas gangrene. Benzylpenicillin is given one hour preoperatively and continued 6-hourly for 3–5 days.

Meningitis

Patients with compound skull fractures and technically compound basal skull fractures involving the paranasal sinuses, the mastoid air cells or the middle ear are at risk of developing meningitis. Ampicillin and flucloxacillin are given for several days. The antibiotic cover for basal fractures is continued until cerebrospinal fluid rhinorrhoea or otorrhoea ceases.

Prevention of endocarditis

Patients with congenital, rheumatic or degenerative valve disease, septal defects, or prosthetic heart valves are at risk of bacterial colonization if bacteraemia occurs. Before any operation that might expose them to such a risk they are given prophylactic antibiotics to cover the following procedures.

For dental treatment under local anaesthesia outside hospital, amoxycillin 3 g orally one hour before the procedure, and a second oral dose of 3 g 6–8 hours after treatment, is recommended. If the patient is allergic to penicillin, erythromycin 1.5 g is given orally 1–2 hours before the procedure and 0.5 g orally 6 hours after treatment.

For dental procedures in hospital under general anaesthesia, amoxycillin 1 g by intramuscular injection just before induction of anaesthesia followed by 0.5 g orally 6 hours later is recommended. Penicillin-allergic patients are given erythromycin lactobionate 1 g intravenously before induction and 0.5 g orally every 6 hours in the following 24 hours. Alternatively, vancomycin 1 g given intravenously over 20 minutes (starting 30 minutes before the procedure) provides equivalent cover to a penicillin-allergic patient.

Patients with prosthetic valves should always be referred to hospital for parenteral prophylaxis to cover dental procedures. Amoxycillin 1 g by intramuscular injection plus intramuscular gentamicin 1.5 mg/kg body weight (if renal function is normal) is given just before induction, and a further dose of amoxycillin 0.5 g is given orally after 6 hours. Penicillin-allergic patients in this category are given vancomycin 1 g intravenously over 20 minutes, starting 30 minutes before the procedure, plus intravenous gentamicin (as above).

For prophylaxis before urinary, gynaecological or colonic procedures, intravenous gentamicin is given as above, and amoxycillin 1 g intravenously 30 minutes before the procedure and twice thereafter at intervals of 8 hours. Erythromycin 0.5 g can be given instead of amoxycillin to a penicillin-allergic patient. Some workers add metronidazole cover for gynaecological or colonic procedures.

Before cardiac surgery, intravenous gentamicin should be given as above, and flucloxacillin 2 g intravenously 30 minutes before operation and 6-hourly thereafter for 48 hours. Some workers prefer cefuroxime to the flucloxacillin-gentamicin combination.

Gastrointestinal and genitourinary surgery

Patients undergoing gastrointestinal and genitourinary surgery, whether elective or emergency, are at risk of wound infection, intra-abdominal infection and septicaemia. Many methods have been advocated in the past decade to reduce this risk. A single large dose of antibiotic appropriate for the predicted bacterial flora, and administered intravenously on induction of anaesthesia is probably the most convenient and effective method. Metronidazole alone or in combination with another antibiotic has a good record of success. In heavily contaminated surgery and in emergency surgery, three additional doses at 8-hourly intervals postoperatively may confer further benefit. Antibiotic lavage of the operative field and the incision is another approach to prophylaxis but this is debated and is not universally practised.

Treatment of compound fractures of limbs

As a compound fracture is almost invariably associated with considerable contamination in an area of severely damaged tissue, it is reasonable to give antibiotic cover at once, and preferably before radical wound toilet and debridement if this does not delay essential surgical attention. Opinions differ on the choice of antibiotics. Staphylococci, coliform organisms and anaerobes are likely infecting organisms, often occurring together and with catastrophic potential. Some surgeons rely on penicillin and metronidazole to control at least two of the likely components. Others would use a second or third generation cephalosporin or clindamycin or erythromycin.

Prosthetic implants

Prophylactic antibiotics are obligatory when any prosthetic material is inserted. Staphylococcal infection is the most serious problem, for example in heart valve replacement, cardiac pacemaker insertion, ventriculovenous shunts, aortic grafts, joint prostheses, mammary prostheses or polypropylene mesh repairs of massive abdominal wall defects. However, other bacteria may also be involved, and broad spectrum cover is usually given immediately preoperatively and 8-hourly postoperatively for 24 hours. It is important to have informed bacteriological advice.

Immunosuppressed patients

Patients with suppressed immune mechanisms, either as a result of disease or as a result of therapy (e.g. transplant patients), should receive antibiotic prophylaxis when undergoing surgery. The choice of antibiotic is dictated by individual circumstances. Expert microbiological help should be sought.

Treatment of immunosuppressed patients

Prompt *empirical antibiotic treatment* of suspected bacterial infections in immunosuppressed patients is advisable. A combination of an aminoglycoside with an antipseudomonal penicillin or cephalosporin is often relied upon to cover the range of likely organisms. In these patients, it is also important to be on guard against yeast and fungal and protozoal infections and to be aware of problems posed by viruses such as herpes simplex virus, varicella zoster virus and cytomegalovirus. If antifungal treatment is needed, it should not be delayed.

CONTROL OF HOSPITAL INFECTION

An effective hospital infection control programme depends above all on teamwork, conscientiousness and communication. The possible spread of infection from patient to patient or from patients to hospital personnel should be constantly considered.

Prompt detection and treatment of infection

Day-to-day monitoring in the wards and related areas is essential to ensure that infections are detected and recorded. A wound infection record should be kept in each unit. Ward surveillance is of particular importance in special areas such as intensive care units, baby units, renal units and areas where neutropenic patients are nursed. There must be assured daily links with the laboratory so that the nature of the infecting organisms is known, early notification of a particularly dangerous pathogen is ensured, and trends in antibiotic resistance are monitored. Close cooperation of the control-of-infection officers and control-of-infection nurses with senior staff in the wards, laboratories and associated administrative offices is essential.

Prevention of transmission of infectious agents

Approaches to the prevention of spread of infection in a hospital range from the provision of suitable isolation and containment facilities for those with special infections or at special risk of infection, to the prompt availability of an expert team to mount an immediate investigation and institute necessary changes when the need arises. Prompt diagnosis and treatment of an infection can contribute substantially to the prevention of transmission. Clear policies on such matters as the recording of infection, the correct use of disinfectants, safe disposal of infected material, sterilization of instruments, management of patients who have infections associated with special risks, proper use of antibiotics, and the use of immunizing agents are important in the protection of hospital staff and their patients against cross-infection.

12. Wounds and wound healing

A wound is a disruption of the normal continuity of body structures caused by physical injury. The wound may be *penetrating* (i.e. disrupt the surface epithelium) or *non-penetrating* (the integument remains intact while the force is transmitted to subcutaneous tissues or viscera). In both types of injury, inspection of the body surface may give little indication of the extent of damage to underlying structures.

Wounds may be classified according to the mode of damage.

1. An *incised wound* is caused by a sharp instrument; if there is associated tissue tearing, the wound is said to be *lacerated*.

2. An *abrasion* results from friction damage to the body surface, and is characterized by superficial bruising and loss of varying thickness of skin and underlying tissues.

3. *Crush injuries* are due to severe pressure. The skin may not be breached even if massive tissue destruction is present. Oedema, characteristic of this type of injury, can make wound closure impossible and, by increasing pressure within fascial compartments, may cause ischaemic necrosis of muscle and other structures.

4. *Degloving injury* occurs as a result of shearing forces which cause parallel tissue planes to move against each other (e.g. when a hand is caught between rollers or in moving machinery). Large areas of apparently intact skin may be deprived of their blood supply from rupture of feeding vessels.

5. *Gunshot wounds* may be from shotgun pellets or bullets. Bullets fired from high-velocity rifles cause massive tissue destruction.

6. *Burns* are caused by heat, cold, electricity, irradiation or chemicals. They form a distinct variety of wound requiring special consideration (see Ch. 13).

PRINCIPLES OF WOUND HEALING

The essential features of the healing process are common to wounds of almost all soft tissues, and result in the formation of a scar. Epithelium, bone and nerve heal in distinct ways (see below). Soft tissue healing can be subdivided into three phases according to the development of tensile strength (Fig. 12.1).

Soft tissue healing

Lag phase

The lag phase is the delay of 2–3 days which occurs before fibroblasts begin to manufacture collagen to support the wound. It is characterized by the inflammatory response to injury. Capillary

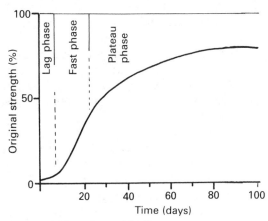

Fig. 12.1 Phases of wound healing

permeability increases and a protein-rich exudate (from which collagen is later synthesized) accumulates in the wound. Inflammatory cells migrate into the area (polymorph neutrophil leucocytes appear early but most are quickly lysed), dead tissue is removed by macrophages (which also trigger fibroblast production) and capillaries at the wound edges begin to proliferate.

Incremental phase

During the incremental, or proliferative, phase there is progressive collagen synthesis by fibroblasts and an increase in tensile strength. Fibroblasts arise from perivascular connective tissue and migrate into the wound along fibrin strands. High lactate levels resulting from ischaemia provide a local stimulus for their invasion of the wound. The increased turnover of collagen in remote areas suggests that there may also be a systemic stimulus. The synthesis of collagen increases over a period of about 3 weeks during which the gain in tensile strength accelerates. Old collagen undergoes lysis while new collagen is laid down. The tensile strength of the healing wound is determined by the balance between these two processes.

Proline and lysine are essential for collagen formation. They are hydroxylated by oxygen and ascorbic acid and incorporated into tropocollagen, which polymerizes to form collagen fibrils.

Collagen synthesis demands a continuing supply of energy. This is provided by the ingrowth of capillary buds to form fragile capillary arches which bring oxygen and nutrients to the wound. In unapposed wounds new capillary formation is a major feature, the resulting mixture of capillaries, fibroblasts, macrophages and leucocytes forming *granulation tissue*. To the naked eye, healthy granulation tissue is red, granular and friable, and bleeds when touched.

Fibroblasts have other important functions besides collagen manufacture. They synthesize *mucopolysaccharide* ground substance, which forms an ideal environment for alignment and approximation of the tropocollagen monomers prior to polymerization. Some fibroblasts (known as myofibroblasts) contain myofibrils which pull in the wound margins. This *wound contraction*

reduces the size of the defect in unapposed wounds, and must be distinguished from *contracture*, which can be the unfortunate result of healing of a wound which crosses a joint and is associated with shortage of skin. The resultant scar restricts mobility.

The gain in tensile strength in the first 10 days after wounding is usually sufficient to allow removal of skin sutures without wound disruption, but this depends on the site, local stresses, and the physical condition and age of the patient.

Plateau or maturation phase

After 3 weeks there is a levelling-off in the gain in tensile strength as the rate of collagen breakdown first approaches and then surpasses its synthesis. This is the final clearing-up process during which excess collagen is removed and the number of fibroblasts and inflammatory cells declines. Orientation of collagen fibres in the direction of local mechanical forces increases tensile strenth for some 6 months, but this never returns to normal. Thus skin and fascia usually recover only 80% of their original tensile strength.

Healing of specialized tissues

Epithelium

Epithelium heals by *regeneration* and not by the formation of scar tissue. Epithelial cells at the edge of the wound lose their adhesion to each other and migrate across the wound until they meet cells from the other side. As they migrate, they are replaced by new cells formed by division of basal cells near the wound edge. The cells that have migrated also undergo mitosis and the new epithelium thickens, eventually forming a normal epithelial cover over the scar produced by the healing dermis. Wounds may heal by *first intention* if the edges are closely approximated, for example by accurate suturing. In these circumstances epithelial cover is quickly achieved and healing of the apposed dermis and underlying tissues produces a fine scar (Fig. 12.2).

If the wound edges are not in apposition, the defect gradually fills with granulation tissue and restoration of epidermal continuity takes time.

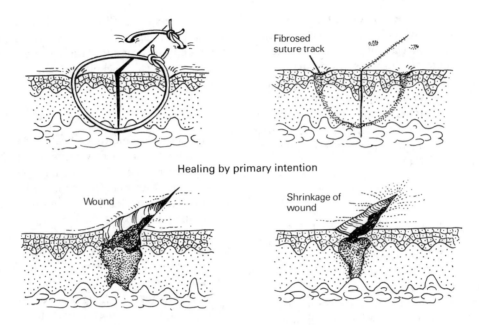

Healing by primary intention

Healing by secondary intention

Fig. 12.2 Wound healing by primary and secondary intention

Continued basal cell division at the wound edges produces sheets of cells which migrate across the denuded area, but their advance is often hindered by infection. This process is known as healing by *second intention* and usually results in delayed healing, excessive fibrosis and an ugly scar.

If a wound has begun to heal by second intention, it may be possible to speed healing by freshening the wound edges and bringing them together or by covering the defect with a skin graft.

Bone

Torn blood vessels produce a haematoma between the fractured bone ends. An inflammatory response similar to that in other tissues leads to an ingress of fibroblasts, collagen formation and the deposition of new bone. If any movement is allowed between the bone ends, a *callus* is formed. This is new bone produced by subperiosteal and intramedullary osteogenic cells. Some cartilage may be formed in relatively ischaemic areas. The callus, at first spongy, gradually shrinks as the new bone between the fractured ends becomes compact and bony union occurs. Strength returns gradually and, as with soft tissue injuries, increases slowly over many months. Extensive remodelling finally obliterates the fracture site.

If the bone ends are rigidly fixed together (e.g. by a compression plate), healing takes place without callus formation. The bone regains a normal appearance more quickly but takes longer to achieve normal strength.

Nerve tissue

Wounds of the nervous system involve both neural and connective tissue. Neural tissue in the central nervous system cannot regenerate. Fibroblasts derived from glial or perivascular cells replace nervous tissue with collagen.

In peripheral nerves, cut axons degenerate distal to the injury but, provided the body of the neural cell survives, the axons of the proximal stump sprout and cross the gap to enter empty Schwann sheaths. Fibroblasts help by forming a connective bridge but this may prove self-defeating if it results in a dense collagen scar. Not all of the axons find their way into Schwann sheaths. Some may end blindly in the surrounding tissue and form a 'neuroma', which can be very painful. Others may find their way into the 'wrong' sheath tube. For example, a sensory neurone may enter a sheath leading to a motor end plate. Nevertheless, useful reinnervation is possible provided the nerve ends are accurately approximated with fine sutures to prevent excessive scarring. Regenerating axons can grow as much as 4–5 mm a day, but the average rate is 1–1.5 mm a day.

Intestine

Damage confined to gut mucosa (as in a gastric erosion) is repaired by re-epithelialization, which leaves no scar. When ulceration extends through the submucosa to involve underlying muscle, a permanent fibrous scar is inevitable.

The stomach and small bowel have a plentiful blood supply and contain relatively small numbers of pathogenic bacteria. Leakage is uncommon following resection and anastomosis, and after one week the anastomosis is usually able to withstand disruptive forces as well as adjoining bowel.

The oesophagus has a weaker wall than stomach and proximal intestine, and a poorer blood supply. The distal colon also has a poor blood supply, while problems of healing are increased by large numbers of pathogenic bacteria in its lumen. Bacteria delay collagen synthesis, and collagenase production can cause excessive lysis. Anastomotic disruption, if it occurs, is usually recognized clinically by the 4th–6th postoperative day.

Surgical technique is of fundamental importance in reducing the incidence of anastomotic leakage and wound infection after gastrointestinal surgery. The connective tissue of the submucosa is the strongest layer of the bowel wall and sutures or staples in this layer maintain apposition until sufficient tensile strength has been regained. In view of the dangers of anastomotic leakage, drains may be left at the site of anastomosis to allow infected material to escape should disruption occur.

FACTORS INFLUENCING WOUND HEALING

Many of these factors are interrelated, e.g. the site of the wound, its blood supply and the level of tissue oxygenation. While some are invariable (e.g. the patient's age), others can be modified or eliminated to promote healing (e.g. nutritional status, surgical technique and intercurrent disease).

Blood supply

Wounds of ischaemic tissue heal slowly, are prone to infection and frequently break down. When this occurs, the ischaemic wound may not be able to sustain the metabolic demand for healing by second intention. Partial pressure of oxygen in arterial blood (Pao_2) is the important determinant of the rate of collagen synthesis. Anaemia per se does not impair healing if the patient has a normal blood volume and arterial oxygen tension.

Crude surgical technique, such as crushing tissue with forceps, dragging wound edges together under tension or tying sutures too tightly, can render well-vascularized tissue ischaemic and lead to wound breakdown.

Infection

Both general and local factors may be responsible for infection of a surgical wound.

General factors. The risk of wound infection is increased in the elderly, in patients with cardiovascular, respiratory and nutritional disorders, and in the presence of intercurrent infection.

Local wound factors. The most important of these is bacterial contamination. This can be minimized by careful skin preparation and meticulous aseptic technique. The type of operation obviously affects the degree of likely contamination. Operative wounds are classified as clean, clean-contaminated or dirty (see below).

Despite every precaution, some bacteria will gain access to the wound during operation. They may enter from the surrounding atmosphere, from internal foci of sepsis, or from the lumen of transected organs. In some cases, contamination occurs in the postoperative period. Provided contamination is not gross and local blood supply is good, the natural defences are usually able to deal with incoming bacteria and prevent overt infection. Devitalized tissues, haematoma, and the presence of foreign material (e.g. sutures and prosthetic materials) favour bacterial survival and growth.

Common infecting organisms are staphylococci, streptococci, coliforms and anaerobes. The latter grow in ischaemic tissue.

Overcrowding of surgical wards and excessive use of operating theatres increase the bacterial population of the atmosphere and thus the risk of wound infection (see Ch. 8 and Ch. 11).

The role of prophylaxis. When wound contamination is anticipated, topical antibacterial chemicals or topical and systemic antibiotics can be used for prophylaxis. For example, lavage of the wound with the antibacterial agent providone-iodine reduces the incidence of wound infection after appendicitis. Antibiotics are used widely to prevent infection during elective colon surgery (the current emphasis is on short courses of therapy to cover the period of operation). However, apart from tetanus prophylaxis, antibiotics are not normally necessary for acute traumatic wounds, provided prompt and thorough surgical treatment is undertaken.

Age

Wounds in the elderly may heal poorly because of impaired blood supply, poor nutritional status or intercurrent disease.

Site of wound

Surgical incisions placed in the lines of least tissue tension are subject to minimal distraction and should heal promptly, leaving a fine scar. In the face, these lines run at right angles to the direction of underlying muscles and form the lines of facial expression.

Wounds of the head and neck heal quickly so that sutures or skin clips can usually be removed within 3–5 days. Wounds of the leg and foot heal slowly and sutures may have to be retained for 14 days. These differences reflect the importance of blood supply — warm vascular areas generally heal more quickly than cool extremities.

Nutritional status

When competing for body resources, a wound has high priority over unwounded tissue. Malnutrition

has to be severe before healing is affected (see below). Protein availability is most important, and wound dehiscence and infection are common when the serum albumin is low. Healing problems should be anticipated if recent weight loss exceeds 20%.

Ascorbic acid is essential for proline hydroxylation and collagen synthesis. The number of fibroblasts is not reduced in scorbutic states. Zinc is a component of enzymes involved in healing and zinc deficiency retards healing. Supplements of ascorbic acid and zinc are effective in patients with known deficiencies, but do not improve healing in normal subjects.

Intercurrent disease

Healing may be affected by the disease itself or by its treatment. *Cachectic patients* with severe malnutrition (as seen in advanced cancer) have marked impairment of healing.

Diabetes mellitus impairs healing by reducing tissue resistance to infection and causing peripheral vascular insufficiency. Peripheral neuropathy with diminished peripheral sensation may add to the problem by allowing trauma to the healing wound.

Haemorrhagic diatheses increase the risk of haematoma formation and wound infection.

Obstructive airway disease lowers arterial Po_2 and so affects healing. Abdominal wound dehiscence is commoner in patients with respiratory disease because of the strain on the wound during coughing.

Corticosteroid therapy reduces the inflammatory response, impairs collagen synthesis and decreases resistance to infection. The effect of steroids on wound healing is most marked if they are given within 3 days of injury.

Immunosuppressive therapy impairs healing by reducing resistance to infection. Such patients are already compromised by their underlying disorder.

Radiotherapy greatly reduces the vascularity of the tissues, and healing of wounds in irradiated areas is often impaired.

Surgical technique

Skin incisions are placed where possible in the line of least tissue tension. Meticulous aseptic technique is essential to avoid wound infection and poor healing. Gentle tissue handling is mandatory. Crushing with tissue forceps, failure to achieve haemostasis, excessive use of diathermy and crude ligatures all contribute to wound devitalization.

Potentially infective sites (e.g. the gut lumen during colon surgery) should be isolated from the wound by additional sterile drapes, and spillage of contents avoided by correct use of occlusion clamps. Particular care must be taken in areas where there is reduced resistance to infection (e.g. bones and joints), where prosthetic implants are being inserted, or where infection would have particularly serious consequences (e.g. neurosurgery).

Accurate apposition of wound edges favours healing by first intention. Dead spaces in the depth of the wound are avoided, as bleeding and accumulation of exudate encourage infection. Correct suturing of the deeper layers often allows the skin edges to fall together without tension so that skin apposition can be achieved by superficial sutures or adhesive tape. Any potential dead space should be obliterated by deep sutures. If this is not possible, the space must be drained. Drains should also be used in contaminated wounds and those where a great deal of exudate is expected. They may be connected to a suction apparatus or allowed to drain by gravity.

Choice of suture and suture materials. The choice of suture materials is important. Foreign material in the tissues predisposes to infection. The finest sutures that will hold the wound edges together should be used. A wound must never be closed under tension.

Wounds are often subjected to stress postoperatively and while 5/0 or 6/0 sutures are appropriate for the face, stronger sutures (3/0 or 4/0) are needed for incisions near joints and still stronger ones for the abdominal wall. The suture should be strong enough to support the wound until tensile strength has recovered sufficiently to prevent breakdown. Absorbable materials are preferred for buried layers, but non-absorbable sutures may be needed in some situations, e.g. in the aponeurotic layer of an abdominal paramedian wound. Non-absorbable sutures should be inert, retain strength, and preferably be monofilamentous, without interstices which might favour bacterial growth.

Suture materials are designed to pass through the tissues with as little trauma as possible. To this end, sutures are no longer threaded through a wide needle eye but are usually bonded to the needle without any increase in bulk (atraumatic suture). The needle may be round-bodied or triangular on cross-section. The round-bodied needle is used when tissue resistance is low (e.g. for intestinal suture), while a triangular needle is preferred when sharp cutting edges are needed to facilitate passage through tough tissues such as skin and aponeurosis.

To avoid wound devitalization, sutures should not be placed too close together or too near the wound margin, nor should they be tied too tightly. When there is an increased risk of abdominal wound dehiscence, closure used to be reinforced with 'deep tension sutures' which pass through all layers of the abdominal wall except the peritoneum. These sutures were of strong (gauge 1) non-absorbable material and were threaded through a length of plastic tubing to avoid cutting into the abdominal wall. However, many surgeons now prefer a mass closure technique in which non-absorbable sutures are placed through all layers of the abdominal wall except skin. Others use a continuous suture of monofilament non-absorbable material to reapproximate the anterior rectus sheath.

PROBLEMS IN WOUND MANAGEMENT

Postoperative wound infection

Surgical procedures can be classified according to the likelihood of contamination and wound infection.

Clean procedures are those in which wound contamination is not expected and should not occur. An incision for a clean elective procedure should not become infected provided no infective focus is encountered and no viscus is entered which might contain pathogenic bacteria (e.g. colon). Subtotal thyroidectomy, parietal cell vagotomy and meniscectomy are examples of clean operations in which the wound infection rate should be less than 1%.

Clean-contaminated procedures are those in which no frank focus of infection is encountered but where a significant risk of infection is nevertheless present. Cholecystectomy, subtotal gastrectomy and prostatectomy are examples of operations in which wound infection occurs occasionally. Infection rates in excess of 5% denote breakdown in ward and operating theatre routine.

Contaminated or 'dirty' wounds are those in which gross contamination is inevitable and the risk of troublesome wound infection is high. Emergency surgery for perforated diverticular disease and drainage of a subphrenic abscess are examples of procedures in this category.

Clinical features

Postoperative wound infection usually becomes evident 3–4 days after surgery. Commonly the first signs are superficial cellulitis around the wound margins or swelling of the wound with some serous discharge from between the sutures. Fluctuation is occasionally elicited when there is an abscess or liquifying haematoma, and crepitus may be present if gas-forming organisms are involved. In some cases of deep infection there are no local signs although the patient may have pyrexia and increased wound tenderness. Systemic upset is variable, usually amounting to only moderate pyrexia and leucocytosis. Toxaemia, bacteraemia and septicaemia can complicate serious wound infection.

The differential diagnosis includes other causes of postoperative pyrexia, wound haematoma and wound dehiscence. Wound haematoma may result from reactive bleeding during the first 24–48 hours after operation. It causes swelling and discomfort but only minimal pyrexia and few systemic signs. As a haematoma is liable to become infected, it should be evacuated. Wound dehiscence is considered separately later in this chapter.

Prevention

The risk of wound infection is reduced by careful preparation of the patient, prophylactic use of antibiotics in high-risk patients and meticulous attention to good operative theatre techniques. To avoid cross-contamination, wounds should be dressed postoperatively in a separate treatment or dressing room and not in the general ward.

Severely contaminated wounds are sometimes best closed by *delayed primary suture*. For example, after emergency operation for perforated appendicitis or resection of gangrenous bowel in a strangulated hernia, the peritoneum and aponeurotic layer may be closed but the skin and subcutaneous tissues left open. Skin sutures may be inserted at this time but are not tied for several days, until it is clear that infection has been avoided.

Antibiotic therapy is essential for grossly contaminated wounds, the aim being to achieve high tissue concentrations as soon as possible. The choice of antibiotics is determined by the nature of the infection.

Antibiotics which achieve excellent concentrations in the wound include crystalline penicillin, flucloxacillin, ampicillin and cephalosporins. Gentamicin, carbenicillin and oxacillin achieve only modest concentrations and are used only when indicated by tests for bacterial sensitivity.

Following emergency surgery for faecal peritonitis, a combination of penicillin and either gentamicin or lincomycin was commonly used to reduce the dangers of peritonitis, wound infection and septicaemia. For the destruction of anaerobes, metronidazole (e.g. Flagyl) is now added routinely. Topical agents such as povidone-iodine may also be used to combat infection in contaminated wounds.

Although antibiotic treatment is a valuable and important part of management of the contaminated wound, it is no substitute for careful surgical management. Radical excision of the wound margins, thorough mechanical cleansing and delayed suture are the true foundations of success.

Treatment

Trivial superficial cellulitis can be managed expectantly. The area of redness is 'mapped out' with an indelible pen so that its extent can be monitored. Spreading cellulitis is an indication for antibiotic therapy.

Deeper and more serious infections can often be aborted by the removal of one or more skin sutures to allow free drainage of infected material from the suture track or wound. Failure to provide free drainage promotes infection in the hypoxic closed space and can lead to abscess formation. If removal of skin sutures does not result in free discharge of infected material, the wound should be probed gently with sinus forceps under aseptic conditions.

If pus is believed to be present but adequate drainage has not been provided, the patient should be returned to theatre for a full exploration of the wound under general anaesthesia. Following evacuation of pus and debris the wound is left open or packed lightly to prevent premature closure of the skin edges. Otherwise infection may persist in the depths of the wound.

Many infected wounds heal rapidly without further surgery, particularly if the original skin incision is placed in the line of least tissue tension. The problem is often to keep the wound open rather than to achieve closure. If it appears that spontaneous wound closure will take a long time, *secondary suture* or skin grafting can be considered to speed healing, but only once it is clear that infection has been eradicated. The presence of clean healthy granulation tissue in the wound is usually a good indication that closure can be undertaken.

In all infected wounds a wound swab or specimen of pus is sent routinely for bacteriological culture and sensitivity determination. Although antibiotics are not usually required when the infection is limited and free drainage has been established, they are indicated when there is spreading cellulitis, severe deep infection or persistent pyrexia. It is therefore important to know the sensitivity of the causative organism. In urgent cases a Gram-stain of a smear of material from the wound will give guidance as to the initial choice of antibiotic. If in doubt, a combination of a penicillin, a cephalosporin and metronidazole is reasonable.

Abdominal wound dehiscence

Most general surgical units have an overall incidence of abdominal wound dehiscence of about 1%. Wound dehiscence is particularly troublesome in obese patients, and in those with chest complications, abdominal distension due to ileus or ascites, or a debilitating disease such as cancer. The risk can be minimized by careful preoperative preparation, including chest care and cessation of smoking for at least 2 weeks before surgery, and by prompt treatment of any postoperative respiratory tract infection.

Signs of dehiscence are frequently delayed for 7–10 days after surgery. A profuse serosanguineous discharge of peritoneal fluid from the wound is often the first clinical sign and indicates dehiscence unless proved otherwise. The patient may be unaware that dehiscence has occurred, or may have felt 'something go' after a bout of coughing or sudden exertion. Although the surface of the wound may appear intact, disruption of the deeper layers can be demonstrated by contraction of the abdominal wall. This is best done by asking the patient to cough or to lift his head or straight legs from the bed. In some cases, protrusion of bowel or omentum through the wound makes it clear that dehiscence has occurred.

Immediate operative repair is mandatory when dehiscence is complete. Partial dehiscence of the deep layers can be treated conservatively, but only if operation is contraindicated by the patient's general condition. The patient is provided with an elastic or adjustable abdominal support which can be tightened by him during coughing or exertion. With careful management, the wound may then heal but an incisional hernia is inevitable and may require subsequent repair.

Surgical repair is carried out under general anaesthesia using 'through-and-through' sutures which pass through all layers of the abdominal wall.

Traumatic wounds

The state of immunity against tetanus is assessed and appropriate action taken (see Ch. 11). The wound is inspected carefully under good illumination to determine whether it is contaminated, and to assess the extent of devitalization and injury to vital structures. It is important to appreciate that a small, apparently innocent wound may conceal extensive damage to deeper structures. Body cavities may have been penetrated, or tendons, nerves and blood vessels divided.

Damage to muscle, tendon or nerve is assessed by checking relevant motor and sensory function. If the injury involves a limb, the distal circulation is checked. Where appropriate, X-rays will help to establish whether peritoneal, pericardial or pleural cavities have been entered. A decision is made whether the wound can be dealt with under local (or regional) anaesthesia in the casualty department or whether there is any possibility of damage to deep structures requiring more extensive exploration under general anaesthesia in an operating theatre. Provided there is no obvious deep damage, small, relatively uncontaminated wounds should be treated under local anaesthesia on an outpatient basis. The wound margins are cleaned with a mild antiseptic such as cetrimide and the wound is irrigated copiously. Any devitalized tissue is removed, deep tissues are sutured with absorbable material and the skin margins are closed.

More extensive or severely contaminated wounds usually require inpatient treatment with exploration and debridement under general anaesthesia. The wound and its margins are cleansed, and pieces of grit, soil and other obvious foreign material are picked out. All devitalized tissue is trimmed back until bleeding occurs. This process is known as debridement. In areas of poor vascularity such as the leg, or if there is severe contamination, crushing or a fracture, the wound margins are formally excised (Fig. 12.3). Bleeding from the wound margin is not a certain indication of its ultimate survival, as impaired venous drainage can lead to progressive necrosis, particularly after a crushing or degloving injury (see p. 142). If there is any doubt, the wound should not be sutured and a 'second-look' dressing applied under anaesthesia after 48 hours.

Primary closure should also be avoided if there is significant delay in treating a grossly contaminated wound (i.e. more than 6 hours without antibiotic cover). If this is attempted, wound infection and breakdown are likely and there is a risk of anaerobic infection which may threaten both life and limb. It is also too late for formal excision, as bacteria will have penetrated the tissues, but foreign bodies and dead tissue should be removed in the usual way. The wound is dressed and antibiotics are started. The dressing is changed daily, and if the wound is clean in 2 or 3 days *delayed primary suture* may be carried out. If

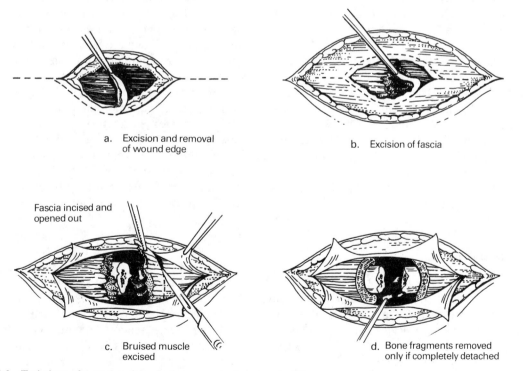

a. Excision and removal of wound edge

b. Excision of fascia

Fascia incised and opened out

c. Bruised muscle excised

d. Bone fragments removed only if completely detached

Fig. 12.3 Technique of wound excision in the presence of a compound fracture

closure is delayed until granulation tissue has formed, this is usually excised and *secondary suture* performed. If this is not possible, split skin grafts (see below) can be applied over the granulations.

Provided that surgical treatment is carried out early, prophylactic antibiotics (often used for tetanus) are not required except for deeply penetrating wounds such as dog bites or those caused by nails where adequate debridement may be impossible. However, the early use of antibiotics in situations where delay in surgical treatment is anticipated may allow primary suture of wounds after 8–12 hours, an interval that is normally considered safe.

Devitalized skin flaps

A common emergency problem is posed by the patient, usually an elderly female, who falls and raises a triangular flap over the surface of the tibia. In many cases the flap is blue-black in colour and obviously non-viable; in most, viability is uncertain. Similar injuries can occur elsewhere in the body.

The wound must be cleansed and all non-viable tissue excised. No attempt should be made to suture the flap back into place. Because of the post-traumatic oedema this would only be possible under tension and lead to death of the flap. If the defect is small, it can be treated conservatively on an outpatient basis. The wound is dressed, an elastic supporting bandage is applied to the leg and the patient is kept ambulant. The wound will normally take several weeks to heal. Alternatively, and this is essential if the defect is large, a split skin graft can be applied either immediately or as a delayed primary procedure. The patient must be kept in bed with the leg horizontal until the graft has taken.

Wounds with skin loss

The aim of wound care is to obtain skin cover and healing as soon as is safely possible, either by primary or by delayed primary closure. If skin has been lost as a direct result of trauma, or following excision of a tumour or necrotic tissue, direct suture will not be possible. If the skin defect is small and at a functionally or aesthetically unimportant site, it may be allowed to heal by secondary intention, but it is often better to speed healing by importing skin to close the wound. This may be by means of a *skin graft* (which requires a vascular bed as it has no blood supply of its own) or a *flap*.

Skin grafts

These may be *split skin* or *full thickness*. Split skin grafts are cut with a special, guarded freehand knife or an electric dermatome, leaving behind the deeper layers of the epidermis. The donor site heals by re-epithelialization aided by cells from the dermis (the bases of hair follicles and sweat ducts) within 2–3 weeks, so that large sheets of skin can be taken. To cover very large areas the graft can be expanded by 'meshing'. The thinner the graft, the more easily it will take on a bed of imperfect vascularity, but the poorer the quality of skin the more it will shrink. Split skin grafts are used to cover wounds after acute trauma, granulating areas and burns, or when the defect is large.

A full thickness graft leaves a donor defect (which needs to be sutured or grafted) as large as the one to be filled and requires a well-vascularized bed to survive. However, such grafts are strong, do not shrink and look better than a split skin graft. They are rarely needed after acute trauma but are commonly used in reconstructive surgery to close small defects where strength is needed (e.g. on the palm of the hand) or a good cosmetic result is important (e.g. on the lower eyelid). An area where there is skin to spare is chosen for the donor site (e.g. the groin for the former and the area behind the ear for the latter).

Other tissues such as bone, cartilage, nerve and tendon can be grafted to restore function and correct deformity after tissue damage or loss.

Flaps

While grafts require a vascular bed to survive, flaps bring their own blood supply to the new site. They can therefore be thicker and stronger than grafts and can be applied to avascular areas such as exposed bone, tendon or joints. They are used in acute trauma only if closure is not possible by direct suture or skin grafting, and are more usually reserved for the reconstruction of surgical defects

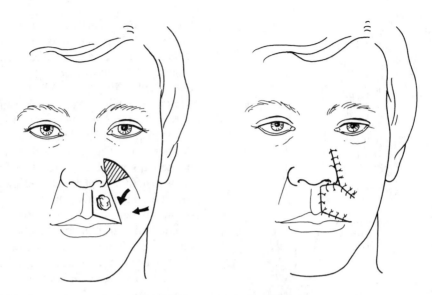

Fig. 12.4   Local skin flap used to repair the defect left after excision of a facial tumour

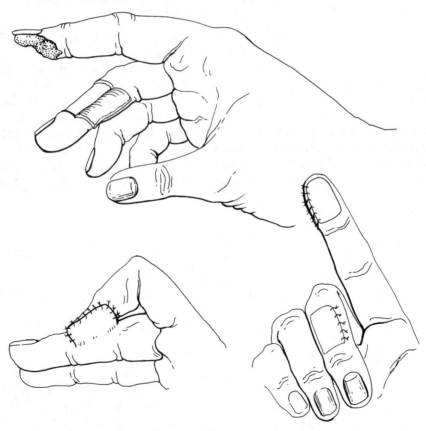

Fig. 12.5   Example of a pedicled skin flap used to cover a defect on the tip of the index finger. Once a blood supply is established, the pedicle is divided

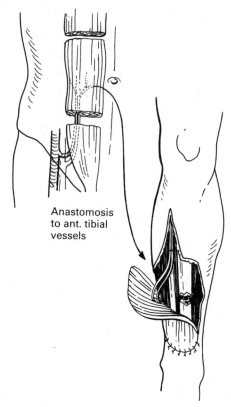

Anastomosis
to ant. tibial
vessels

Fig. 12.6   Example of free tissue transfer based on inferior epigastric vessels.

and for secondary reconstruction after trauma.

The simplest flaps use local skin and fat and are often a good alternative to skin grafting for small defects such as those left after excision of facial tumours (Fig. 12.4). If enough local tissue is not available, a flap may have to be brought from a distance and remain attached temporarily to its original blood supply until it has picked up a new one locally (Fig. 12.5). This usually takes 2–3 weeks, after which the pedicle can be divided.

Advances in our knowledge of the blood supply to the skin and underlying muscles have led to the development of many large skin, muscle and composite flaps which have revolutionized plastic and reconstructive surgery. One example is the use of the latissimus dorsi musculocutaneous flap for reconstruction of the breast (see Fig. 17.20).

The ability to join small blood vessels under the operating microscope now allows the surgeon to close defects in a single stage, even when there is no local tissue available, by *free tissue transfer* (Fig. 12.6).

Crushing and degloving injuries, gunshot wounds

Wounds of this type should never be closed primarily, as tissue destruction is always much greater than appears at first. After thorough irrigation and removal of any obviously dead tissue and foreign material such wounds should be lightly packed and dressed. Dressings are removed 48 hours later under anaesthesia and further excision is carried out if necessary. The wound is closed by suture, skin grafting or flap cover once it is clear that all dead tissue has been removed.

13. Burns

As burns affect principally the skin, a knowledge of the structure and function of skin is central to an understanding of burn injury.

STRUCTURE AND FUNCTIONS OF SKIN

Skin consists of epidermis and dermis. The epidermis is a layer of keratinized, stratified squamous epithelium (see Fig. 18.1). The hair follicles, sweat glands and sebaceous glands are epithelial appendages within the dermis. Due to their deep location, the appendages escape destruction in partial thickness burns, and are a source of new cells for reconstitution of the epidermis.

The skin area is approximately 0.25 m^2 at birth, and is 1.5–1.9 m^2 in adults. Skin accounts for some 15% of lean body mass and is one of the largest organs of the body. It prevents excessive water loss, helps control body temperature and provides a barrier against infection.

For further details of skin anatomy see Chapter 18.

TYPES OF BURN

Burn injuries cover a wide spectrum of severity. Severe burns pose a major threat to life, involve a long stay in hospital, and carry a risk of permanent disfigurement or impairment of function. The majority of burns follow accidents in the home and could be prevented by basic safety precautions.

Injurious agents

Burns may be caused by flames, hot solids, hot liquids or steam, or by physicochemical agencies such as irradiation, electricity or chemicals. Toddlers are particularly liable to scalding by hot liquids in kitchen accidents, and unguarded fires are a threat to all children. Severe disfigurement of the face and neck can result from clothing catching fire, although the incidence of this type of injury has been reduced by use of less flammable clothing materials. Burns sustained in house fires are often accompanied by smoke inhalation with injury to the lungs. Impaired mobility, poor coordination and diminished awareness of pain increase the incidence of burns in the elderly and infirm. Alcohol is a very common contributing factor.

Sunburn is the commonest irradiation injury but is rarely a major problem. Industrial accidents account for most physicochemical burns, although accidental or deliberate ingestion of caustic or corrosive chemicals is still an occasional cause of domestic burn injury. The extent of injury caused by high-tension electrical cables is easily underestimated, as surface damage may be small despite extensive deep injury.

THE EFFECTS OF BURN INJURY

Local effects

The local effects result from destruction of the more superficial tissues and an inflammatory response of those lying more deeply. Destruction of the epidermis allows loss of fluid from the surface, the magnitude of which depends on the extent of injury; this fluid is often trapped in blisters. Instead of the normal insensible loss of 15 ml/m^2 body surface per hour, as much as 200 ml/m^2 per hour may be lost during the first few hours. Loss of the epidermis also removes the barrier to bacterial invasion and opens the door to infection.

In its least severe form, the dermal inflammatory response consists of capillary dilatation, as in the erythema of sunburn. Following more severe burns, the damaged capillaries become permeable to protein, and an exudate forms with an electrolyte/protein content only slightly less than that of plasma. Lymphatic drainage fails to keep pace with the rate of exudation and interstitial oedema results, leading to a reduction in circulating fluid volume. An increase of 2 cm in the diameter of a lower limb represents accumulation of over 2 litres of interstitial fluid. Exudation is maximal in the first 12 hours, capillary permeability returning to normal within 48 hours. With more severe injury, the epidermis and dermis are converted into a coagulum of dead tissue termed *eschar*. Contamination of the burn surface may occur at any time and wound care should commence at the time the patient is first seen. Sepsis delays healing, increases the patient's energy (caloric) needs, and in a large burn, forms a new threat to life just when the dangers of hypovolaemia have been overcome.

General effects

The general effects of a burn depend on its size. A large burn leads to hypovolaemia, water and salt loss, and increased catabolism. Circulating plasma volume falls as oedema accumulates and fluid leaks from the burned surface. In large burns the effect is compounded by a generalized increase in capillary permeability as oedema becomes widespread. Some red cells are destroyed by a full thickness burn, and many more are damaged but not destroyed immediately. However, red cell losses are small in comparison to plasma loss in the early period, and haemoconcentration is reflected in a rising haematocrit (packed cell volume). Hypovolaemic shock ensues if plasma volume is not restored. The effects of the shifts in water and electrolytes are ultimately shared by all body tissues.

Following a large burn there is an increase in the metabolic rate partly explained by excessive water loss from the burned surface which causes expenditure of calories through heat of evaporation. In severe burns some 7000 kcal may be expended daily and weight loss of 0.5 kg/day is not unusual unless steps are taken to prevent it.

CLASSIFICATION OF BURNS

Burns are classified according to their depth as partial or full thickness skin loss (Fig. 13.1). In a partial thickness burn, epithelial cells survive to restore the epidermis. Full thickness burns destroy all the epithelial elements.

Partial thickness burns

The most superficial injuries involve only the epidermis. Pain and swelling subside within 48 hours and the superficial epidermis peels off within a few days. New epidermal cover is provided from undamaged cells of the basal germinal layer and the final cosmetic result is perfect.

In more severe injury, the epidermis and superficial dermis are destroyed. Restoration of the epidermis then depends on intact epithelial cells within the appendages. Pain, swelling and fluid loss are marked. Partial thickness burns can be subdivided according to their severity. *Superficial partial thickness* burns heal in less than 3 weeks and do not leave scars. *Deep partial thickness* or *deep dermal* burns take longer than 3 weeks to heal, as fewer epithelial elements survive, and the attenuated surviving dermis heals with the production of ugly hypertrophic scars. Infection will delay healing and can cause further tissue destruction, converting the injury to a full thickness one.

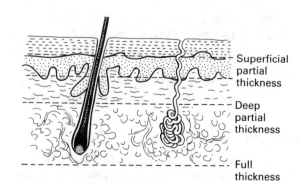

Fig. 13.1   Diagram of skin showing categories of burn depth

Full thickness burns

A full thickness burn destroys the epidermis and underlying dermis, including the epidermal appendages. The destroyed tissues undergo coagulative necrosis and form an eschar which usually begins to lift off the underlying tissues within 2–3 weeks. Unless the raw area is grafted, epidermal cover can only occur through laborious inward movement and growth of cells from the intact skin around the burn margin, and by contraction of its base. Fibrosis and ugly contracture are thus inevitable in all but small injuries.

Determination of burn depth

There is no foolproof method for determining the depth of a burn in the early period after injury, and even experienced plastic surgeons may not be able to make an accurate assessment for days or even weeks following the injury.

Scalds from liquids below boiling point usually produce partial thickness injury, whereas scalds from boiling water and burns due to electricity or contact with hot metal usually produce full thickness injury. Flame burns can be of mixed depth but nearly always include areas of full thickness loss.

Erythema denotes that epidermal damage is superficial, and blanching on pressure confirms intact dermal capillaries and a partial thickness injury. A *dead white appearance* frequently indicates full thickness injury, although at least some of these burns prove to be deep dermal. A *dry leathery mahogany-coloured* eschar with visible thrombosed veins denotes full thickness destruction.

Intact cutaneous sensation implies that the epidermal appendages have survived, as they lie at the same level as cutaneous nerve endings in the dermis. Superficial burns are thus very painful. In practice, anaesthesia to pinprick can be misleading and does not always indicate full thickness loss.

Blisters are accumulations of fluid at the junction of epidermis and dermis and suggest partial thickness damage. They may continue to appear several hours after injury and are often broken by the time the patient is seen by the doctor.

PROGNOSIS AFTER BURN INJURY

Prognosis depends on the following factors.

Age and general condition. Infants, the elderly, alcoholics, and those ill from other disease fare less well than healthy young adults.

Extent of the burn. Extent can be estimated in the adult by using the 'rule of nines' (Fig. 13.2), but tables are available for more accurate calculation. The patient's hand with fingers together accounts for about 1%. The rule of nines cannot be used in children because of the relatively large size of the head, which accounts for about 20% of body surface at birth, whereas each lower limb accounts for only 13%. Hypovolaemic shock is anticipated if more than 15% of the surface is burned in an adult, or more than 10% in a child. If the sum of an adult patient's age and percentage body area of full thickness burn comes to more than 80 there is a high risk of a fatal outcome.

Depth of the burn. Following successful resuscitation, superficial burns of whatever size should, if properly treated, heal within 3 weeks leaving no scars. Full thickness burns, on the other hand, will inevitably become infected unless excised early; if they are large, the infection may be life-threatening.

Site of the burn. Burns involving the face, neck, hands, feet or perineum are particularly liable to threaten appearance or function. They require inpatient management.

Associated respiratory injury. This is now extremely common in victims of house fires and is usually due to inhalation of the smoke produced by burning plastic foam upholstery. It is frequently fatal.

MANAGEMENT OF THE BURNED PATIENT

First aid

Prompt effective action prevents further damage, and may save life or avoid months of suffering. The principles of first aid are to arrest the burning process, ensure an adequate airway and avoid wound contamination.

Arrest the burning process. Burning clothing is extinguished by smothering the flames in a coat or carpet. The victim must be placed flat on the ground to avoid flames rising to burn the head and neck with inhalation of smoke and fumes. The heat within clothing can continue to burn the body

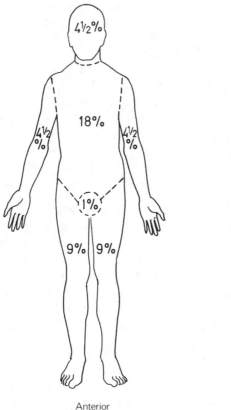
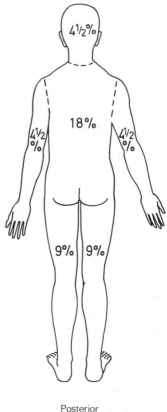

Anterior   Posterior

Fig. 13.2 The 'rule of nines' for estimating extent of burn

for many seconds after flames have been extinguished, so that clothing must be removed immediately or doused in cold water. Similarly, clothing soaked in scalding water will continue to cause damage until it is removed. Cool water is an excellent analgesic and can dissipate heat but common sense must be used in its application. Immersing a child with a large burn in cold water or covering a patient with cold soaks can cause hypothermia, and cooling can counteract the heat of the burn only if applied immediately after the injury.

Chip pan fires are a common cause of domestic accident. It is dangerous to attempt to remove the burning pan from the kitchen. The source of heat must be turned off and the top of the pan covered with a lid, a fibreglass firemat (if available) or a damp dish towel to exclude all air and extinguish flames.

Chemical burns require copious irrigation with water for several minutes. If the eyes are involved, prompt and prolonged irrigation may save the patient's sight.

Electrical burning is arrested by switching off the current source, not by pulling the patient free. If this is not feasible, the patient is pushed free from the contact with a non-conductor such as a wooden chair.

Ensure an adequate airway. If the patient is in a smoke-filled room, it is essential to move him as quickly as possible into a smoke-free atmosphere. Smoke and fumes cause asphyxia, often contain poisons and can precipitate respiratory arrest. Mouth-to-mouth ventilation is commenced if necessary. If cardiac arrest follows electrocution, resuscitation should be instituted.

Avoid wound contamination. The burn should be covered with a clean sheet or 'cling' film. On no account should traditional 'household remedies' be applied. At best they are messy and interfere with subsequent care; at worst they can be positively destructive, converting partial to full thickness injuries.

Transfer to hospital

The patient should be transferred to hospital as soon as possible, unless the burn is obviously trivial. Severe burns are best treated from the outset in a specialized burns unit. Hypovolaemia takes time to become manifest, and it is easy to misjudge the severity of injury, thus missing the opportunity for uncomplicated transfer. Transfer of a patient with a large burn between hospitals should be avoided during the first 8–24 hours after injury. Patients embarking on a journey expected to take more than 30 minutes should ideally be accompanied by a trained person, and an intravenous infusion should be commenced if the burn is extensive.

Full thickness burns are often relatively painless. Partial thickness injuries can be excruciatingly painful and opiates may be needed for pain relief. Analgesics should be given intravenously; the dose and route of adminstration must be recorded.

Arrival in the accident and emergency department

Adequate ventilation

Maintenance of an adequate airway remains the first priority. A patent airway on admission is no guarantee that the patient will remain free from airway problems, and no patient who has been exposed to smoke in a closed room should ever be sent home but should be admitted for observation. Respiratory tract injury is suggested by dyspnoea, coughing, hoarseness, cyanosis and coarse crepitations on auscultation, and by the presence of soot particles around the nostrils, in the mouth or in the sputum. Endotracheal intubation is advisable if there is anxiety about airway patency. Tracheostomy is never undertaken lightly in view of the danger of infection of burned tissues around the stoma.

Initial assessment and management

Once airway patency is assured, the time of injury, type of burn and its previous treatment are established. The extent and depth of the burn are assessed to determine whether shock can be expected. If the burn is over 15% in extent (or 10% in a child), an intravenous infusion is commenced, and blood is withdrawn for cross-matching and determination of haematocrit and blood urea and electrolyte concentration. Blood gas analyses are performed if there is concern about the airway. Establishing an intravenous infusion takes priority over a detailed history or full physical examination. Intravenous therapy may be required for many days, but the number of available veins is often reduced by the extent of the injury and they must be treated with great respect. It is best to start with the most peripheral available vein in the upper limb, as lower limb veins tend to go into spasm. Vasoconstriction is often marked and it may be necessary to insert a cannula into the internal jugular or subclavian vein. Once intravenous infusion is established, regular recording of pulse, blood pressure, peripheral circulation (temperature, venous filling and capillary return) and hourly urine output is commenced. In patients with burns involving over 20% of body surface it is necessary to insert a catheter into the bladder to obtain an accurate measurement of urinary output.

Severe pain is relieved by intravenous injection of opiates. Tetanus can rarely complicate burns, and if the patient has not recently received tetanus toxoid this should be given.

In general, patients with burns involving more than 10% of the body surface should be admitted to hospital, as should all patients whose site of injury poses particular management problems and those with significant full thickness skin loss.

Prevention/treatment of burn shock

The aim of management is to prevent shock by prompt fluid replacement. Some workers favour colloid solutions for resuscitation, while others prefer electrolytes or a mixture of the two, but whatever solution is used must contain sodium. Salt-free fluids should never be used, as they will cause water intoxication. Assessment and management of the shocked patient is discussed in general terms in Chapter 3. Various 'formulae' are available to help calculate fluid requirements in burned patients, but whichever formula is used it is essential to remember that it is merely a guide and that the amounts often need to be modified according to the patient's response. The most commonly used regimen in the UK is based on the Muir and Barclay formula. The first 36 hours after the burn are divided into six successive periods of 4, 4, 4, 6, 6 and 12 hours. In each of these periods the volume of plasma to be infused is calculated using the following equation:

$$\frac{\text{Burn area (\%)} \times \text{body weight (kg)}}{2}$$

i.e. 0.5 ml/kg for each percent burn.

The originally described formula contained reconstituted freeze-dried plasma as the colloid. This is no longer available and is usually substituted by a purified protein solution (PPS). There have been suggestions that greater volumes of PPS may be needed but this is not always the case. The need for fluid is greatest in the early hours, and lasts for up to 36–48 hours.

Despite renal retention of sodium after injury, there is a tendency to hyponatraemia in the first 2–3 days due to secretion of antidiuretic hormone and sequestration of sodium in interstitial oedema. As inflammatory oedema is reabsorbed, the serum concentration returns to normal, and unless water intake is maintained there is a danger of hypernatraemia. Tissue destruction releases large amounts of potassium into the extracellular fluid, but hyperkalaemia is largely prevented by increased renal excretion of potassium as part of the metabolic response to injury (Ch. 1). Once the first few days have passed, continuing potassium losses can produce hypokalaemia in a patient unable to eat and drink normally.

Water replacement. A 5% dextrose solution is used to replace the normal daily water losses. Excessive evaporation continues until the burn has re-epithelialized, and a high water intake must be maintained. Although most burned patients are thirsty, paralytic ileus is common for several days in those with very large burns, and oral fluids may cause gastric distension, vomiting and aspiration.

However, the majority of patients are able to drink normally after 48 hours and it is important that they are encouraged to do so as soon as they can.

Blood transfusion. Blood should not be given in the first 24 hours, but will be needed in the second 24 hours after a large full thickness burn. Continuing red cell destruction in deep burns with suppression of the bone marrow leads to anaemia, and haemoglobin concentration and haematocrit (packed cell volume) should be monitored frequently. Repeated blood transfusions may be necessary.

Organ failure complicating the management of burn shock

The problems of organ failure in shock have been discussed in detail in Chapter 3 and only those respiratory and renal problems specific to burn shock are considered here.

Respiratory problems

Patients with head and neck burns are best nursed sitting up to encourage dispersal of oedema. Physiotherapy is essential to clear bronchial secretions after inhalation of smoke and fumes. Continued observation is mandatory, and blood gas analysis and chest X-rays are repeated regularly in patients with ventilation problems. Arterial hypoxaemia is proof of inadequate ventilation. Oxygen therapy, endotracheal intubation and assisted ventilation may be needed and antibiotics should be prescribed. Tracheostomy may occasionally be unavoidable despite the problems associated with its management. Encircling eschar impairing chest or abdominal expansion must be incised or excised as soon as it is recognized.

Renal failure

Acute tubular necrosis is a potential complication of extensive burns. The risk is especially high in the elderly, those with pre-existing renal disease and patients developing haemoglobinuria or myoglobinuria. These pigments appear in the urine after massive red cell destruction or extensive muscle damage (particularly after electrical injury) and can damage the tubules and obstruct urine flow by forming pigment casts.

Hourly urine output must be maintained at between 30 and 50 ml an hour in the adult. A falling output reflects either inadequate resuscitation or the onset of renal failure. Measurement of urine specific gravity or osmolality and the response to small test infusions will distinguish between them. Diuretics are used only if oliguria persists after adequate fluid replacement, when 20% mannitol (1 g/kg) should be infused over half an hour.

Nutritional management

Evaporation from open wounds is a major cause of excessive energy expenditure following a severe burn, as is wound sepsis. Energy losses are reduced if the patient is nursed in an environmental temperature of 30–32°C. A high caloric intake is impracticable during the period of hypovolaemic shock, but is encouraged as soon as the patient can drink. An adequate intake for adults can be calculated from the following formula:

Calories: 20 kcal/kg   body   weight   plus 70 kcal/percent burn

An appropriate amount of protein must also be provided, again according to the weight of the patient and the extent of the burn.

In large burns it is necessary to supplement oral intake by feeding via a fine-bore nasogastric tube (enteral feeding), with the aim to supply the patient's total calculated normal daily energy and protein requirements. If this is done, weight loss can be limited to less than 10%, which is acceptable. Parenteral nutrition is only rarely required, e.g. in patients with prolonged paralytic ileus. Vitamin supplements and iron must be provided after severe injury.

Sepsis

Septicaemia is a constant threat to the burned patient until skin cover has been fully restored. Resistance to infection is low, the wound provides a continuing reservoir of infecting organisms, and intravenous cannulae, indwelling urinary catheters and tracheostomy wounds are all potential sources of infection. The incidence of septicaemia has been reduced by use of topical antibacterial agents and by early excision and grafting but the risk remains high with large burns. Prophylactic antibiotics should be avoided as superinfection with resistant organisms is almost inevitable. Regular monitoring by blood cultures is essential but antibiotics are reserved for invasive infection and a positive culture is an absolute indication for systemic antibiotic therapy.

Curling's ulcer and stress ulceration

Acute ulceration of the duodenum (Curling's ulcer) and multiple gastric erosions (stress ulceration) may follow major burns. The early institution of feeding reduces their incidence, but an H_2-receptor antagonist such as cimetidine or ranitidine should be prescribed prophylactically.

LOCAL MANAGEMENT OF THE BURN

Care of the burn wound begins at the time of injury and continues until epithelial cover has been restored. Infection poses the major problem and is the main threat to life once the first 48 hours have passed.

Principles of wound management

Initial cleansing and debridement

The burn is cleaned meticulously with a mild detergent containing antiseptic and saline as soon as possible after admission, and adherent clothing and loose devitalized tissue are removed. An aseptic technique is essential, and cleansing must be carried out in an operating theatre or clean dressing room. Blisters should be punctured and serum expressed, and any broken blisters must be completely deroofed. General anaesthesia may be necessary, but in most patients pain is best relieved by intravenous opiates. In shocked patients, the wound is covered with a clean drape, and further local care is postponed until the circulatory state has stabilized.

Prevention of contamination

The burned patient is particularly susceptible to

infection. The protective epidermis is destroyed and, in a full thickness injury, thrombosis of cutaneous vessels impairs the normal response to infection. In a large burn both cellular and humoral immune mechanisms are depressed. Organisms readily colonize the burn wound and, if dead tissue is present, multiply rapidly and can soon invade the surrounding tissues.

Improved wound care and topical antibacterial agents have greatly reduced the risk of burn sepsis. Staphylococci remain by far the most common infecting organisms and *Pseudomonas aeruginosa* remains troublesome in most burn units. Haemolytic streptococci are feared because they can convert superficial into deep burns and can cause a severe systemic illness. Once contaminating organisms have been cleared from the burn surface, mechanical protection against further contamination and infection can be provided in a number of ways. The following methods are not mutually exclusive and more than one technique may be employed as the needs of the patient alter. All personnel coming into contact with the burned patient must wear a cap and mask, and all dressings are applied using meticulous aseptic technique.

Evaporative dressings. These dressings prevent contamination, allow exudate to evaporate and provide comfortable support. After the initial cleansing, the burn is covered by a layer of sterile paraffin gauze dressing, a layer of cotton gauze swabs, a bulky layer of cotton wool or Gamgee Tissue, and an outer retaining crepe bandage. The dressing is reviewed daily but should be left in place for 8–10 days. However, if exudate soaks through to the outside, the dressing must be changed down to the inner layer, for bacteria traverse a soaked dressing in hours.

Exposure. Following initial cleansing and debridement, burns of a single surface may be exposed to the air. Evaporation of the protein-rich exudate leaves a dry, adherent crust which, as long as it remains intact, is an effective barrier to bacterial invasion. Exposure is particularly useful for burns of the face and neck, and can be used for burns of the trunk and extremities, but as it is extremely difficult to use this technique properly, it should be left to units that are familiar with the method. Badly performed 'exposure' is a recipe for infection.

Topical antibacterial agents. Silver sulfadiazine cream (Flamazine) and povidone iodine (Betadine) are valuable local antibacterial agents in treating large burns. They are often used for minor burns but are not necessary as long as proper initial surgical debridement is performed and evaporative dressings are applied. To be effective they must be reapplied daily, which is not cost-effective for small injuries and is painful and time-consuming.

Plastic film dressings. These have the advantage of making the burn pain-free. 'Cling' film has been used as a first aid measure but it leaks and is too messy to be useful as a definitive dressing. *OpSite* is an adhesive film which is effective for small superficial burns but it, too, may leak initially and should be covered with a well-padded dressing for 48 hours. Thereafter it can be patched or replaced if necessary.

'Hand bags'. Commercial polythene bags of the 'snappy' type are sterile when taken from the roll, are very cheap and are useful for treating superficial burns of the hands. The hands are smeared with silver sulfadiazine cream and the bags kept in place with a bandage at the wrist. The bags must be changed daily, the hands washed and the antiseptic cream reapplied, but the effort is worthwhile in this situation, as it prevents stiffness and allows the patient to use the hand.

'Biological' dressings. Xenografts such as porcine skin are now available in the freeze-dried state and can be reconstituted for use as a temporary occlusive 'biological' dressing, but they are very expensive. Amnion and stored homograft skin used to be popular alternatives but with the increasing danger of infection with human immune deficiency virus (HIV) it is likely that they will become less widely used.

Relief of constriction (escharotomy)

The dangers of progressive respiratory embarrassment from eschar in encircling burns of the chest have already been mentioned. Increasing oedema beneath encircling eschar in the limbs may imperil the circulation, and relieving incisions (escharotomies) which run from top to bottom of the circumferential deep burn may then be required in the first few hours after the injury.

Restoration of epidermal cover

Full thickness and deep dermal burns of less than 10% are suitable for primary excision of eschar under general anaesthesia within a few days of the accident. *Tangential excision* is used for deep dermal burns. This consists of shaving away the outer dead layers of skin down to the deep dermal layer and applying a split skin graft immediately. In this way tissue that otherwise would have died can be preserved. Primary excision and grafting is not feasible for more extensive burns except in a few highly specialized centres. However, the burn can be partially excised and grafted soon after the injury and the remaining areas of skin destruction treated by delayed grafting. Eschar begins to separate spontaneously after some 2 weeks, the process being accelerated by infection. Topical antibacterial agents delay separation by inhibiting bacterial growth. As the slough separates, healthy granulation tissue should be revealed and, when all the slough has gone (helped if necessary by the surgeon's scalpel), the burn should be ready for grafting. The β-haemolytic streptococcus is a troublesome cause of graft lysis, and grafting should never be carried out when it has infected the burn. If it is grown from wound swabs, the patient must be treated with intramuscular penicillin and barrier-nursed until three successive swabs are clear.

Avascular tissues such as bone, tendon, or open joints may not provide sufficient nourishment for free grafts, so that a vascularized flap may be required to provide skin cover.

Free skin grafts may be full thickness or partial thickness (split skin), but only split skin grafts are used to cover acute burns. They may vary in thickness from epidermis only (Thiersch grafts) to almost full thickness, but medium thickness grafts are most commonly used. The donor site forms a new epidermis from remaining islands of epithelium and, if necessary, more skin can be harvested after 14 days. Excess skin can be stored at 4°C for up to 3 weeks.

Full thickness grafts are used for secondary reconstruction in cosmetically important areas where contraction has to be avoided or in areas such as the palms of the hands, which are subjected to repeated trauma.

A graft will not 'take' if there is movement between it and the recipient area, or if the graft is floated off by accumulation of blood or serum. Large flat surfaces are covered by sheets or strips of skin which may be held in place by occasional sutures or staples. Accumulation beneath the graft is prevented by multiple small perforations. Grafts can be *meshed* in a special machine which cuts small slits so that they can be expanded up to nine times their size to allow cover of very large areas (Fig. 13.3). The interstices of the mesh epithelialize from its edges. In practice, expansion to more than three or four times is rarely used as the quality of the healed skin is poor.

Non-meshed grafts are exposed if feasible, but in many areas a bulky firm dressing is needed to protect the area. Meshed grafts need to be dressed to prevent the interstices drying out. Shearing can be prevented by leaving the sutures long and tying them over the dressing (a 'tie-over' dressing).

Functional and cosmetic result

With energetic treatment it is usually possible to restore skin cover to even the most extensive

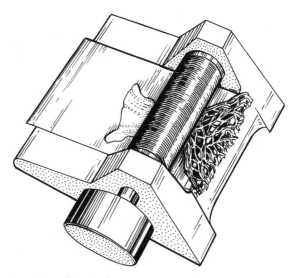

Fig. 13.3 Skin mesher

injury within 3 months, but wound closure is not the end-point in management. Skin grafts and donor sites must be kept soft and supple by applying a moisturizing cream several times a day for many months. Splints may be needed to prevent contractures, and physiotherapy is necessary to mobilize joints. Elastic pressure garments should be worn to prevent the build-up of hypertrophic scars. In spite of all this care, reconstructive procedures may be required over many years to correct contractures or rebuild missing or distorted features. The severely burned patient may have a difficult struggle coming to terms with permanent disfigurement and limitation of his way of life. Long-term support with counselling from his surgeon and other staff is then necessary.

14. Multiple injury

Patients with multiple injuries present a major challenge, as survival depends not only on competent care at the site of the accident but also on careful transport, and skilled resuscitation and surgical treatment. In particular, rapid and accurate decision-making in the initial diagnosis and assessment of treatment priorities of individual injuries demands wisdom and experience.

Legislation on the wearing of seat belts and crash helmets has helped to reduce the number of fatalities in road traffic accidents, and the severity of head, facial and thoracic injuries.

Yet in the United Kingdom, road traffic accidents remain a major cause of death and severe multiple injury, the latter constituting as great a problem as all industrial, domestic, criminal and sporting injuries taken together. Each year some 7000 people are killed and 350 000 injured on British roads. In one-third of those who are killed the blood alcohol level exceeds the legal limit.

More than one region of the body is injured in 80% of those who die, compared to only 20% of those who survive road accidents. Injuries of the head are the most frequent cause of death, while the thorax is affected in one-half and the abdomen in one-quarter of fatal cases. Spinal or pelvic fractures and fracture-dislocations are present in one-fifth of those who are killed.

MECHANISM OF INJURY

Although there are many components to the forces that injure the body in violent accidents, the resulting injury can usually be classified as either 'blunt' or 'penetrating'. Blunt injuries typically result from civilian accidents, whereas penetrating injuries tend to be associated with armed conflict, whether military or civilian.

Blunt injuries

Blunt injuries usually result from forces such as crushing, shearing or torsion. For example, in a head-on collision a car driver who is inadequately restrained by his seat belt may receive a direct blow to the chest from the steering wheel, shearing injuries to his small bowel and its mesenteric attachments as a result of sudden compression of his abdomen by the seat belt, and a whiplash injury of the cervical spine as his head is flung backwards and then forwards.

Both solid and hollow viscera are susceptible to blunt injury. Hollow viscera are especially vulnerable when distended. For this reason, drunken drivers are particularly at risk from rupture of the stomach or bladder.

Penetrating injuries

These are characteristically the injuries of wartime, terrorism and interpersonal violence. Firearm injuries, although common in the United States, remain rare in the United Kingdom apart from Northern Ireland. However, their incidence is increasing, and stabbing injuries are now commonplace in most inner city areas and seaside resorts at holiday time.

While damage caused by stabbing is confined to the track of the offending weapon, that from bullets and shrapnel is disseminated as their kinetic energy passes through the body (Fig. 14.1). The resulting damage to the body is proportional

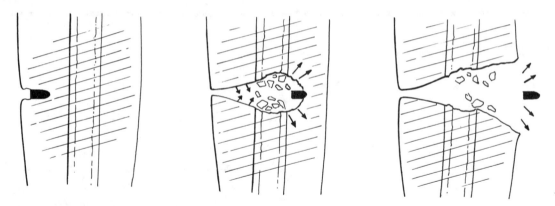

Fig. 14.1 Missile with shock waves from track. Note that the exit wound is larger than the entry wound

to the size and shape of the missile and, more importantly, its velocity. Low-velocity bullets fired from a revolver cause less damage than the small, high-velocity bullets used in modern rifles such as the Armalite, which travels at 1000 m/s.

Such high-velocity missiles produce a shock wave which causes cavitation and disruption of tissues irrespective of the presence of the bullet itself. A bullet trajectory is initially stable, and if of low velocity may traverse the tissues cleanly. If its path is deflected (e.g. by bone), it becomes unstable and its energy is transferred to the surrounding tissues, with subsequent disruption. A low-velocity bullet which is 'tumbling' when it hits the body may carry foreign material into the wound.

Blast injuries

Blast injuries may occur as a result of fireworks, domestic or industrial explosions, but are most commonly due to bomb explosions. Bomb injuries combine the effects of shrapnel and flying debris (from fragmentation of the shell) with those of the pressure wave radiating from the explosion which commonly causes damage to ears and lungs. If the victim is close to the explosion, the 'blast' wave can cause extensive damage by blowing off extremities or other parts of the body. One quarter of those killed by bomb injuries have traumatic amputations.

Assessment of a missile injury requires inspection of both the entry and the exit wound. Absence of an exit wound means that the missile is still in the body. Exit wounds vary according to

the velocity of the missile: high-velocity missiles do not always produce large exit wounds but are much more likely to do so than those of low velocity.

PATTERNS OF INJURY

Patients with multiple injuries, particularly those involved in road accidents, frequently have a characteristic pattern of injury. Recognition of the different patterns can be useful in detecting lesions that might otherwise be missed. For example, an unrestrained car driver involved in a head-on collision may present with a horizontal forehead laceration from contact with the driving mirror, a circular imprint on the chest from the steering wheel, and a horizontal cut on the knee (sometimes combined with an upper tibial fracture) from contact with the dashboard. With experience, an increasing number of patterns of injury will be recognized.

Car occupants involved in road traffic accidents should always be examined carefully for cervical spine injury, myocardial contusion, liver injury and posterior dislocation of the hip joints, all of which may be asymptomatic at first assessment but are common injuries in this type of accident. Detection of these and other injuries becomes even more difficult in patients who are unconscious or confused. In such circumstances it is wise to remember the general rule that if injuries can be detected in two separate areas (e.g. the head and lower limbs), there is a high chance of further injury to the area in between.

Table 14.1 Priorities in the management of multiple injury

FIRST PRIORITY: deal with any *immediate threat of life*
Ensure patent airway
Maintain ventilation
   relieve tension pneumothorax
   seal open chest wounds
   assist ventilation
Maintain circulation
   control haemorrhage
   relieve cardiac tamponade
   monitor and treat shock
Relieve increased intracranial pressure

SECOND PRIORITY: treat conditions which pose an
ultimate threat to life or an *urgent threat to function*
Debride cerebral wounds
Repair gastrointestinal perforations
Explore thoracic and abdominal wounds
Relieve pressure on spinal cord
Repair vascular injuries
Reduce, debride and immobilize compound fractures
Immobilize single fractures

THIRD PRIORITY: treat conditions *not threatening life or
posing an urgent threat to function*
Reduce dislocations
Reduce closed fractures
Debride soft tissue injuries (with or without closure)
Repair peripheral nerve injuries

TREATMENT PRIORITIES

The first priority in managing any patient with severe injuries, be it at the scene of the accident, during transport to hospital or in the emergency ward, is to deal with any problems which pose an immediate threat to life. This usually means ensuring patency of the airway and stopping any external haemorrhage. Once this has been achieved, the priority changes to measures which will prevent other injuries from getting worse, and so avoid deterioration of the patient. The treatment priorities in patients with multiple injuries are summarized in Table 14.1.

Establishing a patent airway

Securing patency of the airway is usually straightforward. If the patient is conscious and has a good cough reflex he can remain in any position that he finds comfortable. If he is unconscious, irrespective of the state of his reflexes, he should be rolled into the three-quarter prone or recovery position, provided his injuries allow this to be done (Fig. 14.2). This ensures that, should he

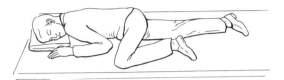

Fig. 14.2 Nursing of an unconscious patient in the three-quarter prone position

vomit, he will not inhale foreign material into his respiratory tract. If the airway is obstructed, the tongue should be pulled forward and the pharynx cleared of debris and saliva. An airway can then be inserted to hold the tongue forward. If the patient is deeply unconscious, intubation of the trachea may be necessary. Should breathing cease, artificial respiration is commenced immediately either by mouth-to-mouth techniques or ventilation through an airway or endotracheal tube (Fig. 14.3) using an Ambu bag.

While paying attention to the airway, consideration should be given to the possibility of injury to the cervical spine. If this is suspected, a collar should be applied. Special care is needed to protect the neck when moving the patient.

If patency of the airway cannot be maintained because of severe facial injuries or other reasons which prevent intubation, direct temporary access to the trachea can be obtained by incision of the cricothyroid membrane. The gap between thyroid and cricoid cartilage is easily palpable. The incision can then be held open by the handle of a scalpel and a tube inserted (Fig. 14.4).

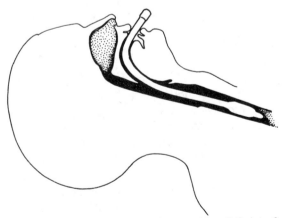

Fig. 14.3 Cuffed endotracheal tube in position. Inflation of the balloon will prevent aspiration into the respiratory tract.

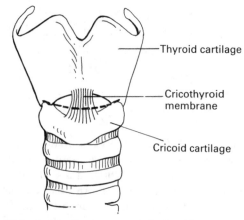

Thyroid cartilage

Cricothyroid membrane

Cricoid cartilage

Fig. 14.4   Incision for emergency cricothyroidotomy

Exposure of the trachea lower in the neck (emergency tracheostomy) should be avoided. This almost invariably causes severe haemorrhage from the congested veins in the neck associated with respiratory obstruction.

Any tension pneumothorax must be decompressed urgently. This is best done by insertion of a wide-bore needle through the second intercostal space. If air escapes, a tube attached to a water-sealed drain should be inserted (see p. 168).

Sucking chest wounds which communicate with the thoracic cavity should be occluded by a dressing or any other available material such as a handkerchief. Flail segments in the thoracic wall should be stabilized by hand pressure or by bandaging of the chest wall sufficiently firmly to stop the segment moving. The patient is placed on the injured side so that the unaffected lung is uppermost.

Maintenance of circulation

Control of haemorrhage and maintenance of the circulation is often readily accomplished by simple manoeuvres. External haemorrhage can usually be stopped by direct pressure on the bleeding vessel. To stop bleeding from the depths of a wound, it may be necessary to pack the wound cavity with gauze rolls. Occasionally, when bleeding is profuse and difficult to control (e.g in patients with extensive scalp lacerations), mass suture of the wound

with interrupted sutures through the skin and subcutaneous tissues will control the haemorrhage. Attempts to apply artery forceps to retracted blood vessels are usually ineffective and lead only to further blood loss.

Bleeding around fractures can be minimized by immobilizing the injured limb, preferably with pneumatic splints. Haemorrhage into body cavities often ceases spontaneously due to a combination of natural haemostatic mechanisms and pressure on the confined haematoma (tamponade). Gentle handling of the patient and avoidance of unnecessary movement will aid this process.

Intravenous fluid replacement is essential to maintain the circulation. As soon as possible, preferably at the scene of the accident, the patient should receive an intravenous infusion of saline or plasma substitute such as dextran or a gelatin-based solution. This can be delivered through a peripheral vein in the arm or leg. On arrival in hospital additional lines can be placed in major veins, such as the subclavian, if this is considered necessary. Blood should be taken for crossmatching. Resuscitation should be aggressive, with rapid administration of intravenous fluid and oxygen by a face mask. It is particularly important to continue resuscitation while the patient is being assessed and investigated — a patient may die in the X-ray department if resuscitation is interrupted. Occasionally, where blood loss has been massive, the use of pneumatic trousers (MAST) is advocated to compress vessels in the lower limbs and thus maintain cardiopulmonary and cerebral circulation. Their value remains a matter of dispute.

Clinical examination

Following stabilization of the patient, a detailed clinical examination is carried out, commencing at the head and working down to the feet. Both the front and back of the patient must carefully be examined. All injuries are documented and assessed with regard to urgency of treatment. Simultaneous operative treatment of more than one site may be necessary, for example in a patient with an expanding extradural haematoma and rapid bleeding from an abdominal viscus.

SPECIFIC INJURIES

HEAD INJURY

Head injury sufficiently severe to warrant admission to hospital occurs in 200 persons per 10 000 population each year. About 12 (6%) of these are serious injuries producing coma. Road traffic accidents account for half of all head injuries; conversely, two-thirds of road traffic accident victims have head injuries.

Mechanism and effects of head injury

Primary brain damage

Primary brain damage at the time of injury commonly results from displacement and distortion of brain tissue. The extent of damage depends on the plane and direction of the applied force and on its velocity and magnitude. The brain is suspended within the cranium and can move along an anteroposterior axis while its lateral movement is limited by the falx cerebri and falx cerebelli. Blows to the front or back of the head thus produce maximal displacement of the brain, the cerebral hemispheres being displaced relative to the less mobile brainstem. The resulting tearing and shearing can cause loss of consciousness, and if extensive may prove fatal.

Concussion is a disordered state of consciousness due to diffuse neuronal and axonal injury. There is no obvious gross brain damage. Injury of greater severity causes *contusion* or *laceration* of brain substance at the point of impact or at the diametrically opposed pole due to the brain being driven against the skull or dural septum — the so-called 'contre-coup' injury (Fig. 14.5). Diffuse shearing lesions in the white matter are another common finding. Gross brain damage also follows tearing of the small vessels of the brainstem, with consequent ischaemia and interruption of nervous pathways.

Injuries from penetrating missiles are much less common than closed head injuries. Missiles traversing the brain drive bone fragments along their path and produce widespread brain damage. A tangential missile path can cause a 'gutter' fracture, driving bone fragments into the brain and producing profuse bleeding from torn vessels.

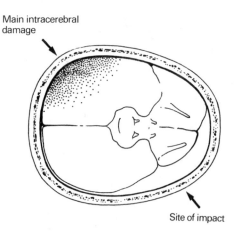

Main intracerebral damage

Site of impact

Fig. 14.5 Contre-coup injury

Increased intracranial pressure

Increased intracranial pressure within the unyielding cranium leads to cerebral compression and is a major cause of death in patients who survive the primary injury. The increase in pressure results primarily from brain swelling and less commonly from intracranial bleeding or a combination of the two. Intracranial bleeding may be extradural, subdural, subarachnoid, intracerebral or intraventricular (see Ch. 40).

Skull fractures

The skull may be fractured by compression, local indentation, or tangential injury. Compression usually produces closed linear *fissure fractures* which pass through the thinner areas of the skull and skirt bony buttresses (Fig. 14.6). Linear fractures of the vault frequently extend into the base of the skull, and may cross foramina to damage cranial nerves or become compound through involvement of the middle ear, air sinuses and cribriform plates. Such compound fractures can allow passage of cerebrospinal fluid (CSF) through the ear (CSF otorrhoea) or nose (CSF rhinorrhoea) and thus permit entry of infection.

Depressed fractures are produced by indentation of the vault (Fig. 14.7) and may be compound or closed, depending on whether the scalp remains intact or not. Compound fractures are complicated by infection in 5–10% of cases. The inner table of

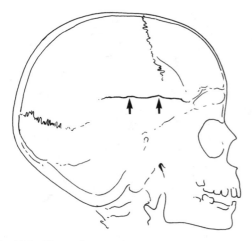

Fig. 14.6 Fissure fracture of skull

the skull is driven through the dura to lacerate and contuse the underlying brain in 50% of cases. There is an increased risk of epilepsy if the depressed fracture has been complicated by cerebral contusion, haemorrhage or infection.

Tangential injury may cause wide separation of large fragments of skull and lift them off the underlying dura (Fig. 14.8). Surprisingly, there may be little or no primary brain damage despite the alarming X-ray appearances.

Skull fracture may occur without significant brain damage. Conversely, the absence of a fracture on X-ray does not exclude brain injury or compression. This is particularly true in young children.

Principles of management

Immediate management

Adequate ventilation is of prime importance. Hypoxia, which is present in 30% of comatose head-injured patients, increases brain swelling and intracranial pressure. If the patient is deeply unconscious, an endotracheal tube should be passed and ventilation assisted as necessary. Blood pressure, heart rate and the state of the peripheral circulation are then assessed and immediate measures taken to treat shock.

In view of the risk of aspiration, a nasogastric tube should be passed if the patient is unconscious (unless he is bleeding from the nose, in which case the tube is passed through the mouth) to keep the stomach empty. Conscious patients are not given anything by mouth until it is certain that operation is not needed.

Assessment of injury

The cause and time of head injury are established, and the level of consciousness is assessed by separately noting eye opening, motor and verbal responses. The level of consciousness cannot be assessed reliably in patients who are shocked or hypoxic. The patient may have remained conscious throughout, been unconscious since the time of the accident or suffered a transient loss of consciousness followed by recovery. Rapid recovery does not imply trivial injury. On the con-

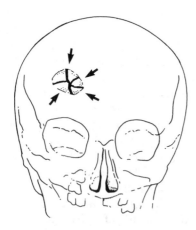

Fig. 14.7 Depressed fracture of skull

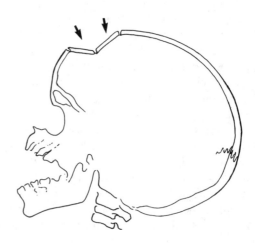

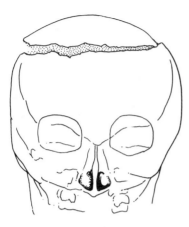

Fig. 14.8 Effect of tangential injury

trary, recovery may be short-lived and the patient become unconscious again after a 'lucid' interval. This sequence of events suggests cerebral compression from intracranial haemorrhage, but can be due to other factors such as hypoxia from a missed chest injury.

Continuing assessment of the level of consciousness is the key to the early diagnosis of cerebral compression, and sedation must be avoided. Care is indicated in patients who have taken drugs or alcohol, as depression of the level of consciousness may be wrongly ascribed to these agents. When in doubt, it must always be assumed that depression of consciousness is the result of brain injury.

The head and neck are examined carefully and the neurological evaluation is then completed. The size, shape and light response of the pupils is noted. Limb movement and power, deep tendon reflexes and plantar responses are checked. Pulse rate, blood pressure, respiration rate and temperature are measured and recorded on a special head injury chart (Fig. 14.9). Regular reassessment at 15–30 minute intervals is essential if neurological deterioration is to be detected in time to allow effective surgical treatment. The head injury chart is commenced on admission and the following variables are monitored.

Level of consciousness. As indicated above, repeated monitoring of the level of consciousness is essential to assess the patient's progress. For example, a rapid deterioration in his condition

should alert the surgeon to the possibility of a space-occupying lesion which may have resulted in herniation of the brain through the tentorium, thus placing the patient's life at grave risk. Various scales have been used to define the level of consciousness. The Glasgow coma scale (Table 14.2) is now officially accepted as the international standard for assessment of consciousness level and is used in many accident and emergency departments.

Size and reaction of pupils. Unilateral cerebral compression causes a transitory constriction of the pupil on the side of the lesion, followed by dilatation, loss of light response and ptosis. These changes are caused by prolapse of the temporal lobe through the tentorium, with consequent irritation and compression of the oculomotor nerve on the side of the lesion (Fig. 14.10). As intracranial pressure continues to rise, similar changes develop in the pupil of the opposite side. Bilateral fixed and dilated pupils indicate advanced cerebral compression. Bilateral small fixed pupils are an indication of intrinsic brainstem damage.

Movement, muscle tone and reflex function. Pressure on the motor cortex causes progressive paresis on the opposite side of the body. Herniation of the temporal lobe through the tentorium may distort the ipsilateral cerebral peduncle and cause contralateral paresis. Increasing pressure is followed by extensor or 'decerebrate' rigidity. In

Table 14.2 Glasgow coma scale

Eyes open	spontaneously	4
	to verbal command	3
	to pain	2
	no response	1
Best motor response to verbal command	obeys verbal command	6
to painful stimulus	localizes pain	5
	flexion withdrawal	4
	abnormal flexion (decorticate rigidity)	3
	extension (decerebrate rigidity)	2
	no response	1
Best verbal response	orientated and converses	5
	disorientated and converses	4
	inappropriate words	3
	incomprehensible sounds	2
	no response	1
Total number of points (minimum 3, maximum 15)		—

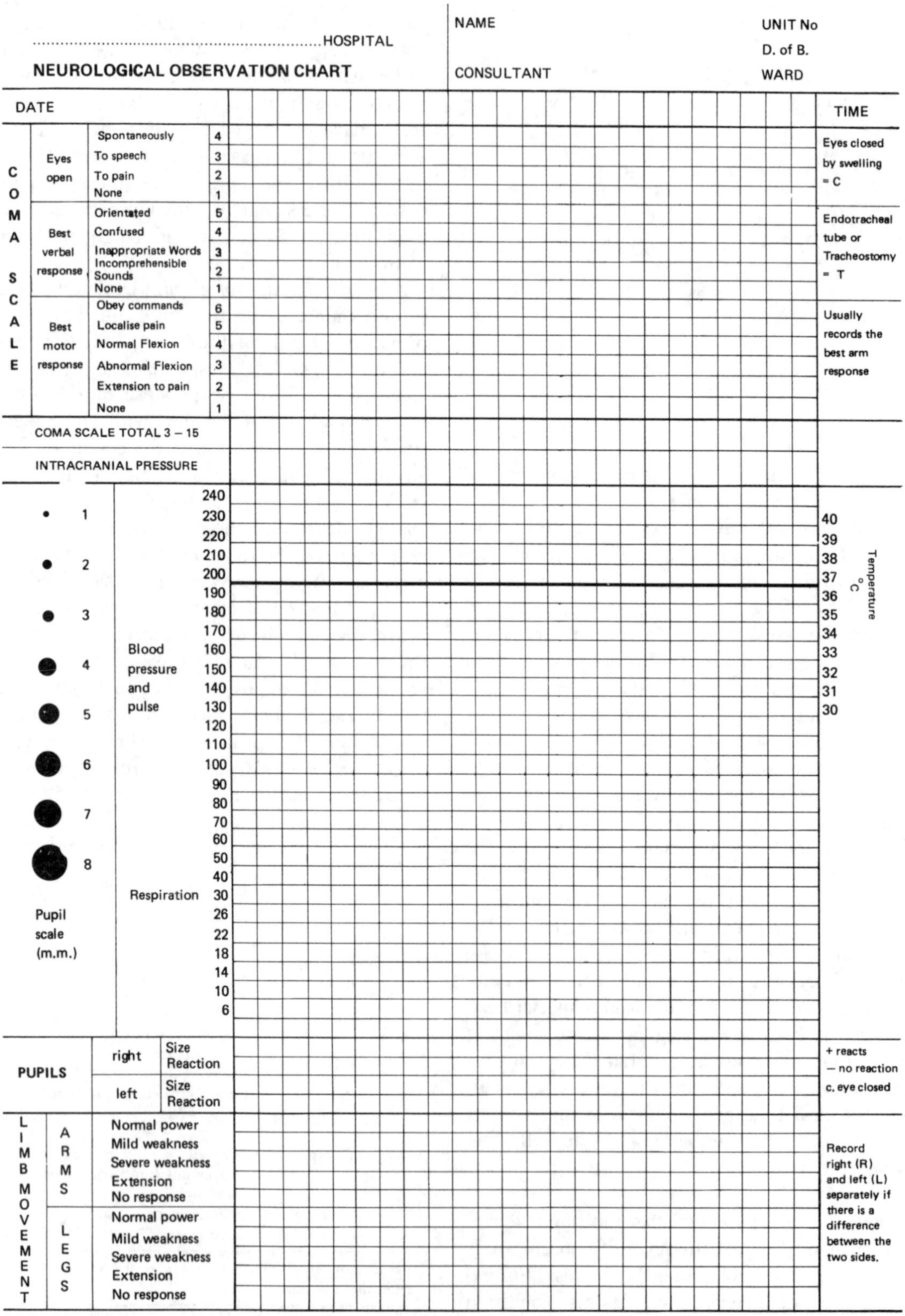

....HOSPITAL

NEUROLOGICAL OBSERVATION CHART

NAME

CONSULTANT

UNIT No

D. of B.

WARD

DATE				TIME

COMA SCALE

Eyes open	Spontaneously	4	
	To speech	3	
	To pain	2	
	None	1	
Best verbal response	Orientated	5	
	Confused	4	
	Inappropriate Words	3	
	Incomprehensible Sounds	2	
	None	1	
Best motor response	Obey commands	6	
	Localise pain	5	
	Normal Flexion	4	
	Abnormal Flexion	3	
	Extension to pain	2	
	None	1	

Eyes closed by swelling = C

Endotracheal tube or Tracheostomy = T

Usually records the best arm response

COMA SCALE TOTAL 3 – 15

INTRACRANIAL PRESSURE

Pupil scale (m.m.)
1, 2, 3, 4, 5, 6, 7, 8

240 230 220 210 200 190 180 170 160 150 140 130 120 110 100 90 80 70 60 50 40 30 26 22 18 14 10 6

Blood pressure and pulse

Respiration

Temperature °C
40 39 38 37 36 35 34 33 32 31 30

PUPILS	right	Size			
		Reaction			
	left	Size			
		Reaction			

+ reacts
— no reaction
c. eye closed

LIMB MOVEMENT

	ARMS	Normal power			
		Mild weakness			
		Severe weakness			
		Extension			
		No response			
	LEGS	Normal power			
		Mild weakness			
		Severe weakness			
		Extension			
		No response			

Record right (R) and left (L) separately if there is a difference between the two sides.

Fig. 14.9 Head injury chart

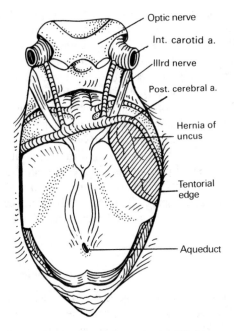

Fig. 14.10 Temporal lobe prolapse causing IIIrd nerve irritation and palsy

some instances, e.g. when there is a chronic subdural haematoma, the brainstem is forced against the opposite edge of the tentorium, compressing the contralateral motor tract and causing hemiplegia on the side of the lesion.

Pulse, blood pressure, respiration rate and temperature. Further increases in pressure force the midbrain through the tentorium (midbrain coning), and the medulla oblongata and portions of cerebellum through the foramen magnum (Fig. 14.11) with consequent distortion of vital centres in the medulla. This produces an increase in blood pressure, bradycardia and decreased respiration rate. These signs appear late in the coma of brain compression unless the lesion is in the posterior fossa. Damage to the hypothalamus or pons leads to hyperpyrexia.

Further investigations

Skull X-rays. Skull X-rays are ordered in all cases of head injury and should include anteroposterior, right and left lateral, and Towne's views. Towne's views are taken anteroposteriorly at an angle of 30° so that the occipital bone is shown (Fig. 14.12).

Open-mouth X-rays to show the odontoid process and facial views to show the sinuses and sites of related fractures may also be required. X-rays are inspected for fractures and foreign bodies. If the pineal gland is calcified, it may be displaced from the midline by a unilateral increase in pressure ('pineal shift').

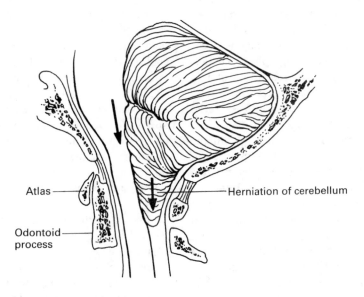

Fig. 14.11 Foraminal coning

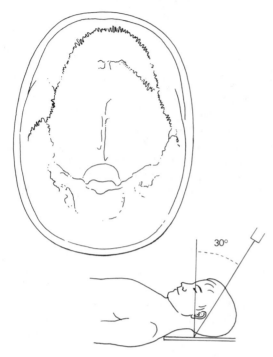

Fig. 14.12 Towne's view to demonstrate the base of the skull

In comatose patients a lateral view of the cervical spine should also be taken.

CT scanning. Computerized axial tomography has revolutionized the diagnosis of intracranial lesions. It is non-invasive and sufficiently sensitive to reveal cerebral oedema as well as intracranial haemorrhage (see Ch. 40). CT scanning has rendered obsolete previously used imaging techniques such as echoencephalography and angiography. As the patient must remain absolutely still during the investigation, general anaesthesia may be required if the patient is restless. Serial examinations can be performed.

Pressure monitoring. The pressure within the subarachnoid space is a useful and precise indicator of intracerebral pressure, especially when the patient is sedated or on a ventilator. Repeated measurements allow treatment to be monitored and may reveal late haemorrhage. An increase in pressure is an indication for a repeat CT scan. Continuous recording can be arranged by screwing a threaded bolt into a small burr hole in the skull.

Exploratory burr holes. These are rarely necessary nowadays and are indicated only when neurological deterioration due to suspected intracranial haemorrhage is extremely rapid or when facilities for CT scanning or angiography are not available (see Ch. 40). The dura and brain surface must be exposed so that extracerebral haemorrhage can be detected and dealt with.

Pneumoencephalography, ventriculography and electroencephalography have *no* place in the assessment of acute head injury. Lumbar puncture is dangerous in patients with head injuries. If intracranial pressure is high, coning of the brain is favoured by reducing the pressure in the spinal subarachnoid space. The only indication for lumbar puncture is suspected meningitis.

Management of the unconscious patient

Sedation must be avoided even if the patient is restless. A cause for the restlessness can usually be found. Hypoxia from airway obstruction, hypotension due to haemorrhage or a full bladder are all common and correctable causes of restlessness. The patient must be positioned on his side. Prophylactic anticonvulsants are sometimes given to patients with intracranial haematomas or contusions. The skin over pressure points is protected by frequent changes of posture, and by the use of a ripple mattress or soft sheepskin.

Hyperpyrexia is common and should be corrected, as it promotes brain swelling and increases intracranial pressure. It also increases the metabolic rate of the brain. It is controlled by surface cooling with fans, wet sheets or ice packs, or administration of the antihistamine promethazine.

The bladder should be drained by an indwelling Foley catheter. This avoids retention of urine, keeps the bed dry and, most important of all, allows accurate monitoring of urinary output. Involuntary micturition at a later stage can be managed by attaching a length of Paul's tubing around the penis and leading it into a collecting bag.

A nasogastric tube keeps the stomach empty and is used for feeding if coma is prolonged for more than 3–4 days.

Intravenous fluids are given to maintain fluid balance. Care must be taken to avoid overhydration, and the use of 5% dextrose solution should

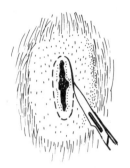
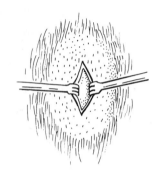
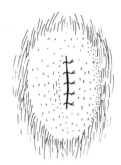

Fig. 14.13   Suture of scalp wound

be avoided. Brain swelling occurs if the serum sodium falls below 120 mmol/l.

H$_2$-receptor antagonists can be used to prevent the development of stress ulceration of the duodenum.

Management of specific head injuries

Scalp injuries

Scalp lacerations bleed profusely but heal well. Temporary haemostasis is achieved by compression of the wound edge or mass suturing. Definitive repair can be undertaken later on when, under good conditions, the area around the laceration is shaved, and the wound is debrided, cleaned and then sutured in layers (Fig. 14.13).

Skull fractures

Although patients with simple fractures of the vault do not require active treatment, they are at increased risk of intracranial complications and must be admitted to hospital for observation to exclude intracranial bleeding.

Depressed fractures of the vault are compound, i.e they communicate with the exterior, in 90% of cases. The surface wound is usually small and can be debrided and closed. If there is extensive skull depression on X-ray, a formal skin flap is raised and reflected so that the fracture can be fully exposed (Fig. 14.14). Loose pieces of bone are removed or elevated. The dura is left intact unless intracranial bleeding is suspected. If the dura has been breached, the wound is cleaned and devitalized brain tissue is removed by suction. The dura

is closed if possible, defects being filled with grafts of pericranium. Larger bone fragments are replaced as a mosaic and the scalp flap is sutured without drainage. Extensive skull defects can be covered 3–6 months later with plates of acrylic resin or metal.

Simple depressed fractures can be left untreated, provided the inner table is depressed only a few millimetres. Depressed fractures which overlie a major venous sinus are also treated conservatively, as operative interference can cause major bleeding.

Fractures of the base of the skull are usually compound into the ear or nose. They are managed conservatively at first, including antibiotic cover. If discharge of cerebrospinal fluid persists for more than 1–2 weeks, the torn dura is repaired with a fascial graft. This is more often necessary in frac-

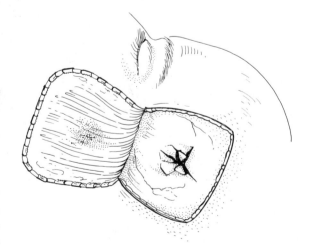

Fig. 14.14   Exposure of a depressed skull fracture

tures involving the anterior rather than the middle fossa.

Extradural haemorrhage

In 70% of patients with extradural haemorrhage (Fig. 14.15) bleeding is due to rupture of the middle meningeal vessels during temporal bone fracture. In the remainder the haematoma is located frontally over the vertex or in the posterior fossa. (In young children the skull is sufficiently thin and pliable to permit extradural haemorrhage without a fracture.) Primary brain damage is usually not severe and the classical history is one of transient loss of consciousness followed by an apparent return to normality. A bruise or 'bogginess' in the temporal region of a patient with X-ray evidence of an underlying fracture should always signal the possibility of extradural bleeding. Following the 'lucid' interval there is deterioration in the level of consciousness which may be extremely rapid. Signs of tentorial herniation appear, followed by slowing of the pulse and respiration rate, and an increase in blood pressure. As soon as any deterioration is suspected, a CT scan should be obtained and urgent surgical treatment instituted. The 'classical' picture described above is seen in only a minority of cases and the

best aid to detection is a high index of suspicion in all patients with skull fractures, whether awake or in coma.

At operation, the clot is evacuated through a temporal burr hole. The opening is enlarged by craniectomy and the bleeding point is coagulated.

Extradural haemorrhage can also follow injury to dural venous sinuses, in which case the clinical course of the syndrome is protracted.

Subdural haemorrhage

Subdural haematomas are more common than extradural haematomas. Although conventionally classified as acute or chronic, both are the result of acute injury with laceration of the brain substance and its vessels leading to accumulation of blood in the subdural space (see Fig. 14.15). This is particularly likely to occur at the temporal pole.

Acute subdural haemorrhage. Cerebral compression by clotted blood may be acute or subacute. In its acute form, subdural haematoma simulates extradural bleeding but skull fracture is less common. Craniotomy is required to allow removal of the mass of subdural blood clot, and to define and arrest the source of haemorrhage.

Chronic subdural haemorrhage. This form of subdural bleeding is particularly common in older

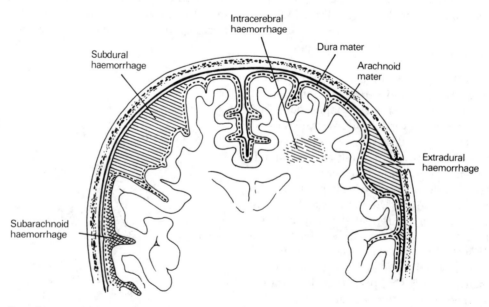

Fig. 14.15 Sites of intracranial haemorrhage

patients, possibly because brain atrophy facilitates displacement. Then little force is needed to tear the veins passing from the cerebral hemisphere to the venous sinuses, and the initial injury may be trivial. Signs of cerebral compression may be delayed for weeks or months after the initial injury. This is due to the gradual enlargement of the 'chronic' subdural haematoma by the entry of fluid to balance hypertonicity.

Headache, apathy and gradual deterioration in consciousness level are associated with localizing signs and evidence of an increase in intracranial pressure. A CT scan will reveal the haematoma. Following CT localization appropriate burr holes are made to allow evacuation of the liquid haematoma. The prognosis is excellent provided surgery is undertaken before severe compression occurs.

Subarachnoid haemorrhage

The commonest cause of subarachnoid haemorrhage is trauma. Subarachnoid bleeding does not produce a circumscribed haematoma (see Fig. 14.15). Blood in the cerebrospinal fluid is irritant and produces headache, neck stiffness, photophobia and irritability.

Conservative management is indicated, but the possibility of confusing this clinical picture with that of meningitis must be remembered. A lumbar puncture is diagnostic.

Intracerebral haemorrhage

Cerebral contusion can prove fatal if there is extensive damage and profuse intracerebral bleeding (see Fig. 14.15). A large haematoma causes cerebral compression and localizing signs which reflect the area involved. The haematoma may rupture into the ventricular system. The temporal lobes are the commonest sites for traumatic intracerebral haematoma, followed by the frontal lobes. Surgery is indicated only if compression occurs or the CT scan shows a large haematoma. The clot is evacuated and devitalized brain tissue is removed.

Brain swelling

Brain swelling can increase intracranial pressure and cause clinical deterioration without localizing neurological signs. It is usually due to congestive distension of cerebral blood vessels. Brain oedema is much less common, and after head injury is usually limited to the zones of the brain in the vicinity of extra- or intracerebral haematomas or brain contusions. The diagnosis may be suspected after head injury, but is only accepted after intracranial bleeding has been excluded by CT scan. Brain swelling is best managed by hyperventilation and diuretics (e.g. mannitol 0.5–1.0 g/kg body weight given as a rapid intravenous infusion). The patient's progress should be monitored by intracranial pressure recording. Glucocorticoid therapy has no place in the management of brain swelling after head injury.

Facial injuries

Although facial lacerations are dramatically obvious, facial fractures are easily overlooked, especially when associated with head injuries.

Lacerations. Injuries of the soft tissues of the face are rarely life-threatening, although they can cause respiratory obstruction, especially in the unconscious patient. They can bleed furiously. Careful repair is essential, as badly repaired facial lacerations may result in lifelong psychological problems. The best time to repair such lacerations accurately is at the time of presentation. Wounds must be carefully explored to detect any damage to deeper layers, which must also be repaired. In the case of the nose and eyelid, damage to the cartilage must be sought and repaired. Penetrating lacerations of the lip are examined to ensure that they do not involve both inner and outer surfaces.

Most such injuries can be repaired under local anaesthesia, but if there are multiple lacerations, it is kinder to the patient to administer a general anaesthetic. In the face, wound excision should be confined to the minimum necessary to allow neat apposition of skin edges with multiple fine sutures such as 6/0 monofilament synthetic sutures.

Fractures. Fractures of the facial skeleton are easily missed because haematoma formation around the orbit may be attributed to basal skull fractures rather than to local injury. Systematic palpation of the bones of the orbit and face will help to detect these fractures.

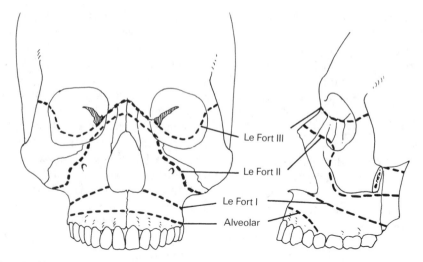

Fig. 14.16   Le Fort classification of maxillary fractures

Fractures of the maxilla are classified as Le Fort I, II and III (Fig. 14.16). A Le Fort I fracture involves only the maxilla and runs through the base of the antrum on either side and across the nasal floor through the septum. A Le Fort II fracture passes across the base of the nose through the posterior wall of the maxillary antrum and across the orbit. A Le Fort III fracture separates the facial skeleton from the cranium, fracturing both zygomatic arches. An alveolar fracture is also described. All these fractures produce mobility of the facial skeleton which can be detected by gentle pressure of a finger on the hard palate. Other reliable signs are anaesthesia in the distribution of the infraorbital nerve, malocclusion of the teeth, diplopia, a change in the level of the eyeballs and effusions into the maxillary antrum (visible on facial X-ray.)

Mandibular fractures are easier to diagnose. They are nearly always compound because of laceration of the gums, and cause malocclusion and loose teeth. The three major points of mandibular fracture are (1) the neck of the condyle or coronoid process, (2) the angle of the mandible, and (3) the ramus (Fig. 14.17). Fracture of the body of the mandible may also occur.

Injuries of the facial bones can only be reliably detected by X-rays of the area(s) involved. A skull X-ray does not provide adequate views of the facial bones. Once diagnosed, fractures are

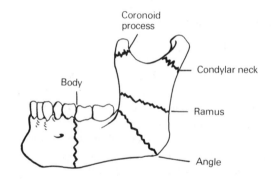

Fig. 14.17   Common sites of fractures of the jaw

reduced as necessary, and fixed by plates, wires and splinting of the teeth.

CHEST INJURY

Only the general principles of the management of chest injuries are discussed in this chapter. For further details of specific conditions see Chapters 19 and 20.

Injuries to the chest occur as a result of penetrating (bullet and stab) wounds and blunt trauma. Crush injuries of the chest are particularly common in accidents involving motor vehicles, either because the driver is compressed against the steering wheel or a pedestrian is 'run over'. In all injuries, attention must first be paid to ensuring a patent airway and unimpaired ventilation of the lungs.

The rib cage is commonly injured. Single or multiple rib fractures occur in all cases of substantial blunt trauma to the chest. Multiple fractures can produce an unstable segment of chest wall (the so-called 'flail chest') by disrupting its attachment to the rest of the rib cage (Fig. 14.18). Unlike the rest of the chest wall which expands on inspiration, the flail segment is sucked in. This 'paradoxical' movement impairs ventilation.

Laceration of the visceral pleura by a penetrating injury or the sharp end of a fractured rib allows air to escape into the pleural cavity, causing a 'pneumothorax'. Sometimes a valve-like effect allows air to enter but not leave the pleural cavity. This produces a 'tension pneumothorax' which displaces the mediastinum to the opposite side, impairing ventilation and venous return. This has potentially fatal consequences. Air may also escape into the chest wall, producing surgical emphysema, or into the mediastinum, producing a pneumomediastinum. Both are visible on chest radiography. Bleeding into the pleural cavity results in a 'haemothorax'. Contusions and lacerations of the lung may cause pulmonary oedema.

Severe trauma to the chest can have even more serious effects. Laceration of the trachea or a main bronchus may cause both massive pneumothorax and gross surgical emphysema, the latter giving rise to the typical 'Michelin man' appearance. Because of the rigidity of the bronchus, the hole will not seal and leakage of air continues despite decompression of the pleural cavity. The heart is also prone to injury, and myocardial contusion or bleeding into the pericardial sac can have dangerous consequences. Rising pressure within the pericardium causes 'cardiac tamponade', which impairs venous filling of the heart to the extent that cardiac failure and death may ensue. Rupture of the aorta may occur as a result of rapid deceleration. The oesophagus, thoracic duct and diaphragm can all be damaged by severe crushing injury.

Evaluation

The severity of a chest injury is easily underestimated and a thorough examination must be carried out in all cases. Signs of respiratory distress include dyspnoea, stridor and cyanosis. All clothing must be removed and chest movements carefully observed, noting asymmetrical expansion, paradoxical movement and indrawing of the intercostal muscles. Bruising is sought and may point to the severity of the trauma. For example, the imprint of the hub of a steering wheel over the sternum should alert the surgeon to the possibility of serious injury to mediastinal vascular structures. The position of the trachea is noted: any deviation indicates mediastinal displacement.

Gentle palpation may reveal tenderness over the ribs or sternum at the site of fracture, unstable segments of chest wall, or the 'crackling' sensation of subcutaneous emphysema. Percussion may detect hyperresonance due to air or dullness due to blood in the pleural cavity. Auscultation is essential in all cases. Coarse crepitations indicate accumulation of secretions, while diminished or absent breath sounds indicate areas of underventilation or fluid in the pleural cavity.

If there are any signs of respiratory distress, arterial blood is withdrawn for blood gas estimations.

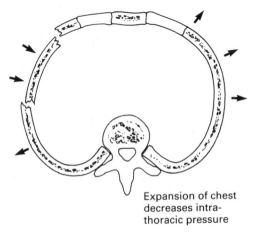

Atmospheric pressure causes flail segment to move inwards

Expansion of chest decreases intra-thoracic pressure

Fig. 14.18 Flail chest injury showing indrawing of flail segment during inspiration

Immediate action

Attention to the airways always has priority. In a

patient with respiratory distress, hyperresonance, inaudible breath sounds and tracheal displacement, a *tension pneumothorax* must be suspected and the pleural cavity decompressed *immediately* by inserting a wide-bore needle through the second intercostal space in the midclavicular line. If air escapes under pressure, the clinical diagnosis is confirmed and a tube can be inserted either at the needle site or laterally in the fourth intercostal space. Underwater-seal drainage is established to allow continued escape of air from the pleural cavity and expansion of the lung (Fig. 14.19). Continuing major escape of bubbles on inspiration in the water seal ('clunking') suggests damage to a bronchus.

If there is a defect in the chest wall which is larger than the diameter of the trachea, air will move in and out of the defect with each attempted breath in preference to passing down the trachea.

This is a called a *sucking wound*. The situation is alleviated when the lung on the side of the injury collapses or if the patient is placed so as to lie on the affected side. Such wounds should immediately be packed with gauze and the patient positioned to compress the injured side until definitive closure can be obtained.

A *flail segment*, while undoubtedly causing pain and some respiratory distress, rarely needs urgent treatment. However, if associated with paradoxical movement, it requires urgent intubation of the trachea with a cuffed tube and assisted ventilation.

Falling arterial blood pressure, distended neck veins and diminished heart sounds are signs of *cardiac tamponade* and demand urgent evacuation of the blood. With the patient in the supine position, a wide-bore needle is inserted at the junction of the left lower costal cartilage and xiphisternum, and passed at an angle of 45° to the skin towards

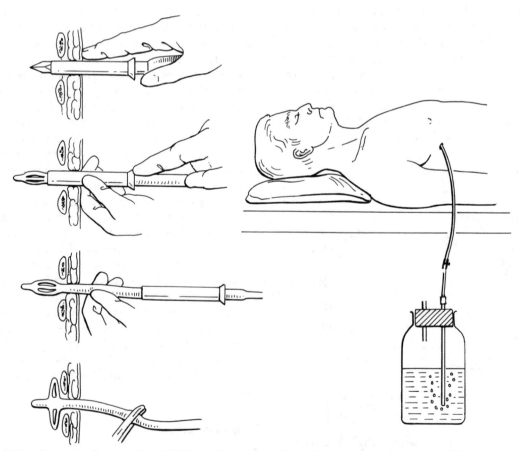

Fig. 14.19 Treatment of pneumothorax (Malécot catheter inserted in the fourth intercostal space laterally)

the tip of the right scapula. If blood is obtained, the pericardial sac should be opened as a matter of urgency and the blood evacuated. This life-saving measure should be followed as soon as possible by operation to arrest the source of the bleeding.

Chest X-ray

Provided there are no such life-threatening injuries, a posteroanterior X-ray of the chest is obtained and scrutinized as follows.

1. The rib cage is examined rib by rib. Particular emphasis is placed on the first rib, as any fracture here implies severe thoracic injury. Additional local views may be needed if fracture is suspected. Surgical emphysema appears as streaks of air in the tissue planes of the chest wall.

2. Evidence of a pneumothorax should be sought in all cases. Lung markings may be absent, or the edge of a partially collapsed lung may be seen. A shift of the trachea or mediastinum to the opposite side associated with a pneumothorax indicates a tension pneumothorax. Accumulation of fluid in the pleural cavity first causes opacification of the costophrenic angle, but as much as 500 ml of fluid can accumulate without radiological abnormality. Larger amounts of fluid cause more extensive opacification.

3. Mediastinal widening, particularly if associated with pleural fluid, suggests bleeding from major vessels and is an urgent indication for angiography. Mediastinal emphysema (air streaks) and surgical emphysema in the tissue planes of the neck suggest damage to the oesophagus.

4. An enlarged cardiac shadow suggests tamponade. However, as little as 50 ml of blood in the pericardial sac can obstruct venous return. This amount will not be radiologically visible.

5. Foreign bodies may be detected if radio-opaque.

6. Loops of air-filled bowel in the chest indicate rupture of the diaphragm.

Definitive management

The management of the various complications of chest injury is described in Chapter 19.

ABDOMINAL INJURY

Mechanisms of injury

Non-penetrating trauma of the abdomen is more common than penetrating injury. Assessment of the likelihood of internal injury requires considerable judgement. Even minor blows can cause serious injury if the anterior abdominal muscles are relaxed at the moment of impact or if the underlying viscera are distended or pathologically enlarged. There may be few outward signs of internal injury.

Penetrating trauma can also be deceptive in that the full extent of injury may not become apparent until the abdomen is explored. This is particularly so with injuries from high-velocity missiles. Penetrating wounds of the chest, loin, flank, buttocks and perineum may all extend into the abdomen. Knives still in place should not be removed until the patient is in the operating theatre.

Sudden deceleration or direct compression are the common causes of blunt injury to viscera. The spleen and liver are relatively protected by the rib cage, but a direct blow to the lower chest may cause rib fractures and so rupture these organs. The kidneys are frequently damaged by blows in the loin, and the full bladder is particularly liable to damage from falls or blows to the lower abdomen. Pelvic fractures are commonly associated with bladder and urethral injury.

The gut and its mesentery may be damaged directly by penetrating injury or torn by the shearing forces of sudden deceleration. The gut tears most frequently at the junction of fixed and mobile parts such as the duodenojejunal flexure and the ileocaecal junction.

Bleeding is the main danger after trauma to solid organs, whereas peritoneal contamination is the prime danger after rupture of hollow viscera. Trauma to the pancreas can cause massive bleeding; transection may occur at the point where it crosses the vertebral column. Pancreatitis and subsequent pseudocyst formation can follow lesser degrees of injury.

Evaluation of abdominal injury

Repeated examination of the abdomen and regular

monitoring of vital signs are the basis of assessment of injury and determine the need for surgery.

Clinical examination

Abdominal pain may be due to bruising of the abdominal wall or to peritoneal irritation by blood or intestinal contents. Occasionally abdominal pain may be referred from spinal or chest wall injuries. The absence of pain or lessening of its severity does not rule out serious injury. Pain may be masked by associated neurological injury or shock. Pain at the shoulder tip suggests diaphragmatic irritation and is most often due to intraperitoneal bleeding after rupture of the spleen or liver. Rupture of a hollow viscus may give surprisingly little pain in the early stages. Analgesia should be withheld, if possible, until the abdomen has been examined by the surgeon who will be responsible for the further care of the patient.

Bruising of the abdominal wall is a useful guide to the site and severity of injury. If the pattern of clothing, seat belt or steering wheel is imprinted on the bruised area, severe compression has occurred.

Tenderness and guarding are the most reliable signs of injury, but their absence does not exclude intra-abdominal damage. Increased muscle tone is a reflex response to peritoneal irritation and is one of the few signs preserved in unconscious patients. Board-like rigidity, such as occurs with a perforated peptic ulcer, is uncommon after abdominal trauma.

Abdominal distension may reflect major haemorrhage. Sequential measurement of girth is often advised but is of doubtful value. Leakage of bowel content, pancreatitis, retroperitoneal haematoma and spinal cord injury can all produce distension from intestinal dilatation due to ileus.

Digital rectal examination may reveal 'bogginess' in the pouch of Douglas due to accumulation of blood. Perirectal surgical emphysema is occasionally detectable and suggests colonic or rectal injury. Blood on the examining finger raises the suspicion of contusion or laceration of the bowel.

Urinalysis is essential. Haematuria indicates urinary tract injury (see Ch. 39).

Radiographic investigation

X-rays of the chest and abdomen are ordered unless signs of massive bleeding demand immediate operation. The standard supine anteroposterior view of the abdomen does not disturb the injured patient. Useful radiological signs include:

1. free intraperitoneal gas on the erect chest X-ray, indicating perforation of a hollow viscus or, less commonly, penetration of the abdominal wall;
2. retroperitoneal gas (shown by streaking) signifying duodenal, colonic or rectal injury;
3. obliteration of the psoas outline by retroperitoneal bleeding;
4. fracture of the lower ribs, raising the suspicion of hepatic, splenic or renal damage;
5. loops of bowel in the chest, indicating rupture of the diaphragm; and
6. demonstration of radio-opaque foreign bodies.

Intravenous pyelography is essential if renal damage is suspected. A *Gastrografin* meal or enema may be useful if there is doubt regarding the integrity of the gastrointestinal tract. Many surgeons now regard *selective arteriography* as mandatory if rupture of the liver or kidney is suspected.

Laboratory investigation

As indicated above, urinalysis is essential to detect haematuria which may indicate urinary tract injury. Others laboratory tests are seldom of diagnostic value in the early course of abdominal trauma. The haemoglobin concentration and packed cell volume (haematocrit) reflect blood loss only after blood volume has been restored by haemodilution, which may take several hours or days. An increased serum amylase activity is helpful in indicating trauma to the pancreas or duodenum.

Abdominal lavage

Abdominal lavage is now performed in many centres to determine whether there has been leakage of blood or intestinal contents into the peritoneal cavity. One litre of warm sterile saline is run into the peritoneal cavity through a needle or tube inserted in the midline below the umbilicus. The fluid is then recovered by lowering the container to below the level of the abdomen (Fig. 14.20). The presence of bile or significant amounts of blood (obscuring vision through the effluent fluid) indicates the need for exploration. Although false positive or false negative results are rare with peritoneal lavage, clinical examination remains of prime importance in assessing the need for exploration.

Ultrasound, CT scanning and laparoscopy are increasingly being used in the early assessment of patients with abdominal injury.

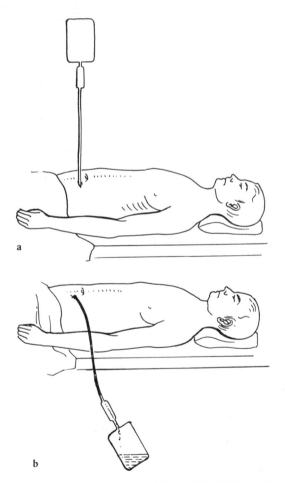

Fig. 14.20 Abdominal lavage. (a) 500–1000 ml of 'normal' (isotonic) saline is run into the abdominal cavity. (b) Saline allowed to reflux back into the bag and presence of blood noted

Principles of management of abdominal injury

Resuscitation

Massive intraperitoneal bleeding requires urgent laparotomy, as blood volume can be restored only after the source of bleeding has been controlled. In most patients there is time for resuscitation before laparotomy, but, if continuous bleeding is suspected, operation should not be unduly delayed.

Indications for operation

Careful and repeated assessment of the patient is the key to management. In contrast to former teaching, isolated stab wounds are now treated expectantly unless there are specific indications for laparotomy, such as spreading peritonitis or recurrent hypovolaemia and shock. Larger wounds likely to be associated with multiple injury, e.g. those caused by firearms, require laparotomy followed by debridement and excision of the penetrating wound. When there is gross wound contamination, the superficial tissues should be left open and delayed primary suture performed 72 hours later.

Laparotomy is indicated in cases of blunt abdominal trauma if there are signs of major blood loss or peritoneal irritation; if there are localizing signs within the abdomen; or if free gas is shown on abdominal X-ray films. Laparotomy is also indicated if there is unexplained clinical deterioration in a patient with minimal abdominal signs or if the requirements for resuscitation exceed those suggested by the known extent of injury. If the integrity of the abdominal viscera is in doubt, it is usually better to operate than to await further clinical deterioration. Otherwise, one may miss the opportunity to deal effectively with the problem before complications develop.

Principles of operation

The abdomen is opened through a long midline incision. Any blood in the peritoneal cavity is removed so that bleeding sites can be identified, clamped with artery forceps or compressed by gauze packs. Open wounds of the intestine are occluded with light clamps.

Injuries are then dealt with systematically. An injured spleen is removed or repaired, an injured liver repaired or partially resected. Any injured gut is repaired, resected or exteriorized. A final careful palpation and inspection of all organs and viscera, including the pancreas, is carried out to make certain that no injury has been missed. If the peritoneal cavity has been contaminated, it is lavaged with saline and the abdomen closed with appropriate drainage.

Specific abdominal injuries

Haematoma formation

Intraperitoneal haematomas are evacuated, and bleeding vessels are clamped and ligated. Insertion of a drain is advisable if oozing continues or if tissue damage is extensive. Retroperitoneal haematomas are left undisturbed, unless they are in close proximity to the duodenum or pancreas. In this case exploration is necessary, as such haematomas are invariably secondary to duodenal or pancreatic rupture. If bleeding continues postoperatively, aortography is indicated to determine further management.

Injury to the spleen

The spleen is one of the organs most frequently damaged by abdominal trauma. It is particularly susceptible to injury when pathologically enlarged, as in infective mononucleosis or malaria. The degree of splenic damage varies. There may be rupture of the spleen; a tear beneath the capsule (which remains intact) with a subcapsular or intrasplenic haematoma; or avulsion from its pedicle (Fig. 14.21). Rupture and avulsion are the common forms of injury. They cause immediate intraperitoneal bleeding with related clinical signs. Delayed rupture occurs in approximately 5% of splenic injuries and is thought to be due to gradual enlargement of a subcapsular haematoma which then bursts through the capsule. In such cases, rupture and free bleeding usually occurs within 2 weeks of injury, but this may be delayed for months or even years.

The classical clinical features of splenic rupture are pain, tenderness and guarding in the left upper quadrant of the abdomen, pain in the left shoulder-tip, and signs of blood loss. Associated fractures of the lower left ribs are found in about 20% of patients. As blood spreads through the peritoneal cavity, peritonism increases and hypovolaemic shock may develop.

In doubtful cases, ultrasonography may confirm splenic enlargement or haematoma. This investigation has superseded splenic scans with ^{51}Cr-labelled red blood cells or ^{99m}Tc colloid. Splenic arteriography is valuable when haematoma or delayed rupture is suspected.

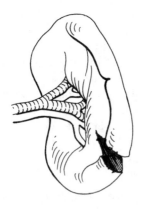
Rupture

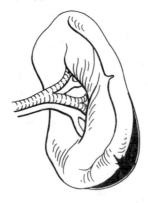
Tear with subcapsular haematoma

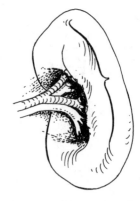
Avulsion of vascular pedicle

Fig. 14.21 Types of splenic injury

Splenectomy used to be the standard form of treatment for all forms of splenic rupture, but in view of the risks of systemic infection following splenectomy, especially in children, there is now a growing tendency to conserve splenic tissue by partial splenectomy or by suture of small capsular tears. A novel method of conserving the injured spleen is to wrap it in a polyglycolic acid (Dexon) mesh. Provided modern scanning techniques are available, a child with a ruptured spleen who remains physiologically stable can be treated without operation. If splenectomy is necessary, prophylactic measures are taken to avoid infection. These include penicillin and pneumococcal vaccines.

Injury to the liver

Blunt trauma. Damage to the liver is more commonly due to blunt trauma than to penetrating injury. Bleeding from a superficial laceration has usually stopped by the time the patient comes to laparotomy and no more than abdominal drainage is required. On the other hand, there may be extensive hepatic disruption, which can be difficult to assess particularly when the superior and posterior surfaces of the organ are affected (Fig. 14.22). Haematomas within the liver substance often escape detection on palpation. However, they are readily revealed by ultrasound and CT scanning. Occasionally, selective angiograms are useful in evaluating chronic haematomas. Severe bleeding can sometimes be controlled temporarily by occlusion of vessels in the free border of the lesser omentum. Bleeding from torn hepatic veins cannot be controlled in this way. Packing of the torn liver is only justified for temporary control during laparotomy, or if the surgeon decides to transfer the patient to a specialist liver surgical unit.

The principles of management are: adequate exposure, if necessary by extending the abdominal wound into the chest or anterior mediastinum; debridement with removal of devitalized tissue; and suture-ligation of torn vessels and bile ducts. Extensive damage may require hepatic lobectomy. Multiple abdominal drains are essential after all forms of hepatic trauma to prevent collection of blood and bile which may later become infected.

Penetrating trauma. Stab wounds and injuries caused by low-velocity bullets can be managed by abdominal drainage if the liver wound is not bleeding actively at laparotomy, but the possibility of residual intrahepatic haematomas must be kept in mind (Fig. 14.23). Damage to a large vessel is repaired by direct suture of the vessel whenever possible. Buttresses of ox fibrin are a useful means of preventing sutures from cutting through the liver substance. High-velocity bullets cause extensive liver damage and hepatic resection is usually required.

Operations for all forms of hepatic trauma may be complicated by the occurrence of jaundice due to temporary hepatic insufficiency or biliary obstruction, hypoalbuminaemia, hypoglycaemia or coagulation disorders in the postoperative phase.

Injury to the biliary tract

Biliary tract damage is a rare complication of

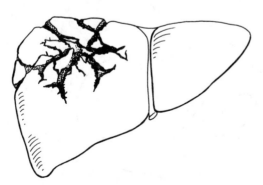

Fig. 14.22 Severe hepatic laceration

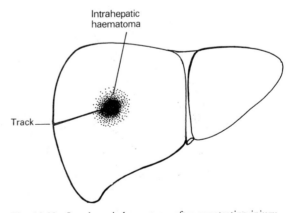

Fig. 14.23 Intrahepatic haematoma after penetrating injury

penetrating trauma. Gallbladder damage is treated by cholecystectomy, while bile duct injuries are repaired (if possible) by direct suture and temporary T-tube drainage. Extensive injury to the bile duct may necessitate choledochojejunostomy.

Injury to the gastrointestinal tract

Stomach. Injury to the stomach is rare and is usually due to penetrating trauma. Blunt injury occasionally causes rupture if the stomach is distended. Escape of gastric juice causes peritoneal irritation, as in perforation of a peptic ulcer. In most cases the gastric wound can be excised and sutured.

Duodenum. Damage to the duodenum is more serious and usually follows severe crushing which also damages the pancreas. Rupture of the duodenum is often retroperitoneal and is usually overlooked at laparotomy unless the duodenum is formally mobilized. Small wounds may be excised and repaired; larger defects can be occluded with a loop of jejunum acting as a patch (Fig. 14.24). Duodenectomy and partial pancreatectomy may be required if damage is extensive.

Small bowel. The small bowel may be damaged at several sites by penetrating trauma. Rupture due to blunt trauma most often occurs at the duodenojejunal flexure. Clinical signs of injury may be minimal in the early stages, and a high index of suspicion is required. Small wounds can usually be sutured after debridement, but resec-

tion is indicated if damage is extensive or if the bowel has been devitalized by tears in its mesentery.

Large bowel. The large bowel is frequently damaged by penetrating wounds of the abdominal wall or perineum. Faecal contamination of the peritoneum is usual and the traumatized bowel is often devitalized. Primary suture is justified only if the wound is small, as in a knife wound. The damaged bowel is usually resected with exteriorization of the cut ends (Fig. 14.25). Intestinal continuity is restored at a later date following appropriate bowel preparation.

Injury to the pancreas

The pancreas may be damaged by penetrating or blunt abdominal trauma. Because of its fixed position as it crosses the vertebral column, the gland is at risk of injury from heavy blows to the upper abdomen and is especially vulnerable in the region of its neck (Fig. 14.26). Pancreatic injury is a particular risk in children suffering crush injuries such as blows to the epigastrium caused by bicycle handlebars. The close relationship of the pancreas to major blood vessels makes haemorrhage the major cause of death in pancreatic trauma. If blood and enzymes escape into the retroperitoneal tissues, a palpable swelling may be felt. Injuries to other organs may divert attention from the pancreas, which must always be carefully

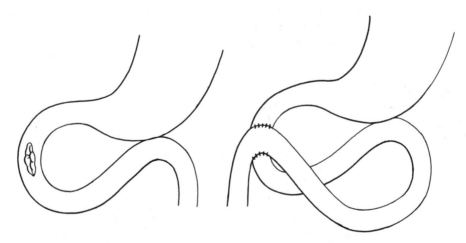

Fig. 14.24 Jejunal patch for duodenal tear

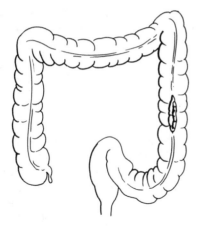
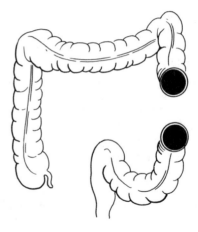

Fig. 14.25 Treatment of large bowel laceration

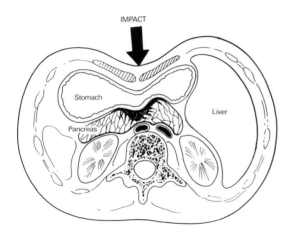

Fig. 14.26 Mechanism of pancreatic rupture

examined as part of an abdominal exploration for trauma.

Diagnosis. Diagnosis of pancreatic trauma may be difficult and abdominal signs are sparse in the early stages. The indication for laparotomy is often haemorrhage or rupture of another viscus. During the laparotomy it is vital that the pancreas is mobilized and carefully inspected. A rise in serum amylase after abdominal trauma suggests pancreatic injury and, if associated with increasing abdominal signs, necessitates laparotomy. Sometimes the diagnosis of pancreatic trauma is missed and the patient presents later with a pseudocyst.

Surgical treatment. Haemorrhage is first controlled to allow adequate examination of the gland.

Further management then depends on whether there is major duct injury. If there is no duct injury, adequate drainage of tissues surrounding the pancreas should be provided.

If the duct is damaged in the body and tail, distal pancreatectomy is indicated. If the head of the pancreas is badly damaged, pancreatico-duodenectomy may be needed, particularly if there is also major damage to the duodenum. If the duodenum is intact and haemorrhage can be controlled, it may be wiser to provide adequate drainage to the region and monitor progress. In many such patients the gland heals without serious dysfunction and further operation is unnecessary.

Injuries to the urinary tract

Blunt trauma to the flank may cause contusion, laceration or rupture of the kidney. Sporting injuries are a common cause of renal trauma. In motor traffic accidents, rapid deceleration, by throwing the kidney forward, may tear or transect the renal pedicle. Penetrating wounds of the kidney are relatively rare. On the other hand, damage to the ureter, although rare, is almost exclusively due to this cause.

The urinary bladder is susceptible to injury when distended. The degree of trauma required is usually severe and will have caused associated fractures of the pelvis. Rupture of an overfilled bladder may occur with relatively minor trauma. Rupture may be either into the peritoneal cavity (intraperitoneal) or, when the peritoneum remains intact, into the perivesical tissues (extraperitoneal). Extravasated urine spreads along the tissue planes and is limited only by fascial attachments. About 80% of extraperitoneal ruptures are associated with fracture of the pelvis.

Laceration or rupture of the male urethra may also complicate a fractured pelvis. This commonly affects the prostatic or membranous portions. Injury to the anterior urethra is less common and follows direct damage to the penis or perineum, classically as a result of a straddle injury. In contrast to injuries of the bladder, extravasation of urine is not prominent unless the sphincteric mechanism is disrupted.

The management of injuries to the urinary tract is fully discussed in Chapter 39.

INJURY TO THE EXTREMITIES

Most injuries to the extremities do not pose an immediate threat to life and, unless complicated by major haemorrhage, have a low priority in management. However, the injured limb should be immobilized to prevent further blood loss from movement at the fracture site.

Penetrating wounds are cleansed, debrided and explored. Meticulous cleansing minimizes the risk of infection; wide debridement prevents tetanus and gas gangrene; and exploration uncovers unsuspected injury to major vessels, nerves and tendons. The principles of wound management are discussed in Chapter 12.

Vascular injury

Almost 90% of all vascular injuries follow penetrating trauma. If major, they may threaten life by haemorrhage or threaten limb survival by devascularization.

Injury to an artery may result in contusion, laceration or transection. Contusion with occlusion of flow is due to damage of the intima and is the most common result of injury. Arterial lacerations usually continue to bleed, as the intact portion of the vessel prevents retraction. With transection, retraction can occur and bleeding may cease.

Venous injury may be due to penetrating trauma

or to compression and occlusion by adjacent arterial bleeding or soft tissue injury. Oedema and distal venous congestion may then obstruct arterial inflow and lead to gangrene. Penetrating wounds involving arteries or veins often lead to an arteriovenous fistula.

It is important in all injuries involving the limbs to evaluate the state of the peripheral circulation by checking peripheral pulses and temperature, and assessing pallor and capillary and venous filling. A cold, pale, pulseless limb indicates interruption of arterial blood supply and is easily recognized. It should never be mistaken for a sign of spasm in an injured vessel. It must also be remembered that the peripheral circulation is reduced by shock. Repeated assessment after resuscitation is therefore essential if vascular injuries are not to be misread. Haematomas are common after all injuries; if expanding or pulsatile, arterial injury must be suspected.

Principles of management

The principles of management of suspected vascular injuries are as follows.

1. Control of bleeding by application of direct pressure to the wound.

2. Resuscitation to relieve shock.

3. Evaluation of the vascular supply to the limbs.

4. If there is evidence of ischaemia, urgent angiography is indicated unless there are fractures and dislocations which may contribute to arterial damage, or there is a penetrating wound. In these patients immediate reduction of the fracture and/or exploration of the wound is essential. In others angiography will determine the need for action.

5. In closed fractures or dislocations which are associated with ischaemia, an angiogram should be obtained after reduction to confirm that the vascular supply is intact.

The management of individual vascular lesions is discussed in more detail in Chapter 21.

Fractures and dislocations

Fractures and dislocations, unless complicated by neural or vascular injury (see below), have a relatively low priority in the management of multiple injuries. Associated blood loss usually poses a more immediate problem, and temporary splinting of fractures can provide pain relief while more pressing injuries are assessed and treated.

Fractures and dislocations complicated by neural or vascular injury, although not life-threatening, constitute a serious threat to limb survival and function. Treatment is undertaken as soon as life-threatening injuries have been dealt with.

Compound fractures

Compound fractures are defined as fractures which communicate directly or indirectly with a body surface. All such fractures are potentially infected. All fractures caused by bullets· must be treated as compound fractures, however small the entry wound.

Treatment of compound fractures has a very high priority once life-threatening conditions have been attended to (see Table 14.1). Delayed or inadequate treatment may allow infection of the wound and fractured bone, leading to delayed or non-union and osteomyelitis.

Extensive debridement and meticulous cleansing of the wound are essential. Primary skin closure is preferred unless the viability of deeper tissues is in doubt or the wound is grossly contaminated. Reduction and immobilization of the fracture can usually be achieved immediately; internal fixation is inadvisable because of the risk of infection. Antibiotics are given routinely and prophylaxis against tetanus is essential (see Ch. 11).

Peripheral nerve injuries

Peripheral nerve injuries are usually the result of penetrating trauma, but can occur in association with fractures and dislocations.

Neuropraxia

This is the transient loss of physiological function after slight injury. There is no loss of nerve continuity and no nerve degeneration. The prognosis is excellent and recovery within 6 weeks is usual.

Treatment is the same as for axonotmesis (see below).

Axonotmesis

This more serious injury follows compression or traction damage. Continuity of the nerve sheath is maintained but there is Wallerian degeneration of nerve fibres distal to the point of injury. Recovery requires that the axons regenerate and grow down into the intact sheath. This can occur at a rate of 3–4 mm a day. Excessive fibrosis may hinder growth so that reinnervation is delayed and the final functional result less than perfect.

Both neuropraxia and axonotmesis are managed conservatively. Passive exercises and careful splinting prevent fixed contractures and preserve joint mobility. Protection of anaesthetic skin is essential. Sequential electrical testing of muscle activity and nerve conduction are used to monitor progress of return of function.

Neurotmesis

Neurotmesis denotes division of a nerve. It is usually caused by penetrating trauma but may result from fracture in blunt injury. Fibrous tissue forms between the divided nerve ends and, although the divided axons attempt to grow distally, reinnervation of end organs is unusual.

Complete interruption of nerve function causes loss of cutaneous sensation and flaccid paralysis in the area supplied by the affected nerve.

Operative repair is required if function is to be restored. Clean lacerations are repaired immediately by end-to-end suture of the nerve sheath. If the wound is contaminated, delayed nerve suture is preferred. The cut nerve ends are marked with non-absorbable sutures and secondary nerve suture is undertaken once the original wound has healed soundly, usually within 2–3 weeks. Nerve suture gives variable results in that fibrous tissue formation hinders growth of the axons. Many axons are diverted from their course and fail to enter the appropriate neurilemmal sheath. Taking into account the various periods of delay during initial recovery of nerve cell function and restoration of myoneural activity, the overall time for recovery is unlikely to be less than one day for each millimetre of growth required.

Limb replantation

Using microsurgical techniques it is now possible to replant an entire limb or one of its constituent parts. Digital replantation can be carried out if the severed digit is sound, and the big toe can be transferred to the hand to replace a severely damaged thumb. Replantation of the arm or leg is also feasible. The severed limb is immersed in a container of iced water to reduce metabolism, the arteries are perfused with a combination of low molecular weight dextran, heparin and saline, and operation is performed as soon as possible after resuscitation. These procedures are highly specialized and best results are achieved by teams specifically trained in their application.

15. Organ transplantation

The transplantation of simple and relatively inert tissues from one human to another is now an established technique. Avascular tissues such as cartilage and cornea survive well in a new host and are used freely by plastic and ophthalmic surgeons. More complex tissues such as arteries and bones survive initially but are slowly rejected or degenerate. For this reason non-biological materials such as silicone polymers, nylon and polyester (e.g Terylene), which elicit no reaction, are preferred for the provision of a conduit, valve or supporting structure.

Organ transplantation is much more complicated. To be successful, the organ must not only be accepted in its new environment, it must also remain capable of normal function. Although organ transplantation can theoretically be used to treat all manner of organ failure, technical and biological constraints limit its practical application to the kidney, liver, heart, lung and, more recently, the pancreas.

In this chapter the general principles of organ transplantation as applied to the kidneys will be discussed. The current status of liver, heart and other organ transplantation will be noted.

Bone marrow transplantation, now a recognized part of the treatment of lymphomas and some genetic abnormalities, is primarily a medical procedure and only briefly considered here.

RENAL TRANSPLANTATION

In the treatment of chronic renal failure, long-term dialysis and transplantation are complementary. In most renal centres, transplantation is regarded as the prime method of management. It allows full rehabilitation of the patient without reliance on a machine and the chance of long-term survival is greater than in those treated by chronic dialysis. Transplantation is also cheaper, demands less manpower, and frees dialysis machines for the long-term support of patients unsuitable for transplantation.

Sufficient donors are not yet available to meet the needs of all potential recipients. As a result many suitable patients are denied the opportunity of a transplant.

Successful renal transplantation depends on a number of factors. These include a good kidney, technical expertise, meticulous post-transplantation care of the patient, prompt recognition and management of complications, and control of the allograft reaction.

Preservation of donor kidneys

The more complex an organ, the less it can withstand deprivation of its blood supply. The time of deprivation is termed the 'total ischaemic time'. This is inversely proportional to the likelihood of speedy recovery of function following revascularization. The effect of ischaemia is markedly reduced by lowering the temperature of the organ. Pretreatment of the donor with heparin, adrenergic blockade and induction of a diuresis are desirable. Following removal of the kidney, it is immediately flushed out with 20 ml of 0.5% lignocaine together with 250 i.u. heparin at room temperature to relieve vessel spasm and prevent clotting. Perfusion with a chilled (5°C) electrolyte solution through the renal artery is then commenced and continued until the venous effluent is blood-free and the kidney surface pale.

The simplest method of storing the ischaemic

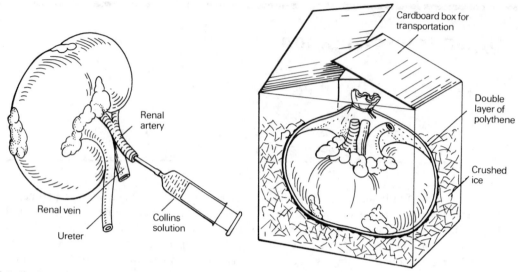

Fig. 15.1   Perfusion and storage of donor kidney

kidney is in a plastic container, immersed in the electrolyte solution used for perfusion. This is kept at 5°C by placing the container in crushed ice (Fig. 15.1).

Alternatively, especially if the time between loss of blood supply and cooling exceeds 45 minutes, the renal artery can be connected to a perfusion machine which allows continuous pulsatile hypothermic perfusion with a suitable colloid solution (usually albumin) to which nutrients and electrolytes have been added. The preferred solution is 4.5% albumin with added hydrocortisone, benzylpenicillin, magnesium, potassium and glucose at a flow rate of 100–300 ml/min and a temperature of 8°C. As these machines are portable, cold perfusion can be maintained during transport of the kidney.

The total ischaemic time is thus composed of a period of 'warm ischaemia' (i.e. the time from donor cardiac arrest to the time cold perfusion is started) and a period of 'cold ischaemia' (i.e. the time from the start of the cold perfusion to the time of connection of the graft to the recipient). Restoration of renal function is possible after a maximum of 1 hour of warm ischaemia and 4 days of cold ischaemia. For early onset of graft function (i.e. within 3 days of transplantation) the warm ischaemic time should not exceed 40 minutes, or the cold ischaemic time 8 hours. The transportation of

kidneys from a donor in one city or country to a recipient in another is now commonplace.

Source of donor kidneys

The type of donor and manner of death affect the warm ischaemic time and the state of the kidney. Preferably a donor should be young, fit, and not suffering from any condition likely to impair renal function. Most suitable donors have been involved in road traffic accidents.

For many years British practice determined that potential donors had to be pronounced dead from circulatory failure before the transplantation team could remove the kidney. The resultant delay meant that the limits of warm ischaemic time were frequently exceeded. For this reason the success rates of renal transplantation in this country were relatively poor. With the legal acceptance of 'brain death' and continuation of circulatory support until the donor organ is removed, ischaemic time should now be minimal. The diagnosis of brain death is not legally accepted in all countries, but is becoming the norm in those offering transplantation programmes. In recent years, kidneys from living donors have been increasingly used for transplantation. This has a number of advantages: graft survival is enhanced, transplantation can be arranged at an optimum time, the number of available organs is increased, and immunological matching is often more satisfactory. The mortality of unilateral nephrectomy is now less than 0.1% and there are no long-term sequelae of note.

The recipient

Clinical assessment includes a full physical examination, full blood count, and liver function tests to identify patients in whom cyclosporine metabolism may be abnormal. Antigen tests for hepatitis B and HIV are essential. Bladder function should also be assessed.

Before dialysis was readily available, recipients of renal transplants were often in poor general condition and liable to overhydration, anaemia, hyperkalaemia and acidosis. Dialysis now ensures that recipients are in better condition although fluid and electrolyte disturbances are still a problem. In patients with bilateral renal failure and hypertension or with chronic bilateral renal infection, bilateral nephrectomy used to be carried out before transplantation, but because of the high morbidity this is now indicated only in those with persistent upper urinary tract infection. Infections must be treated prior to transplantation and prophylactic antibiotic therapy instituted.

Pretransplant blood transfusion

The beneficial effect on graft survival of previous blood transfusion has now been confirmed in many centres. It is believed that this effect is due to generation of suppressor cell activity or an anti-idiotypic antibody. It was also thought that donor-specific blood transfusions (rather than those from random donors) might confer additional benefit, but this is now known not to be the case. Approximately 3–5 units of blood are usually given before admission for transplantation.

The operation

The operation itself is technically not difficult (Fig. 15.2). The new kidney is implanted in an extraperitoneal pocket in the iliac fossa. The renal artery is anastomosed first, either end-to-end to the internal iliac artery or end-to-side to the external iliac artery. The renal vein is then implanted

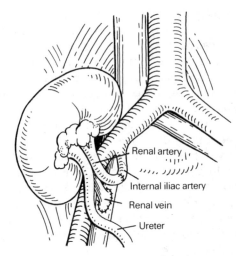

Fig. 15.2 Anastomoses in renal transplantation

into the side of the external iliac vein and the ureter is implanted into the bladder.

The allograft reaction

The main obstacle to renal transplantation in the past was the allograft reaction which, if uncontrolled, led to rejection of the organ. The first recorded allograft rejection was in a young boy who had received his mother's kidney (in 1952 in Paris). Foreign antigens from donor kidney cells sensitize the host, who then mounts a cell-bound and humoral attack on the foreign organ. In the absence of continuous immunosuppressive therapy, a transplanted organ will survive only if identical in antigenic composition to the host tissues. This situation is found only in identical twins. The first successful kidney transplantation was performed in identical twins in 1954 in Boston.

Although blood group antigens of ABO type are carried on all cells and affect graft survival, the main histocompatibility antigens are of the HLA series. So far four loci have been defined (A, B, C, DR), each of which carries many separate alleles. In all, some 150 different antigens have been recognized. Most belong to the HLA-A and HLA-B subgroups. There are two main classes of HLA antigens: class I, which are present on all cells except erythrocytes; and class II, which are present only on B lymphocytes and other antigen-presenting cells, including activated T cells. It is these latter, class II, antigens which initiate the immunological cascade to activate cytotoxic T cells, which are of prime importance in acute rejection. Specific typing sera are obtained from parous women and used to determine HLA type of donor and recipient (Fig. 15.3).

In the past, tissue compatibility was also tested by culturing lymphocytes from the prospective donor with those of the recipient (mixed lymphocyte culture) to see whether activation led to the formation of blast cells. This test is no longer routinely performed. However, the degree of sensitivity of the recipient can be assessed by using a panel of T and B lymphocytes to test for circulating antibodies.

Although ideally a perfect match should be achieved in all cases, the number of tissue antigens makes this a practical impossibility except in identical twins. When using a living donor it is essential that at least two HLA antigens belonging to HLA-A and B subgroups are correctly matched. Good matching is less important for cadaver kidneys but a two-antigen match (one in each main subgroup) is preferred. Compatibility of ABO blood groups between recipient and donor is always sought.

Immunosuppression

Until recently the standard drugs used to suppress immune reaction in the recipient were azathioprine (Imuran) and prednisone. Azathioprine inhibits lymphocyte proliferation and suppresses both

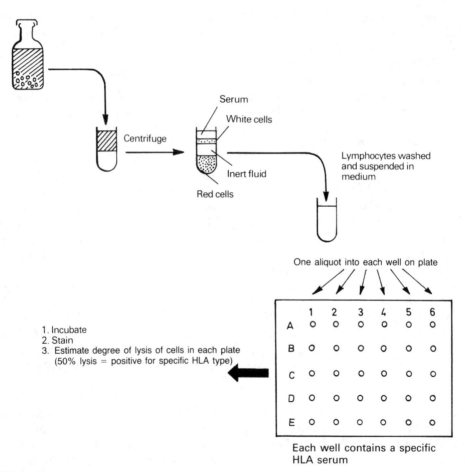

Fig. 15.3 HLA typing

cellular and humoral immunity. It is given in large doses (5 mg/kg per day) for the first few days after transplantation and then gradually reduced to a maintenance dose of around 2 mg/kg per day. The dose of azathioprine is adjusted to keep white cell counts around $8 \times 10^9/l$. Overdosage leads to diminished graft function.

Glucocorticoids have a complementary effect and many consider that prednisone is the most important adjunct to transplantation. It inhibits synthesis of immunoglobulins and reduces the effect of antigen-antibody complexes on the enzyme systems of the transplanted organ. The initial dose of 200 mg per day is gradually reduced to a maintenance dose, which should be kept as low as possible (10–15 mg/day).

The development of cyclosporine, a new immunosuppressive agent of fungal origin, has been a major breakthrough in transplant surgery. By blocking humoral and cellular effector mechanisms it interferes with lymphocyte activation, 'blunting' the overall effect of T cell proliferation. The liberation of suppressor-cell inducing factors is not affected, so that a 'tolerant' state is induced. The introduction of this agent has increased 1-year cadaver graft survival from 50 to 90%, but as it is itself nephrotoxic and hepatotoxic, some surgeons prefer to change immunosuppressive therapy to azathioprine after 3 months. Cyclosporine is now the drug of choice for immunosuppression at the time of transplantation. It is given initially by continuous infusion but converted to oral administration after a few days. Blood levels are monitored. It is usually combined with prednisolone.

Other methods of enhancing immunosuppression include antilymphocytic serum, antilymphocytic globulin and extracorporeal irradiation of the recipient's blood. Monoclonal antibodies to lymphocyte determinants are now also available.

Following transplantation, the new kidney does not function for a few days. Copious quantities of dilute urine are then passed as the graft gradually reassumes full function. Provided maintenance immunosuppressive therapy is satisfactory, function should continue for many years. 'Rejection crises' may occur from time to time (see below).

Complications of renal transplantation

Renal transplantation is likely to be followed by a number of complications. These relate mainly to the previous ill-health of the patient and to the need for continuous immunosuppressive therapy.

1. Bacterial, viral and fungal infections are frequent and occur at some time in 40% of transplant recipients. Early recognition and prompt treatment are essential.

2. As many of the patients accepted for transplantation have systemic arterial disease and advanced uraemia, cardiovascular and cerebrovascular complications are common (25% of cases) and account for one-third of deaths. Pulmonary embolism is also common. For some reason this is more frequent when the warm ischaemic time has been prolonged.

3. Gastrointestinal complications include peptic ulceration, gastrointestinal haemorrhage, pancreatitis and hyperamylasaemia. In patients with a previous history of peptic ulceration, acid secretion should be reduced prophylactically by administration of an H_2-receptor blocker such as cimetidine.

4. Like other patients receiving long-term steroid therapy, renal transplant patients develop metabolic complications such as diabetes and osteoporosis. The maintenance dose of steroid should therefore be kept as low as possible.

5. Hypercalcaemia is a particular problem. Secondary hyperparathyroidism is common during the period of renal failure and frequently develops into a 'tertiary' autonomous phase unrelieved by correction of the renal state. Patients with severe hypercalcaemia should be treated by subtotal parathyroidectomy before a new kidney is transplanted.

6. Long-term immunosuppressive therapy increases the risk of developing cancer. Malignant disease develops in approximately 7% of transplant patients and may affect any site. Reticulum cell lymphoma of the brain is particularly common; its incidence in transplant patients is 250 times that of the normal population.

7. The operation itself may give rise to complications which may threaten the graft. These include anastomotic haemorrhage, ischaemia with

non-function of the kidney, and ureteric leakage. Lymphatic leakage with the formation of lymphoceles, renal artery stenosis and outflow obstruction are late complications which demand prompt attention to avert graft failure.

8. Long-term function of the graft may be impaired by several factors, including primary glomerular disease, urinary tract obstruction, and graft rejection. The latter is the most important cause, prevention of which depends on continuous successful immunosuppressive therapy.

Graft rejection

Three types of rejection are described.

1. *Hyperacute rejection* is due to the presence in the recipient of circulating antibodies to donor antigen and occurs immediately after the operation, usually within 24–48 hours. Graft function ceases, the kidney becomes swollen and tender and there is fever, leucocytosis and thrombocytopenia. Sensitive cross-matching and testing for circulating cytotoxic antibodies have virtually eliminated this complication, which is generally refractory to treatment.

2. *Acute rejection* most commonly occurs during the first month after transplantation and is a cell-mediated reaction. The patient usually recognizes its onset by feeling unwell, with flu-like symptoms. The other clinical features depend on the type of immunosuppressive therapy used. In patients treated with azathioprine there is fever, graft tenderness and deterioration of renal function with falling urine volume, hypertension and rising creatinine concentration. In those receiving cyclosporine, these symptoms are attenuated, so that functional impairment over a few days, mild hypertension and occasional fever may be the only signs. As these may be confused with the nephrotoxic effects of cyclosporine, measurement of cyclosporine levels and needle biopsy of the graft are necessary investigations.

Acute rejection is treated by parenteral administration of steroids or, if resistant, by anti-lymphocytic globulin or monoclonal antibodies.

3. *Chronic rejection* is a late phenomenon. There is gradual deterioration in graft function, together with proteinuria and hypertension.

Careful monitoring of graft function is essential following transplantation, and should include measurement of urine volume and serum creatinine; ultrasonography to detect urinary obstruction; scintigraphy to study renal blood flow and tubular function; and sequential fine-needle aspiration to assess the inflammatory response. Facilities for these investigations should be available in every transplant unit. Monitoring of the immunological response is an important adjunct.

Results of renal transplantation

The results of renal transplantation in any centre depend on the availability of good kidneys with minimal periods of warm ischaemia, recipients in good health, reasonable matching and, cyclosporine therapy. With cadaveric transplantation, 80–90% of grafts survive for one year and 70% for three years. Even better results are obtained with related living donors. If function of the graft is well stabilized at three years, prospects of prolonged survival are excellent, particularly if the patient is under 50 years of age and has no cardiovascular disease.

LIVER TRANSPLANTATION

While dialysis has been outstandingly successful in renal failure, there is no easy way of removing noxious substances from the circulation in patients with liver failure. Attempts have been made to remove these substances by dialysis over dextran-coated charcoal, but with disappointing results. Alternatively, an animal liver can be connected extracorporeally to the patient to serve as a 'dialysis machine'. Experimentally, baboon livers have been shown to carry out both synthetic and excretory functions on prolonged perfusion without immunological or other clinical reaction. Studies in man are still limited. Other approaches include the establishment of cross-circulation with a living baboon, a human volunteer, or a cadaver human liver.

Surprisingly, the lack of an effective 'artificial' liver has not proved to be an obstacle to the development of liver transplantation, which, with the introduction of cyclosporine, has become an acceptable form of therapy for all benign causes of

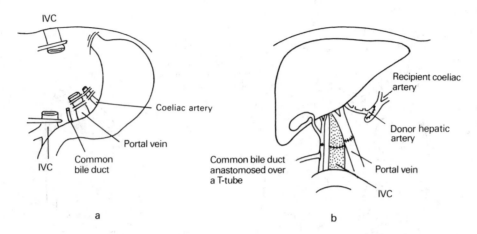

Fig. 15.4 Liver transplantation. (a) Liver removed from recipient with section of the inferior vena cava (IVC). (b) Orthotopic liver transplant with drainage of bile via choledochodochostomy over a T-tube

liver failure. These include post-necrotic cirrhosis, sclerosing cholangitis, primary biliary cirrhosis, Budd-Chiari syndrome, biliary atresia, and some inborn errors of metabolism in infants and children. Liver transplantation is now rarely performed for hepatocellular carcinoma or cholangiocarcinoma (which are better treated by resection when possible) and is usually regarded as contraindicated in alcoholics.

The technique of liver transplantation is now well established. Because of its size, the new liver is best placed orthotopically, i.e. in the bed of the excised organ (Fig. 15.4). Heterotopic transplantation is also described. The regenerative powers of the liver are great so that even small remnants can attain normal liver function. Most postoperative problems are due to stasis in the biliary tract, with accumulation of sludge and, in some cases, a biliary fistula from a leaking anastamosis.

HEART TRANSPLANTATION

Heart transplantation is now regularly performed in this country. In one centre alone, over 1000 transplants have been carried out so far. The heart must be removed from the donor while still beating, which is now legally permissible in brain-dead individuals maintained on a respirator. Initially, long-term survival was poor, but with the introduction of cyclosporine it has improved dramatically and now equals that of kidneys.

It is important that the warm ischaemic time is kept as short as possible. After clamping of the vena cava, cold cardioplegic solution is infused into the aortic root to cool the heart and induce diastolic arrest. The heart is then removed and immersed in cold (4°C) saline solution, which is kept cold by storing the container in ice. It should be reimplanted within 3–4 hours.

The recipient's heart is excised, leaving a shell of right and left atrial walls posteriorly to which the new heart is anastamosed. The pulmonary artery and aorta are reconnected (Fig. 15.5). On receiving coronary flow, rhythmic activity restarts, although initial fibrillation may require electric shock defibrillation. In some patients a pacemaker may also be required.

Endocardial biopsy through a cardiac catheter is used to monitor suspected rejection, although with cyclosporine therapy this is now rare.

LUNG TRANSPLANTATION

For the treatment of respiratory failure, single-lung transplantation is unsatisfactory, as it leaves an end-diseased lung in situ which causes shunting and imbalance of ventilation and perfusion. Further, the transplanted bronchus has no blood supply and leakage at the site of anastamosis is a problem. These disadvantages are avoided by using a combined heart-lung transplant which provides a circulation to the bronchi through the

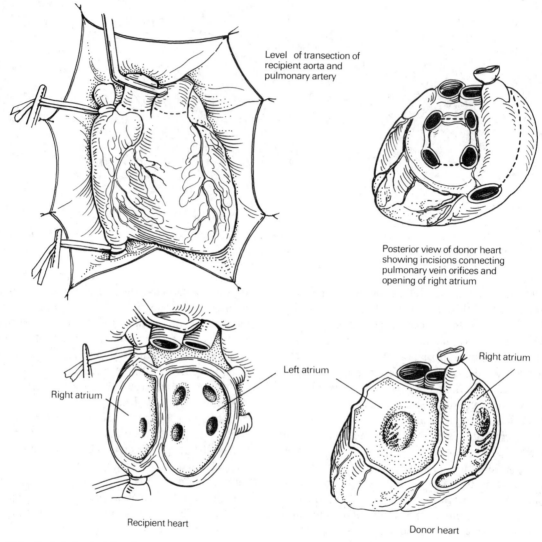

Level of transection of
recipient aorta and
pulmonary artery

Posterior view of donor heart
showing incisions connecting
pulmonary vein orifices and
opening of right atrium

Right atrium

Left atrium

Right atrium

Recipient heart

Donor heart

Fig. 15.5   Technical principles of cardiac transplantation

coronary-bronchial anastamoses. This procedure is now the preferred transplant option for irreversible and terminal pulmonary failure with or without cardiac involvement; initial results are encouraging.

PANCREATIC TRANSPLANTATION

In insulin-dependent diabetic patients, insulin therapy controls the day-to-day needs for carbohydrate. Although its use prolongs life, it does not prevent the long-term complications of the disease. It is believed that this is due to failure to restore the control of homeostatic responses which require variations in the secretion of insulin over short periods of time. The availability of genetically manufactured human insulin and micropumps which can alter dosage according to need may improve the situation, but at present patients with insulin-dependent diabetes are 25 times more prone to blindness, 17 times more prone to renal disease, 5 times more prone to gangrene and 2 times more prone to heart disease than the general population. Transplantation of functioning islet tissue is therefore of therapeutic relevance. This may be achieved by a free vascularized graft of the pancreas or by the infusion of isolated resuspended islets. Only the former is of proven value in man.

Either the whole pancreas can be transplanted or a segment of body and tail. The blood supply is connected to the iliac vessels, and the exocrine secretions are diverted either into a loop of bowel or into the urinary tract. Alternatively, the duct system can be injected with a polymer to seal it. Graft survivals of 60% at one year (up to 80% in living HLA-identical siblings) have been reported.

Grafts of pancreatic islet cells, obtained by dispersal of the human pancreas following the injection of collagenase into the duct system, can reverse diabetes in rodents but not yet in man. A potential advantage is that they can be implanted in privileged sites (e.g. within the testicle, under the renal capsule or enclosed in an artificial membrane) in which rejection is less likely to occur.

SMALL INTESTINE

Transplantation of the small intestine has been at-tempted for treating mesenteric vascular occlusion, massive volvulus, and short bowel syndrome following multiple resections. Even with cyclosporine, there have only been a few long-term survivors in animal experiments. The problem is the large quantity of lymphatic tissue in the small gut which causes graft-versus-host disease, and the inability to restore the gut's complex motor and hormonal functions.

BONE MARROW TRANSPLANTATION

The experimental finding that mice could be protected against lethal irradiation by intravenous infusion of marrow cells suggested that bone marrow transplantation might be used for victims of radiation accidents and patients with immunological deficiency disorders. Bone marrow transplants are also used to treat severe aplastic anaemia and to facilitate the treatment of leukaemia by whole-body irradiation or high-dose chemotherapy. As bone marrow contains immunologically competent cells, the problems of histocompatibility are compounded by reaction of donor cells against host tissues. This syndrome of graft-versus-host disease may affect the skin, gastrointestinal tract and liver. It presents as a skin rash, followed in a few days

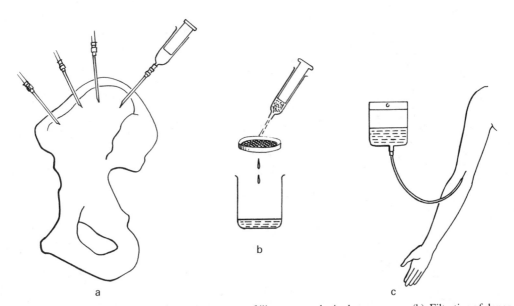

Fig. 15.6 Bone marrow transplantation. (a) Multiple puncture of iliac crest to obtain donor marrow. (b) Filtration of donor marrow and addition to heparin. (c) Intravenous infusion of processed marrow

by diarrhoea, abdominal pain and distension, and an increase in liver enzymes. Diagnosis is confirmed by skin biopsy.

Bone marrow cells are obtained by multiple aspirations from the iliac crests of histocompatible donors and are sieved to make a single-cell suspension which is infused intravenously (Fig. 15.6). As, following colonization of the marrow, it takes some 3 weeks before function is restored, the patient will be leucopenic and thrombocytopenic in the interval and will require platelet and granulocyte infusions. Infection is a major hazard and special care must be taken to protect the patient by isolation in a laminar-flow ventilated room and administration of broad spectrum antibiotics. Viral interstitial pneumonia poses a continuing threat. Patients with an immunodeficiency syndrome need no immunosuppressive therapy but all others will have to be immunosuppressed, usually with cyclophosphamide methotrexate. Graft-versus-host disease is treated with antilymphocytic globulin and cyclosporine.

Prevention of graft-versus-host disease by prior irradiation of the marrow is currently under study; ultraviolet radiation has recently been described to be effective in experimental animals.

16. Principles of surgery for cancer

THE NATURE OF A NEOPLASM

A neoplasm or new growth consists of a mass of cells which proliferate in an atypical and relentless way, and serve no useful function. The mechanism by which this abnormal activity is induced is not known; a prime event is the induction of change in genetic protein by a virus or other carcinogens. Amino acid sequences identical to those found in transforming viruses have been identified in the genome of normal cells. If activated, these 'oncogenes' may induce transformation and therefore initiate the first step in the formation of a neoplasm.

Neoplastic transformation of cells does not necessarily result in a tumour. Transformations occur continuously, but because of immune surveillance or simple wastage, i.e. loss of cells from the surface, mutant cells are destroyed before they proliferate. For persistence of growth these protective mechanisms must break down to allow the neoplastic cells to reproduce within the tissues of their host. It may also be that for the formation of a tumour the stem cells must be transformed so that they can constantly replicate in mutant form (Fig. 16.1).

Environmental agents in the host are also needed for the 'promotion' of tumour growth. A good example are the 'hormone-dependent' cancers such as those of the breast, prostate and endometrium, which require a 'correct' balance of hormones secreted from the endocrine glands of the host for their continued growth (Fig. 16.2).

Types of neoplasms

Neoplasms may be *benign* or *malignant*. The essential difference is the capacity to invade and metastasize. The cells of benign tumours do not invade surrounding tissues but remain as a local

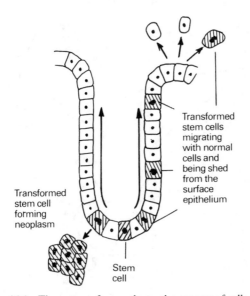

Fig. 16.1 The nature of a neoplasm: the concept of cells transforming and either being released to the surface or forming a tumour

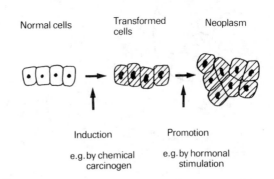

Fig. 16.2 Induction and promotion of tumour growth

conglomerate. Malignant tumours are invasive, and their cells enter blood and lymphatic channels to be deposited in remote sites. These deposits form 'secondary' or 'metastatic' tumours similar in cell type to the original, 'primary', site. Malignant tumours are fatal because of their ability to metastasize.

The distinction between simple and malignant tumours is fundamentally clinical, but must be confirmed by histopathological examination.

Tumours are also classified according to:

1. tissue of origin, e.g. skin, gastrointestinal tract, breast, lung or nervous system;

2. gross appearance, e.g. ulcerating, proliferating, fungating, cicatrizing; and

3. microscopic appearance and cellular origin: tumours arising from epithelial or endothelial cells are known as *adenomas* if benign and as *carcinomas* if malignant; those from mesenchymal or connective tissues are named after their tissue of origin, e.g. *lipoma, fibroma, myoma, angioma* if benign, and *liposarcoma, fibrosarcoma, myosarcoma, angiosarcoma* if malignant.

Mechanisms of spread

Traditionally, a malignant tumour was believed to spread initially by local *permeation*, i.e. by direct centrifugal extension along tissue spaces and by *embolization* of lymphatics to the regional lymph nodes. Metastasis to these regional lymph nodes was regarded as the first step in the dissemination of a tumour which thus could be contained as a regional disease. The second step, that of dissemination by the blood stream, followed later (Fig. 16.3).

It was this theory which led to the general belief that cancer was 'curable' provided that it had not spread beyond the regional nodes, and to the development of 'curative' radical operations designed to eradicate all malignant cells in the primary tumour and its related lymph nodes.

This theory is no longer tenable. It is now believed that even at the earliest stage tumour cells invade both the lymphatic and the blood vessels which carry them to regional and distant sites to form widespread micrometastases. Regional lymph node involvement is no longer regarded as a stage in the progression of the disease but as an indicator that widespread dissemination has occurred (Fig. 16.4). It is this concept which has led to a reappraisal of the role of local treatment, and to recognition of the need for systemic treatment for long-term control of the disease.

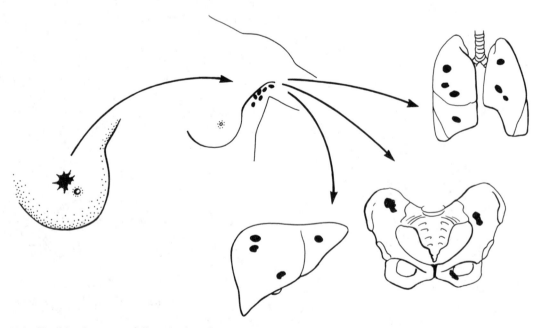

Fig. 16.3 Traditional concept of dissemination of cancer

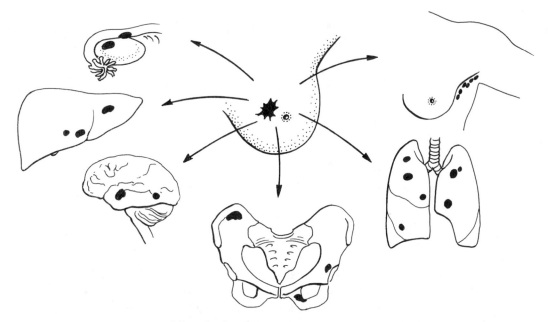

Fig. 16.4 Modern 'explosive' concept of dissemination of cancer

The mechanisms of invasion and metastasis are obscure (Fig. 16.5). Malignant cells secrete a number of factors or 'tumour-secretory' products which may determine their biological behaviour and promote growth both at primary and metastatic sites. Examples are the 'angiogenesis factor', which stimulates surrounding capillary growth; proteolytic enzymes, which digest surrounding fibrous tissue; and prostaglandins, which induce osteolysis and allow development of skeletal deposits.

The natural history of a tumour is also related to its growth rate. Some tumours grow rapidly, and quickly outpace the resistance of normal tissues. Others are slow-growing and years may pass before deposits reach a size which threatens normal tissue function. The reason for this difference is ill-understood but the degree of differentiation of the tumour cells is one relevant factor. Tumours which histologically are composed of primitive 'anaplastic' cells are more aggressive than well differentiated tumours. A whole host of cellular functions have now been identified which influence the likely behaviour of a tumour and can be used to determine its prognosis.

Natural history and estimate of cure

Benign tumours rarely threaten the life of the patient. They are usually self-limiting but may cause functional abnormalities.

Because they invade and metastasize, malignant tumours relentlessly replace normal tissues, causing destruction of supporting structures, disturbance of function, and eventually death. Calculations based on an exponential model of growth suggest that three-quarters of the lifespan of a tumour is spent in a 'preclinical' or occult stage (Fig. 16.6) and that the clinical manifestations of

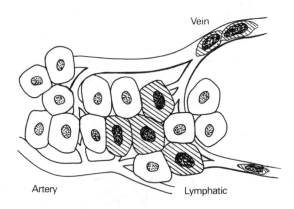

Fig. 16.5 Mechanism of invasion

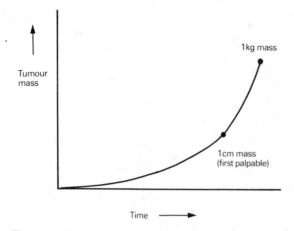

Fig. 16.6   Exponential model of tumour growth

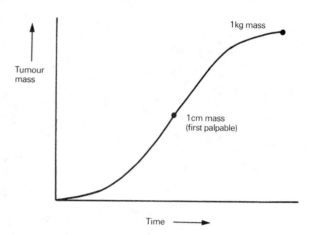

Fig. 16.7   Gompertzian model of tumour growth

the disease are limited to the final quarter. The number of cell divisions (or 'doublings') which can take place is finite. The duration of the 'doubling time', i.e. the time needed for each cell to duplicate itself, determines the total duration of a tumour, assuming that this time remains constant. It is estimated that 45 doublings are required for a single cell to grow into a tumour of 1 cm in diameter, and that a further 15 doublings will result in a tumour of 1 kg (1 billion cells), which is likely to be fatal. The faster the cell cycle, i.e. the shorter the time between each doubling, the more rapid is the course of the disease and the shorter the expected survival.

These estimates of tumour growth do not take account of the variations which may occur as a result of periods of accelerated or retarded growth. It is now believed that the best mathematical model for tumour growth is not exponential but 'Gompertzian' (Fig. 16.7).

Definition of cure and survival

For cure every malignant cell must be eradicated. Not only should there be no recurrent tumour during the patient's lifetime, there should also be no evidence of residual tumour at death. This rigid definition of curability can rarely be applied. A normal duration of life without further clinical evidence of disease is generally accepted as evidence of cure even though microscopic deposits of tumour may still be present.

'Cure' rates of individual cancers are assessed by survival rates at various times after treatment. Conventionally, 5 and 10 year intervals are used. Cumulative survival curves (life-tables) can be constructed for individual cancers and compared with those of age-matched healthy subjects of the same population (Fig. 16.8). Divergence of these two curves indicates that patients with cancer are dying faster than their normal counterparts, while parallel curves indicate that patients with the disease are dying at no greater a rate than their age-matched controls. The point after primary treatment at which these two curves become parallel is the time at which statistical cure can be assumed.

Cure rates vary according to the aggressiveness of the disease and the success of treatment. In

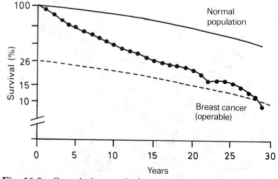

Fig. 16.8   Cumulative survival curve in operable breast cancer (●–●–●). At 20 years the curve begins to parallel that of the normal population. (From Brinkley & Heybittle 1981, Yorkshire Breast Cancer Group Symposium)

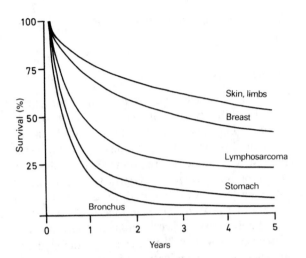

Fig. 16.9 Survival curves for different malignant neoplasms

some cancers, e.g. those of the stomach and lung, metastases grow rapidly and cause death within a few years of clinical presentation of the disease. In others, e.g. cancer of the breast and melanoma, many years may elapse before metastatic spread becomes evident and even when metastases have occurred life may be long (Fig. 16.9). It is for this reason that five-year survival rates cannot provide a satisfactory estimate of cure for all tumours.

Many regard the treatment of a malignant tumour as a matter of extreme urgency. When one considers the natural duration of a cancer, a week or two spent in careful investigation and planning of treatment is good practice. However, this period must not be unduly delayed: patients with cancer are naturally worried and wish their initial treatment to be completed within a reasonable time. But, equally, time spent on counselling is usually well spent.

THE MANAGEMENT OF CANCER

There are three main steps in the management of the patient with cancer.

1. Diagnosis of the disease
2. Determination of its extent (staging)
3. Treatment.

In many cancers it is also important to know the histological type of the tumour and the presence or absence of functional biological markers.

CLINICAL FEATURES AND DIAGNOSIS

Benign tumours often remain unrecognized during life or may cause symptoms due to local or general effects.

Malignant tumours vary in their clinical effects. Some cause a rapidly progressing and debilitating illness; in others local effects predominate.

Local effects

A tumour which lies on the body surface or within a hollow viscus may bleed or discharge excess mucus or pus. In the gastrointestinal tract diarrhoea is often a manifestation.

A hollow viscus or duct may be obstructed. Bronchial obstruction and pulmonary collapse can be caused by a tumour of the lung, intestinal obstruction by a tumour of the bowel, and jaundice by a tumour of the bile ducts or pancreas.

A tumour within a closed space may cause pressure symptoms. For example, increased intracranial pressure may complicate intracerebral tumours, and paraplegia may result from a tumour of the spinal cord. Invasion of an organ by tumour may compromise its normal functions and cause organ failure. Invasion of tissues such as the pancreas, bone or nerves can cause severe pain. A cancer can also mimic the pain of benign disease. For example, cancer of the stomach can produce dyspeptic symptoms similar to those of a benign ulcer.

Systemic effects

Anorexia, asthenia, lassitude and general debility are classical symptoms of cancer. In part these may be explained by chronic anaemia or inanition, but secretion of abnormal proteins and peptides by the tumour is also believed to contribute, for example by inhibiting appetite.

The secretory products of some tumours produce characteristic clinical syndromes. These products may be appropriate to the organ of origin (Fig. 16.10). A tumour of the adrenal cortex may secrete excess corticosteroid and cause Cushing's syndrome; a parathyroid tumour may secrete excess parathormone and cause hypercalcaemia; while an islet cell tumour of the pancreas may secrete excess insulin and cause hypoglycaemia.

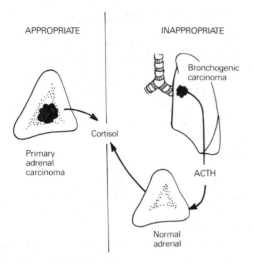

Fig. 16.10 Examples of appropriate and inappropriate tumour secretion

Secretory products may also be inappropriate to the site of a tumour (Fig. 16.10). Such 'ectopic' secretion occurs predominantly in tumours of neuroendocrine origin and produces a variety of endocrine syndromes (Table 16.1).

Clinical signs

A tumour on the surface of the body is obviously visible; those within a body cavity or hollow viscus may be seen through an endoscope. Tumours of subcutaneous tissues or superficial organs, e.g. the breast, may form a visible swelling but are more likely to be found by palpation.

Many tumours are without clinical signs. Lying deep within the body, they are best diagnosed by imaging techniques. Simple radiology may demonstrate a soft tissue tumour, e.g. of the lung or bone, but for tumours of the stomach or intestine barium and/or air contrast studies are necessary. For some deep-seated tumours, e.g. of the pancreas or brain, other methods of imaging are needed. These include angiography, radioactive scintiscans, ultrasonography, computerized tomography and magnetic resonance imaging.

Tumours may also cause functional disturbances which can often be demonstrated by the resultant physical (e.g. electroencephalographic) or biochemical abnormalities. For example, abnormal liver function may indicate invasion of the liver by tumour.

Presymptomatic diagnosis

It is now recognized that by the time a tumour is first clinically apparent it may already be far advanced. This has led to the introduction of 'screening' of normal populations, with the result that many tumours are now diagnosed at a presymptomatic stage. Air contrast barium studies and endoscopy can be used to detect mucosal cancers of the stomach; mammography to detect impalpable breast cancer; cytological examination of urinary deposits to detect cancer of the bladder; and cytological examination of vaginal secretions to detect cancer of the cervix. As screening is costly, its effectiveness and cost must be critically evaluated before routine use. In the UK cervical cytology and mammographic screening are available as a national service.

Histological diagnosis

Neoplastic disease can be detected cytologically, e.g. by the demonstration of malignant cells in secretions, in washings, from hollow viscera or in needle aspirates. However, a definitive histological diagnosis is required in most cases of suspected cancer. No major mutilating procedure for cancer should ever be carried out without cytological or histological proof of malignant disease. The suggestion that a preliminary biopsy can facilitate the spread of cancer is not supported by fact, and punch, needle and drill biopsies are now established techniques (see Ch. 6).

Initial cytohistological diagnosis allows further investigation and treatment of the disease to be planned on the basis of a proven diagnosis.

STAGING

The aim of 'staging' is to define the extent of the disease and assess its likely prognosis. The International Union against Cancer (UICC) has described a system of staging (TNM) in which three components of the disease are assessed. These are the extent of the primary tumour (T), the absence or presence and extent of metastases

Table 16.1 Ectopic hormone production

Hormone produced	Neoplasms responsible	Main clinical features
ACTH, MSH (adrenocorticotropic hormone, melanocyte stimulating hormone	1. Oat-cell carcinoma of lung 2. Non-beta islet-cell carcinoma 3. Carcinoma of pancreas 4. Thymomas 5. Carcinoid tumours 6. Other: tumours of thyroid, adrenal cortex, liver, prostate, breast, ovary, parotid, phaeochromocytoma, paragangliomas, gangliomas	Cushing syndrome: hypertension, hypokalaemia, oedema, acne and hirsutism (in women), impaired glucose tolerance, occasionally obesity and striae. Dark pigmentation.
LH (luteinizing hormone)	1. Hepatoma 2. Mediastinal teratoma 3. Various lung tumours	Precocious puberty in children. Gynaecomastia in men
ADH (antidiuretic hormone)	1. Carcinoma of lung 2. Carcinoma of duodenum 3. Carcinoma of pancreas	Weakness, confusion, incoordination, nausea and vomiting; hyponatraemia (part dilutional, part secondary to increased urinary sodium loss; plasma osmolality <260 mmol/l)
PTH (parathyroid hormone)	Carcinomas of lung, pancreas, liver, colon, adrenal, parotid, ovary, vagina, uterus, bladder and kidney	Lethargy, weakness, nausea, vomiting, confusion, coma progressing to death; short Q-T interval on ECG and arrhythmias; peripheral neuropathy; rarely, bone resorption and renal calculi
TSH (thyroid stimulating hormone)	1. Choriocarcinoma 2. Hydatidiform mole	Symptoms of hyperthyroidism, e.g. tremor tachycardia, sweating, weight loss
Insulin	1. Malignant bronchial carcinoid 2. Fibrosarcoma; liposarcoma	Attacks of tachycardia, sweating, tremor, loss of concentration and diplopia, especially during fasting; relieved by carbohydrate ingestion
Erythropoietin	1. Phaeochromocytoma 2. Hepatoma 3. Cerebellar haemangioma	Raised red-cell mass, features of polycythaemia, headache, high blood pressure, ruddy face, DVT

DVT = deep venous thrombosis

in regional lymph nodes (N), and the absence or presence of distant metastases (M). The addition of numbers to each of these three components indicates the extent of malignant disease.

In the initial TNM system only clinical, radiological and endoscopic investigations were used (Table 16.2). Such clinical staging is still important in defining the extent of local disease, but its value in detecting the extent of metastatic spread is limited. For example, the palpability of regional lymph nodes is a poor indicator of their involvement by tumour. Impalpable nodes may still contain metastases, while palpable nodes are not necessarily involved by tumour. Reactive hyperplasia in regional lymph nodes occurs with many tumours. Lymphangiography may aid in the detection of metastases in regional nodes in some types of cancer, but, in general, histological assessment is the only certain method. Similarly, small deposits of tumour in viscera and bones cannot be detected by routine radiology. Even the resolution of radioisotope scintiscans, ultrasonograms and CT scans is insufficient to detect small deposits. Many patients who on clinical and radiological grounds appear to have localized disease (M0; see Table 16.2) have in fact unrecognized widespread microscopic deposits of a tumour. For this reason the TNM system has now been modified to include

Table 16.2 TNM pre-treatment classification (post-treatment histopathological classifications have also been defined)

T — Primary tumour

Tis	Pre-invasive carcinoma (carcinoma-in-situ)
T0	No evidence of primary tumour
T1, T2, T3, T4	Evidence of increasing degrees of size and/or local extent of primary tumour
TX	The minimum requirements to assess the primary tumour cannot be met

N — Regional lymph nodes

N0	No evidence of regional lymph node involvement
N1, N2, N3	Evidence of increasing degrees of involvement of regional lymph nodes
N4	Evidence of involvement of juxtaregional lymph nodes (where applicable)
NX	The minimum requirements to assess the regional lymph nodes cannot be met

M — Distant metastases

M0	No evidence of distant metastases
M1	Evidence of distant metastases

Pulmonary:	PUL	Bone marrow:	MAR
Osseous:	OSS	Pleura:	PLE
Hepatic:	HEP	Peritoneum:	PER
Brain:	BRA	Skin:	SKI
Lymph nodes:	LYM	Other:	OTH

MX	The minimum requirements to assess the presence of distant metastases cannot be met

not only a pre-treatment clinical classification but also a post-surgical histopathological classification denoted pTNM. Excision of regional lymph nodes is one way to provide such information. In some tumours even more accurate staging is possible by additional surgical procedures. For example, assessment of lymphomas may now include bone and marrow sampling and a full laparotomy, at which the spleen is removed for histological examination and biopsies are taken of retroperitoneal lymph nodes and liver. In some melanomas and skin tumours, and in cancer of the bladder and large bowel, histological assessment of the depth of penetration provides important information about the extent and prognosis of the disease.

Biochemical 'markers' which reflect functional abnormalities from invasion of organs or tissues are seldom helpful. Although metastases in the liver may cause elevation of liver enzymes, and metastases in bone an increase in urinary excretion of collagen breakdown products (hydroxyproline), such tests are rarely of value in detecting occult

metastatic disease. Of more importance are specific markers of tumour burden (Table 16.3) which can be used to detect residual tumour after removal of the primary lesion. These are available for prostatic cancer (acid phosphatase), chorionic carcinoma (human chorionic gonadotrophin; HCG) and to some extent for cancer of the colon (carcinoembryonic antigen; CEA) and liver cancer (alphafetoprotein; FP). Elevation of these substances indicates significant tumour burden. CEA and FP are two of the so-called 'oncofetal antigens'. These are secreted by fetal tissues and some tumours. Other markers reflect the turnover of nucleoproteins, e.g. the levels of polyamines and methylated nucleosides in the urine. The main value of biological markers is not in early disease but later on, to monitor the progress of recurrent disease by serial assay.

The prognosis of a tumour is also affected by its biological characteristics. Its size, contour, degree of nuclear and cellular anaplasia and the extent of lymphocytic infiltration all influence outcome. Lymphomas with cell surface receptors for

Table 16.3 Some 'specific' tumour markers

Marker	Likely tissue of origin
Human chorionic gonadotrophin	Chorion Testis
Acid phosphatase	Prostate
Carcinoembryonic antigen	Colon and rectum Breast Liver Bronchus Pancreas
Fetoprotein	Liver Testis
Thyrocalcitonin	Thyroid
Tyrosinase	Melanoma Breast
Creatine kinase BB	Prostate Breast
β-glucuronidase	Leptomeninges
Breast-cyst fluid protein	Breast
Pancreatic oncofetal antigen	Pancreas

immunoglobulins respond better to systemic chemotherapy than those without; breast cancers which contain cytoplasmic protein with a high affinity for binding oestrogen (oestrogen receptors) are more likely to respond to hormonal measures and have a better prognosis than those without.

The degree of reactivity of regional lymph nodes to the tumour, as indicated by the appearance of sinus histiocytosis, also correlates with prognosis. Tumours associated with marked reactive changes fare better than those associated with inactive lymph nodes. This reactive change may represent a host–tumour response.

TREATMENT

Benign tumours

Provided sufficient surrounding tissue is excised to ensure complete removal, a benign tumour is cured by local excision. Some benign tumours, e.g. pleomorphic adenomas of the parotid, extend beyond their apparent macroscopic limits. Removal of the involved segment of the gland or organ is then the only sure way to cure.

Malignant tumours

Local treatment

Primary tumour. Some malignant tumours grow slowly, have little tendency to recur and may be cured by local excision. In many cancers, however, local treatment is used primarily to control local disease and prevent local and regional recurrence. Reduction of tumour burden may contribute to the success of systemic treatment, which is aimed at controlling the disease as a whole.

The extent of the local treatment required for a malignant tumour depends on its natural history, in particular the likelihood of local recurrence and multifocal deposits. Anatomical considerations are also important, as damage to nearby tissues must be avoided. The establishment of a balance between relief of symptoms and morbidity is often difficult, and it is important to remember that the quality of life is as important as survival.

The general aim is to excise the primary tumour with as wide a margin of normal tissue as is practicable. In most sites this requires removal of the organ of origin.

During any operation for cancer care is taken to try and avoid spillage of malignant cells. In some sites (e.g. testes, large bowel) it is usual to ligate the main vessels draining the area before the tumour is mobilized so that the shedding of malignant cells into the circulation is avoided.

Before handling a tumour of the bowel, a ligature is placed around the bowel proximally and distally to prevent spillage of cells into the lumen of remaining bowel which may cause recurrence at the anastomotic site. Many surgeons now irrigate the wound or body cavity with 1:500 cetrimide to destroy 'free floating' cells and thus reduce the likelihood of local recurrence. There is little evidence that this is of value.

Radiotherapy is a useful alternative to surgery in some forms of cancer (Fig. 16.11). The development of high-energy irradiation with megavoltage X-rays, accelerated electrons and beams of heavy particles permits more effective irradiation of the tumour with less damage to the skin and surrounding tissues. Techniques to increase tumour sensitivity to X-rays are under

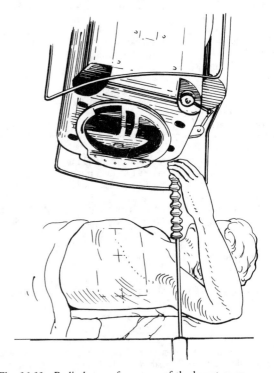

Fig. 16.11 Radiotherapy for cancer of the breast as an alternative to surgery

study. These include hyperbaric oxygenation and radio-sensitizing drugs. Many tumours are resistant to all forms of radiation.

Radiotherapy is also used to increase the local control achieved by surgery. Examples are irradiation of the pelvis in rectal carcinoma and of the breast or chest wall and lymph node areas in breast cancer.

Regional lymph nodes. The management of regional lymph nodes depends on the site and type of the tumour. With some tumours, e.g. those of the gastrointestinal tract, breast and testes, regional lymph nodes are routinely resected or irradiated irrespective of their involvement. In others, e.g. malignant melanoma, head and neck cancer, regional lymph nodes are treated only if they are proven to contain metastatic growth. This difference in treatment has arisen from considerations of technique and morbidity rather than from any logical plan of management. In general, nodes which can readily be removed in continuity with the primary tumour are treated by primary block excision. Removal of uninvolved nodes has no therapeutic advantage. By contrast, removal of involved nodes is a rational way to reduce tumour burden and prevent progression of regional disease. Prior sampling of lymph nodes for histological examination is indicated particularly in sites where node dissection causes severe morbidity, e.g. the neck and groin.

Radiotherapy may also be used to treat regional lymph nodes and so prevent continued growth of lymphatic deposits. This is routinely done in some radiosensitive tumours, e.g. seminoma of testis.

Table 16.4 Analgesics used in cancer therapy

	Preparations	Dosage	Contraindications	Side effects
MILD TO MODERATE PAIN				
Non-narcotics				
Aspirin	tabs 300 mg	300–900 mg 4-hourly	peptic ulcer anticoagulants	gastric irritation
Paracetamol (Panadol)	tabs 500 mg syrup 120 mg/5 ml	0.5–1 g 4-hourly	hepatic impairment	hepatotoxic
Naproxen (Naprosyn)	tabs 250, 500 mg syrup 125 mg/5mg suppositories 500 mg	250 mg 6-hourly	–	mild
Mefenamic acid (Ponstan)	caps 250 mg tabs 500 mg	500 mg three times daily	hypersensitive states	diarrhoea dizziness
Ibuprofen	tabs 200, 400, 600 mg syrup 100 mg/5 ml	2 g daily	–	mild gastrointestinal upset
Narcotics				
Codeine phosphate	tabs 15, 30 mg syrup 25 mg/5 ml injection 60 mg/ml	10–60 mg 4-hourly	hepatic impairment respiratory disease	constipation dizziness
Dihydrocodeine tartrate (DF 118)	tabs 30 mg	30 mg 4-hourly	hepatic impairment respiratory disease	constipation dizziness
Pentazocine (Fortral)	caps 50 mg tabs 25 mg injection 30 mg/ml suppository 50 mg	25–100 mg 4-hourly		hallucinations
Dextropropoxyphene hydrochloride plus paracetamol (e.g. Distalgesic)	tabs 32.5 mg plus paracetamol 325 mg	2 tabs three times daily		respiratory depression

Systemic therapy

'Adjuvant' systemic therapy is now advised for many types of cancer. Its aim is the control of occult metastatic disease but effective agents are still lacking, particularly for solid tumours. Controlled therapeutic trials to assess the value of chemotherapeutic agents are an essential prerequisite to their routine clinical use. Chemotherapy is toxic: morbidity and the quality of life must always be considered before advising this form of treatment.

The recognition that different chemotherapeutic agents act at specific points in the cell cycle has led to the development of combinations of cell-cycle dependent and independent drugs. These compounds, which may be administered for months or even years, have revolutionized the treatment of lymphomas but are as yet of little proven value in solid tumours except those of the testis and ovary and, to a lesser extent, the breast.

Other methods of systemic therapy, e.g. suppression of circulating hormones or stimulation of the immune system, are under study. For example, the anti-oestrogen tamoxifen may be used as adjuvant therapy in primary breast cancer, where it has been shown to be of benefit.

Follow-up

Most cancer patients attend follow-up clinics in hospital where their clinical condition is kept

Table 16.4 (Cont'd)

	Preparations	Dosage	Contraindications	Side effects
SEVERE PAIN				
Narcotics				
Methadone hydrochloride (Physeptone)	tabs 5 mg/ml injection 10 mg	5–10 mg 6- hourly	– nausea	constipation nausea
Pethidine hydrochloride	tabs 25.5 mg injection 50 mg/ml	50–150 mg 4-hourly	renal impairment	nephrotoxic
Phenazocine hydrochloride (Narphen)	tabs 5 mg	5 mg 4-hourly	poor respiratory reserve mono-amine oxidase inhibitor therapy asthma increased intracranial pressure	constipation nausea respiratory depression urinary retention
Buprenorphine (Temgesic)	tabs 200 μg (sublingual) injection 300 μg/ml	200–400 μg 8-hourly	poor respiratory reserve mono-amine oxidase inhibitor therapy asthma increased intracranial pressure	constipation nausea respiratory depression urinary retention
Diamorphine hydrochloride (heroin)	tabs 5, 10 mg injection 5 mg, 10 mg/ml suppositories 10 mg	5–10 mg 4-hourly	poor respiratory reserve mono-amine oxidase inhibitor therapy asthma increased intracranial pressure	constipation nausea respiratory depression urinary retention
Morphine	tabs 10 mg, 30 mg injection 10, 30 mg/ml elixir 8.4 mg/ml suppositories 15 mg	10–20 mg 4-hourly	poor respiratory reserve mono-amine oxidase inhibitor therapy asthma increased intracranial pressure	constipation nausea respiratory depression urinary retention
MST Continus (morphine sulphate)	tabs 10 mg	10–20 mg twice daily	as above	as above

under review. In general, it is wasteful to carry out sophisticated investigations for metastatic disease in asymptomatic patients. More important in most solid tumours amenable to surgical treatment is to check that there is no local recurrence of disease and that the patient is symptom-free.

Palliation of advanced cancer

The terminal stages of malignancy can be prolonged, and pain and other distressing symptoms are frequent. Effective palliation is achieved by: (1) local and/or systemic therapy to induce tumour regression; and (2) non-specific treatment which does not affect tumour growth but relieves symptoms.

Specific therapy

Tumour regression can be induced by local radiotherapy or by systemic hormone or chemotherapy according to tumour type. Surgery has little place in the palliation of advanced malignant disease. However, local excision of an ulcerating or fungating tumour may prove worthwhile, and palliative resection of gastric or rectal tumours spares considerable discomfort. Surgery may also relieve functional upsets caused by tumours, e.g. dysphagia, intestinal obstruction or impending paraplegia.

When a palliative operation is performed the patient and his relatives should understand that its object is to prevent additional suffering and not to attempt cure.

Symptomatic care

Pain relief. A wide range of analgesic and narcotic drugs are available to relieve pain. The choice depends on the type of pain, its severity and the stage of the illness. The aim is to achieve complete analgesia without impairing mental clarity or inducing side effects. Some commonly used agents are shown in Table 16.4. It is essential never to let the patient 'wait' for his or her next dose of analgesic. Schedules of administration are planned to *prevent* rather than treat pain. When pain is severe, narcotic drugs should be used; fear of addiction is irrelevant.

A useful narcotic mixture is morphine sulphate (starting with 5–10 mg) with prochlorperazine (5 mg) in chloroform water. This is as effective as the traditional Brompton cocktail, and doses of morphine up to 60 mg every 4 hours can be given in this way. For parenteral therapy, diamorphine is the drug of choice. The initial dose is 5 mg given at 4-hourly intervals. This can be increased as required.

Pain due to intracerebral or nerve root compression can often be helped by dexamethasone (8 mg daily in divided doses). Pain may also be reduced by neurosurgical procedures (see Ch. 40). Supplementation of analgesics with antiemetics (e.g. prochlorperazine/Stemetil 5–10 mg) and tranquillers (e.g. chlorpromazine/Largactil 25–50 mg) prevents nausea and relaxes the patient.

Vomiting is caused by mechanical obstruction of the stomach or intestine, by drug toxicity, or by anxiety and fear. Reassurance, attention to diet, sedatives and/or antiemetics may help. Obstructive vomiting may require surgical relief.

Dysphagia due to oesophageal obstruction is distressful, as the patient cannot swallow his own saliva. Relief can be provided by the insertion of a prosthetic tube by means of an endoscope. Gastrostomy and jejunostomy do not relieve dysphagia but add to the patient's discomfort. They are seldom indicated.

Dyspnoea can be helped by a bronchial dilator, e.g. salbutamol or aminophylline. Diffuse lymphangitic permeation of the lungs can cause severe respiratory distress which may be relieved by prednisone 10–15 mg three times daily. Purulent sputum may indicate the need for antibiotic therapy. Episodic bouts of acute dyspnoea terrify the patient, particularly at night. Adequate sedation is therefore essential. Excess bronchial secretions can be controlled with atropine.

The majority of patients with terminal cancer develop a monilial infection (*thrush*). Nystatin suspension usually leads to considerable improvement in appetite and well-being. Sucking a slice of fresh pineapple is a good way to clean the mouth.

The smell of a *fungating lesion* is distressing, and may be minimized by isolating the patient in a well ventilated cubicle and using deodorant aerosols or fumigators and frequent dressings of eusol and 4%

povidone (Betadine) in liquid paraffin or proflavine emulsion. Adequate *sleep* is essential. Nitrazepam (Mogadon) is best, except for the elderly in whom chlormethiazole (Heminevrin) is preferred.

Care of the dying

Death from malignant disease is usually a gradual process of withdrawal. A sympathetic doctor can greatly help the patient and his relatives. A dying patient must never feel abandoned on a surgical ward: doctors and nursing staff must be prepared to spend time to help the patient die with dignity.

It is not usual to tell a patient that he or she is dying from malignant disease, but relatives must be kept informed. In some cases, a frank but kind discussion with the patient and his relatives can do much to restore confidence and prepare everyone for the inevitable outcome.

The attention of a doctor must not cease after the death of a patient. Words of sympathy from a member of the surgical staff can give great comfort to the bereaved relatives.

17. The breast

ANATOMY AND PHYSIOLOGY

The breast is an appendage of skin and is a modified sweat gland. It contains some six to eight segments of glandular tissue, each drained by a duct opening on to the nipple. The primary secretory unit is a group of saccular alveoli draining into a ductule, the 'terminal duct–lobular unit'. In the resting state this secretes watery fluid which is believed to be reabsorbed through the walls of larger ducts (Fig. 17.1).

The alveoli and ducts are lined by a single layer of epithelial cells, the last centimetre of the main ducts by stratified squamous epithelium. Myoepithelial cells surround the ducts, but not

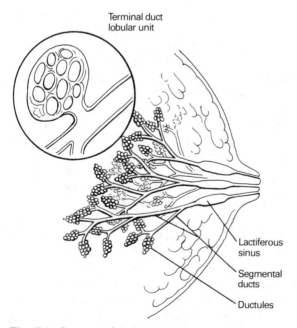

Terminal duct lobular unit

Lactiferous sinus

Segmental ducts

Ductules

Fig. 17.1 Structure of the breast and its secreting unit

the lobules. They are contractile and move secretions along the duct system.

The shape of the female breast is due to fat contained within fibrous septa. In adolescents and young adults the breast is firm and prominent; with age the glandular and fibrous elements atrophy, the skin stretches and the breast sags.

The breast lies between the skin and pectoral fascia to which it is loosely attached. It extends from the 2nd to 6th ribs and from the lateral border at the sternum to the midaxillary line. A prolongation of parenchymatous tissue, the axillary tail, runs upwards between the pectoralis major and latissimus dorsi muscles to blend with the fat of the axilla. The breast has an excellent blood supply. Laterally this comes from branches of the lateral thoracic artery and perforating branches of the intercostal vessels, medially from perforating branches of the internal mammary artery. Its veins follow the same course. The lymphatics are profuse and run within the substance of the breast medially to the internal mammary nodes (which lie under the medial ends of the ribs close to the internal mammary artery) and laterally to nodes along the lateral thoracic vessels (pectoral group) and subscapular vessels (subscapular group). From these nodes, lymph passes up through the central and apical axillary nodes to the subclavian trunk. A few lymphatics pierce the pectoral fascia and enter the chest with the perforating vessels, some draining into occasional nodes lying between the pectoral muscles. Although lymph from the medial part of the breast may drain medially, lymph from all parts of the breast drains laterally through the axillary lymph nodes, which are generally regarded as the main route of lymphatic spread of malignant disease (Fig. 17.2).

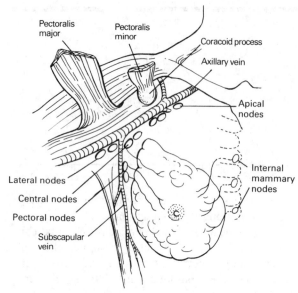

Fig. 17.2 Axillary and internal mammary nodes draining the breast

Development of the breast

Early in uterine life two 'milk ridges' form on a line from midclavicle to groin. These consist of differentiated ectodermal cells which form the buds of the mammary glands. The number and position of these glands vary in different species but small 'accessory' buds of breast tissue may lie anywhere along the milk lines. In women there are two pectoral buds. Solid cords of cells extend into the subcutaneous tissues which later develop into the alveoli and ducts of the adult breast.

Apart from a transient burst of activity in the newborn due to circulating hormones of maternal origin, the breast remains dormant until puberty. Then the onset of cyclical hormonal activity stimulates growth, branching of ducts, and formation of ductules and primitive terminal duct lobular units. The size and shape of the post-pubertal breast is not determined by the amount of glandular tissue but by fat.

Although in the resting state terminal duct lobular units can be recognized microscopically, lobular development is only marked during pregnancy. Secretions can be obtained by suction from the nipple in some 75% of young women. After the menopause lobules normally disappear and secretions become sparse.

Hormones and breast development

Breast development is the result of stimulation by hormones of the endocrine system. Studies in rodents suggest that oestrogen, adrenocortical steroids and growth hormone promote development of ducts, that prolactin is essential for alveolar formation, and that a growth tetrad of oestrogen, progesterone, prolactin and growth hormone is required for full lobulo-alveolar development such as that found in late pregnancy. During pregnancy the placenta is an important source of these hormones.

During pregnancy, the high levels of ovarian and placental steroids inhibit lactation. Following delivery, reduction of oestrogens increases sensitivity of the mammary epithelium to the lactational complex (prolactin, growth hormone and cortisol). Suckling stimulates release of prolactin and oxytocin. Oxytocin stimulates the myoepithelial cells to eject milk into the terminal ducts. These effects are reversed with weaning.

Normal and abnormal growth

Enlargement of one or both breasts may be observed in the newborn. This may be associated with secretion of a colostrum-like fluid ('witches milk') from the nipple. These changes are due to stimulation by hormones of maternal origin and are temporary.

As puberty approaches, the breast enlarges again, initially as a firm 'button' of breast tissue beneath the nipple. At first this may be unilateral and a cyst or fibroadenoma may be suspected. One should never interfere surgically with developing breasts lest serious distortion of their eventual form is caused, or even inadvertent mastectomy is performed. The only exception to this rule is unequivocal evidence of malignancy, which in this age group is exceedingly rare. Early skin fixation and ulceration are characteristic.

During the menstrual years the breast undergoes cyclical changes which can cause heaviness, discomfort and increasing nodularity during the latter part of the menstrual cycle.

Excessive growth of connective tissue and fat in one or both breasts can cause discomfort and embarrassment. Reduction mammoplasty may be required but should not be advised until the breasts have fully grown. This operation is designed to remove a portion of the normal breast, thus restoring a small youthful shape. The nipple requires to be transposed to a new site.

Small breasts can also cause embarrassment. Various methods of enlarging the breast have been tried. These include massage with hormonal creams and injection of paraffin wax or silicone (see p. 210) but safe augmentation can only be achieved by inserting a silicone rubber prosthesis behind the breast tissue or under the pectoral muscles.

Complete failure of development of both breasts at puberty may be due to ovarian agenesis. In Turner's syndrome this is associated with infantilism, short stature, web-neck and cubitus valgus. Failure of breast development may be accompanied by absence of the pectoral muscle or can result from inappropriate surgery during puberty. The ease of reconstruction depends on the availability of tissues and the size of the opposite breast. In its simplest form it requires no more than insertion of a silicone-rubber prosthesis.

EXAMINATION OF THE BREAST

History

The patient should be asked if she has any symptoms referable to the breast and in particular whether she has noted any discrete abnormality or areas where the texture is different from normal. Premenstrual discomfort, nipple discharge, recent retraction or distortion of the nipple are enquired about.

It is important to determine whether the patient has had any previous breast complaint, has attended a breast clinic, had a mammogram or biopsy, or whether there is a family history of breast cancer. Routine enquiries include number of children and whether breast fed, the patient's age at first pregnancy, her menstrual status and date of last menstrual period.

Physical examination

It is necessary to have a strict routine for examination of the breast (Fig. 17.3). The patient is undressed to the waist and sits facing the examiner. The breast is inspected from in front while the patient's arms are first placed by her side, then raised above her head, and finally placed upon her hips. The examiner looks for assymetry, visible lumps, flattening, skin tethering, abnormal fixation of the breast, or retraction and altered axis of the nipples. The patient is then asked to place her hands on the examiners shoulders and to lean forward. The breasts are again inspected and gently palpated. The fingers are slid behind the outer border of the pectoralis major to seek enlarged pectoral lymph nodes.

Further palpation of the breast is best carried out with the patient lying down and with each shoulder supported in turn by a small pillow. If the arm is raised and the hand tucked behind the patient's head, the breast 'flows' over the chest wall. The patient should be asked to point to any abnormality and this area is examined first. Thereafter each quadrant of each breast is examined in turn by careful palpation between the fingers and underlying chest wall.

Palpation is repeated with the patient's arms at her side. The axillary, central, apical and subscapular axillary lymph nodes are then palpated, the arm being supported to relax the axillary muscles. Subscapular and supraclavicular nodes are best palpated from behind.

Should a lump be felt, its position, size (measured by a calliper), consistency and discreteness must be carefully recorded. It is particularly important to decide whether a lump is smooth, roughened or nodular and whether it is separate from surrounding breast tissue or integrated within it. Fixity to skin is sought by pinching up the skin overlying the mass, fixity to the pectoral muscle by assessing the mobility of the mass first with the pectoral muscles relaxed then with them contracted. Contraction is achieved by asking the patient to place her hands on her hips and press.

If the patient complains of discharge from the nipple, an attempt should be made to reproduce this, to determine whether it arises from one or several ducts and to test it for blood. Pressure is applied to the alveolar margin with the finger 'around the clock', palpating for a dilated duct or nodule and observing if the discharge can be produced (Fig. 17.4). If this is unsuccessful, the breast tissue immediately under the nipple is picked up and gently compressed.

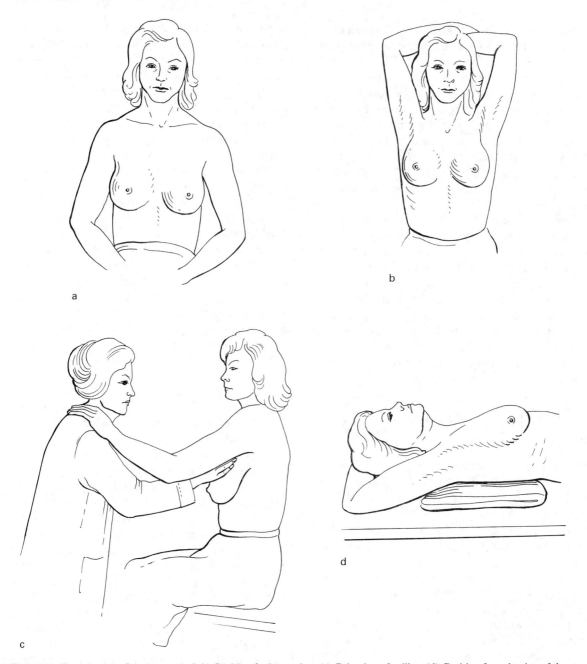

Fig. 17.3 Examination of the breast. (a & b) Position for inspection. (c) Palpation of axillae. (d) Position for palpation of the breast

The discharge is tested for blood with a Clinitest strip and a smear is made for cytological examination. If it arises from one duct, note should be made of the position of that duct and whether its orifice is dilated.

Ancillary investigations

Needle aspiration

Needle aspiration of a breast lump is carried out in the clinic using a 10 or 20 ml syringe and a 21-

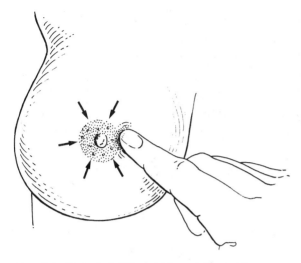

Fig. 17.4 Method of differential 'round-the-clock' palpation to induce discharge

gauge or smaller needle. A special handle is available which holds the syringe and allows the operator to apply constant suction using only one hand (Fig. 17.5). This allows the mass to be steadied between finger and thumb while the needle is inserted into it through the overlying skin. The 'consistency' of the mass gives useful information. The sudden relief of resistance on entering a cyst, the tough rubbery feel of fibrocystic breast tissue, and the grittiness of a cancer are typical.

A cyst is emptied of fluid (see below). If the lesion is solid, an aspiration biopsy is taken by applying suction at constant pressure and advancing

and withdrawing the needle several times through the centre of the tumour. The pressure on the syringe is then released and the needle and syringe are removed. The contents of the needle are expressed onto a slide and smears are prepared for staining and examination.

Mammography

Mammography (soft tissue radiology of the breast) uses high-resolution fine-grain film, high-intensity screens and X-rays of low penetrating power. With modern systems the dose of radiation is small (0.5–2.0 mGy per film).

In some clinics xeromammograms are preferred, as they highlight changes of density by a 'brush' effect, show calcifications clearly, and can be read in reflected light. The dose of radiation is larger than with mammography, and most radiologists now prefer film-screen combinations which allow good imaging with a smaller dose. This is particularly important in the screening of well women.

A mediolateral oblique view taken from upper medial to lower lateral aspects is now standard and includes the whole of the breast on the film (Fig. 17.6). It may be combined with a craniocaudal view, although if the patient is asymptomatic a single oblique film is now considered adequate by many. This is particularly relevant to screening programmes. In symptomatic women, mammography is generally reserved for those over 35 years of age.

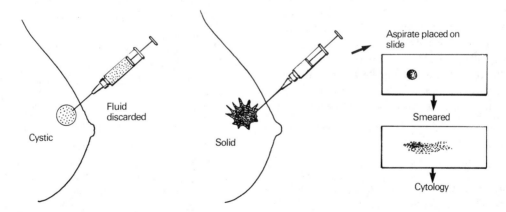

Fig. 17.5 Needle aspiration of a breast mass

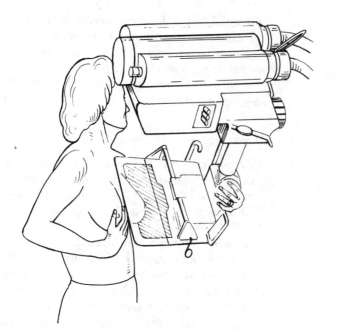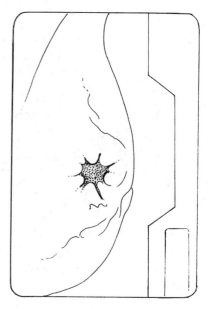

Fig. 17.6   Mediolateral oblique mammography

Thermography

Once popular for examining the breast, thermography has limited diagnostic value and is now seldom used (see Ch. 6).

Histology

Traditionally information about the histology of breast lesions is obtained by excision biopsy, often combined with frozen section examination. Closed biopsy methods are now standard in specialist breast clinics. The simplest device is a Tru-cut needle with which a core of tissue is removed; a biopsy gun is also available. However, a combination of clinical examination, high quality mammography and fine-needle aspiration cytology carried out by an experienced aspirator and skilled cytologist will now most often provide a precise diagnosis.

Breast biopsy

Surgical removal of a benign lesion from the breast is a common operation. If the lesion is superficial, biopsy can be performed under local anaesthesia;

otherwise a general anaesthetic is used. Incisions should be placed transversely, following the curve of the breast and avoiding distortion of the breast contour. The breast tissues are divided and the lesion is carefully dissected out with a little surrounding normal breast tissue.

A frozen section may be used to give an immediate histological diagnosis but this is by no means essential. The availability of the other investigative procedures described above allows a precise diagnosis to be made preoperatively so that the patient can be further investigated and counselled before definitive treatment needs to be carried out.

Removal of mammographically visible but impalpable lesions poses particular problems. Some surgeons simply perform wide local or segmental resection of the area concerned, but this is not good practice. It is better to localize the lesion radiologically before operation using either a hooked wire inserted through a needle (Fig. 17.7) or injection of a radio-opaque and visible dye. Following excision the specimen must be X-rayed to confirm that the lesion has been removed.

Frozen section examination of small mammographic lesions is not advised. Considerable

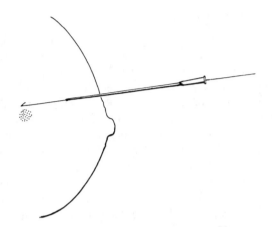

Fig. 17.7 Localization of non-palpable mammographic lesion

experience and expertise are needed for their pathological assessment, which requires radiological as well as histological methods of examination.

INFLAMMATORY DISEASE OF THE BREAST

Acute and chronic mastitis

Inflammation of the breast may accompany systemic infection. Acute mastitis can complicate mumps, while causes of chronic mastitis include tuberculosis, hydatid disease, syphilis and actinomycosis. These are rare. The common form of acute mastitis is staphylococcal infection of local origin and occurs most frequently during the puerperium. Infection usually gains access through a cracked nipple and improved hygiene has done much to reduce its incidence.

Acute mastitis starts as a localized area of inflammation which is painful, red, indurated and tender. It may resolve spontaneously or spread through the breast, which becomes swollen, hot and oedematous. Fever and toxicity occur. Necrosis and pus formation cause a multilobular abscess. Fluctuation may be elicited but only if the abscess is superficial. The involved skin is then glazed and thin. If the abscess lies deeply within or behind the breast, fluctuation is absent.

Antibiotics can prevent the full development of acute mastitis but must be given early in the disease and in adequate doses. The type and sensitivity of the organism(s) can be determined by fine-needle aspiration of the infected area. Until this is known the choice of antibiotic is based on the likely sensitivity of the organisms. For domiciliary practice a combination of penicillin and flucloxacillin may prove satisfactory; in hospital a cephalosporin or erythromycin are preferable. Cessation of breast feeding is normally advised. Firm support may be all that is needed. Alternatively, bromocriptine 2.5 mg twice daily may be given.

An abscess should be drained surgically. Indications for drainage are a fluctuant mass, glazed red oedematous skin, or persistence of local signs of infection for more than 5 days or of severe systemic upset for more than 48 hours after full antibiotic treatment.

At operation, loculi are broken down to form a single cavity, which is then drained. A curved transverse incision is made, the abscess is opened and a finger is inserted to break down the septa. A biopsy is taken from the abscess wall and a tube drain brought out through the wound or at the most dependent part of the breast (Fig. 17.8).

Pus is sent to the laboratory for identification of the organism and its sensitivity. Antibiotic therapy is continued for a few days and the drainage tube removed when drainage ceases. Some surgeons prefer to excise small abscesses under antibiotic cover rather than to drain them.

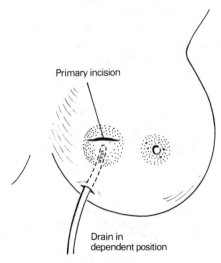

Primary incision

Drain in dependent position

Fig. 17.8 Drainage of a breast abscess

Inadequate antibiotic therapy alters the natural history of the disease. Necrosis and pus formation is retarded, fibrosis is increased and the breast becomes chronically thickened and honeycombed with pus. The resemblance to an inflammatory cancer can be startling. Treatment consists of multiple incisions and drainage. Biopsy of several areas of breast tissue is mandatory.

Non-lactational mastitis

In young women an episode of inflammation may occur in a segment of the breast, forming a peri-areolar red tender and oedematous swelling. At first diffuse, it may localize at the areolar margin to form a peri-areolar abscess. Initial treatment consists of antibiotics. As anaerobes are frequently present, e.g. bacteroides species, metronidazole should be combined with a penicillin. Flucloxacillin 250 mg four times a day plus metronidazole 200 mg four times a day for five days is commonly prescribed.

If an abscess forms, this will need to be opened through a small circumareolar incision even though this is likely to result in a subsequent mammillary fistula.

Granulomatous mastitis

This is a rare process of unknown aetiology which is characterized by granuloma formation associated with non-specific inflammatory changes. It is a cause of recurrent chronic inflammatory masses in the breast associated with sinus formation, usually some distance from the nipple. It can be confused with cancer.

Mammillary fistula

This condition of young women is associated with peri-areolar sepsis. Some believe it may arise from blockage of a lactiferous sinus in the nipple by a keratin plug. The sinus becomes dilated, its epithelium undergoes squamous metaplasia and infection leads to a subareolar abscess. This may burst spontaneously (or is incised) to form a fistula opening at the areolar margin (Fig. 17.9).

Recurrent attacks of acute inflammation and intermittent discharge of pus through the 'mammillary fistula' follow. Treatment consists of surgical exploration with excision of the wall of the lactiferous sinus, its related cavity and in some cases a segment of breast tissue. Alternatively, as in operation for fistula-in-ano, the lactiferous sinus between the fistula and the orifice of the duct may be deroofed and the lining excised. The wound may be allowed to granulate or delayed primary suture can be performed. Antibiotic cover (as above) is advised.

Paraffin and silicone granulomas

The current desire for large breasts has led many women with small breasts to seek augmentation. Initially liquid paraffin was injected into the submammary space. Unfortunately, paraffin migrated into the breast tissues, causing an intense low-grade inflammatory reaction and formation of abscesses and chronic sinuses. Organic polymers of silica (silicones) of glue-like consistency were then developed and these were also injected into the submammary space. Pure silicones are inert, but the use of inferior grades to which irritants were added to prevent migration resulted in

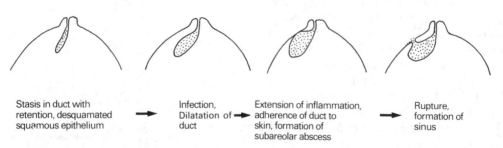

| Stasis in duct with retention, desquamated squamous epithelium | → | Infection, Dilatation of duct | → | Extension of inflammation, adherence of duct to skin, formation of subareolar abscess | → | Rupture, formation of sinus |

Fig. 17.9   Stages in the formation of a mammary fistula

inflammatory reactions. Multiple painful lumps ('silicone granulomas') developed throughout the breast; the overlying skin became inflamed and often broke down to form multiple sinuses. Systemic reactions such as granulomatous hepatitis also occurred from absorption of the chemical. Mastectomy is the only possible treatment.

It is now recognized that even 'medical grade' silicone should not be injected. If mammary augmentation is indicated, it should be performed by insertion of a prosthesis consisting of silicone gel enclosed in a silicone-rubber envelope.

BENIGN EPITHELIAL TUMOURS

Fibroadenoma

A fibroadenoma is the commonest breast mass of young women. It arises from a breast lobule and is an aberration in lobular development. It is not neoplastic. It forms a well-defined, small, painless, smooth firm swelling which is clearly demarcated from the surrounding breast tissue and is characteristically mobile, hence the term 'breast mouse'. Frequently fibroadenomas are multiple. Mammography may reveal a round or ovoid density with a radiolucent halo from compression of surrounding fat. However, its density may be similar to that of breast tissue and it may not be detectable. In later life it may form a dense coarsely calcified mass.

On gross examination a fibroadenoma is clearly demarcated from surrounding breast tissue, which suggests encapsulation. Its cut surface is granular, whitish-brown and glistening and bulges outward. Interweaving clefts form dark lines.

Microscopically there are two components: proliferation of fine connective tissue ('fibrosis') and an abnormal multiplication of ducts and acini ('adenoma'). These two components are present in varying degrees and produce a wide range of histological appearances. However, 30% of clinically diagnosed 'fibroadenomas' are but areas of fibrocystic change which microscopically cannot be classified as true single fibroadenomas.

A typical fibroadenoma is slow-growing and self-limiting. It takes some 6–12 months to double in size and usually stops growing when about 3 cm in diameter.

If untreated, it may undergo hyalinization and merge with surrounding tissue or it may form a hard calcified mass. Many consider it wise to excise all fibroadenomas. A primary carcinoma may be indistinguishable and, although rare, cancer does occur in the young. However, provided fine-needle aspiration cytology reveals no malignant cells, the decision to excise a fibroadenoma can safely be delayed in young women (under 35 years) provided careful follow-up is arranged. A small proportion of such tumours will disappear and some remain static, but many continue to grow. If persistent or if the patient is concerned, the mass should be excised, usually under local anaesthesia.

A fibroadenoma may grow during pregnancy. There is always a risk of later malignant change but this is rare.

Soft fibroadenoma. A variant of fibroadenoma with more rapid growth is found in older women. This is softer in consistency than the typical lesion of the young patient but is still quite benign and is cured by excision with a small margin of surrounding breast tissue. Care must be taken to differentiate this from cystosarcoma phyllodes.

Giant fibroadenoma. This is a distinct entity in young adolescent females. It is rare in Britain but common in some African countries, appearing a few years after puberty and growing rapidly to a very large size. The girl usually complains that one breast has become larger than the other. On examination the involved breast is distended by a large softish lobular tumour in which clefts can be palpated. The skin is thin with distended veins, yet the tumour is not fixed to skin or deeper tissues. Mammography demonstrates a large well-defined opacity within the breast.

These tumours are quite benign and cured by local excision, provided this is complete.

Cystosarcoma phyllodes

This tumour is so called because of the leaf-like masses of tumour tissue which project into cystic cavities and the 'sarcomatous' appearance of the connective tissue stroma on microscopy. The term is, however, a misnomer and many now prefer the term 'phyllodes tumour'. The tumour is fibroepithelial in origin, the deep elongated clefts which typify it being lined by epithelial cells.

Some believe that it originates in a fibroadenoma. Myxomatous degeneration and metaplastic formation of fibrous and fatty elements are common. If the stroma becomes frankly malignant (3–12%), metastases may occur. These are of sarcomatous type.

Clinically the tumour presents as a rapidly growing unilateral mass in women aged 40–50 years. Typical are its irregular 'bosselated' surface, palpable deep clefts and the shiny stretched thin skin containing grossly dilated veins (Fig. 17.10). Lymph node enlargement is rare.

Treatment consists of total mastectomy combined with axillary node sampling. As local recurrence is the main problem, wide removal of skin and breast tissue is advised. Replacement by a musculocutaneous flap may be necessary. Radiotherapy is of no value.

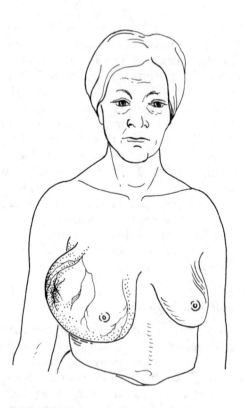

Fig. 17.10 Clinical appearance of a phyllodes tumour (cystosarcoma phyllodes)

CYSTIC DISEASE AND EPITHELIAL HYPERPLASIA

Definitions

Cystic disease. This is regarded as a disease of the breast lobules with dilatation and coalescence of breast acini. Dilatation of the duct system is known as duct ectasia. The two conditions may coincide. Thus, inspissated secretions may exude from dilated ducts during operation for cystic disease.

Cystic disease is a condition of late premenopausal and menopausal women. Unlike cancer, its incidence does not increase with age and it is rare in postmenopausal women. It is probably a disorder of involution of the fine connective tissue within a breast lobule. This allows the acini to dilate and form small cysts visible only on microscopy (microcysts). These small cysts coalesce to form large cysts lined by epithelium which may show metaplastic transformation to apocrine (sweat gland) type. If the outflow tract becomes obstructed, a large tension cyst forms which is filled with clear yellow or brownish fluid.

Benign epithelial hyperplasia. This is commonly associated with cystic disease and may consist of adenosis or epitheliosis. Adenosis is non-neoplastic glandular hyperplasia in which all epithelial units within a lobule are hypertrophied and lie within fine connective tissue stroma. Epitheliosis is solid epithelial hyperplasia occurring within small ducts, ductules and even acini. When extensive, this forms finger-like projections of epithelium which some call papillomatosis. If adenosis is accompanied by marked proliferation of fibrous tissue, the condition is called 'sclerosing adenosis'. The epithelial elements are distorted and strangled by this proliferation, and microscopically the lesion may resemble a scirrhous cancer.

Clinical presentation and diagnosis

Diffuse cystic disease may affect the whole breast, which becomes heavy, thickened and lumpy (Fig. 17.11). Pain and discomfort are common, particularly in the premenstrual phase of the cycle. On mammography the breast parenchyma is dense, and ductal and vascular shadows are

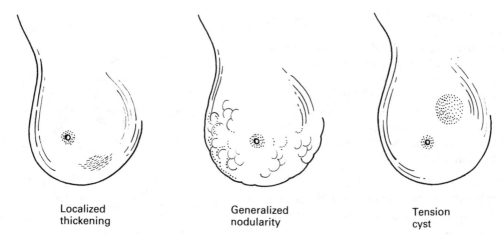

| Localized | Generalized | Tension |
| thickening | nodularity | cyst |

Fig. 17.11 Cystic disease and its clinical presentation

obscured. The edges of cysts and fibrotic nodules form so-called 'curvilinear' shadows.

Treatment of the painful nodular breast is unsatisfactory. Reassurance that the lesion is not cancerous may be all that is required, but, if discomfort is severe, antihormone treatment with the gonadotrophin inhibitor danazol (Danol) may be prescribed. Cancer is difficult to detect in a 'knobbly' breast and ideally the patient should be kept under review.

Localized thickening (see Fig. 17.11) is caused either by a conglomeration of small cysts or by fibrosis. The patient notices that a segment of one breast differs in texture from the rest. This area may have become particularly prominent towards the end of a menstrual cycle, but unlike the rest of the breast does not resolve and soften after the period finishes.

On clinical examination the area feels rubbery, thickened and nodular. It is more readily palpated by the fingers than with the flat of the hand. Mammography is essential and any suggestion of discrete opacity or microcalcification indicates the need for fine-needle aspiration cytology or biopsy. Provided the mammograms do not show such change, the patient may be kept under review. Clinical suspicion of a discrete nodule within the area indicates the need for fine-needle aspiration cytology; if this is not available, a biopsy is mandatory.

Sclerosing adenosis gives rise to a firm mobile nodular mass which may suggest malignant disease. On needle aspiration it feels tough and rubbery, rather than hard and gritty. Biopsy is the only safe course of action. Because the microscopic appearances can resemble scirrhous cancer, careful examination of the gross specimen (a greyish-white nodular mass) and of multiple paraffin sections is desirable to avoid inappropriate mastectomy.

A tension cyst (see Fig. 17.11) forms a firm or hard mass in the breast. This may be well demarcated, smooth and mobile, or integrated into an area of fibrocystic disease, when its surface feels irregular. The clinical differentiation of a cyst from a cancer is not always easy; absence of fixation to the skin is a helpful guide.

The diagnosis can readily be confirmed by fine-needle aspiration. The needle traverses the wall of the cyst to enter the fluid-filled cavity, from which typical yellow, green or brown cyst fluid is aspirated. Usually a cyst contains 5–15 ml of fluid, but much larger amounts can occur.

Needle aspiration is a safe method of treating a breast cyst, provided certain precautions are taken.

1. The breast must be palpated carefully after aspiration. A hollow may be felt at the site of the cyst so that the surrounding breast tissue is more clearly palpable. There should be no residual discrete mass.

2. The cyst fluid should be examined for blood.

Cytological examination of the cyst fluid is unhelpful.

3. Mammograms should be requested. These may show additional cysts in one or other breast but no signs of cancer.

4. The patient should be re-examined in 3–4 weeks' time to determine whether the cyst has remained empty. If it has refilled, one further aspiration may be done. Refilling thereafter is a definite indication for removal.

Indications for excision biopsy are: a residual mass after aspiration, significant blood in the cyst fluid, a suspicious mammogram, and repeated re-filling of the cyst.

Risk of malignancy

The risk of developing cancer in women with cystic disease is reported to be two to three times higher than normal. These estimates are based on retrospective studies. There are no good prospective studies in which women with cystic disease have been matched with normal controls, both being meticulously followed over a long period of time.

As epithelial elements are believed to be at risk, attempts have been made to classify atypical appearances of ductal and lobular epithelium. These are difficult to interpret and require detailed study. A breast must never be removed solely on the basis of a frozen section report of epithelial atypia.

BENIGN DISEASES OF THE DUCTS

Duct ectasia

This condition is characterized by dilatation of the major ducts, which fill with inspissated pultaceous creamy secretion, and is associated with a periductal inflammatory reaction in which round cell infiltration predominates (Fig. 17.12). It is not known whether the dilatation of the ducts occurs first and is followed by leakage of secretions which initiate the periductal reaction or whether, conversely, periductal reaction occurs first, destroying elasticity and allowing duct dilatation.

Duct ectasia may be completely asymptomatic or 'occult', being recognized only in mastectomy

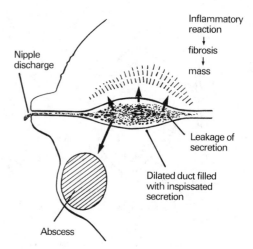

Fig. 17.12   Duct ectasia and its clinical presentation

specimens or at post-mortem examination, or it may be associated with one or more of the following clinical signs.

1. Discharge from the nipple (bloody, serous or creamy) arising from one or more ducts.

2. Retraction or inversion of the nipple due to shortening of the ducts.

3. An episode of acute inflammation affecting a segment of the breast which may lead to a non-lactational abscess or a mammillary fistula (see p. 210).

4. Chronic inflammation of a localized area or segment of the breast (plasma cell mastitis). This forms a hard craggy area within the breast which may be associated with tethering and dimpling of overlying skin, and with nipple retraction. Its similarity to cancer may lead to inappropriate mastectomy.

Duct ectasia is treated by excision of the involved ducts and surrounding breast tissue. When there is discharge or nipple inversion, the major duct system is excised with or without eversion of the nipple.

Nipple discharge

Discharge from the nipple may be from a single duct or from several ducts, a fact which can be ascertained by clinical examination. The discharge may contain blood; its colour varies from clear through yellow and green to dark brown. Examination should include clinical palpation, paying particular attention to the peri-areolar region; biochemical testing for blood; cytology for red cells and malignant epithelial cells; mammography; and possibly ductography (X-ray following the injection of a water-soluble contrast medium into the duct orifice). The likely causes of multiple duct discharge, which may contain blood, are pregnancy and duct ectasia. Provided mammography does not indicate any localized disease, no action is required.

If the discharge is profuse and the patient is concerned, a microdochectomy is indicated. A circumareolar incision is made and the nipple and areola are retracted, allowing removal of a cone-shaped core of tissue from the central area of the breast which includes the main ducts. These must be removed close to the undersurface of the nipple, which is then everted and held in place with a purse-string suture.

Single-duct discharge is commonly bloody and most frequently due to a duct papilloma (see below). Bleeding from a single duct is an indication for its excision together with the related segment of the breast. This can readily be carried out through a small circumareolar incision. The involved duct can be identified more easily if the orifice has been sealed by application of a transparent plastic dressing (e.g. Nobecutane spray) to the nipple on the previous evening. A non-bloody discharge from a single duct is not an indication for surgery unless there is a clinical or mammographic abnormality in the related segment of the breast, or the patient is seriously concerned.

Duct papilloma

Benign papillomatous growths can form from the epithelial linings of the main ducts. They may be pedunculated or sessile, and are situated within 1 cm of the nipple. Bleeding from the nipple is characteristic and originates from a single duct, the orifice of which is dilated and slit-like. The papilloma may be felt as a small nodule at the areolar margin. Pressure at that point reproduces the discharge (Fig. 17.13).

Mammography shows a dilated duct and/or a

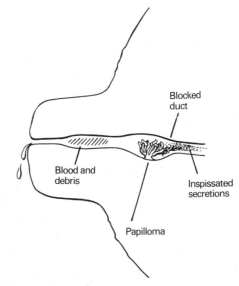

Fig. 17.13 Duct papilloma

small round opacity close to the nipple, and on ductography a filling defect is demonstrated. Treatment consists of surgical excision of the involved duct.

THE PAINFUL BREAST

Pain, discomfort and heaviness in the breasts are common symptoms which, if severe, can interfere with the normal sex life of a woman and cause irritability and depression. Breast pain may be cyclical, occurring predominantly in the premenstrual phase, or non-cyclical, when its occurrence has no relationship to the menstrual cycle. The former is frequently associated with tender nodularity and fullness of the breast, which is most pronounced in its upper outer quadrant. This is generally assumed to be of hormonal origin. Non-cyclical pain may be associated with inflammatory disease of the breast or with duct ectasia, or it may be a symptom of neurosis.

The breasts should be carefully examined. In women over 35 years, a mammogram should be obtained. Most patients have no local disease, but if cysts are present they should be aspirated, and tender fibrous nodules may require excision.

Many patients with breast pain are helped by reassurance that there is no serious disease present. If cyclical symptoms are severe, the antiprolactin bromocriptine or the anti-oestrogen tamoxifen may give relief.

Non-cyclical pain is not helped by such measures. If the breasts appear normal, a psychiatric opinion may be required.

MISCELLANEOUS TUMOURS

Connective tissue tumours

Benign connective tissue tumours. Lipomas, angiomas, leiomyomas and neurofibromas are all rare. A lipoma of the breast forms a soft lobulated mass which on mammography is radiolucent. Its importance lies in the possibility of its confusion with a 'pseudolipoma', the soft fatty mass which can surround a small scirrhous carcinoma and is caused by indrawing of surrounding fat by fibrous spicules.

Malignant tumours. Fibrosarcoma, lympho-sarcoma, rhabdomyosarcoma, angiosarcoma and osteogenic sarcoma are all rare. Unlike the phyllodes tumour (see above), these tumours contain no epithelial elements. A sarcoma presents as a rapidly enlarging breast mass. Spread occurs predominantly by the blood stream and gives rise to metastases in lungs and other viscera. Treatment consists of radical local surgery. Sarcomas of the breast are radioresistant.

Lymphoma

The breast may be the site of a lymphomatous deposit. This forms a smooth discrete and firm mass resembling a fibroadenoma. Axillary lymph nodes are typically rubbery and discrete.

Secondary tumours

Metastases can occur within the breast and form a well-defined discrete mass which mammographically is also usually well defined. Primary sites are most commonly a bronchus, the thyroid, a malignant melanoma or cancer of the opposite breast.

SCREENING FOR BREAST CANCER

The recognition that breast cancer presents fre-quently at an incurable stage has led to interest in earlier detection of the disease. Programmes of education and 'self-palpation' have been instituted in which women are encouraged to seek advice for the smallest abnormality. With the development of mammography, it soon became apparent that small cancers of less than 1 cm in diameter could be visible radiologically before they became clinically palpable. Small discrete opacities, areas of disturbed breast architecture, clusters of irregular small (micro-) calcifications and asymmetry of parenchymal density between the breasts may point to a cancer months or even years before it becomes clinically obvious. Controlled trials in New York and Sweden, supported by case-control studies in Holland, indicate that regular mammographic screening of women over the age of 50 years reduces mortality from breast cancer by one-third. A national programme has now been set up in the UK to perform mammography (by a mediolateral oblique view of each breast) every three years in women aged 50–64 years.

Facilities for the assessment of mammographic abnormalities are essential to an efficient screening programme. This should include clinical examination, sophisticated mammography (including magnification views), ultrasonography, and fine-needle aspiration to differentiate solid from cystic lesions. For solid lesions fine-needle aspiration cytology is a valuable investigation, and stereotactic equipment is now available to guide a fine needle into an impalpable mammographic lesion. The training of skilled 'assessment teams' to support screening programmes is essential if these are to be effective.

Should a surgical biopsy be indicated, localization techniques are required to guide the surgeon to the site of an impalpable lesion. This may be done either by insertion of a hooked wire marker into the breast under radiological control or by injection of a small quantity of methylene blue combined with a contrast agent so that it is both visible on an X-ray and to the surgeon exploring the breast. In both instances X-rays are taken after insertion of the localizing material to define the lesion for the surgeon.

It is also critical that the surgeon confirms that the lesion has been removed. This requires immediate radiology of the specimen, and dedicated apparatus is now available to permit this to be carried out in the operating room.

Considerable experience and expertise are required for the histopathological examination of these small lesions. Rapid diagnosis by frozen section is not satisfactory; the pathologist must define the site of the lesion by slicing the specimen and if necessary X-raying the slices. He will also wish to examine relevant areas of normal tissue by microscopy.

As screen-detected lesions are small and therefore well-suited to methods of treatment conserving the breast, they are best managed by surgeons and radiotherapists experienced in these techniques.

Radiation can induce breast cancer. It has been calculated that for each 0.01 Gy of radiation received by the breast there will be six extra cancers per million women, starting after a latent period of 10 years. Radiation dose must therefore be kept low. With modern systems of sensitive film-screen combinations a complete two-view examination of the breast can be performed with a dose to the breast of a fraction of 0.01 Gy.

CANCER OF THE BREAST

Cancer of the breast is an adenocarcinoma arising from epithelium lining the ducts and acini. Cancers arise in the terminal-duct-lobular unit and are divided into ductal and lobular types. Both ductal and lobular cancers may be invasive (infiltrating) or non-invasive (non-infiltrating) or in situ. Only invasive cancers metastasize.

Types of invasive cancer

Duct cancers

About 80% of all invasive cancers of the breast are of the ductal type of 'nondescript histological pattern'. However, ductal cancers with specific histological features do occur. Those of greatest importance are described below.

Medullary cancer. This is a well-delineated tumour accounting for 5% of cancers. Microscopically it is sharply and completely circumscribed. It consists of syncytial sheets of large neoplastic cells with a substantial diffuse infiltrate of mononuclear lymphoid cells. Its prognosis is better than that of a typical duct cancer.

Tubular cancer. This is a well-differentiated tumour which accounts for some 10% of invasive breast cancers and is typified by proliferation of small tubular duct-like structures which are haphazardly arranged in a loose cellular stroma. It is this type of cancer which may be confused with sclerosing adenosis. Its prognosis is better than average.

Mucoid cancer. Like medullary cancer this is well circumscribed. It is a rare tumour characterized by a copious matrix of mucinous tissue. It also has a relatively good prognosis.

Lobular cancer

Lobular invasive cancer accounts for 5–10% of breast cancers. It is typified by the bland homogeneous nature of its small cells. As with ductal carcinoma, various histopathological types are described, including cribriform, solid and tubular types. The differentiation between lobular and ductal cancers is not easy and there is no single criterion by which they can be identified.

Carcinoma-in-situ

Non-invasive cancers of the breast are confined to the ducts and acini and have not penetrated the basement membrane of the epithelial cell layer. Lobular carcinoma-in-situ is usually an incidental finding in biopsy specimens of postmenopausal women. There is total infiltration of one or more lobules with small neoplastic round cells.

Intraduct carcinoma is usually detected as microcalcifications on mammography. The epithelial cells of otherwise normal ducts and lobules undergo malignant change and either cling to the duct wall or form papillary masses with the ducts. Both lobular cancer and intraduct carcinoma-in-situ have a long natural history and a good prognosis. This is further considered below.

Biology and natural history

Spread of breast cancer

Invasive breast cancer spreads by lymphatic and blood streams (Fig. 17.14). The regional lymph

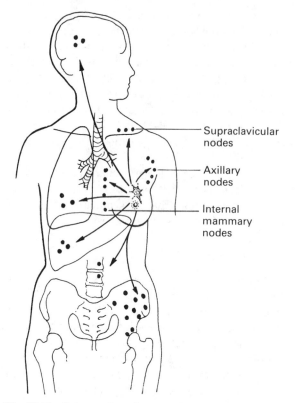

Fig. 17.14 Common sites of spread of breast cancer

nodes most commonly involved are the axillary nodes and those lying in relation to the lateral thoracic (the pectoral nodes) and subscapular vessels (the subscapular nodes). From these nodes the disease spreads to those lying along the axillary vein (the central group) up to the level of the first rib (apical group). Supraclavicular nodes may also be affected.

Although tumours in all parts of the breast can give rise to axillary node metastases, those in the medial half may also spread to the internal mammary group of nodes lying along the internal mammary vessels within the mediastinum. This is most common when the axillary lymph nodes are also involved and only occasionally are the internal mammary nodes the sole route of spread. Internal mammary node involvement is a bad prognostic sign and usually indicates spread to mediastinal nodes and pleural cavities.

While it used to be believed that breast cancer spread in two distinct steps with initial spread to the regional lymph nodes and only then to distant organs, it is now known that tumour cells can bypass the node 'filter' and that spread by both lymphatic and blood streams occurs from the start. Systemic spread can occur to any site but metastases are particularly common in the skeleton, lungs, liver, brain, the ovaries and peritoneal cavity.

Aetiology

Breast cancer is the commonest cancer affecting females in Western countries. In the UK at least 7% of women develop the disease. In Japan, Africa and South America its incidence is one-sixth of that in Europe and North America. The difference in incidence is particularly marked in postmenopausal women. The cause for the geographical variation in the incidence of the disease is unknown; some believe that dietary factors (particularly fat) are important.

There are certain other factors which increase the risk of developing breast cancer. Early age at menarche, late age at first pregnancy, nulliparity, late age at menopause, upper social class, a previous history of certain types of benign breast disease and a family history of breast cancer are all associated with an increased risk. Some of these factors have been examined alone and in combination to determine whether they can be used to select women at high risk for regular screening. However, they are not sufficiently sensitive for this purpose. Nevertheless they may have a place in determining the frequency of examination in individual women.

Only women who have already been treated for breast cancer (whose opposite breast is at risk) or who have a mother or sister who has been treated for the disease justify special surveillance.

The relationship between atypical changes in the breast epithelium and later development of breast cancer is under study. At present only frank in situ cancer and atypical hyperplasia of the breast associated with a family history of the disease are proven antecedents of invasive cancer.

Natural history

The risk of breast cancer increases with age, but because of the number of women at risk it is most common in women of 50–60 years. There is a fall-off in incidence during the menopause (Fig. 17.15) which has led some to believe that there are two distinct types of breast cancer, affecting premenopausal and postmenopausal women respectively. This is unproven.

Breast cancer is a slow-growing chronic disease and metastases may develop many years after apparently successful local treatment. The length of recurrence-free interval and survival time are affected by the extent of the disease at the time of presentation. The larger a tumour and the more extensive the local spread the worse its prognosis. Lymph node involvement also affects survival adversely. The larger the number of lymph nodes involved the worse the prognosis. Only 30% of women with four or more invaded axillary lymph nodes will survive for 5 years.

Biological factors also affect the aggressiveness of the disease. These include the type of tumour and tumour-host relationship. The histological grade of differentiation (based on the degree of tubule formation and the regularity of nuclear size and shape), tumour contour, degree of periductal elastosis and lymphocytic infiltration, and reactive changes in the regional lymph nodes all affect prognosis. Tumours which are well differentiated, have a smooth contour, exhibit elastosis or marked lymphocytic infiltration and evoke reactive enlargement of regional lymph nodes have a better prognosis than poorly differentiated lesions with a spiculated contour, no lymphocytic infiltration and no reaction in regional nodes.

Recently it has been found that tumours expressing differentiation antigens, rich in oestrogen receptor (ER) activity and with a greater proportion of diploid cells have a more favourable prognosis than undifferentiated, ER-negative and aneuploid tumours. The factors influencing the prognosis of breast cancer are summarized in Table 17.1.

Curability

Recent reports on the long-term follow-up of women with breast cancer treated only by local surgery and radiotherapy indicate that 'cure' (define as survival for a normal lifespan free from disease) is achieved in less than 30% of patients with so-called 'operable' disease. If those considered inoperable when first seen are also included, the 'cure' rate is less than 20% (Fig. 17.16). Even 30–40 years after primary treatment, women with breast cancer have an excess mortality from metastatic disease compared to the normal population.

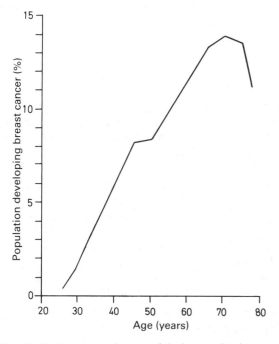

Fig. 17.15 Prevalence of cancer of the breast related to age

Table 17.1 Factors influencing the prognosis of breast cancer

Biological factors	Extent of disease
TUMOUR	Size of tumour at time of presentation
Histological type Grade Contour	Involvement of regional lymph nodes
Necrosis Lymphocytic infiltration ER concentration Degree of elastosis DNA (ploidy)	Distant metastases
NODES Reactive changes	

ER = oestrogen receptor

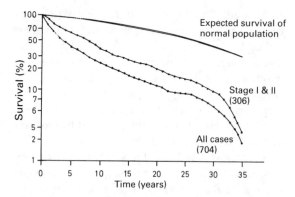

Fig. 17.16 Survival curve of women with breast cancer. Long-term follow-up of 704 patients with breast cancer. (From Brinkley & Heybittle 1984, Lancet)

Diagnosis

Clinical examination of the breast

Breast cancer usually presents as a lump which is painless or at most associated with a tingling discomfort. It most commonly occurs in the upper outer quadrant of the breast and may have caused recent nipple retraction. The breast should be carefully examined for visible signs of fixation. These include asymmetry of the breast, flattening of its contour, dimpling or puckering of the overlying skin and retraction or altered axis of the nipple. These signs are more evident when the patient is sitting with her hands raised above her head or when she places her hands on her hips and pushes out her chest.

The mass is readily palpable. Classically it is hard with an irregular surface which merges into the surrounding breast tissue. Cancer in a fatty breast may be deceptively soft due to 'packaging' of surrounding fat by the contraction of the fibrous framework of the breast. This may even be mistaken for a lipoma (pseudolipoma).

It is important to appreciate that *any* discrete lump, no matter how small or mobile, can be a cancer. This is particularly important in young women with a glandular breast, in whom cancer cannot be distinguished clinically from a small fibroadenoma.

Some patients present with advanced local disease and exhibit skin ulceration, infiltration, oedema or fixity and in some instances obvious contraction of the whole breast to the chest wall. Then the diagnosis should not be in any doubt.

The regional lymph nodes in the axilla and supraclavicular fossa are carefully palpated and the findings recorded. It should he noted whether nodes are palpable and if so whether they are soft, hard, mobile, matted or fixed to surrounding structures.

It is hoped that with the introduction of mammographic screening an increased number of breast cancers will become evident in the preclinical phase.

Needle aspiration

The most important point when dealing with a breast mass in a middle-aged woman is to distinguish between a cancer and a cyst. Aspiration with a fine (21-gauge) needle is attempted. If no fluid is obtained, an aspirate of the tumour is prepared for cytological examination. This is done by repeatedly advancing the needle through the tumour while suction is applied. On withdrawal, the tissue aspirated into the needle is expressed onto a slide, fixed and stained. The demonstration of malignant cells provides unequivocal evidence of cancer.

Radiology

In expert hands mammography has an accuracy of diagnosis of cancer (sensitivity) of 95%. A cancer appears as a dense opacity containing small clustered microcalcifications and has an indefinite outline from which irregular spicules (or spikes) jut out into the surrounding breast. Secondary signs of tumour include thickening of the overlying skin, a distorted duct and vascular pattern, and dilated veins (Fig. 17.17). Mammography is of less diagnostic value in young women, in whom the density of the lesion differs little from that of the surrounding parenchymatous tissue. Mammography is important for the full examination of both breasts and may detect additional (multifocal) tumour deposits in one or other of the breasts.

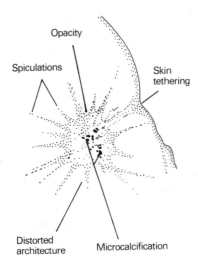

Opacity

Spiculations

Skin tethering

Distorted architecture

Microcalcification

Fig. 17.17 Mammographic signs of breast cancer

Tru-cut biopsy

The final diagnosis of cancer rests on histo-pathological examination. This used to be made at the time of definitive surgery by examining a specimen of tumour by frozen section, but the use of fine-needle aspiration cytology and Tru-cut biopsy has obviated the need for this step. Tru-cut needle biopsy provides a small core of tissue suitable for examination by standard histological techniques.

Staging

The international TNM system of classifying breast cancer allowed grouping of the disease into *clinical stages* which traditionally determined curability by local treatment. It was considered that if the growth was confined to the breast and regional (axillary) lymph nodes it could be eradicated by mastectomy and axillary lymph node clearance or by a combination of surgery and regional radiotherapy. This is no longer accepted.

Nevertheless careful clinical staging allows comparison of patients treated in different centres and defines those patients whose local disease is unsuitable for surgical treatment. Its two main drawbacks are that:

1. palpability of axillary lymph nodes is not synonymous with tumour involvement; and

2. clinical methods are insufficiently sensitive to detect small 'micrometastases' in viscera and bones.

The first drawback has been resolved by acceptance of the need for histological examination and the institution of pathological TNM stages. Removal of some or all of the axillary nodes for histopathological examination is now regarded as a necessary part of breast cancer surgery.

It was hoped that the development of more sensitive methods of detecting occult metastatic disease would resolve the second problem. However, the use of radionuclide, ultrasonic and CT scans and of sophisticated tests of organ function has not proved of great value.

At present, routine examination of a patient with early breast cancer for occult metastatic disease need include only X-rays of chest, haematological examination and liver function tests. A bone scan is frequently also performed (particularly in special units concerned with the conduct of therapeutic trials), but in operable disease the yield of positive scans is low.

The current system of staging is shown in Table 17.2.

Table 17.2 Summary of TNM classification of breast cancer

Primary tumour

Tis	Pre-invasive carcinoma (carcinoma-in-situ) Paget's disease (no tumour)
T0	No evidence of primary tumour
T1	Tumour ≤2 cm ⎫ a. no fixation to underlying pectoral fascia and/or muscle
T2	Tumour 2–5 cm ⎬ b. fixation to underlying pectoral
T3	Tumour >5 cm ⎭ fascia and/or muscle
T4	Any size with direct extension to chest wall or skin a. fixation to chest wall b. oedema, lymphocytic infiltration, ulceration of skin or satellite nodes c. both of the above

Regional lymph nodes

N0	No palpable homolateral axillary lymph nodes
N1	Moveable homolateral axillary nodes a. not considered to contain growth b. considered to contain growth
N2	Fixed homolateral axillary nodes
N3	Homolateral supraclavicular or infraclavicular nodes or oedema of arm

Distant metastases

M0	No evidence of distant metastases
M1	Evidence of distant metastases

Treatment

Until recently the orthodox treatment of cancer limited to the breast and axillary lymph nodes was either 'radical mastectomy', in which the breast was totally removed and the axilla cleared of all lymph nodes, or 'simple mastectomy', in which only the breast was removed and radiotherapy given to 'sterilize' the lymph nodes and skin of the chest wall. Realization that these procedures resulted in long-term cure in only a minority of patients led to a reappraisal of the objectives of treatment and to the introduction of systemic as well as local methods of control.

Local therapy

Stages I and II. For tumours which are 5 cm or less in size with no skin involvement or chest wall fixation (T1, T2, a or b) there are two accepted methods of local treatment.

1. *Mastectomy* is still considered by some to be the treatment of choice. Provided the axillary lymph nodes are not fixed to each other or to surrounding structures (N0, N1), the axilla may either be surgically cleared of all nodes or the nodes can be sampled. Sampling entails removal of the pectoral or lower axillary nodes for histological examination.

There is no need for postoperative radiotherapy if the axilla has been surgically cleared of lymph nodes even if node histology is positive. However, if *sampled* nodes are involved by tumour, radiotherapy is advised to control possible residual disease in the unremoved nodes. In this case, radiotherapy is given to the chest wall, axilla and supraclavicular and internal mammary lymph node regions in a dose of approximately 45 Gy. This selective policy has the advantage that high surgical dissection of the axilla or radiotherapy are avoided in node-negative patients.

2. Recently there has been a swing towards *conservation of the breast* and, for tumours of less than 4 cm in diameter, local excision of the mass combined with radical radiotherapy to the remaining breast and nodal region gives local and systemic control equal to that of a mastectomy. For tumours of 4–5 cm in diameter mastectomy is still

preferred. The axilla is either dissected completely, with clearance of all or most lymph nodes, or it may simply be sampled, three to four nodes being obtained from the lower axilla for histological examination.

Radical radiotherapy requires megavoltage (6 MV) equipment to deliver high doses of radiation to the breast, surrounding chest wall and nodal regions (the axilla being excluded if a full dissection has been carried out). Using fractionation, a dose of 60 Gy can be delivered without severe reaction in the overlying skin. Irradiation of the tumour area may be boosted by an external beam of electrons or by lengths of iridium-90 wire 'after-loaded' into plastic tubes which are inserted into the tumour bed at operation. In this way a further 20–30 Gy can be delivered to the region of the breast involved by the tumour.

Conservation treatment is contraindicated if the cosmetic result is likely to be unsatisfactory (e.g. in a small breast with a large tumour); if there is evidence of multifocal disease; if the tumour is insufficiently excised and extends to the margin of the excision specimen; or if there is extensive in situ malignancy surrounding it. Re-excision may be advised, rather than proceeding to a mastectomy. Evaluation by preoperative mammography and careful examination of the excised tumour and surrounding breast is essential.

It is uncertain whether radiotherapy is required in all cases and studies are being conducted to determine whether some small tumours may be treated by local excision and axillary dissection alone.

Stage III. Provided there is no skin involvement or deep fixation, tumours over 5 cm in size may still be suitable for mastectomy but this should be followed by radiotherapy. If there is skin involvement or deep fixation (T4), surgery is contraindicated but local control can be achieved by radiotherapy.

Clinical lymph node status affects the choice of local treatment only when nodes are fixed. In this event surgical treatment of the axilla is contraindicated.

Studies are being conducted to determine the place of primary systemic therapy in these large tumours.

Adjuvant systemic therapy

The aim of systemic therapy is to inhibit the growth of micrometastases. The best indicator of the existence of established systemic spread and its likely aggressiveness is axillary node status.

Clinical trials suggest that chemotherapy with cyclophosphamide, methotrexate and 5-fluorouracil (CMF) reduces recurrence and improves survival of premenopausal women with involved axillary nodes. The effect in post-menopausal women is less clear and chemotherapy is not generally advised as a routine.

As breast cancer may be dependent on oestrogens, ovariectomy and ovarian irradiation have been recommended in premenopausal women at the time of initial primary treatment and appear to give similar benefit, particularly if low-dose prednisolone (5 mg daily) is also given. Comparisons are being made with the benefit achieved by chemotherapy.

The role of hormone therapy in older women is also under study, and the results of numerous controlled randomized trials indicate that long-term administration of the anti-oestrogen tamoxifen (20 mg daily) increases survival of those with involved lymph nodes. Treatment with this drug is now regarded as rational in such patients. Evidence that tamoxifen similarly benefits women with negative lymph nodes is less convincing, but patients with tumours of bad prognosis, e.g. large anaplastic carcinomas, or with lymphatic and intra-vascular invasion should be considered for tamoxifen therapy even if node-negative.

The role of oestrogen receptor activity in the tumour in determining the type of systemic therapy to be given as adjuvant treatment in primary disease is being studied (see later).

Complications of treatment

Radiotherapy

Following radiotherapy the skin must be kept dry during the erythematous reaction. The patient is advised not to wash and a light talc is applied. If moist desquamation occurs, zinc and castor oil ointment is applied. The reaction to radiotherapy usually lasts 5–6 weeks. Patients must avoid direct sunlight on the area for several years or serious sunburn may result.

Lymphoedema of the arm

A troublesome complication of breast cancer is lymphoedema of the arm. This may be due to malignant infiltration of axillary lymphatics but more commonly it is a complication of surgery and radiotherapy. Radical removal of the lymph nodes in the axilla interrupts lymph drainage from the arm and this effect is intensified by postoperative irradiation. Lymphoedema is more common when infection has complicated surgery. Thrombotic occlusion of the axillary vein may also occur. Lymphatic and venous obstruction together cause massive arm swelling.

Oedema is usually first noted in the hand and forearm, which become heavy. The condition spreads up the arm and if untreated the whole arm gradually becomes swollen, tense, brawny, hard, heavy and painful. Infection from minor injuries leads to attacks of cellulitis and lymphangitis, usually of streptococcal origin, which extend lymphatic obstruction. In rare cases small nodules of tumour appear in the skin; these have been described as angiosarcomatous but more frequently are metastatic (of breast cancer origin).

Lymphoedema is best treated by intermittent compression with an inflatable arm cuff (Fig. 17.18) and a supportive elastic arm stocking. The patient is warned to avoid minor trauma and should wear gloves when carrying out rough work or gardening.

Surgical treatment of lymphoedema is unsatisfactory. Flaps of latissimus dorsi have been used to form a lymphatic conduit from the arm but are of uncertain value.

Microsurgical techniques now allow lymphatico-venous anastomoses to be performed. To be successful these must be carried out at several sites as soon as lymphoedema is suspected. However, as thrombosis of the anastomoses is common, long-term results are disappointing. Occasionally lymphoedema is so severe that the limb becomes massive and an intolerable burden to the patient. In these rare cases forequarter amputation may be indicated.

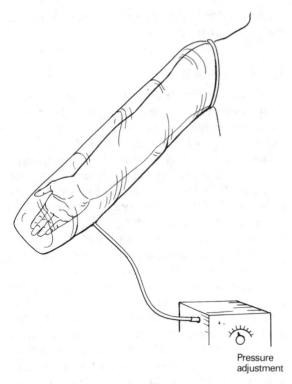

Pressure
adjustment

Fig. 17.18 Pneumatic compression to treat lymphoedema of the arm

Psychological effects of mastectomy

Cancer of the breast induces great psychological stress. Following mastectomy one-third of patients have moderate or severe anxiety and depression and are in need of psychiatric help. The symptoms include intolerance of body image, concern about its effect on husband and family, and anxiety about relationships with other people. As a result a patient may withdraw from her normal social relationships, and radically alter her domestic and sexual activities.

While many of these problems are related to the mutilation from mastectomy, fear of the disease and uncertainty about the future play an equally important role. Thus, even patients treated by local excision and radiotherapy may develop psychological disturbances.

Good counselling is essential. While in theory this is an important role of the surgeon, in practice it is difficult to achieve and in many specialist units nurse counsellors are now employed. Not only are they responsible for keeping the patient informed of the nature of her disease and its treatment, they also give advice on the best type of prosthetic support and are trained to recognize those patients who may develop serious psychiatric disturbances and require psychiatric support.

If a patient is completely intolerant of her mastectomy, breast reconstruction may be considered. In its simplest form this consists of insertion of a silicone gel prosthesis under the pectoral muscles. Symmetry is difficult to achieve, but 'expansion' prostheses are now available which can be 'topped up' each week through a reservoir implanted in the axilla until they reach the size of the other breast. They are then replaced by a standard prosthesis. Where loss of tissue or post-radiation fibrosis is marked it may be necessary to advance a musculocutaneous flap of latissimus dorsi to form new skin covering for the false breast (Fig. 17.19).

In some specialized centres these methods of reconstruction are now offered to patients requiring mastectomy as a primary procedure. Two surgical teams are an advantage, one to perform the mastectomy, the other to mobilize the musculocutaneous flap.

Follow-up

Following treatment for primary breast cancer, patients are reviewed at regular intervals (usually 3-monthly for the first 2 years, 4-monthly for the next 3 years and annually thereafter). Attention is paid to local control. In those treated by mastectomy the chest wall and regional node areas are carefully examined. In patients with breast conservation, detection of recurrence in the breast is not easy and yearly mammograms are necessary. Because lymphoedema of the breast may follow radiation therapy, mammograms are not always satisfactory. Fine-needle aspiration cytology of the irradiated breast is equally unreliable.

A search for metastatic disease is not profitable and in asymptomatic patients routine investigations are a waste of resources. Because of the incidence of cancer in the other breast (1% per year) annual mammography of the contralateral breast is advised.

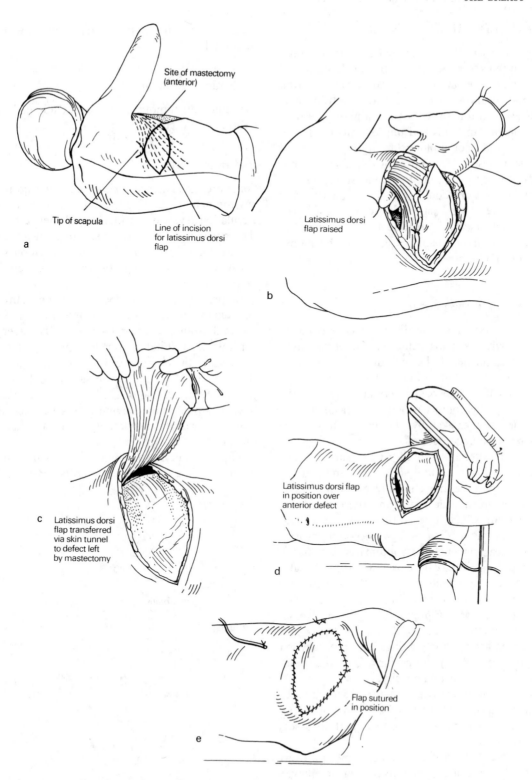

Fig. 17.19 Latissimus dorsi flap for reconstruction of the breast. (A silicone prosthesis may be inserted under the flap.)

ADVANCED BREAST CANCER

In its later stages breast cancer can cause distressing symptoms, e.g. discomfort from ulcerating and fungating lesions on the chest wall, dyspnoea from lung and pleural involvement, and pain from bone metastases. At this stage the main aim of treatment is to relieve symptoms and improve the quality of life; one must not prolong life at the expense of increasing misery. As control of the disease is important for reducing symptoms, measures to effect tumour regression should normally be instituted as soon as overt metastatic disease is recognized. These include local treatment by surgery or radiotherapy and systemic treatment by hormones or by chemotherapy.

Assessment of the patient

When treating metastatic disease it is essential to measure what is being achieved. Otherwise ineffective treatment may be prolonged unnecessarily and cause more discomfort than the untreated disease itself. Three parameters are relevant: the tumour, the symptoms which arise from it, and the morbidity caused by the treatment. These must be separately assessed.

Various criteria are used to measure tumour regression. These require serial measurements of tumour deposits either clinically or from X-rays. Responses are not clear-cut, and there is a 'grey area' within which it is difficult to be certain whether a tumour is regressing or becoming worse.

The 'measurement' of symptomatic response is even more difficult. Various self-assessment scales are available by which the patient can grade her symptoms and from which it can be determined whether they are improving or getting worse. Typical symptoms are pain, breathlessness and fatigue. Similarly, activity ratings have been devised in which the ability to perform day-to-day activities is expressed numerically.

The morbidity of treatment varies according to the methods used. Structured questionnaires can be used to determine side effects and to assess their progress.

Any form of treatment takes time to exert benefit. In general 2–3 months should be allowed before therapy for advanced breast cancer is regarded as ineffective and new treatment instituted.

Systemic treatment

Systemic anti-tumour measures include endocrine treatment and chemotherapy.

Endocrine therapy

Some breast cancers are sensitive to their hormonal environment (Fig. 17.20), and measures to alter circulating levels of hormones and their action on the cancer cell have been used to treat advanced disease for many years. The main hormones implicated in promoting breast cancer are the oestrogens.

In premenopausal women the main source of oestrogens are the ovaries, where they are synthesized from precursor C-19 steroids under the control of pituitary gonadotropins. After the menopause the ovary atrophies and oestrogen synthesis depends on the conversion of C-19 steroid precursors of adrenal origin in fat, muscle and the liver by aromatasing enzymes. Breast cancer tissue also has aromatasing activity and can therefore manufacture its own oestrogens.

The action of oestrogen on target tissue depends on its binding to specific receptor protein. The

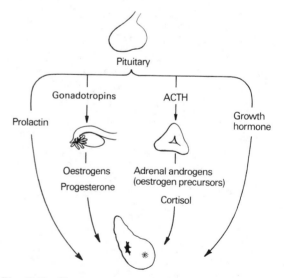

Fig. 17.20 Hormones which may influence breast cancer

resulting complex acts on the genome to stimulate protein synthesis and cell proliferation. About 60% of human breast cancers possess oestrogen receptor activity. This can be estimated biochemically on cytosol preparations by saturation with 31, 1-oestradiol, separation of bound and unbound steroid using dextran charcoal, and scintillation counting of these fractions. The recent development of specific monoclonal antibodies to oestrogen receptor protein has allowed enzyme-linked immunoassay on cytosol and immunochemical assay on intact cells. This can now be performed on cytological aspirates obtained by fine-needle aspiration.

A variety of methods are available to reduce the levels of circulating oestrogen or inhibit its action.

Surgical endocrine ablation. In premenopausal women surgical oophorectomy or ovarian irradiation effectively reduces circulating oestrogen levels, and effects a remission in approximately one-third of young women with advanced breast cancer. The average duration of remission is 18 months. In older (postmenopausal) women in whom the ovaries have ceased to function, oophorectomy is of no value. However, levels of circulating oestrogens can be reduced by removing the source of C-19 steroid precursors by bilateral (total) adrenalectomy. Alternatively, secretion of corticotropin (ACTH), which stimulates production of adrenocortical steroids, can be abolished by removal of the pituitary or by its destruction by insertion of radioactive yttrium (^{99}Y) into the pituitary fossa.

These procedures require life-long replacement therapy with cortisone and have largely been superseded by pharmaceutical agents.

Pharmaceuticals. A variety of agents are used to inhibit oestrogen action. These act either by preventing the synthesis of oestrogen or by interfering with its peripheral effects.

Gn-RH analogue agonists. Gonadotropin secretion from the pituitary is normally stimulated by pulsatile 'spurts' of gonadotropin-releasing hormone (Gn-RH) of hypothalamic origin. If the pituitary is bombarded continuously with large amounts of Gn-RH, it becomes desensitized to this normal mechanism and gonadotropin secretion is inhibited. Analogues of the natural releasing hormone which act as potent agonists are now available and can be used to induce 'medical castration' pharmacologically. The analogue can be administered as a nasal spray, by subcutaneous injection or (most conveniently) in delayed-release polymer capsules which are implanted into the abdominal wall. Initial results in patients with advanced breast cancer are encouraging.

Aromatase inhibitors. Aminoglutethimide is an anticonvulsant which inhibits aromatase activity and, in postmenopausal women, also reduces oestrogen synthesis. As it also acts on hydroxylating enzymes in the adrenal cortex, it inhibits the synthesis of cortisol. It must therefore be administered together with hydrocortisone (40 mg). In a dose of 0.5–1.0 g daily it gives similar remission rates in advanced breast cancer to surgical adrenalectomy (30%).

Side effects of the drug can be troublesome and include lethargy, skin rash, gastrointestinal upset and occasionally thrombocytopenia and leucopenia. For this reason aminoglutethimide is usually reserved for 'second-line' endocrine therapy. To minimize the side effects, smaller doses (250–500 mg) may have to be used.

A new generation of aromatase inhibitors are now being synthesized. One of these, 4-hydroxyandrostenedione, is currently undergoing clinical trials and good remission of disease has been reported.

Tamoxifen. This triphenylamine acts by binding to the oestrogen receptor protein. Not only does this form an ineffective complex, it also prevents access of natural oestrogen to its receptor. In a dose of 20 mg daily it produces remissions of advanced breast cancer equal to those achieved by other endocrine means (30%). Its great advantage is that it has few side effects, and although thrombocytopenia, jaundice and vaginal bleeding have been described these occur only occasionally and are not of consequence. Tamoxifen is without doubt the endocrine treatment of choice in postmenopausal women. In premenopausal women it is not clear that it is as effective as ovarian ablation or Gn-RH agonists.

Other agents. In the past, high doses of oestrogen, androgen and progesterone were used to treat advanced breast cancer and induced remission of disease in a proportion of patients. Only two progestogens are now commonly used. These are medroxyprogesterone acetate (Provera), which is given either by mouth (in a dose of up to 1.5 g daily) or by intramuscular depot injection (in doses varying from 250 mg weekly to 1.0 g daily), and megestrol acetate (Megace) 160 mg daily by mouth. These are usually given as 'second-line' therapy.

Prolactin inhibitors (levodopa and bromo-ergocriptine) and the gonadotropin inhibitor danazol have also been used by some.

Chemotherapy

Single-agent chemotherapy is relatively ineffective in breast cancer. Combinations of cell-cycle dependent and independent drugs are now preferred. These include alkylating agents (cyclophosphamide) and antimetabolites (methotrexate and 5-fluorouracil). Doxorubicin (Adriamycin) is the most effective of these drugs, and most courses of treatment for advanced disease now include this agent. Its total dose is limited by its cardiotoxic effects.

Cyclical combination chemotherapy will cause remission in 60% of patients. The duration of remission is relatively short, averaging 6 months. Typical regimens are given in Table 17.3.

Selection of therapy

The availability of oestrogen receptor assays has rationalized anti-tumour therapy in breast cancer.

Tumours with low concentrations of receptor are refractory to endocrine treatment; conversely, those which are receptor-rich have a 50% chance of response.

In premenopausal women with a receptor-positive tumour removal of functioning ovaries should still precede other forms of endocrine treatment. Not only is this the most effective method of reducing oestrogenic influences, but patients who respond positively to oophorectomy are also likely to gain further benefit from other agents (e.g. aminoglutethemide or progestogens) when their tumour subsequently relapses. Those who fail to respond to oophorectomy are likely to remain unresponsive to other endocrine measures. It is for this reason that gonadotropin-releasing hormone analogues, which have a profound but reversible effect, offer an exciting alternative to oophorectomy.

In postmenopausal women a trial of tamoxifen (20 mg daily for 2–3 months) is usual, and many surgeons will give this treatment irrespective of receptor status, knowing that a small proportion of patients with tumours low in oestrogen receptors will gain worthwhile benefit from tamoxifen. Others use the drug only for tumours which are rich in oestrogen receptor.

In a responding patient the drug is continued until relapse, when 'second-line' endocrine therapy is initiated. This may either be amino-glutethimide with hydrocortisone or high-dose progestogen therapy. If considered necessary,

Table 17.3 Examples of chemotherapy regimens used in the treatment of advanced cancer

CMF			
Cyclophosphamide	750 mg/m^2	i.v.	
Methotrexate	50 mg/m^2	i.v.	3-weekly
5-Fluorouracil	600 mg/m^2	i.v.	
VAP			
Vincristine*	1.4 mg/m^2	i.v.	
Adriamycin (doxorubicin)**	50 mg/m^2	i.v.	3-weekly
Prednisolone	10 mg	four times/day for 5 days, by mouth	
CHOP			
Cyclophosphamide	1 g/m	i.v	
Hydroxyadriamycin (doxorubicin)	50 mg/m^2	i.v.	3-weekly
Oncovin (vincristine)*	1.4 mg/m^2	i.v.	
Prednisolone	10 mg	four times/day for 5 days, by mouth	

* Maximum dose 2 mg.
** Mitozantrone is a possible substitute for Adriamycin which is potentially less cardiotoxic. Alopecia, nausea and vomiting are not a major problem. It is given by intravenous infusion over 15–30 min in a dose of 14 mg/m^2 at 3-weekly intervals.

these may be used sequentially. The new generation of aromatase inhibitors are likely to be preferred in time.

For women with proven receptor-negative tumours and those who fail to respond to endocrine therapy, chemotherapy is the only alternative option. In advanced disease it is usual to use a regimen which contains Adriamycin. In some life-threatening situations (e.g. severe bone marrow depression, pulmonary lymphangitis, liver metastases), immediate chemotherapy is the preferred option irrespective of the receptor status of the tumour.

If the response is good, the drug should be continued. On relapse, or if there is no response, further treatment will depend on the fitness of the patient and the oestrogen-receptor status of the tumour. A trial of aminoglutethimide is worthwhile; if this is successful, hypophysectomy or adrenalectomy may be considered. Otherwise the only useful alternative is chemotherapy.

General support

Care of the patient with advanced breast cancer requires more than control of the tumour. Palliation includes control of symptoms and is particularly important in those who fail to respond to endocrine treatment or chemotherapy. The methods which are available are outlined in Chapter 16.

Treatment of special problems

Certain types of metastatic disease require special methods for their control.

Pleural metastases. Pleural effusions in those with a history of breast cancer are regarded as malignant until proven otherwise. Symptoms of severe dyspnoea demand aspiration. This is best carried out by tube thoracostomy, a small chest drain being inserted through the 8th and 9th space in the midaxillary line and connected to waterseal drainage to which suction is applied (at 25 cm water). Fluid should be sent for cytology.

Pleural effusions usually respond well to systemic therapy. If not, local instillation of a cytotoxin may be required, bleomycin being the preferred agent. Following tube thoracostomy, 60–120 mg dissolved in 100 ml saline is injected. The tube is clamped while the patient lies supine, prone and on either side. The clamp is removed after 24 hours and the tube reconnected to an underwater seal with suction to empty the chest completely.

Lung metastases. Discrete lung metastases do not cause severe symptoms. Lymphangitis carcinomatosa, in which the pulmonary lymphatics are infiltrated by cords of tumour, causes bronchospasm and severe dyspnoea. This may be relieved by steroid therapy (prednisolone 30 mg daily) and bronchodilators (e.g. salbutamol). Chemotherapy is the preferred treatment.

Hypercalcaemia. Transient increases in serum calcium concentrations occur in 40% of patients with bone metastases. More severe hypercalcaemia (over 3 mmol/l) associated with gastrointestinal, renal and neuromuscular symptoms occurs in 10% and can develop rapidly following hormone or diuretic therapy. The most prominent symptoms are nausea, constipation, thirst and polyuria, personality change and muscle weakness, these usually being associated with increasing bone pain.

Persistent levels of over 3 mmol/l must be reversed. Infusions of sodium chloride correct dehydration and promote excretion of calcium; diuretics are given to maintain a urine output of 3–5 litres/24 hours and steroids (prednisolone 60 mg daily) to enhance bone resorption and reduce serum calcium. Oral and intravenous phosphate will predictably lower serum calcium according to the dose given but this sequesters calcium, and precipitation in the kidneys, blood vessels and soft tissues is a long-term problem. Oral phosphate (1–3 g daily) is usually given but can cause diarrhoea. New preparations of diphosphonates are becoming available.

Mithramycin 25 mg/kg rapidly reduces serum calcium by interfering with osteoclastic function but is toxic. Effective anti-tumour therapy is an essential part of management.

Bone metastases. These are usually of osteolytic type. The majority of patients with widespread bone metastases have severe pain and are disabled. Systemic therapy is essential but local radiotherapy (20 Gy over 5–7 days) can relieve pain and promote healing. Recalcification of osteolytic lesions is particularly valuable in weightbearing bones and may prevent pathological fracture. It may also prevent vertebral collapse and paraplegia. If fracture occurs, orthopaedic reinforcement may be required. This can include total hip replacement. Oral phosphates are reported to confer additional benefit.

Spinal cord compression. Compression of the spinal cord by extradural tumour is common in breast cancer. The condition must be recognized early and treatment instituted promptly. Patients with back pain who develop neurological symptoms are treated as surgical emergencies. A myelogram is performed to determine the site and extent of compression. The spinal column is surgically decompressed and postoperative irradiation arranged. The duration of symptoms prior to treatment is the most important guide to recovery and delay must be avoided.

Brain metastases. Rising intracranial pressure and neurological dysfunction associated with intracerebral metastases cause severe problems. As soon as cerebral secondaries are suspected, high-dose steroid therapy with dexamethasone (10 mg intravenously, followed by 4 mg intramuscularly at 6-hourly intervals) should be instituted and a CT scan arranged. Treatment can be continued with oral dexamethasone 2 mg three times a day.

Whole-head irradiation (30 Gy over 3 weeks), although accompanied by loss of hair, is worthwhile. Neurosurgical excision is rarely indicated unless an apparently single lesion is demonstrated on CT scan. In this case removal may give striking palliation.

Liver metastases. Progressive liver failure and jaundice result from infiltration of the liver by metastatic disease. Occasionally endocrine treatment can induce dramatic shrinkage but this is rare and liver metastases are generally regarded

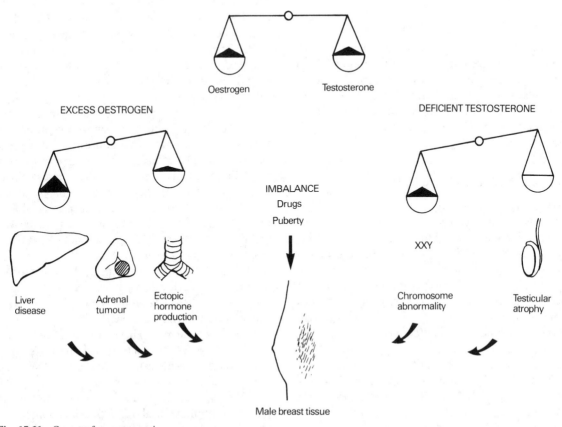

Fig. 17.21   Causes of gynaecomastia

as an indication for chemotherapy. They are often rapidly fatal. Steroid therapy may improve well-being.

THE MALE BREAST

Gynaecomastia

Enlargement of the male breast is becoming increasingly common. Histologically the swelling consists of duct and fibroepithelial elements; alveolar formation is rare. Although clinically it is usually unilateral, mammograms will normally show hypertrophy of both breasts. Irritation and tenderness of the nipple may be a feature.

Gynaecomastia must be differentiated from cancer. Helpful guides are its concentricity and firmness and the lack of skin fixation or ulceration. A cancer is eccentric in relation to the nipple, stony hard and fixed.

Gynaecomastia results from excessive hormonal drive (Fig. 17.21). It is a physiological event at puberty and at the 'male menopause'. In these older men it may be associated with testicular atrophy, low testosterone and high gonadotropin levels.

Drugs are another important cause of gynaecomastia (Table 17.4). Digitalis, spironolactone, phenothiazines and cimetidine are the most common. As spontaneous resolution may occur, there is no need to stop the treatment unless pain and tenderness are severe or the patient is unduly disturbed by his enlarged breast. Increased levels of circulating oestrogens are an obvious cause of gynaecomastia and may be due either to administration for therapeutic purposes (e.g. in the treatment of cancer of the prostrate) or to excess

Table 17.4 Some drugs commonly associated with gynaecomastia

Amphetamines	Oestrogens
Adrenocorticosteroids	Phenothiazines
Androgens	Radioactive iodine
Bendrofluazide	Reserpine
Cimetidine	Salbutamol
Digoxin	Spironolactone
Marihuana	

production (e.g. in testicular feminization or as a result of an oestrogen-secreting tumour of the adrenal gland). Ectopic hormone production by a bronchial carcinoma or other tumour can also cause the condition.

Failure to metabolize steroid hormones, e.g. in chronic liver disease, may also result in gynaecomastia. When due to excess hormonal stimulation, gynaecomastia is usually bilateral.

Provided there is no endocrine cause, a gynaecomastic breast can be removed by a simple operation preserving the nipple and overlying skin.

Cancer

Cancer of the male breast is rare. Because of the lack of breast tissue it rapidly becomes fixed to the skin and chest wall and ulceration is common. Treatment is similar to that for the female. Metastatic cancer in the male follows a similar pattern to that in women but is frequently hormone-sensitive. Excellent regression of disease has been noted following orchidectomy or tamoxifen therapy, and aminoglutethimide can be used as 'second line' therapy.

18. Skin, connective and soft tissues

Structure of the skin and its appendage

Skin

The skin of an adult covers a surface area of some 1–1.8 m². It is thinnest on the glans penis and eyelids and thickest on the palms, soles and back. Skin consists of two elements (Fig. 18.1). The *dermis* is composed of collagen, elastic fibres and fat which support blood vessels, lymphatics, nerves and the epidermal appendages. The *epidermis* is avascular and consists of several layers of keratin-producing cells (keratinocytes) at different stages of differentiation and degeneration. The junction between epidermis and dermis is undulating. Projections of dermis push upwards into the epidermis to form 'dermal papillae' which carry capillaries and lymphatic channels which nourish the epidermis and permit fluid exchange. The dermal papillae are separated by ridges of epidermis, the 'rete pegs'.

The deepest layer of epidermal cells contains the basal germinal cells which produce the keratin-producing cells. The basal layer also contains pigment cells (melanocytes) which donate melanin to the developing keratinocytes, which are believed to be neuroectodermal in origin. As the epidermal cells migrate to the surface they become increasingly keratinized and are eventually shed. The whole process takes around 28 days. Production of new epidermal cells (prickle cells) equals

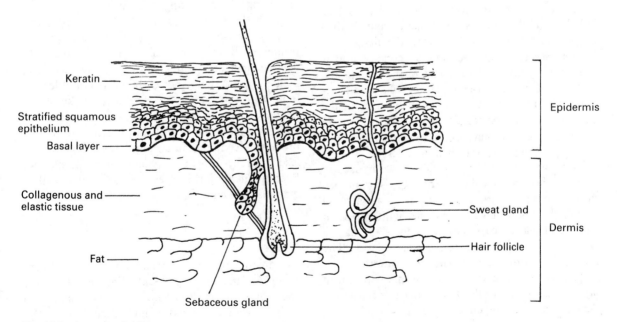

Keratin

Stratified squamous epithelium

Basal layer

Epidermis

Collagenous and elastic tissue

Sweat gland

Dermis

Hair follicle

Fat

Sebaceous gland

Fig. 18.1 Anatomy of skin

the rate of loss of fully keratinized cells, so that the thickness of the skin normally remains constant.

It is estimated that there are about 2000 million melanocytes in the human skin. They secrete melanin, which is synthesized from tyrosine and phenylalanine by cytoplasmic enzymes. They can be demonstrated histochemically by the DOPA (dihydroxyphenylalanine) reaction, which depends on the presence of an oxidative enzyme to convert dihydroxyphenylalanine to melanin.

The pigment granules can be demonstrated by silver stains. They are formed in the cytoplasm of melanocytes and pass along dendritic processes to enter neighbouring epithelial cells. As the cells migrate towards the surface, the melanin within them forms a layer of pigment which protects the germ cells of the basal epidermis and the melanocytes from the effects of ultraviolet light.

The *skin appendages* (hair follicles, sebaceous glands and sweat glands) arise from the epidermis and grow down into the dermis and in some sites to the subcutaneous tissues. The *hair follicle* is a downgrowth of epidermal cells. At its end is a small papilla containing vessels and nerves to nourish and sensitize the hairs. The colour of the hair is due to pigment which is produced by melanocytes in the hair follicle.

The *sebaceous glands* secrete sebum into the hair follicles. This contains fatty acids and hydrocarbons and lubricates the skin and hairs.

The *sweat glands* are simple coiled tubular glands lying in the dermis and opening onto the surface. They are of two types. *Eccrine* glands secrete salt and water over the entire surface of the skin, while *apocrine* glands (which are present in the axilla, breast and genital regions) secrete a musty-smelling fluid into hair follicles.

The *nails* are flat horny structures composed of keratin whose proximal part (the root) is implanted into a groove of skin. They arise from a matrix of germinal cells which appears as a white crescent (the lunula) at its base. On avulsion of the nail, a new nail will grow from this germinal layer. The rate of regrowth is about 3 mm per month.

The nail bed is composed of dermis with a thin layer of epidermal cells. If the matrix of a nail is destroyed, so that regeneration cannot occur, these epidermal cells form a thick keratinized protective layer.

Subcutaneous tissue

The subcutaneous tissue is composed of a supporting structure of collagen and elastic tissue containing fat, blood vessels, nerves and lymphatics. It is interposed between skin and the underlying muscles and is enclosed by the superficial fascia.

Diagnosis of skin swellings

Three questions should be asked when examining a swelling which is visible on the surface.

1. *Is it in the skin or subcutaneous tissues?* This is determined by 'pinching up' the skin over the swelling and attempting to move it from side to side. If the swelling is in the skin, neither can be moved independently.

2. *Is it epidermal or dermal?* The stretched normal epithelium overlying a dermal swelling may look glossy but normally remains smooth. It may ulcerate from pressure necrosis, but only when the swelling is large. An epithelial lesion causes roughening of the skin surface, papilliform growth or ulceration even while still small.

3. *Is the lesion pigmented?* Melanin produces black to brown pigmentation while haemosiderin produces brown to yellow pigmentation. In general, melanin pigmentation is characteristic of melanocytic activity, but certain other skin lesions (e.g. basal cell carcinoma or seborrhoeic keratosis) may also show melanin pigmentation within constituent epidermal cells. Any warty growth is prone to bleeding, and accumulation of blood may lead to red, brown or yellowish pigmentation. Such pigmentation is a feature of vascular malformations (haemangiomas).

CYSTS

Two main types of cyst occur in the skin and subcutaneous tissues (Fig. 18.2). The sebaceous (or epidermoid) cyst lies *within* the skin and is a dermal swelling covered by normal epidermis. The

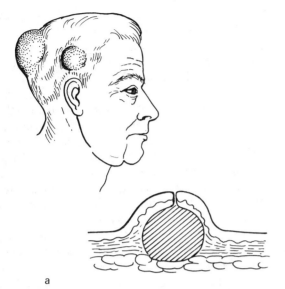
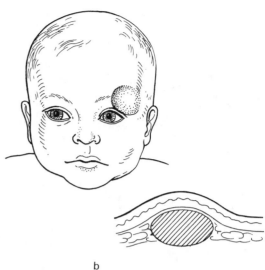

a b

Fig. 18.2 Types of cyst. (a) Sebaceous cyst. (b) Dermoid cyst

dermoid cyst lies in the subcutaneous tissues and is covered by normal skin.

Sebaceous cysts

A sebaceous cyst has a thin wall of flattened epidermal cells and contains cheesy white material composed of epithelial debris and sebum which has a characteristic sweet musty smell. Originally believed to be a retention cyst of a sebaceous gland, it is now believed to arise from a hair follicle. It is common on hair-bearing areas, i.e. the scalp, face, ears, neck, back and scrotum, where it forms a hemispherical smooth soft swelling which lies within the skin. The skin cannot be moved over it. The overlying epithelium is normal but a small punctum marking the site of the involved hair follicle is common.

A sebaceous cyst may become infected. The overlying epidermis then becomes hot, red and glazed, and the cyst may discharge spontaneously.

Treatment. An uninfected cyst is removed by excision. Following infiltration of the skin and surrounding tissues with local anaesthetic, a small ellipse of skin is incised over the cyst. This allows traction to be applied so that the cyst can be dissected from the surrounding dermis and subcutaneous tissue without rupture (Fig. 18.3).

An infected cyst is incised. Excision is delayed until the inflammation has completely resolved. It may not always be necessary as the inflammation may destroy the lining of the cyst.

Dermoid cysts

Dermoid cysts (see Fig. 18.2) arise from a nest of epidermal cells in the subcutaneous tissues. These occur either as an embryological anomaly or by implantation of epidermal cells from the skin as a result of puncture. Congenital cysts are found at sites of embryonic fusion and are most common on the face around the forehead, base of the nose and occiput. Implantation dermoids occur at sites of minor injury such as the plantar surface of the fingers and hands.

A dermoid cyst is lined by squamous epithelium and contains sebum, degenerate cells and sometimes hair. A soft rubbery swelling forms deep to the skin. The cyst may be fixed deeply, particularly when situated on the face.

Treatment. Implantation dermoids can be removed under local anaesthesia. As congenital cysts may extend deeply, they require formal dissection under general anaesthesia. *External angular dermoid* is the commonest congenital dermoid. It is situated at the junction between the outer and

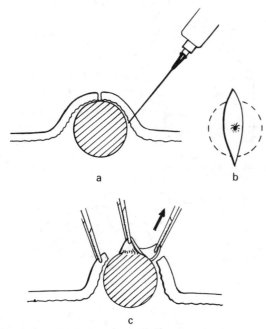

Fig. 18.3 Removal of sebaceous cyst. (a) Infiltration of local anaesthetic. (b) Ellipse of skin incised around punctum. (c). Cyst removed together with attached skin ellipse

upper margins of the orbit at the line of fusion of maxilla and frontal bones (see Fig. 18.2). Diagnosed in infancy, the cyst is best removed when the child is a few years old. As the presenting cyst may be only the outer part of an hourglass dermoid with intracranial extension, the operation may prove to be extensive. It should be preceded by a skull X-ray and a CT brain scan.

TUMOURS OF THE SKIN

These may arise from the epidermis or dermis. Epidermal tumours arise from basal germinal cells or from melanocytes. Dermal tumours may arise from any component of the dermis.

EPIDERMAL NEOPLASMS

Benign epidermal tumours

Papillomas and warts

Benign warts (or papillomas) are particularly com-

mon. Two main types are seen: infective warts (verruca vulgaris), which are viral in origin, and senile warts (seborrhoeic keratosis).

Infective warts. These are found most commonly on the hands and fingers of young children and adults (*verruca vulgaris*). They are greyish-brown, round or oval, elevated lesions with a filiform surface and keratinized projections, and may be studded with spots of blood pigment (Fig. 18.4a). They spread by direct inoculation and are commonly multiple. The natural history is one of spontaneous regression but, if troublesome, they can be treated by caustics or freezing (acetic acid, liquid nitrogen or CO_2 snow).

Plantar warts (*verruca plantaris*) are particularly troublesome and are spread by contagion in swimming pools and showers. They are usually found under the heel or heads of the metatarsals (Fig. 18.4b). Flush with the surface, they are covered by a thickened layer of epithelium and are intensely painful. If persistent, they can be removed by curettage or freezing with liquid nitrogen.

Infective warts may also occur in the perineum and on the penis and may be of venereal origin. Cauliflower-like bulky papillomatous growths (condylomata acuminata) may occur in the perineum in syphilis, lymphogranuloma and in immunosuppressed patients. They may be associated with infection by human immunodeficiency virus (HIV).

Senile warts (seborrhoeic keratosis). These are basal cell papillomas which occur in older people. They form a yellowish brown or black greasy plaque with a cracked surface which falls off in pieces and has been likened to the end of a dirty paint brush. Senile warts are often multiple, occur particularly on the upper back and trunk, and are best treated by curettage.

Pedunculated papilloma. Simple non-infective papillomas can occur at any site. They form flesh-coloured spherical warty masses which hang on a stalk of surrounding normal epithelium (Fig. 18.4c). If small, they can be removed by snipping the pedicle with scissors or induced to necrose and drop off by tying a thread around them. If large, the papilloma and its pedicle are removed together with an ellipse of normal skin.

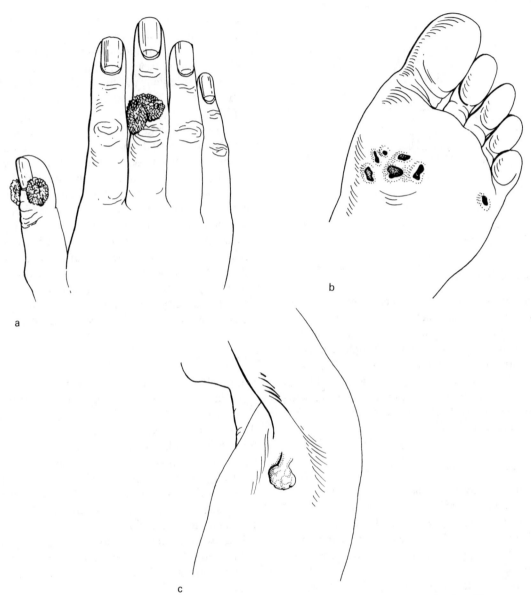

Fig. 18.4   Some types of warts and papillomas. (a) Verruca vulgaris. (b) Plantar warts. (c) Pedunculated papilloma

Keratoacanthoma (molloscum sebaceum)

This lesion is important because of the likelihood of confusion with a squamous cancer. It occurs most commonly on the face, where it forms a hemispherical nodule with a mushroom-like friable red centre crusted with keratin (Fig. 18.5). It is infective in origin, occurs mainly in those over 50 years of age and may grow at an alarming rate. It is self-limiting and heals after shedding of its central core. It is cured by curettage.

Benign melanoma

Benign moles and naevi are described later in this chapter.

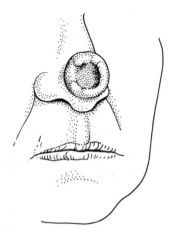

Fig. 18.5 Keratoacanthoma

Premalignant keratoses

Actinic or solar keratosis is characterized by the development of small single or multiple firm warty spots on the face, back of the neck and hands particularly of older, fair-skinned people who have been exposed excessively to sunlight. The scaly lesions drop off, leaving a shallow premalignant ulcer. They are best treated by freezing following biopsy to confirm the diagnosis and exclude malignant change.

Intraepidermal cancer (carcinoma-in-situ)

This inactive form of cancer is non-invasive. It forms a discrete, often solitary, raised brown or red fissured plaque which is keratinized. Histologically, the lesion consists of hyperplastic epithelial cells which have atypical forms but remain in situ.

When on the skin, the condition may be referred to as *Bowen's disease*. In-situ cancer of the glans penis, which is rare, is also known as 'erythroplasia of de Queyrat'.

Epidermoid cancer

Skin cancer occurs primarily on exposed areas and in those with poor natural protection against sunlight. It is rare in negroes and other dark- and yellow-skinned races. Albinos and those with *xeroderma pigmentosa* (a congenital defect leading to undue sensitivity to sunlight) are particularly at

risk. Chronic skin irritation by arsenic, tar or soot is a well established cause of skin cancer. Other established causes include chronic ulceration (e.g. from old burns, scars or varicose ulcers) and therapeutic radiation, which causes an intense skin reaction with erythema and blistering leading to atrophy, loss of appendages, pigmentation, telangiectasis, fibrosis and scarring. In those exposed to chronic radiation such changes may pass unnoticed and lead to skin cancer. Fissuring of the fingers is a warning sign which must not be ignored.

Skin cancer may occur at any age but is more common in men over 50 years. There are two distinct pathological forms: basal cell carcinoma (rodent ulcer) and squamous cell (or epidermoid) carcinoma. These two types of cancer behave very differently. A rodent ulcer is very slow-growing, is only locally malignant, and seldom metastasizes; a squamous carcinoma grows more rapidly and metastasizes early to regional lymph nodes.

Basal cell cancer (rodent ulcer)

Almost all rodent ulcers arise on the midportion of the face, typically on the nose, inner canthus of the eye, forehead and eyelids (Fig. 18.6). Rodent ulcers are rare in other sites; they never occur on the palms or soles of the feet. They occur at an earlier age than squamous cell cancers. Microscopically, a rodent ulcer consists of club-shaped projections of basal epidermal cells which extend downwards into the dermis and are surrounded by an inflammatory reaction.

The earliest clinical lesion is a hard pearly nodule, dimpled in its centre and covered by thin telangiectatic skin. If there is cystic degeneration,

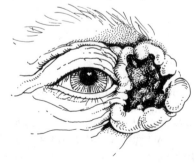

Fig. 18.6 Rodent ulcer

the neoplasm becomes raised and translucent (*cystic basal cell carcinoma*).

Characteristically, a rodent ulcer grows very slowly. Over a period of years the lesion repeatedly scales over and breaks down before the patient expresses concern. Spread may be of the 'field fire' type in which the edges spread actively while the centre is apparently burnt out. In some cases the tumour is highly invasive and burrows deeply despite little apparent surface activity. For this reason all suspicious lesions must be excised or biopsied.

Treatment. Definitive treatment consists of surgical excision or radiotherapy. Radiotherapy is contraindicated if the lesion is close to the eye or overlies cartilage. Occasionally patients are seen at a stage where deep extension necessitates radical excision and complex reconstuctive surgery.

Squamous cell cancer

This tumour can occur anywhere on the surface but is particularly common on exposed parts, i.e. the ears, cheeks, lower lips, back of hands (Fig. 18.7). All cancers arising from stratified squamous epithelium are also of this type. Chronic skin changes induced by chemical irritation, irradiation or ulceration are a predisposing factor, and squamous cell carcinomas usually develop in a pre-existing area of epithelial hyperplasia or keratosis. In the mucosa, e.g. of the lips, the analogous change is leukoplakia (see Ch. 25). The lesion starts as a hard erythematous nodule which proliferates to form a cauliflower-like excrescence

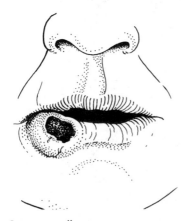

Fig. 18.7 Squamous cell cancer

or ulcerates to form a malignant ulcer with a raised, fixed, hard edge. Squamous cell cancers grow more rapidly than rodent ulcers but not as rapidly as keratoacanthomas (see above). Metastases to regional lymph nodes occur early in the disease. The nodes become enlarged, hard and fixed.

Histologically, squamous cell carcinomas consist of atypical squamous cells which infiltrate the underlying dermis to form concentric 'pearls' or 'nests'. Keratinization is an obvious feature, and epithelial bridges and prickle cells are numerous.

Treatment. The choice of treatment (i.e. wide excision or irradiation) depends on the size of the tumour, its site and aggressiveness, and whether lymph nodes are invovled. Palpable lymph nodes should be excised by block dissection unless they are fixed, in which case palliative radiotherapy offers the only hope of control. In extensive tumours, treatment with high energy (fast) neutrons has proved superior to orthodox radiotherapy. Bleomycin and other chemotherapeutic agents are of limited value but occasionally effect worthwhile remission of advanced disease.

DERMAL NEOPLASMS

Neoplams arising from the connective tissue of the dermis are rare. Dermal *fibromas*, *lipomas* and *neurofibromas* form nodules in the skin which are covered by normal epidermis. Sweat gland tumours are also rare (see below).

Dermatofibroma

This is a hard dermal nodule, sometimes pigmented, which is most commonly found on the lower legs of women. Histologically it consists of whorls of collagen fibres intermingling with fibroblasts and histiocytes containing haemosiderin, and was previously known as a sclerosing haemangioma. It should be removed.

MELANOCYTE TUMOURS

Benign pigmented moles

The pigment-producing cells, *melanocytes*, lie in the basal layer of the epidermis. The number of melanocytes (approximately 2000 million) is fixed, irrespective of the colour of the person, but the amount of pigment produced by them varies in individuals. As a developmental abnormality, conglomerates of melanocytes may migrate to the dermis or epidermis, forming a mole (shapeless mass) or melanocytic naevus. Such abnormal melanocytes are termed *naevus cells* and, according to their site and activity, cause a variety of pigmented spots and swellings or 'naevi'.

Common moles

Histopathologically, moles are classified according to the site and activity of the clumps of naevus cells. The initial changes occur at the junction of epidermis and dermis — the so-called 'junctional change'. Moles showing active junctional change are common in childhood; all moles on the palms of the hands and soles of feet are of this type. Migration of the sheets or packets of naevus cells to the dermis produces an intradermal naevus; migration to dermis and epidermis produces a compound naevus (Fig. 18.8).

The common mole is a flat or slightly raised brown-black lesion covered by normal epidermis. It has a period of active growth during childhood due to junctional activity but usually becomes quiescent at puberty and may later atrophy. With migration of the naevus cells to the dermis, the lesion becomes firm and raised, and there is often associated aberrant growth of hair. As the epidermis is not involved, the surface of the lesion is smooth. Alternatively, pigmented moles may be soft and rough. This 'fleshy hairy mole' corresponds histologically to the compound naevus.

As only 1 in 100 000 moles becomes malignant, they need not normally be removed except for cosmetic reasons. Active growth during childhood need not cause concern, but growth after puberty demands removal. Increase in pigmentation, scaliness, itching and bleeding also indicate the need for excision. In brief, any mole which has characteristics suggesting malignancy or which has reached 7 mm in diameter should be removed together with at least 1 cm of surrounding normal skin. Further treatment may be necessary once the histological features are known.

Giant hairy mole

Unlike the common mole, this congenital lesion is present at birth. It occupies a wide area, which may correspond to a dermatome. Typical sites are

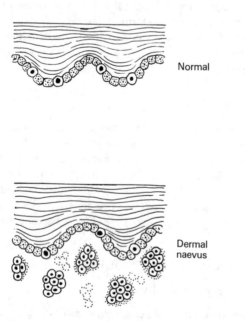

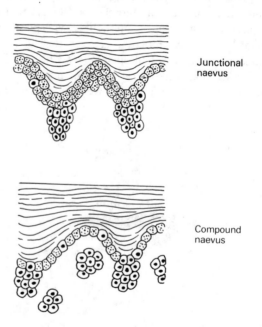

Fig. 18.8 Histopathological types of benign mole

the bathing trunk area and face. Although the risk of malignant change is not great, such moles must be kept under observation. Removal with coverage of the large defect by skin grafting is often necessary for cosmetic reasons.

Histopathologically, the lesion is highly cellular. The cells contain abundant pigment and are confined to the dermis. Neurological elements may be present. These moles are often associated with neurofibromas and other congenital abnormalities.

Blue naevus

This is a deep intradermal naevus in which strap-shaped cells laden with melanin are scattered in the deeper layers of the dermis. The cells may be of mesenchymal origin or may result from faulty migration. The blue colour of the naevus is due to the optical effect caused by the depth of the lesions.

A blue naevus may develop at any time from birth to middle life and may form a blue-black papule (beauty spot) on the face or arms, or ribbon-like areas on the wrist, ankle or buttocks. The Mongolian spot of dark-skinned races is an example. This is a poorly defined brownish area in the skin overlying the sacrum which is present at birth. It later disappears.

Halo naevus

This pigmented naevus is surrounded by a white circle of depigmentation associated with lymphocytic infiltration. This phenomenon is believed to be of immune origin.

Malignant melanoma

Malignant melanomas affect predominantly fair-skinned people. They are rare in negroes except on depigmented areas such as the palms, soles and mucosa. Exposure to sunlight is a precipitating factor. In Scotland the disease incidence per 100 000 population per year is 2.3 compared with 17 in Queensland. Malignant melanomas are commoner in females than males; this is due to an increased incidence on the lower leg of the female.

About half of all malignant melanomas are believed to arise in pre-existing naevi. The average

person has 14 melanocytic naevi, yet the risk of any one of them becoming malignant is very small. However, the greater the number of moles, the greater the risk.

The essential feature of a malignant melanoma is invasion of the dermis by proliferating melanocytes which have large nuclei, prominent nucleoli and frequent mitoses. Three distinct clinical pathological types are described.

Melanotic freckle (lentigo maligna)

One in ten malignant melanomas arises in a melanotic or senile freckle (Fig. 18.9). These occur most commonly on the face of elderly women, affecting particularly the lower eyelids, cheek, side of the nose, forehead or neck. The lesion begins as a brownish-red patch, grows slowly and centrifugally, and advances and recedes over many years. The edge of the lesion is serrated and 'map-like', but the margin with normal skin is abrupt.

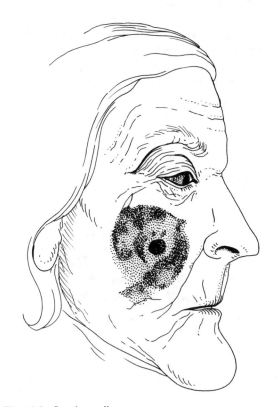

Fig. 18.9 Lentigo maligna

Kaleidoscopic pigmentation of the surface is typical.

During this premalignant phase, which may last for 10–15 years, there are conglomerates of large round melanocytes which extend laterally in the basal epidermis. The first clinical sign of malignancy is the development of a brownish-red papule eccentrically within the freckle. This indicates vertical invasion. Microscopically, abnormal melanocytes extend into the superficial dermis.

Superficial spreading melanoma

This is the commonest type of malignant melanoma (Fig. 18.10). It occurs predominantly on the trunk but is also found on exposed parts. It occurs most commonly in middle age.

During a preinvasive phase, which lasts at most for a year or two, a wave of malignancy spreads in all directions from the basal region of the epidermis. In contrast to the melanotic freckle, the surface of this lesion is slightly raised and its outline indistinct. Pigmentation is again patchy and there may be a wide range of colours.

Vertical invasion of the dermis occurs while the lesion is still relatively small and produces an indurated nodule which soon ulcerates or bleeds. A few longish white hairs may appear at the site of dermal invasion.

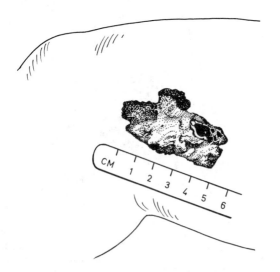

Fig. 18.10 Superficial spreading melanoma

Nodular melanoma

Nodular melanomas can occur at any site and any age. In females they are particularly common on the lower leg (Fig. 18.11). Unlike the above two types, a nodular melanoma is vertically invasive and malignant from its onset. There is no preceding intraepidermal lateral spread and therefore no surrounding pigmented macule. The total width of the lesion rarely exceeds that of two or three rete pegs.

A nodular melanoma starts as an elevated deeply pigmented nodule. It may occur at the site of a pre-existing benign naevus. The nodule steadily enlarges, both on the surface and by centrifugal extension. This expansion is first detected by destruction of the normal skin lines on the surface of the pigmented lesion. It progressively darkens and the surface over the area of active growth becomes jet black and glossy. Bleeding results from even trivial injury and is noted as a 'spotting' of blood on dressing or clothes. Crusting, scab formation and ulceration are typical. Itching and irritation are common.

In neglected tumours, satellite nodules may appear in the surrounding skin.

Other types of malignant melanoma

An *acrolentigerous melanoma* has recently been described which occurs on the volar surfaces of hands and feet and is of the malignant lentigo type.

Not all malignant melanomas are deeply pigmented. *Amelanotic melanomas* do occur and are pale pink in colour. They are usually associated with rapid growth and in pure form are very rare.

A *subungual melanoma* occurs in middle-aged and elderly patients. It most commonly affects the thumb or great toe where it may cause chronic inflammation below the nail, the *melanotic whitlow*, which is commonly misdiagnosed as a paronychia or ingrowing toenail. Pigmentation is not usually visible in the early stages, but a band of pigment may form later around the inflamed area.

Spread

Malignant melanomas (particularly of the nodular type) spread readily by lymphatic and blood

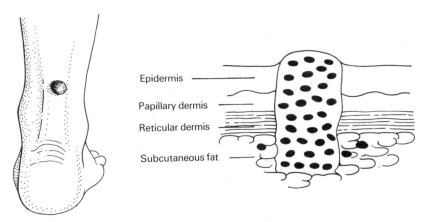

Epidermis
Papillary dermis
Reticular dermis
Subcutaneous fat

Fig. 18.11   Nodular melanoma

streams. 'In-transit' metastases may develop in the subcutaneous or intracutaneous lymphatics and form small painless discoloured nodules in the line of the lymphatics between primary lesion and regional lymph nodes. Lymph node metastases present as a firm enlargement of a single node which remains unattached and mobile. The lesion then spreads to adjacent regional and central lymph nodes. Blood-borne metastases may occur at any site but are found most commonly in the liver, abdominal cavity, lungs, brain, skin and subcutaneous tissues. Extensive metastatic growth may be associated with excretion of melanin or its enzymatic precursor 5-S-cystine L-dopa in the urine. Some 5–8% of malignant melanomas present as metastases without a recognizable primary site.

Prognosis

The most reliable prognostic indicator is the depth of the lesion (Fig. 18.12). The more superficial a tumour the better its prognosis. Depth can be measured either by reference to the normal layers of the skin (Clark) or by a micrometer gauge (Breslow). As normal skin layers are distorted by the tumour so that reference points are difficult to define, the Breslow system is preferred.

Patients with tumours less than 0.7 mm in depth have a normal life expectancy after treatment. The 5 year survival rate in those with lesions 0.7–1.5 mm in depth averages 70%; if the lesion is deeper than 1.5 mm the 5 year survival rate is 30%. A depth of 1.5 mm is therefore taken as the

dividing line between melanomas of good and bad prognosis.

The mitotic activity of the tumour also affects prognosis, and tumours may be graded according to the number of mitotic figures in a microscopic field.

As melanotic freckles and superficial spreading melanomas tend to remain superficial, they are associated with a better prognosis than melanomas of the nodular type.

Treatment of malignant melanoma

Preliminary excision

The first essential step is to reach a diagnosis and, if this is confirmed, to assess the depth of the lesion before proceeding with definitive treatment.

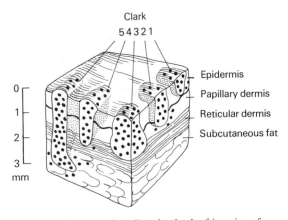

Clark
5 4 3 2 1

Epidermis
Papillary dermis
Reticular dermis
Subcutaneous fat

0
1
2
3
mm

Fig. 18.12   Methods of grading the depth of invasion of malignant melanoma

Small melanomas are therefore excised with a skin margin of 1 cm, usually under local anaesthesia. A large lesion requiring excision under general anaesthesia should be submitted to frozen section examination, which is reliable in 90% of cases.

Curative excision

Tumours of low malignancy, e.g. lentigo maligna, are excised with a skin margin of 1 cm. If there is obvious invasive growth, the margin should be wider (Fig. 18.13). Malignant melanomas of superficial spreading type or, if nodular, of 1.5 mm or less in depth are excised with a skin margin of 3 cm. If deeper than 1.5 mm, removal of at least 5 cm of normal surrounding skin is advised. The tumour and surrounding skin are excised down to, but not including, the deep fascia so that the whole depth of subcutaneous fat is removed.

The defect, if large, will have to be covered with a split skin graft. This is cut before the tumour is excised. In the case of limb melanomas the graft must be taken from the opposite arm or leg. If taken from the same limb, there is a risk that seedling deposits of tumour may develop at the donor site.

Lymph nodes

Block dissection of regional lymph nodes is considered if the primary tumour is in the immediate vicinity of regional nodes, if there is microscopic evidence of deep dermal invasion, if dermal lymphatics are invaded or if the nodes are palpable. In doubtful cases, preliminary lymphangiography may define the state of the nodes. Some surgeons advocate prophylactic dissection of regional nodes if the melanoma is greater than 1.5 cm. in depth.

An alternative method of treating lymph nodes is endolymphatic infusion of radioactive gold or lipiodol which is trapped in the nodes and irradiates them. In Britain, however, it is generally accepted that when there is no evidence of lymph node involvement, prophylactic node dissection or endolymphatic infusion has no advantage.

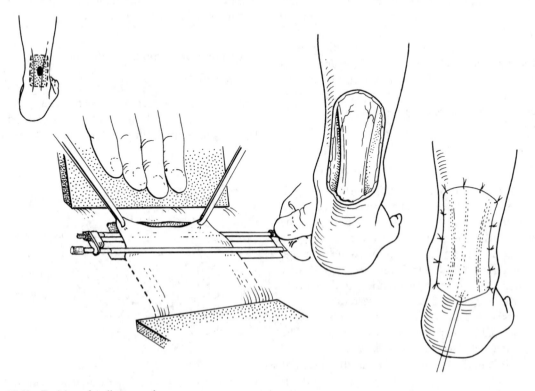

Fig. 18.13 Excision of malignant melanoma

Metastatic disease

The management of metastatic melanoma is unsatisfactory. Occasional short-lived remissions have been reported with chemotherapy using dacarbazine (DTIC; dimethyltriazeno-imidazole-carboxamide), BiCNU (a nitroso urea) and vindesine (a derivative of vincristine). Immune stimulation with BCG (bacille Calmette-Guérin), C-parvum or vaccinia virus, or injection of irradiated melanoma cells has also been used but without proven effect. Systemic therapy has been used as adjuvant treatment for primary disease but there is no evidence that it is beneficial.

Limb perfusion

Recently there has been renewed interest in perfusion of the involved limb with cytotoxins after isolation of its blood supply. In Britain this method of treatment is generally reserved for those with advanced or recurrent local disease.

VASCULAR NEOPLASMS (haemangiomas)

The histological classification of haemangiomas is complex. They are best differentiated by their clinical behaviour, i.e. whether they regress (involute) or persist.

Involuting haemangiomas

These are true tumours arising from endothelial cells. They appear at or within a few weeks of birth and affect predominantly the head and neck. If superficial, an involuting haemangioma forms a bright red, raised mass with an irregular bosselated surface, the so-called 'strawberry naevus'. If deeply situated, it forms a blue-black soft tumour which is covered by normal skin.

Active growth continues for about 6 months. The tumour then remains static until the child is 2–3 years of age, when it shrinks and loses its colour. It usually disappears before the child is 7 years of age. Such involuting haemangiomas should always be left alone.

Non-involuting haemangiomas

These are hamartomas due to abnormal formation of blood vessels. There are two main types.

Port wine stain. This is a bright red patchy lesion, often overlying the area of distribution of a peripheral nerve. Microscopically there are enlarged capillaries in the dermis which are lined by active-looking endothelial cells. However, the lesion neither grows nor involutes. It is removed if small, but large lesions are best treated by tattooing with a skin-coloured pigment. Treatment with neodymium laser is under trial.

Cavernous haemangioma. This appears as a bluish-purple elevated mass which empties on pressure and slowly refills. Unlike the strawberry naevus, it does not appear until early childhood. Histologically it consists of mature vein-like structures which lie in a fibrous stroma and are lined by flat endothelial cells. It is treated by excision.

Cirsoid aneurysm. This is a variant of a cavernous haemangioma in which the mass of vein-like structures is fed directly by arterial blood and becomes tortuous, dilated and pulsating. A common site is the scalp. Pressure from the pulsating vas-

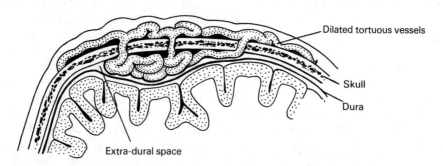

Fig. 18.14 Cirsoid aneurysm

cular mass erodes the skull. Penetrating channels may connect the superficial lesion with a similar malformation in the extradural space (Fig. 18.14).

The most effective treatment is complete excision following ligation of all feeding vessels. As serious haemorrhage may complicate the operation, preliminary angiography is essential to show the distribution of the lesion and outline its arterial supply. Preliminary embolization by injecting clot or metal beads into the feeding vessels may prove helpful.

Granuloma pyogenicum. This acquired condition is due to formation of a capillary haemangioma in a traumatized or infected area. There is a localized superficial polypoidal mass which is devoid of epithelium and resembles granulation tissue. The surface is fragile and bleeds easily. The differential diagnosis includes malignant melanoma and vascular metastases from a renal cancer. Demonstration of a pedicle is a good diagnostic guide. The condition is self-limiting in most cases. The lesion should be excised if the diagnosis is in doubt.

TUMOURS OF NERVES

Neurilemmoma

This is an encapsulated solitary benign tumour which originates from the Schwann cells of a nerve sheath and forms a subcutaneous swelling in the course of the nerve. On clinical examination it is laterally mobile but fixed in the direction of the nerve (Fig. 18.15). It may cause radiating pain in the distribution of the involved nerve. Most neurilemmomas occur superficially in the neck or limbs. They grow slowly, have no malignant potential, and are readily treated by excision.

Neurofibroma

This is regarded as a hamartoma of nerve tissue. Such lesions may be solitary but more commonly they are multiple and associated with von Recklinghausen's disease (neurofibromatosis). This is a genetically transmitted autosomal disorder condition present at birth or becoming apparent in early childhood. Multiple dermal and subcutaneous nodules arise from peripheral nerves

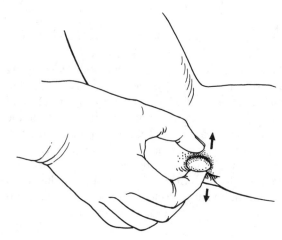

Fig. 18.15 Neurilemmoma showing characteristic lateral mobility

and are associated with patches of dermal pigmentation called 'café-au-lait' spots. The tumours cause bony deformities particularly of the spine. It is important that this syndrome is recognized, as the tumours are potentially malignant. Increase in size of existing swellings or appearance of new swellings suggests malignant change.

TUMOURS OF MUSCLE AND CONNECTIVE TISSUES

Lipoma

A lipoma is a slow-growing benign tumour of fatty tissue which forms a lobulated soft mass and is enclosed by a thin fibrous capsule. Large lipomas occasionally undergo sarcomatous change.

Although lipomas can occur in the dermis, most lipomas are subcutaneous and arise from the fatty tissue between the skin and deep fascia. Typical features are their soft fluctuant feel, their lobulation and the free mobility of overlying skin.

Lipomas may also arise from fat in the intermuscular septa, where they form a diffuse firm swelling under the deep fascia which is more prominent when the related muscle is contracted. They may cause discomfort.

As lipomas are radiolucent, soft tissue X-rays can be diagnostic but are only indicated when the diagnosis is in doubt and removal may pose problems. Unless small and symptomless, a lipoma should be removed.

Liposarcoma

Liposarcoma is the commonest sarcoma of middle age. It may occur in any fatty tissue but is most common in the retroperitoneum and legs. Wide surgical excision is the best initial treatment. This is difficult for retroperitoneal tumours, and postoperative radiotherapy and chemotherapy are advised but of doubtful worth.

As the growth rate of most liposarcomas is slow, recurrence may take a long time to develop.

Fibrosarcoma

This tumour may arise from fibrous tissue at any site but is most common in the lower limbs or buttocks. It forms a large deep firm mass. Wide excision is the initial treatment of choice; radiation therapy may be indicated to palliate recurrence.

Rhabdomyosarcoma

This is a greyish-pink soft fleshy lobulated or well-circumscribed tumour arising from striated muscle. Histologically it resembles primitive (embryonal) striated muscle. A large variety of histological subtypes are described. The tumour is more common in children, is highly malignant, and requires treatment by radical excision and/or radiotherapy. Amputation of a limb may be necessary but should be avoided wherever possible.

MISCELLANEOUS CONDITIONS

DISORDERS OF SWEAT GLANDS

Hidradenitis suppurativa

This is a chronic infection of the apocrine glands in the axilla, perineum or groin. It most commonly affects the axilla of women and is precipitated by shaving, poor hygiene and the use of chemical deodorants. There are multiple intradermal abscesses which lead to sinus formation, fibrosis and a painful diffuse chronic infection of the skin.

As the apocrine glands discharge into the hair follicles, the condition is resistant to local antiseptics. Long-term tetracycline therapy may be successful. If not, surgical excision of the axillary skin with skin grafting is required.

Hyperhidrosis

This is a disorder of the eccrine sweat glands which most commonly affects the axillae of young women. Initial treatment consists of the application of a solution of aluminium chloride. In severe cases the eccrine glands can be scraped away from the undersurface of the skin by inserting a sharp curette through a small incision.

Occasionally excessive sweating of the hands or feet can cause serious social and economic difficulties. Sympathectomy may then be indicated.

Sweat gland tumours

A variety of adenomas of sweat glands are described which give rise to dermal tumours of varying proportions. These are rare.

GANGLION

This is a common cystic swelling arising from the fibrous capsule of a joint or a fibrous tendon sheath. It contains mucoid material within a fibrous capsule and was once considered to be due to herniation of the synovial membrane of a tendon sheath or joint. It is now thought to result from degeneration of collagen.

A ganglion most commonly appears as a smooth tense hemispherical subcutaneous swelling on the dorsum of the wrist or foot (Fig. 18.16). Other sites include the palm of the hand, the palmar surface of a finger over the distal interphalangeal joint, and the lateral side of the knee over the superior tibiofibular joint. Those on the dorsum of the foot are bluish in colour due to the thin overlying skin. So-called 'mucous cysts' arising from the small joints of the hands in older people are believed to be of similar origin. A ganglion should

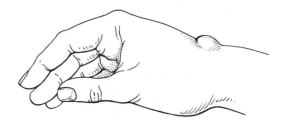

Fig. 18.16 Ganglion in a typical site

be differentiated from a bursa, which is a fluid-filled fibrous swelling overlying a bony exostosis.

A ganglion may be aspirated through a wide-bore needle or dispersed into the surrounding tissue by firm pressure. Recurrence after both procedures is common and excision under general or regional anaesthesia is preferred. A tourniquet is applied to provide a bloodless operating field for careful and complete removal of the swelling.

DISORDERS OF THE NAILS

Onychogryphosis (hooked nail)

This is an overgrowth of a nail which resembles an ox or goat horn. The big toenail is most commonly affected (Fig. 18.17). Simple avulsion of the nail does not prevent recurrence of the deformity, and excision of the nailbed is required. A flap of skin is reflected from the base of the nail and the germinal layer removed. Care must be taken to excise the edges of this layer completely or troublesome spikes of nail continue to grow. An alternative to excision of the nail bed is to cauterize it with phenol.

Ingrowing toenail

This is due to the sharp edges of the nail impinging on the surrounding skin folds (Fig. 18.18). The skin is split and infection follows. The condition is painful and made worse by misguided attempts to cut away the nail.

The patient usually comes for help once infection has occurred. An attempt is made to 'lift out'

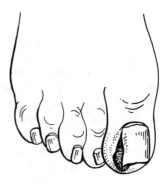

Fig. 18.18 Ingrowing toenail

the ingrowing portion of the nail with a pledget of gauze soaked in antiseptic. The patient is then instructed to cut the nail square, or shorter in the centre than at the edges, and to avoid wearing too narrow shoes.

Once the infection has spread under the nail, or the nail has become deeply embedded, it is best to avulse the nail under general anaesthesia. Antiseptic footbaths then allow the infection to resolve rapidly. The patient is instructed on the correct way to cut the new nail.

Should the condition recur, the nailbed must

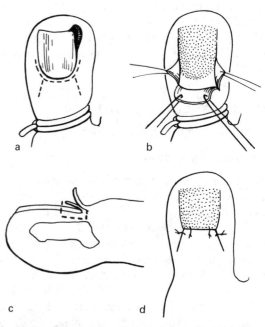

Fig. 18.19 Operation for ablation of the nailbed. (a) Skin incisions. (b) Nail avulsed and skin flaps raised. (c) Excision of nailbed. (d) Skin flaps sutured

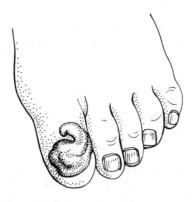

Fig. 18.17 Onychogryphosis

be ablated either surgically or with phenol (Fig. 18.19). Wedge excision of the lateral portion of the nail and underlying nailbed is no longer advised.

Nailfold infections (paronychia)

Pain, redness and swelling at the side and base of a nail are the first signs. This may extend around the nail and when fully developed produce a horseshoe swelling of the nailfold. Extension under the nail and into the underlying pulp space may occur (Fig. 18.20).

A minor paronychia will usually resolve spontaneously, but if the infection is spreading, an antibiotic (penicillin) should be given. The development of a tense shiny swelling indicates suppuration and the need for surgical drainage. A single unilateral incision may suffice, but if the infection extends under the nail, a flap of skin should be reflected from the nailbase, which is then excised to allow free drainage (Fig. 18.21). A simple vaseline gauze dressing is applied.

Failure of an acute paronychia to resolve leads to chronic thickening of the nail fold. Fungal infection is a common cause of chronic paronychia and nail scrapings are essential for diagnosis. The possibility of a subungual melanoma must always be kept in mind.

FIBROSING AND CONSTRICTING CONDITIONS OF THE HAND

Contraction of fibrous tissue occurs in many parts of the body. Symptoms result from secondary

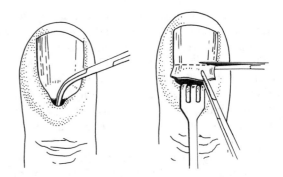

Fig. 18.21 Surgical treatment of paronychia

constriction, and in the hand this may restrict free movement.

Dupuytren's contracture

The palmar aponeurosis is a triangular fibrous structure which covers the tendons in the palm of the hand and prevents their forward dislocation (Fig. 18.22). It originates from the tendon of palmaris longus or flexor retinaculum and is inserted by fibrous bands into the proximal and middle phalanges of the fingers. Thickening and contracture of this aponeurosis is called Dupuytren's contracture. A similar condition affects the plantar

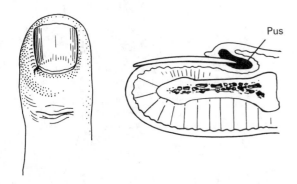

Fig. 18.20 Paronychia. The longitudinal section shows relation of pus to the nailbed

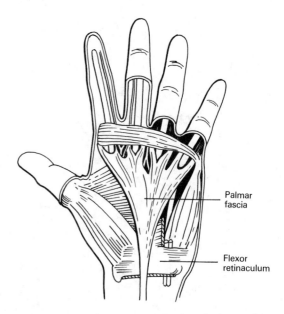

Fig. 18.22 Flexor retinaculum and palmar fascia

fascia of the sole of the foot but, because of constant stretching of the plantar fascia by weightbearing, this often goes unnoticed.

The aetiology of Dupuytren's contracture is obscure. Some cases are familial, while others are associated with alcoholism or chronic ill health, e.g. from pulmonary tuberculosis. Its association with epilepsy is accounted for by the use of phenytoin.

The first sign of the condition is usually a small fibrous nodule or cord just distal to the distal palmar crease in the line of the fourth finger. The medial half of the palmar fascia gradually contracts so that the ring and little fingers become flexed and drawn towards the palm of the hand (Fig. 18.23). This causes a hook-like deformity so that an object once grasped cannot be released. Other fingers progressively become involved. The skin of the palm may fuse with the underlying fascia and become raised and rock hard, or it may become puckered and indrawn. Vessels, nerves and tendons remain free from the fibrotic process.

If the patient is seen at an early stage, he is advised to keep stretching the aponeurosis by passively extending his fingers, e.g. by sitting on the backs of his hands. Once the disease has given rise to contracture this is no longer helpful. If the contracture is localized to a single finger and the overlying skin is still freely mobile, the taut bands of the palmar aponeurosis may be divided by subcutaneous fasciotomy. If several fingers are involved, complete excision of the palmar aponeurosis is required. In severe and long-standing cases the capsules of the metacarpophalangeal and proximal interphalangeal joints become permanently contracted. Capsulotomy is then indicated. Amputation of a severely affected single finger is sometimes necessary.

Stenosing tenosynovitis

Stenosing tenosynovitis is caused by a fibrous stricture in a tendon sheath, usually at the site of a 'pulley' or tunnel through which the tendons pass when changing direction. The tendons predominantly affected are those of the thumb at the level of the radial styloid and those of the finger in the distal part of the palm.

De Quervain's synovitis. This is the name applied to stenosing tenosynovitis affecting the fibrous sheath of the tendons of the thumb (the abductor pollicis longus and extensor pollicis

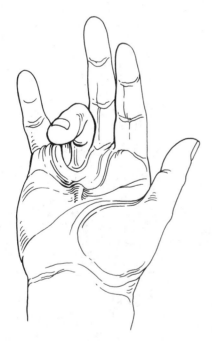

Fig. 18.23 Dupuytren's contracture

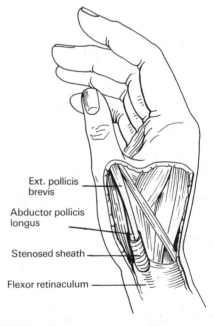

Ext. pollicis brevis

Abductor pollicis longus

Stenosed sheath

Flexor retinaculum

Fig. 18.24 De Quervain's tenovaginitis

brevis) as they run through the tunnel at the tip of the radial styloid process (Fig. 18.24). There is pain and tenderness over these tendons which is exaggerated by active or passive stretching of the tendons. Simple domestic tasks such as wringing clothes or lifting a teapot may cause severe pain.

Trigger finger. This is the more common of the two conditions and is due to thickening of the fibrous flexor tendon sheath at the level of the metacarpophalangeal joint (Fig. 18.25). Pain and tenderness at this site occur on active or passive movements of the affected finger. As the tendon is drawn through the narrowed portion of the sheath it develops a fibrous bulge which may prevent its ready return and 'lock' the finger in flexion. Attempts to extend the finger may require passive assistance which will cause the tendon to 'snap' through the strictured area.

In infants and young children mainly the thumb is affected. Since the child usually does not know how to extend the thumb passively, it remains flexed and may be mistaken for a congenital anomaly. A palpable nodule at the base of the thumb is the clue to the true diagnosis.

These conditions can be corrected permanently by surgical decompression of the fibrous tendon sheath so that the thickened tendon is no longer obstructed.

In Australia a condition known as repeated stress injury (RSI) reached epidemic proportions in keyboard operators. Pain and weakness in wrist and forearm were typical symptoms. The cause is not understood.

Nerve compression syndromes

Nerves, being soft structures, are prone to compression when they run within fibrous or rigid compartments. Examples are compression of the median nerve as it passes under the pronator teres in the forearm, the ulnar nerve as it runs in the groove of the medial condyle of the humerus at the elbow or around the hook of the hamate in the hand, and the lateral cutaneous nerve as it enters the thigh.

The commonest form of nerve compression is the *carpal tunnel syndrome*, in which the median nerve is compressed as it runs below the flexor retinaculum at the wrist (Fig. 18.26). It affects primarily middle-aged women, is a known complication of pregnancy, myxoedema and

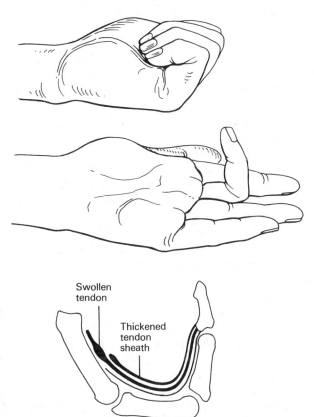

Fig. 18.25   Trigger finger

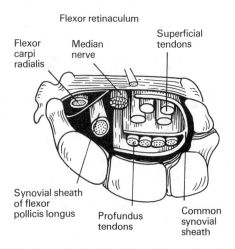

Fig. 18.26   Anatomical relationships of the carpal tunnel

acromegaly, and may be precipitated by local oedema leading to increased tension under the retinaculum. Symptoms include pain, particularly at night, in the thumb and lateral three fingers, disturbance of sensation and wasting of the muscles supplied by the median nerve (first two lumbricals, abductor and flexor pollicis brevis, opponens pollicis).

Splinting of the wrist at night relieves the pain and is a useful diagnostic test. Relief may also be obtained by injection of hydrocortisone succinate under the retinaculum in the line of the nerve. Surgical decompression of the nerve is required if there is muscle wasting or when nerve conduction studies demonstrate a nerve block at the site of the retinacular tunnel. This simple operation can be performed through a small incision using a tenotome (Fig. 18.27).

INFECTIONS OF THE HAND

The hand is particularly prone to minor injury. Even the most trivial puncture wound must be treated with respect, as otherwise infection may enter the anatomical spaces within the hand and lead to the rapid development of lymphangitis and

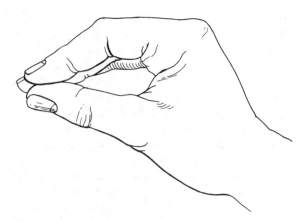

Fig. 18.28 Position of function of the hand

lymphadenitis. The commonest infecting organism is *Staphylococcus aureus*, and prompt and effective therapy is necessary to prevent serious consequences.

In general, the principles of management of a hand infection are systemic antibiotics, elevation of the limb and immobilization of the hand in the position of function, i.e. with the thumb and fingers semiflexed (Fig. 18.28). The choice of antibiotic depends on the likely source of infection. In view of the common frequency of staphylococci, flucloxacillin, which is not inactivated by penicillinase, is usually the first choice. Should streptococcal infection be suspected on account of rapidly spreading lymphangitis, large doses of benzylpenicillin are given. If rapid resolution does not occur, the antibiotic should be changed, e.g. to erythromycin or a second-generation cephalosporin (cefuroxime), and consideration given to draining the infection. Anaerobic or mixed infections of the hand (e.g. from bite wounds) demand urgent attention.

Collar-stud abscess

When a blister becomes infected, a subepithelial abscess forms. If the overlying skin is callous, the abscess spreads by pointing through the dermis into the subdermal fat, forming a so-called 'collar-stud' abscess with subepithelial and subdermal components (Fig. 18.29). Such abscesses may track deeply into the anatomical spaces of the finger and hand. Early surgical treatment by

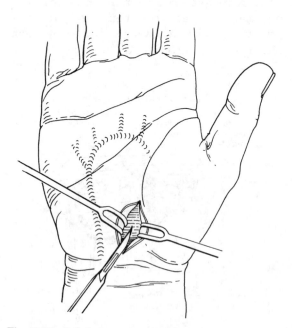

Fig. 18.27 Relief of carpal tunnel syndrome

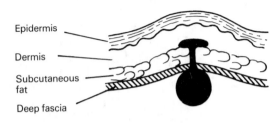

Fig. 18.29 Collar-stud abscess

deroofing the superficial compartment and dilating the dermal tract to allow free drainage of underlying pus is advised.

Pulp space infection

The pulp space lies anterior to the distal phalanx and is divided into loculi containing fat and fatty tissue by septa running from the front of the phalanx to the skin (Fig. 18.30). Infection within the unyielding loculi rapidly builds up painful tension and interrupts the blood supply to the distal phalanx, predisposing to septic necrosis of the bone.

Surgical decompression is therefore performed as soon as an abscess is suspected, i.e. if the pulp is tense, swollen or red, or if the patient complains of throbbing pain. As it is important not to damage digital nerves and vessels, the incisions should be placed longitudinally over the point at which the abscess points, or in the midline anteriorly. Such incisions must not cross the flexor crease over the distal interphalangeal joint for fear of entering the flexor tendon sheath or joint capsule. The spaces over the middle and proximal phalanges may also be infected directly, but this is less common.

Web space infection

The web spaces contain loose areolar tissue and provide a path of least resistance for pus tracking from an infected blister situated distally in the palm or from the lumbrical canals to the fingers. The skin anterior to the web becomes thickened, red and glazed, but swelling is mainly dorsal. If there is a collar-stud abscess in the distal palm, the space is decompressed through this. Otherwise it is best opened through a small dorsal incision.

Midpalmar and thenar space infection

These potential spaces lie in the palm of the hand between the anterior surface of the metacarpals and interossei (midpalmar space), and the adductor pollicis and flexor tendons (thenar space). They may become infected by spread from a web space or tendon sheath, or by direct puncture.

Because the palmar aponeurosis restricts swelling anteriorly, swelling of the hand is disproportionately great on the dorsum, which becomes grossly ballooned. Maximum tenderness is felt anteriorly over those parts of the spaces which are least covered by overlying tissues (Fig. 18.31).

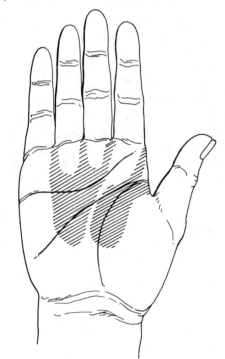

Fig. 18.31 Midpalmar and thenar spaces

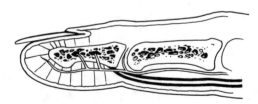

Fig. 18.30 The pulp space

Surgical decompression is achieved by incisions placed over the site at which the infection points. Damage to vital structures is avoided by blunt dissection through the deeper tissues. If there is no obvious site of pointing, the spaces may be opened from the medial or lateral side of the hands.

Acute tenosynovitis

To allow free and frictionless movement of the hand, the flexor tendons are enclosed in two layers of synovium separated by fluid and surrounded by a fibrous sheath (Fig. 18.32). Infection may gain access to these synovial spaces either by spread from contiguous infection or by direct puncture, and then spreads rapidly within their anatomical confines.

Most commonly acute tenosynovitis affects the flexor sheath of a finger, which becomes grossly swollen and semiflexed. Any attempt to move the tendon, either actively or passively, causes severe pain. Such passive movements must be tested gently. Tenderness is maximal just proximal to the crease over the metacarpophalangeal joint where the digital tendon sheath projects into the palm.

Infection of the flexor sheath of the thumb spreads into the radial bursa on the lateral side of the palm of the hand. Infection of the sheath of the little finger may involve the common flexor sheath, in which case there is gross oedema of the whole hand, especially the dorsum. The fingers are held in a semiflexed position and any attempt at moving or stretching the flexor tendons is painful. There is diffuse tenderness over the palm which is maximal on the medial side and may also be elicited in the forearm above the flexor retinaculum.

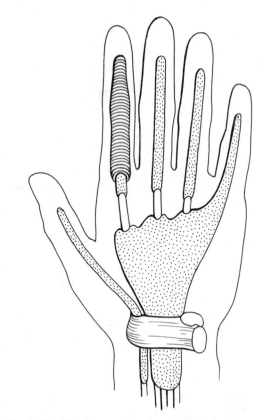

Fig. 18.32 The flexor tendon sheaths of the hand

If there is no immediate response to intensive conservative therapy, surgical decompression of the affected sheath is indicated. Otherwise necrosis of the tendon may occur. Normally two small incisions are made through which pus can be evacuated and soft catheters inserted to allow irrigation and instillation of an appropriate antibiotic.

19. The chest and mediastinum

The respiratory system comprises those organs which bring atmospheric gases into proximity with the blood and permit exchange of oxygen and carbon dioxide. It includes the airways, the lungs with their pleural spaces, and the chest wall. Also in the thoracic cavity, and lying between the lungs, is the mediastinum.

THE AIRWAYS

Air is conducted into the lungs through the upper (nose, pharynx and larynx) and lower (trachea, bronchi and their subdivisions) respiratory tract.

In the upper respiratory tract inspired air is warmed, humidified and filtered. Food, drink, saliva and other secretions do not normally enter the air passages, but are safely directed down the oesophagus during the act of swallowing. If the upper airway is bypassed, as by an endotracheal tube or after tracheostomy (see below), the epithelium of the lower respiratory tract may be injured by drying, making clearance of secretions ineffective and leading to infection. Similarly, if the coordination of the swallowing mechanism is impaired, e.g. by neuromuscular disease or after anaesthesia, the lower airway may be contaminated by aspiration of food or fluid, again with infection as the likely outcome (aspiration pneumonitis).

The trachea is a tube consisting of incomplete cartilage rings joined by fibrous tissue; the cartilage rings are deficient posteriorly. In the adult the trachea is about 10 cm long and lies half in the neck and half in the chest. The cervical part is easily palpable as a midline structure unless deviated by pressure from a mass or movement of the upper mediastinum.

At the main carina the trachea bifurcates into right and left main bronchi. The right main bronchus is more directly continuous with the trachea than the left and therefore is more commonly entered by inhaled foreign bodies. The lobes of the lungs are supplied by lobar bronchi, which in turn divide into segmental bronchi. The

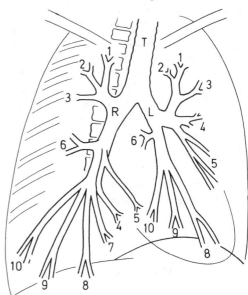

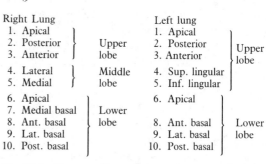

Right Lung		Left lung	
1. Apical	⎫	1. Apical	⎫
2. Posterior	⎬ Upper	2. Posterior	⎬ Upper
3. Anterior	⎭ lobe	3. Anterior	⎭ lobe
4. Lateral	⎫ Middle	4. Sup. lingular	
5. Medial	⎭ lobe	5. Inf. lingular	
6. Apical		6. Apical	
7. Medial basal	⎫ Lower		
8. Ant. basal	⎬ lobe	8. Ant. basal	⎫ Lower
9. Lat. basal	⎪	9. Lat. basal	⎬ lobe
10. Post. basal	⎭	10. Post. basal	⎭

Fig. 19.1 Diagram of bronchial tree as seen on left oblique bronchogram. T = trachea; R = right main bronchus; L = left main bronchus

anatomical arrangement is fairly constant and is shown with its nomenclature in Figure 19.1. As the bronchi continue to subdivide, the cartilage plates in their walls become less prominent, until after 15–20 divisions the resultant small air passages are devoid of cartilage and are known as terminal bronchioles.

The bronchi and bronchioles are surrounded by smooth muscle which can constrict the lumen (as occurs in asthma). The tracheobronchial tree is lined by ciliated pseudo-stratified epithelium. It is three to four cells thick in the upper parts but thins down to a single layer in the bronchioles. Goblet cells in the mucosa and discrete sub-mucosal glands produce a film of surface mucus which is constantly moved up to the larynx to clear away inhaled dust particles by the cilia. Drying of the epithelium interferes with this ciliary clearing action, as does general anaesthesia.

A further protective mechanism for the removal of intrabronchial material is the cough reflex. Stimulation of the sensitive epithelium, especially around the carina, results in forced expiration against a closed glottis. When it opens there is an explosive blast of air which clears secretions or foreign material. Generation of the blast requires adequate muscle strength from the chest wall, which after surgery may be impaired by pain or weakness. Thus general anaesthesia and operations, particularly on the chest or abdomen, lead to retention of secretions and hence a risk of infection.

Management of the airways

Maintenance of unobstructed airways and control of ventilation are important in anaesthesia and surgical conditions affecting the chest. The pumping action of the chest wall is interrupted by muscle relaxants, after major chest injury and during thoracotomy. This necessitates mechanical ventilation, with delivery of a humidified mixture of air and oxygen (and anaesthetic gases) directly into the airway. The gas mixture is under intermittent positive pressure, resulting in cyclical expansion of the lungs similar to that which occurs with normal respiration. A cuffed endotracheal tube (Fig. 19.2) is normally used to deliver the gas; the cuff lies in

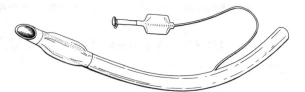

Fig. 19.2 Cuffed endotracheal tube

the trachea beyond the vocal cords and is gently inflated until there is an airtight seal.

With modern low-pressure cuffs, the serious complication of tracheal necrosis is unusual even after many weeks of ventilation, provided over-inflation is avoided. For operations on the lungs a 'double-lumen' tube with a separate limb for each main bronchus is available. This allows one lung to be ventilated and the other to be collapsed. As the intubated patient cannot cough, bronchial secretions will have to be removed from time to time. This should be done gently using a sterile suction catheter.

If prolonged ventilation is required, e.g. after head or chest injury, a tracheostomy may be necessary.

Tracheostomy

If possible, tracheostomy should be performed only when the airway is already controlled with an endotracheal tube. General anaesthesia, a good light and careful aseptic technique are desirable. Emergency tracheostomy is hardly ever required, except in conditions such as severe facial trauma, when an oral endotracheal tube cannot be inserted. Even then cricothyroidotomy is preferred.

For elective tracheostomy a transverse skin incision is made midway between the cricoid cartilage and the sternal notch. This incision is deepened in the midline, splitting the strap muscles. The isthmus of the thyroid may need to be retracted upwards or even divided. The trachea is opened through the second, third and fourth rings either with a vertical slit or as an inverted U-shaped flap. A short, right-angled cuffed tube is then carefully introduced. This allows easy and reliable access to the airway for ventilation or removal of secretions and is much more comfortable than an oral endotracheal tube, which passes through the sensitive larynx and vocal cords. Complications of tracheostomy include drying of secretions (if the inspired air is not humidified), damage to the tracheal wall from the cuff and displacement of the tube into the tissues of the neck.

Examination of the airways

Bronchoscopy

Direct viewing of the airways from the larynx down to the beginning of the segmental bronchi is a routine investigation. Either a rigid or a flexible bronchoscope is used. The rigid instrument (Fig. 19.3) is basically a straight metal tube with a smooth, bevelled end for safer insertion between the vocal cords. It carries a light source near its tip, and a small tube attached to its other end enables a high pressure jet of oxygen to be blown intermittently into the airway. This jet draws in air and ensures satisfactory ventilation of the anaesthetized and paralysed patient. General anaesthesia is preferred, although it is possible to use topical anaesthesia to the larynx. The neck is extended to allow the bronchoscope to be passed gently between the vocal cords and into the trachea. Care must be taken to avoid levering on the teeth. By gently moving the head, each main bronchus can be entered. To examine the smaller bronchi branching off the sides of the main bronchi, a right-angled telescope can be used. This is particularly helpful in the upper lobes. If

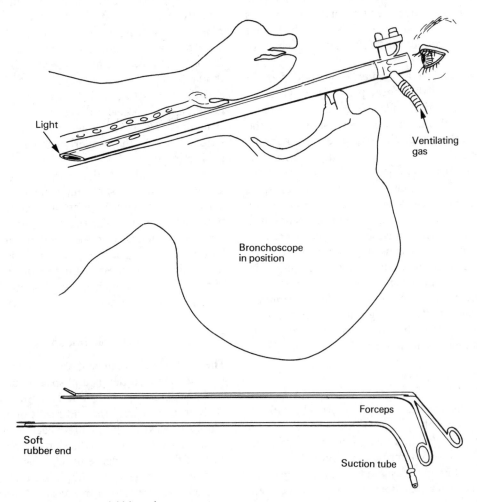

Light

Ventilating gas

Bronchoscope in position

Forceps

Soft rubber end

Suction tube

Fig. 19.3 Bronchoscopy using a rigid bronchoscope

a tumour is identified, it is biopsied with forceps. Those beyond direct reach are brushed with a sponge, and these brushings, together with locally collected secretions, are examined cytologically for malignant cells. Compression or distortion of the bronchi by external masses may also be seen on bronchoscopy. An important example is the widening of the usually sharp carina by enlarged subcarinal lymph nodes (a sign of inoperability in lung cancer).

The flexible bronchoscope can be used more readily with topical anaesthesia and can reach further down the bronchi, at least to segmental level. It is less useful for removing foreign bodies and secretions than the rigid instrument. With an experienced operator, a rigid bronchoscope can also be used to assess the rigidity or deviation of the distal bronchial tree. Rigid bronchoscopy is frequently used postoperatively to suck out inspissated secretions when the cough mechanism is ineffective.

Removal of foreign bodies. The sudden onset of coughing and dyspnoea, particularly when associated with eating, suggests an inhaled foreign body, especially in children. Stridor is often the only physical finding. X-ray may reveal no abnormality or may show obstructive emphysema with evidence of overexpansion on the affected side. Occasionally the foreign body is radio-opaque. With complete blockage there is collapse or shrinkage of a lobe or lung. Urgent bronchoscopy is essential if there is any suspicion of aspiration. The foreign material is usually found in the right bronchial tree. Skilled anaesthesia is required in children, in whom the airway may be almost completely occluded by the object. A firmly jammed object, particularly if neglected, may require thoracotomy and opening of the bronchus (bronchotomy) for its removal.

Bronchography

Although the trachea and main bronchi can be visualized on plain chest X-ray, the distal bronchial tree must first be outlined by coating its walls with a radio-opaque medium (bronchography). This is best done under general anaesthesia. After secretions have been sucked out with a bronchoscope, the medium is injected through an endotracheal tube with the patient positioned so that only one side is coated at a time. Bronchography is used primarily in the investigation of bronchiectasis to outline the extent of dilatation in the distal bronchial tree. As much as possible of the contrast material is sucked out; once the procedure is completed the remainder is coughed up by the patient, without ill-effect, on awakening.

THE PLEURA

The pleura is a thin sheet of connective tissue with a surface mesothelial cell layer which covers the lungs and lines the inside of the cavities (the hemithoraces) which contain the lungs.

Over the lobes of the lungs it is adherent to the underlying parenchyma and is known as *visceral pleura*. It is insensitive to painful stimuli. This visceral pleura is continuous at the lung hilum with the *parietal pleura*, which lines the inside of the thoracic cage as well as covering the diaphragm and the mediastinum. It is sensitive to pain and has the same blood and nerve supply as underlying structures. The parietal pleura can be fairly readily stripped from the underlying chest wall and mediastinum.

In the normal state the two layers of the pleura are in contact. The slight movement which occurs between them with respiration is permitted by a thin film of fluid. The natural elasticity of the lung, which tends to make it collapse towards the hilum, exerts a negative pressure on this 'potential' space. Collection of air or fluid in this space is abnormal and, if significant, must be dealt with in an appropriate manner.

Management of the pleural space

The presence of significant amounts of air, blood, effusion or pus in the pleural space compresses the lung and interferes with function. Any infection is likely to persist, and the end-result of any inflammatory process in the pleural space is obliteration of the space by fibrous adhesions or even entrapment of the lung in dense fibrous scar. Techniques of drainage range from simple needle aspiration, through the insertion of intercostal drains, to open operation (thoracotomy). In all cases the aim

is to achieve full expansion of the lung and obliteration of any space. Not only does this allow
maximal function of the lung, it also prevents re-
accumulation of an abnormal collection.

Aspiration. A fine trocar and cannula attached
via a two-way tap to a syringe (Fig. 19.4) can be
used to aspirate air, remove fluid for diagnostic
tests or to empty the pleural space completely.
The site of aspiration is determined by recent X-
rays and by physical examination. Aseptic
technique and adequate local anaesthesia of the appropriate intercostal space are important. The
needle should pass across the upper border of the
rib below so as to avoid the neurovascular bundle.

Intercostal drainage. Large amounts of air or
fluid, particularly if they reaccumulate, are best
drained continuously through a tube. Ideally this
should be inserted laterally, behind the outer border of pectoralis major but in front of the
midaxillary line, or anteriorly through the second
interspace in the midaxillary line. Prior needle aspiration must always be carried out to confirm the
suitability of the selected site. Local anaesthesia is
again used and the trocar and cannula are inserted
carefully after first incising the skin with a scalpel.
As with needle aspiration, the cannula should pass
just above a rib.

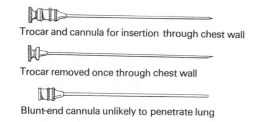

Trocar and cannula for insertion through chest wall

Trocar removed once through chest wall

Blunt-end cannula unlikely to penetrate lung

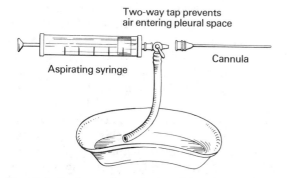

Two-way tap prevents
air entering pleural space

Aspirating syringe

Cannula

Fig. 19.4 Equipment for aspiration of pleural space

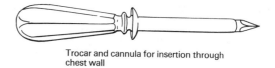

Trocar and cannula for insertion through
chest wall

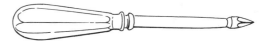

Trocar removed once through chest wall

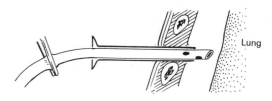

Clamped intercostal tube passed through cannula

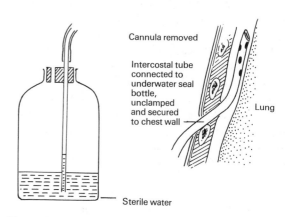

Cannula removed

Intercostal tube
connected to
underwater seal
bottle,
unclamped
and secured
to chest wall

Lung

Sterile water

Fig. 19.5 Intercostal drainage

Once the pleural space is entered, the intercostal
tube is passed through the cannula, which is then
removed. The tube is connected to an underwater
seal bottle which acts as a one-way valve, letting
out air or fluid but preventing either from re-
entering the space (Fig. 19.5).

When drainage is required for long periods
(weeks or even months), as in patients with empyema (see below), rib resection may allow more
efficient drainage. A piece of rib is removed at the
site of drainage to permit a large tube to be inserted and the space to be explored by finger or
forceps. It is more comfortable for the patient and
avoids the risk of the tube eroding into the inter-

costal vessels; they are ligated when the segment of rib is removed.

As the infection fuses the lung to the chest wall, this type of tube can be converted to 'open drainage', as used for any other chronic abscess cavity in the body. There is no risk of producing a pneumothorax.

Pneumothorax

The presence of air in the pleural space is known as pneumothorax. The air usually comes from the lung itself. After penetrating trauma it may come from outside, and occasionally air enters through a perforated oesophagus (e.g. after endoscopy).

Spontaneous pneumothorax

This is the commonest type of pneumothorax. It usually occurs in young adults of either sex who are often tall and thin in build. It presents with pain and dyspnoea, and on examination there is hyperresonance to percussion and reduced breath sounds over the affected side. On chest X-ray there are no lung markings peripherally, and often an ill-defined line marking the border between lung and air (Fig. 19.6). The lung may be collapsed at the hilum. The cause is usually rupture of a tiny bleb or bulla at the apex of the upper lobe.

If the pneumothorax is small, it may need no action other than observation, or it can be aspirated with a needle. If it is large or under tension (see below) or if there is fluid, a formal

intercostal drain should be inserted. As the air comes out of the space, the lung expands and presses against the chest wall, so sealing the site of the leak. Once the drain stops bubbling it can be removed.

Tension pneumothorax

The site of the leak in the lung may act as a flap (one-way) valve, allowing air to enter the pleural space during inspiration and coughing, but preventing it from escaping during expiration, thus raising the pressure within the pleural space. The result of such pressure, or tension, is to compress the lung and then shift the mediastinum towards the other side (see Fig. 19.6). This in turn compresses the normal lung, impairing its function, and may kink and distort the vena cava. The diagnosis should be suspected if there are signs of pneumothorax together with mediastinal shift and perhaps venous obstruction. This is a medical emergency. A large-bore needle plunged into the affected side will, if the diagnosis is correct, be greeted by a hiss of escaping air and relieve the immediate problem. A formal drain should then be inserted.

Recurrent spontaneous pneumothorax

Roughly 30% of spontaneous pneumothoraces will recur. After a second episode the risk rises to 70%. If the same side has been affected twice or more, and particularly if tension has occurred at any time, a definitive procedure should be considered. The most reliable is *pleurectomy*. Through a limited thoracotomy the parietal pleura is stripped off the inside of the chest. Any blebs or bullae can be ligated. The anaesthetist then inflates the lung, causing it to adhere to the raw area on the chest wall. A similar effect can be obtained by blowing an irritant such as iodized talc or kaolin into the pleural space. This induces a chemical pleurisy and obliterates the space. Although simpler than pleurectomy, this procedure (*pleurodesis*) carries the potential risk of introducing foreign (and irritating) material into a body cavity.

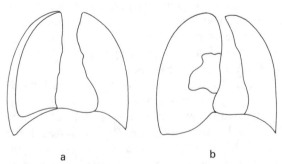

a   b

Fig. 19.6 Radiographic appearance of (a) pneumothorax and (b) tension pneumothorax. (Note the mediastinal shift to opposite side)

Haemothorax

Haemothorax is discussed in detail later in this chapter.

Empyema

The presence of pus in the pleural space is known as empyema. The commonest cause is an underlying pneumonia with spread of infection into an associated effusion. A lung abscess can similarly spread to the pleural space. Infection can also be introduced from outside the chest, e.g. as a result of penetrating injury, or contamination of pleural fluid by poor sterile technique during aspiration. The infection can come from the mediastinum, typically after perforation of the oesophagus; the space left after lung resection can become infected (postoperative empyema); or a subphrenic abscess may spread through the diaphragm (Fig. 19.7). The physical signs of empyema are those of a pleural effusion: dullness to percussion, absence of breath sounds, and evidence of infection such as pyrexia and leucocytosis. On X-ray there is a pleural opacity, classically located posteriorly and with a 'D'-shaped outline.

At the earliest stage pathologically the pleural space is filled with a thin, watery fluid containing pus cells known as a 'purulent effusion'. Later on

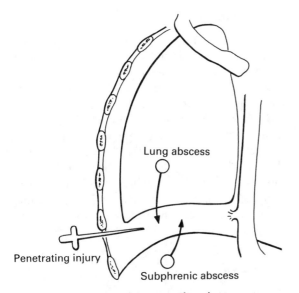

Fig. 19.7 Major causes of empyema thoracis

fibrin is laid down on the lung and parietal pleura, and in time becomes organized as a thick fibrous wall around the cavity. At a very late stage the contained pus may 'point' to the skin surface like an abscess anywhere else in the body. This is termed 'empyema necessitans'.

The aims of treatment are to drain the infection and obliterate the pleural space by encouraging the lung to expand as much as possible. At the stage of purulent effusion, needle aspiration alone may be perfectly adequate. For thicker pus, a tube drain is required, and for a thick-walled abscess, rib resection (see above) allows much better drainage. The cavity then slowly obliterates by fibrous ingrowth, until eventually just the tube tract is left. Although this process may take several months it is safe and effective in the elderly, who now constitute the majority of patients with empyema. In younger patients, open thoracotomy and removal of the walls of the empyema ('decortication') permits full expansion of the lung and more rapid and complete resolution.

THE LUNGS

Each lung is contained within its hemithorax and is attached at the hilum to the mediastinum. The main bronchus, pulmonary artery and pulmonary veins are the major structures at the hilum; lymphatics and lymph nodes, bronchial arteries and autonomic nerves are also present.

The left lung is divided by an oblique fissure into an upper and a lower lobe. The right lung has an oblique fissure from which a transverse fissure runs forward resulting in an upper, a middle and a lower lobe (see Fig. 19.1). The anterior part of the upper lobe on the left is often elongated as the lingula, and corresponds roughly to the right middle lobe. The depth of the fissures is variable, and particularly in older patients the lobes may appear to be completely fused.

The lobes are divided into bronchopulmonary segments by fibrous septa radiating out from the hilum. Each segment has its own bronchus, always with an accompanying artery. Blockage of a lobar or segmental bronchus results in absorption of air beyond the blockage and collapse or atelectasis (airlessness) of the affected lung. Since areas containing no air appear denser than the surrounding lung on chest X-ray, the collapsed segment or lobe can readily be identified.

Bronchopulmonary segments are further divided into lobules, each with its own bronchiole and accompanying pulmonary arteriole, but without fibrous septa. The terminal bronchioles divide into respiratory bronchioles and then alveolar ducts before reaching the alveoli. These last are surrounded by a web of capillaries. Gas exchange occurs across the very thin alveolar epithelial cells, a basement membrane and the equally thin endothelial cells of the capillaries.

Venous drainage is less regular than the pulmonary arterial supply. Veins from the smallest respiratory units eventually drain into segmental veins, some of which lie between the fissures. These in turn are tributaries of the inferior and superior pulmonary veins, which join the left atrium at the hilum. Because the lobes and segments are discrete anatomical units, they can be removed surgically, leaving the remaining lung intact and viable.

Infective lung conditions

Lung abscess

This term implies infection with localized destruction of lung tissue. A lung abscess may occur within an area of pneumonia, although this is unusual if antibiotics have been given. Inhalation of foreign material, e.g. during a period of impaired consciousness, may be followed by abscess formation in the obstructed and contaminated area. The patient is extremely ill with an elevated temperature. If the abscess communicates with the airway, large quantities of foul sputum may be produced. Chest X-ray characteristically shows an opacity with a fluid level. There may be spillage of pus into healthy areas of the lung, or the pleura may be breached, with consequent empyema or pyopneumothorax.

Postural drainage and physiotherapy, together with appropriate antibiotics, will resolve most abscesses. All such patients must be bronchoscoped — the original opacity may have been a cavitating carcinoma or infection may have developed in a bronchus blocked by tumour.

Bronchiectasis

In bronchiectasis parts of the bronchial tree are abnormally dilated. The bronchial walls are abnormal and there is chronic infection in the bronchi and surrounding lung parenchyma. The condition usually follows childhood infections (particularly tuberculosis, measles and whooping cough) in which transient bronchial obstruction is followed by destruction of the bronchial wall and permanent dilatation. It commonly affects the lower lobes, and sometimes the middle lobe on the right or the lingula on the left. It may also be widespread. The main symptom is a persistent cough with production of copious purulent sputum (up to several cupfuls a day). There may also be haemoptysis and recurrent exacerbations of infection. The chest X-ray may be surprisingly normal. Bronchography is required to define the extent and severity of the disease.

Postural drainage and antibiotics given for exacerbations are the mainstay of treatment. If this fails to control symptoms or prevent recurrent severe infection or haemoptysis, surgical resection of the affected segment(s), lobe(s) or even an entire lung may be considered. This can be very successful, but only if the disease is relatively localized. The result of surgery depends on the amount of residual diseased lung.

Benign lung tumours

Benign lung tumours are uncommon. Only bronchial carcinoids and adenoid cystic carcinomas (previously classified as 'bronchial adenomas') are true neoplasms. A number of other non-malignant conditions present as shadows on chest X-ray and must be differentiated from bronchial carcinomas. These include tuberculomas, healed infarcts and hamartomas. Because of the difficulty of proving their benign nature and the importance of not missing a small bronchial carcinoma, many peripheral opacities, or 'coin lesions', are diagnosed only after the suspect area has been surgically removed.

Hamartoma

A hamartoma is a developmental abnormality consisting of a mass of tissue with cartilage, muscle and epithelium. It is firm and mobile within the lung parenchyma, moving around under the surgeon's finger.

Bronchial carcinoid

Bronchial carcinoids account for about 85% of benign lung tumours, and are distantly related to small-cell carcinomas. They typically arise in the major bronchi and cause cough, wheezing or haemoptysis. Unless an airway is blocked, chest X-ray may be normal. Local resection is indicated in all cases. A few may recur and occasionally they develop malignant characteristics and metastasize.

Adenoid cystic carcinoma

This tumour, also known as cylindroma, is even rarer. It should be regarded as being of low-grade malignancy. It commonly occurs in the major bronchi, particularly the trachea, and has a striking tendency to recur even years after initial removal. It is only slightly radiosensitive.

Lung cancer

Lung cancer arises from the epithelium of the bronchial tree. Although men are affected more frequently than women (ratio 4:1 in the UK), it is now the commonest cause of death from malignancy in both sexes. It occurs most frequently between the ages of 50 and 60 years but is increasingly seen in younger patients. Cigarette smoking is the major predisposing factor in nearly all types of lung cancer. A few cases are related to exposure to asbestos, radioactive isotopes, arsenic or chromates.

Pathology

Histologically the tumour may be well differentiated or anaplastic. Well differentiated tumours may be squamous (45–55%) or adenocarcinomatous (20%). Anaplastic tumours are divided into 'large cell' and 'small cell' types. Large cell tumours account for 15% of all types and behave as more malignant forms of the differentiated tumours. Small or 'oat cell' carcinomas account for

20% of all lung cancers and behave as a completely different disease. These cells are believed to be derived from neural crest tissue. They are highly malignant, and many patients have widespread dissemination when first seen.

A lung cancer may be situated centrally, i.e. in a major bronchus, and hence visible at bronchoscopy, or it may lie peripherally. If it is in a major airway, there may be symptoms of cough or bleeding (haemoptysis). Airway occlusion leads to silent collapse of the affected area or, more commonly, infection of the distal airways with consequent pneumonia or lung abscess.

The tumour spreads in the lung by local invasion and along lymphatic channels. Once beyond the lung, it may invade adjacent organs such as the pericardium and heart, oesophagus, chest wall or diaphragm. The aorta is curiously resistant to direct spread.

Lymphatic spread is initially to hilar and mediastinal nodes. Later, supraclavicular nodes may also be involved and are then easily palpable (Fig. 19.8).

Blood-borne metastases occur in most viscera: the commonest sites are the brain, bone, liver,

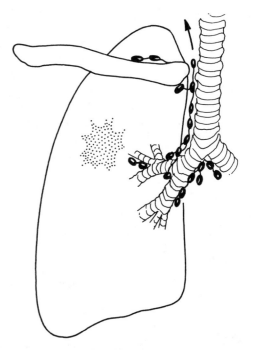

Fig. 19.8 Lymphatic spread of lung cancer

skin and the adrenal glands. Other manifestations of bronchial carcinoma which are not due to metastases are finger clubbing, hypertrophic pulmonary osteoarthropathy, peripheral neuropathy and myopathies, superficial thrombophlebitis and a variety of endocrine disturbances due to inappropriate secretion of hormones.

Presentation

Some tumours are found on routine chest X-rays in asymptomatic patients. A lung shadow in a smoker is always presumed to be a bronchial carcinoma until proved otherwise. More commonly the patient complains of a cough, perhaps with haemoptysis, and often weight loss. Pneumonia which fails to resolve or which recurs in the same area of lung is another suspicious sign and requires further investigation (i.e. by bronchoscopy). Local spread of the tumour within the thorax may cause pain in the chest wall at the site of invasion. If this occurs at the apex of the lung, the brachial plexus and sympathetic chain may be involved. The combination of severe pain (often down the arm), Horner's syndrome and rib erosion is characteristic of the so-called Pancoast syndrome.

Central invasion may affect the recurrent laryngeal nerve (always the left) and cause hoarseness from vocal cord paralysis. Enlarged lymph nodes in the mediastinum may compress the superior vena cava (SVC) and cause engorgement of the face and arms (SVC syndrome). Occasionally bloodborne metastases give rise to the first manifestation of the disease. For example, bone pain, skin nodules or neurological symptoms (e.g. epilepsy) may all point to metastatic disease.

Investigation

A thorough history and physical examination may suggest the diagnosis and give some idea of the extent of spread. The aim of subsequent investigations is to confirm the diagnosis and define the extent of spread both within and outside the chest and to determine appropriate treatment. For nearly all types of lung cancer the only hope of cure is by surgery.

Radiological examination. The commonest findings on chest X-ray are a peripheral opacity,

enlarged hilar or mediastinal nodes or an area of consolidation in the lung. The examination may also reveal bony erosion or secondary deposits in the ribs, and there may be signs of pleural effusion. Other useful radiological investigations are screening of the diaphragm to detect phrenic nerve paralysis (due to invasion of the mediastinum) and barium swallow to determine whether the oesophagus is deviated or indented by enlarged mediastinal lymph nodes. If available, a CT scan of the mediastinum is preferred.

Bronchoscopy. Central tumours can be biopsied directly. Secretions or brushings are collected from segmental bronchi to allow cytological diagnosis of more peripheral lesions. Bronchoscopy can also be used to assess operability. Carinal widening and tracheal invasion are signs of inoperability. Peripheral tumours can be directly biopsied using a percutaneous needle technique under X-ray guidance.

Lymph node sampling. Supraclavicular node metastases indicate inoperability. These nodes can be sampled by direct biopsy or by fine-needle aspiration. Lymph nodes within the mediastinum may be sampled by *mediastinoscopy*. Under general anaesthesia an incision is made in the neck and deepened until a plane beneath the pretracheal fascia is reached. A finger and then an endoscope (similar to a laryngoscope) is introduced as far as the origin of the main bronchi. Involvement of nodes high in the mediastinum or on the opposite side to the tumour denotes inoperability. Routine mediastinoscopy, at least for central tumours, reduces the thoracotomy rate.

Assessment of pulmonary function

When assessing the suitability of a patient with lung cancer for thoracotomy, the surgeon not only has to decide whether the tumour can be resected but also whether the patient has sufficient respiratory reserve to tolerate the operation. As almost all patients will have been smokers, most already have diseased or abnormal lungs. The assessment is based on preoperative fitness (e.g. the ability to climb a flight of stairs), the results of lung function tests and the extent of resection required. Of the large range of pulmonary function tests available, simple spirometry, with measurement of forced expiratory volume in one second (FEV_1) and forced vital capacity (FVC), is the most useful. Postoperative performance obviously depends on the extent of resection, which ranges from a right pneumonectomy, with removal of about 55% of functioning lung tissue, to wedge resection of a slice of lung surrounding a tiny peripheral tumour. Removal of a collapsed lobe is obviously less harmful than removal of one which is fully functional.

Treatment

The principle of surgical treatment is to remove the anatomical unit containing the tumour (segment, lobe or lung) together with its associated lymphatic drainage. Even with apparently curative resection only 35–40% of patients survive for 5 years after the operation. The figure for small peripheral lesions is much better, approaching 90%, and there is worthwhile salvage even if mediastinal lymph nodes have to be removed.

Only a minority of patients with lung cancer are suitable for operation. At presentation, about 50% will already have clinical evidence of spread outside the chest or be unfit for thoracotomy. Further investigation usually rules out another quarter or third of the original group, so that only 20–25% are eventually considered for surgery. For the rest, the outlook is hopeless: the median survival is 8 months, and only 2–3% are alive after 5 years.

Radiotherapy. Some small tumours can be cured by irradiation, but the resulting damage to the surrounding lung is at least as great as that from surgery. Radiotherapy is useful for pain relief from bony metastases. In the chest it can be used to relieve superior vena cava obstruction and reduce tracheal or bronchial compression.

Chemotherapy. Small cell cancers of the lung are relatively responsive to modern chemotherapy. Although cure is rare, median survival may be increased from 3 to 18 months. Other types of lung cancer are not responsive, and chemotherapy is rarely indicated.

Principles of operations to the lung

Opening the pleura to gain access to the lungs or other thoracic structures destroys the usual nega-

tive intrathoracic pressure. In this situation the lung would collapse. Endotracheal intubation and positive ventilation are therefore necessary adjuncts to thoracic surgery. For many operations a standard cuffed endotracheal tube is sufficient. Use of a double-lumen tube allows the lung being operated on to be selectively collapsed ('one-lung anaesthesia'). This is of great help particularly when a bronchus has to be opened during the course of the operation.

Thoracotomy

The patient is placed on his unaffected side on the operating table. For a standard lateral thoracotomy (such as would be used to gain access to the lung) the skin incision runs from between the medial border of the scapula and the vertebral spines forward to the inframammary crease. It is deepened through the fat and fascia before dividing latissimus dorsi and, anteriorly, serratus anterior. To open the chest the periosteum is stripped off the upper border of a rib (usually the sixth) so that the neurovascular bundle is preserved and the pleura divided. The ribs are gently spread apart using a special self-retaining retractor.

Lobectomy

Lobectomy is indicated for tumours or other lesions confined to one lobe. The interlobar fissure is deepened down towards the hilum. The lobar vessels are ligated and divided and the bronchus is divided and closed. Hilar lymph nodes are removed along with the specimen. Small air leaks usually close spontaneously after a few days. Lobectomy has a low mortality and little effect on lung function.

Pneumonectomy

In one-third of cases of tumour, the whole lung must be removed (pneumonectomy). The pulmonary veins and arteries are ligated and divided at the hilum, and the bronchus is divided flush with the carina and closed with non-absorbable sutures or a mechanical stapling device. Breakdown of this closure, leads to 'bronchopleural fistula', which is a serious and potentially lethal complication.

It is usual to drain the pleural cavity via a tube connected to an underwater seal bottle after any operation on the chest to deal with continued air leak and oozing of blood from raw surfaces of the lung.

After lobectomy, the remaining lung expands to fill the space left. Crowding of the ribs, elevation of the hemidiaphragm and movement of the mediastinum all reduce the size of the hemithorax on the operated side so that the pleural space is usually obliterated in a week.

Following pneumonectomy there is no lung to fill the space. The drain is removed after 24 hours, and the space allowed to fill slowly with blood and serum over the next few weeks. This undergoes organization and fibrosis.

THE THORACIC CAGE

The main role of the chest wall and diaphragm is to generate the negative intrathoracic pressure required for ventilation. At rest the diaphragm is the principle muscle involved in inspiration; expiration is normally a passive action. When additional ventilation is required, as during exercise or if there is pulmonary disease, contraction of the intercostal muscles pivots the ribs forwards and outwards, raising the sternum and further increasing the volume of the chest cavity.

Chest wall function may be impaired by damage to the wall itself (e.g. muscle weakness with postoperative pain, fractured ribs) or by pleural disease (e.g. fibrothorax following empyema), both of which restrict lung expansion. Disorders of the lung itself (e.g. pulmonary fibrosis) have similar effects.

Deformities of the chest wall

Pectus excavatum

This is a deformity of the thoracic cage in which the sternum is posteriorly displaced as a result of abnormal development of the costal cartilages. There is a depression in the precordial area, so that the heart is displaced into the left chest. Despite this, the function of the heart is only rarely impaired. Surgery is justified on account of the

distress caused by the cosmetic appearance. The operation involves resection of the costal cartilages and elevation of the sternum, which is kept in its new position by a metal bar which passes behind the sternum and rests in front of the ribs on each side. This bar is removed after a few months.

Pectus carinatum

This is the opposite deformity to that described above, i.e. the sternum is elevated forward as a ridge ('pigeon chest'). Principles of treatment are the same as for pectus excavatum.

Thoracic injury

Blunt injuries to the chest are commonly the result of road traffic accidents. There are frequently other injuries, particularly to the head, abdomen and long bones. The thoracic injury is often a cause of early death, which in many cases could be prevented by appropriate and often very simple steps.

Penetrating injury is almost always the result of stab or gunshot wounds.

Airway obstruction

If the cough reflex is suppressed by unconsciousness or the patient cannot cough because of damage to the chest wall, the airway may become obstructed. Gastric contents, pharyngeal secretions or blood may be aspirated. Provision of an open airway is the first priority when dealing with a patient with a chest injury. This may require a pharyngeal airway or sometimes an endotracheal tube. Emergency cricothyroidotomy or tracheostomy is only required if head and neck or upper airway injury precludes insertion of an endotracheal tube.

Fractured ribs

Pain, made worse by coughing and breathing, is the main problem after simple rib fractures. If there is pre-existing lung disease, such as chronic bronchitis, the inability to cough may lead to retention of secretions and pneumonia. Adequate analgesia (e.g. by local intercostal nerve blocks or thoracic epidural anaesthesia) is essential. Immobilization of the ribs by 'strapping' is contraindicated.

Flail chest

Fracture of a number of adjacent ribs in more than one place results in a flail segment of chest wall. Such a 'floating' segment, if large, may show paradoxical movement with respiration, i.e. it moves outwards with expiration and inwards with inspiration, greatly reducing chest wall function (Fig. 19.9). Contusion of the underlying lung is common. The effect of the injury can be limited by good analgesia, physiotherapy and mild dehydration with diuretics to prevent local pulmonary oedema. Some patients may require artificial ventilation, often for 2–3 weeks, until the injured lung has recovered and the chest wall has become stable.

Traumatic pneumothorax

In blunt trauma, a pneumothorax (see Fig. 19.6) implies lung or, very rarely, oesophageal perforation. Damage is usually due to puncture by the sharp ends of fractured ribs. Penetrating injury, e.g. stab wounds, can have a similar effect. Small pneumothoraces will resolve on their own, but if there is a large space, tube drainage is required. The principal aim, as in any pneumothorax, is to get the lung fully inflated and obliterate the pleural space. Persistent bubbling of air with each inspiration into the underwater seal bottle denotes bronchial rupture.

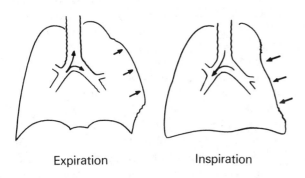

Expiration   Inspiration

Fig. 19.9 Effect of flail segment on chest wall

If the air in the space is under tension, it may track through the wound into the tissues, where it is palpable as a 'crackling' sensation under the skin. This 'surgical emphysema' may cause massive swelling of the chest, neck and face, producing a so-called 'Michelin man' appearance. It always resolves completely once the air-leak seals and never causes any permanent damage.

Haemothorax

Blood in the pleural space may come from the chest wall, lung or mediastinal structures. Fractured ribs may bleed or they may lacerate intercostal vessels, which may also be damaged by penetrating stab wounds, misplaced aspirating needles or chest drains. If the lung itself is injured, bleeding is usually associated with an air leak, leading to a haemopneumothorax. Massive bleeding into the pleura can occur from damage to the heart or the aorta (see below).

The short-term effects are those of blood loss and compression of lung. Blood loss may be insignificant or it can be massive and rapidly fatal: the pleural space can contain most of the circulating blood volume. The compressed lung is unavailable for ventilation, so does not contribute to gas exchange. In the course of time, clot in the pleural cavity may undergo organization and permanently compress (or 'trap') the lung in a fibrous case. If contaminated from the outside, e.g. as the result of penetrating injury, the haematoma is prone to become infected, leading to an empyema.

The principles of management are as for any other fluid in the pleural space, i.e. drainage of the pleural space via a large-bore chest drain connected to an underwater seal bottle, to allow full expansion of the lung and obliteration of the space. If blood loss continues or is excessive, thoracotomy is indicated. The commonest sources of bleeding are the intercostal and internal thoracic vessels. Massive haemorrhage from the heart or great vessels requires immediate repair. It may also be necessary to open the chest to remove large quantities of clot. This should be done early rather than late so that permanent lung compression and empyema are avoided.

Stab injuries to the heart may cause death from tamponade (compression of the heart by blood contained in the pericardium), rather than from exsanguination. Cardiac tamponade rapidly leads to hypotension, tachycardia and elevated jugular venous pressure. Release of tamponade by opening the pericardium through a small anterior thoracotomy often results in dramatic improvement, allowing time for repair of the injury.

Aortic rupture

Severe deceleration injuries may disrupt the aorta. In traffic accidents, rupture typically occurs just beyond the subclavian artery at the start of the descending aorta. In falls from a height (or aircraft accidents) rupture more commonly occurs just above the aortic valve.

About 90% of these patients die at the site of the accident from exsanguination. In the remainder, despite a tear of the aortic intima and media, blood is contained within the adventitia for a few hours or even days. There may be loss of distal pulses or clinical evidence of a left haemothorax. More usually the only clue to the injury is a widened upper mediastinum on chest X-ray, and any patient showing this sign should undergo emergency aortography. Often this will reveal no abnormality, but if there is a disruption the injected dye will show an irregularity of the aorta or even leakage into the surrounding tissues.

Operation should be carried out as soon as possible, as the aorta may rupture completely at any time. On opening the chest the surgeon is confronted by an enormous mediastinal haematoma. The damaged vessel is isolated between clamps and a Dacron tube graft inserted between healthy ends of aorta. As the spinal cord is at risk from ischaemia during this part of the operation, bypass to maintain distal circulation is usually advised. This may be a partial cardiopulmonary bypass (pumping blood from the left atrium to the descending aorta or femoral artery) or, more usually, a temporary bypass of the damaged area by a tube coated on the inside with heparin.

THE MEDIASTINUM

Mediastinal infections

These invariably arise from organs passing through or closely associated with the mediastinum. The commonest cause of mediastinal infection ('mediastinitis') is rupture of the oesophagus. Downward spread of infection from the neck may also occur.

Mediastinal infections spread rapidly through the loosely arranged tissue planes. Clinical features include chest pain radiating to the neck or through to the back, and dysphagia. Pyrexia is invariable. If an air-containing viscus is the source of the infection, surgical emphysema develops. Unless adequately drained, either through the pleura or the neck, such infections are often rapidly fatal.

Mediastinal masses

The mediastinum is a relatively silent area. Mediastinal masses are often first discovered as an incidental finding on chest X-ray. Sometimes pressure on adjacent structures (oesophagus or trachea, superior vena cava or recurrent laryngeal nerve) may cause suspicious symptoms.

Traditionally the mediastinum is divided into four compartments: the superior, anterior, middle and posterior mediastinum. This division is largely artificial and does not correspond to distinct anatomical areas, but it is useful for descriptive purposes. Nor is there any physical division between the mediastinum and the tissue planes of the neck.

Anterosuperior masses

Retrosternal extension of the thyroid is a common cause of a mass at the thoracic inlet. The trachea may be deviated or compressed (causing stridor) and a goitre is usually palpable in the neck. As sudden bleeding into the thyroid can cause acute tracheal compression, retrosternal goitres are best removed.

Aneurysm of the aorta or the vessels arising from the aortic arch can mimic a solid mass in any part of the mediastinum, but are particularly common in the superior part. The wall may be calcified. Aortography or CT scanning with intravenous contrast is indicated to confirm the diagnosis. All aneurysms are at risk of rupture, and if there is evidence of enlargement (pain or erosion of adjacent structures) surgery is advised.

Tumours of the thymus (thymomas) are found in the anterosuperior space. They are usually benign and may be associated with myasthenia gravis. Complete removal of the thymus may result in dramatic improvement, particularly in women with a short history. Surgical removal, which is best done through a median sternotomy, is straightforward, but postoperative ventilation is required.

Lymph node masses may occur at any site in the mediastinum, but most commonly arise at the lung hila, around the lower trachea and in the thymic remnants. They may be the result of benign disease such as sarcoidosis or follow infections, classically tuberculosis. More commonly, however, they are due to malignant disease, either 'primary' disease of lymphoid tissue (as in the various lymphomas) or 'secondary' to spread from other tumour (most usually bronchial carcinoma).

Lymphoid masses often have a lobulated appearance on chest X-ray and, if malignant, may show features of local invasion or compression. Obstruction of the superior vena cava (SVC) causes distension of superficial veins over the trunk, oedema of the arms and head, and a flushed appearance — the SVC syndrome, which is a classical feature of mediastinal invasion from bronchial carcinoma.

Posterior mediastinum

Masses in the posterior mediastinum may originate from local abnormalities of the primitive foregut. Oesophageal duplication may be found at any level in the chest and present as a fluid-filled mass adjoining the oesophagus, often lined with squamous epithelium. A similar abnormality can arise from the respiratory tract forming a bronchogenic cyst which usually lies around the tracheal bifurcation. The wall may contain cartilage and is lined by typical ciliated epithelium. A fluid level visible on X-ray implies communication with the airway, which makes eventual infection inevitable. In children these cysts can rapidly expand and cause respiratory obstruction.

Some cysts are more primitive and cannot be related to the oesophagus or bronchial tree on histological grounds. They are classified as foregut cysts or duplications.

Above the diaphragm, a hiatus hernia may show as a retrocardiac mass containing a fluid level. The gas is in the intrathoracic stomach, and this is the only important situation when a fluid level on chest X-ray does not imply communication with the airway.

Neurogenic tumours are typically found more posteriorly, in the costovertebral recess. The commonest are tumours of nerve sheath origin (neurofibromas) which are usually benign. They may straddle the intervertebral foramen (dumbbell tumours) and require a combined thoracic/neurosurgical approach. In children such tumours are nearly always malignant.

General principles of management

Many mediastinal masses are obviously malignant, secondary to bronchogenic carcinoma, and suitable only for palliation. Some forms of malignant disease are readily treated and cured if properly diagnosed and managed. The best examples are the various lymphomas, where the disease may be limited only to mediastinal lymph nodes. Other masses may be harmless (e.g. benign neural tumours) or non-malignant, but important to detect (e.g. lymph-node enlargement in sarcoidosis). Some benign lesions may progressively enlarge or are at risk of later infection, e.g. foregut-derived cysts. Aneurysms tend to dilate with time and many will eventually rupture, but often they present for the first time relatively late in life.

In some cases, the combination of clinical and radiological features may allow precise diagnosis. For example, a patient with myasthenia gravis and an anterior mediastinal mass is almost certain to have a thymoma. Most frequently, however, the findings of radiological examination are non-specific and careful further investigation is needed to confirm the diagnosis. In practice the safest and most efficient way to achieve this is by contrast CT scanning followed by a biopsy. The CT scan accurately localizes the mass and, combined with intravenous contrast, will detect aneurysms and other vascular lesions. The route of biopsy is determined by the position of the mass. The area around the trachea can be approached by *mediastinoscopy*, the anterior mediastinum via *anterior mediastinotomy*, through a small incision in the second intercostal space on the appropriate side. Posteriorly placed masses require formal thoracotomy.

Large biopsies, ideally of whole lymph nodes, are necessary for accurate diagnosis of lymphomas and thymomas. Fine-needle biopsies are often unsatisfactory.

20. Cardiac disease

Surgery has an important role in the management of many types of heart disease, both congenital and acquired. Ischaemic heart disease is a common cause of morbidity and death. The widespread application of surgery to this type of heart disease in particular has resulted in cardiac surgery becoming one of the major surgical specialties in most Western countries.

Although relatively simple procedures for cure or palliation of congenital heart defects had been developed earlier, it was not until the advent of safe techniques for cardiopulmonary bypass in the mid-1950s that satisfactory correction of intracardiac congenital anomalies became feasible. Replacement or repair of diseased heart valves followed in the early 1960s, and aortocoronary bypass surgery had become widely established by the late 1960s. Surgical techniques are now well standardized and the availability of long-term follow-up in large numbers of patients has clarified the role of surgery in the management of heart disease.

The majority of cardiac operations require the use of an extracorporeal circuit which needs supervision by a trained perfusionist. Surgeons, anaesthetists and operating room staff with specific cardiac surgical training are also required. Patients are usually in the operating room for 3 or 4 hours and intensive postoperative care is necessary for the first 24 hours. Cardiac surgical practice depends heavily on investigative cardiological services, and virtually all preoperative assessment is made by cardiologists and usually requires highly specialized investigations such as echocardiography, cardiac catheterization and angiocardiography.

PRINCIPLES OF SURGICAL TREATMENT

Rational application of surgical treatment for heart disease requires:

1. accurate assessment of the patient;
2. knowledge of the natural history of the condition; and
3. an understanding of the therapeutic possibilities, including techniques and hazards of particular operations.

Assessment of the patient

Patients considered for cardiac surgery are usually first referred to a cardiologist for assessment. They may be referred because of symptoms such as chest pain or dyspnoea, or because of the accidental finding on routine physical examination of an abnormality, usually a cardiac murmur.

The history, physical examination, findings on electrocardiography and chest radiography, and occasionally *echocardiography*, enable the cardiologist to diagnose the cardiac condition with considerable precision. It is important to assess the severity of the disease and the pathological effects it may be having on the heart itself, the lungs or other organs.

Cardiac catheterization and angiocardiography are usually undertaken once surgical treatment is contemplated, and sometimes to aid diagnosis or assess the results of surgery.

Cardiac catheterization is used to record pressures and measure oxygen saturation in the major vessels and cardiac chambers. This permits an assessment of the severity of an obstruction due to a stenotic valve (Fig. 20.1) or calculation of the

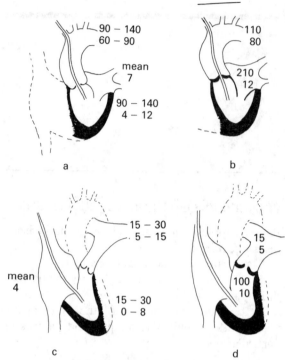

a   b

c   d

Fig. 20.1 Cardiac catheterization. (*Top*) Catheter inserted via systemic artery showing (a) normal left heart pressures and (b) pressure in aortic stenosis. (*Bottom*) Catheter inserted via systemic vein showing (c) normal right heart pressures and (d) pressure in pulmonary stenosis

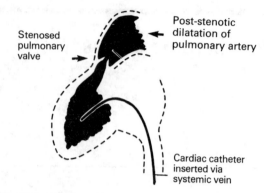

Fig. 20.2   Angiographic appearance of pulmonary valve stenosis

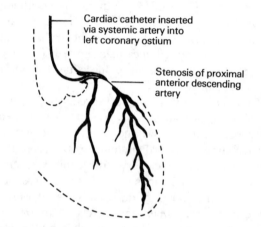

Fig. 20.3   Selective left coronary angiogram

amount of blood 'shunted' through abnormal communications such as ventricular or atrial septal defects.

Angiocardiography (Fig. 20.2) or *selective coronary angiography* (Fig. 20.3), in which radio-opaque contrast medium is injected into a cardiac chamber or coronary artery during cineradiography, allows clear visualization of the morphology of the abnormality.

In addition to obtaining accurate knowledge of the cardiac defect the surgeon must assess the general condition of the patient.

General physical examination may reveal conditions requiring specific investigation and management. Dental sepsis should be treated. Lung function, renal function, hepatic function and coagulation should also be assessed. Lung function is commonly compromised in the elderly by chronic bronchitis, while liver function is impaired in those with long-standing cardiac failure. Patients with coronary artery disease may have

evidence of important vascular disease elsewhere, e.g. a carotid bruit, which merits further investigation.

In some patients requiring valve replacement, long-term anticoagulation may be contraindicated because of concurrent disease, e.g. peptic ulceration, so that the choice of valve prosthesis will have to be modified.

With current techniques of anaesthesia, and operative and postoperative care, only very major abnormalities of other systems jeopardize surgical results sufficiently to make surgery inadvisable. The commonest contraindication to cardiac surgery is malignant disease of poor prognosis.

Natural history

Knowledge of the natural history of any condition

influences the timing and urgency of surgical treatment. For example, symptomatic aortic stenosis carries a poor prognosis, so that early surgery is advised. On the other hand, ventricular septal defects may close spontaneously in childhood and the decision regarding surgery can be deferred provided pulmonary vascular disease is not thought likely to develop. This is the most important hazard of untreated ventricular septal defects with a large pulmonary blood flow. Atrial septal defects usually cause heart failure in middle life, and elective surgical closure is advised in asymptomatic patients.

It is well known that left main coronary artery disease has a poor prognosis with medical treatment alone. Triple vessel disease, particularly when associated with impaired left ventricular function, has a poorer outlook without surgery than single or double vessel disease. For those with single or double vessel disease the prognosis is generally good and is not greatly altered by surgery. Surgery thus improves the outlook of those with left main coronary artery and triple vessel disease to equal that of patients with single or double vessel disease whether they have surgery or not.

Therapeutic possibilities

The surgeon must be familiar with medical measures available to the cardiologist and understand the effects of the drugs used. For example, beta-blocking drugs, which are commonly given for angina, may modify the response of the heart to drugs used postoperatively.

The hazards of any particular surgical procedure also influence decisions about surgery. Closure of atrial septal defects carries a very low risk and surgery can be advised in symptom-free patients for good long-term results. The low risk of mitral valvotomy makes this operation advisable relatively early in the natural history of mitral stenosis. The greater risk of valve replacement and continuing problems with prosthetic valves mean that this operation is less lightly advised.

Aims of surgery

In general terms, surgical treatment of heart disease is undertaken to achieve two goals.

1. *Relief of symptoms* by improving cardiac function. Examples are the treatment of exertional dyspnoea due to mixed mitral valve disease by replacement of the mitral valve, and treatment of angina pectoris by aortocoronary bypass grafting. Mild symptoms well managed by medical measures usually do not warrant surgery, while severe symptoms or poor response to medical measures usually indicate the need for surgery.

2. *Alteration of natural history of the disease.* Examples are (a) resection of aortic coarctation to avoid complications of hypertension; (b) treatment of Fallot's tetralogy to avoid thrombotic complications of polycythaemia or death in cyanotic spells; and (c) treatment of severe aortic stenosis to prevent myocardial damage or death.

The decision to advise surgery for these reasons is not always easy. It requires knowledge of the natural history of the disease and of the long-term results of surgery, and means that surgery may be advised in some symptom-free patients. In practice most patients undergo surgery for the treatment of symptoms and in the expectation that the natural history will be influenced favourably.

CARDIOPULMONARY BYPASS

In principle, cardiopulmonary bypass is a means for removing systemic venous blood from the body, oxygenating it, and returning it to the systemic arterial system at a reasonably physiological pressure, devoid of gas bubbles or solid particles, at a controlled temperature, and at a rate capable of maintaining normal tissue metabolism.

Surgical approach to the heart

Vertical sternotomy is the approach generally used. The sternum is divided longitudinally in the midline and the pericardial cavity is opened to display the heart and major vessels. The ascending aorta and right atrium are now readily accessible for preparation for cardiopulmonary bypass (Fig. 20.4).

Previous cardiac surgery results in adhesions between the heart and pericardial sac or back of sternum, increasing the difficulty of a second operation.

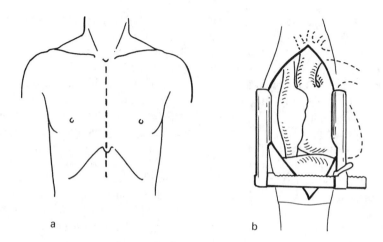

a   b

Fig. 20.4   Surgical approach to the heart. (a) Vertical sternotomy incision. (b) Right atrium and ascending aorta exposed

Cannulation for cardiopulmonary bypass

Systemic venous blood is removed either through two plastic cannulas inserted into the superior and inferior vena cava respectively via incisions in the right atrial wall, or through a single large cannula in the right atrium. Another cannula is inserted high in the ascending aorta to return oxygenated blood from the cardiopulmonary bypass circuit (Fig. 20.5).

Cardiopulmonary bypass circuit

There are a number of commercially available sterile-packed disposable oxygenators which are of two major types. *Bubble oxygenators* achieve gas

exchange by bubbling a mixture of 95% oxygen and 5% carbon dioxide through a column of blood passing through the oxygenator (Fig. 20.6). Defoaming sponge then removes the gas bubbles before the blood runs into a reservoir from which it is pumped back to the patient. *Membrane oxygenators* achieve gas exchange by bringing the blood and the ventilating gas into close proximity, but separated by a thin gas-permeable membrane arranged either as sheets or hollow fibres.

Cooling is inevitable during extracorporeal transit. A heat exchanger is therefore usually incorporated into the oxygenator. The temperature of the circulating water can be adjusted to warm the returned blood back to 37°C, or to induce (and finally correct) systemic hypothermia during cardiopulmonary bypass.

A simple roller pump (see Fig. 20.6) is used to pump blood back to the patient. This gives an even arterial perfusion pressure of between 50 and 100 mmHg with a flow rate of about 2.4 l/m^2 per minute with normothermic bypass. The absence of a physiological pulse pressure for several hours does not appear unduly deleterious. Roller pumps which mimic the normal pulsatile arterial pressure are now also available.

The extracorporeal circuit is filled with an isotonic fluid (e.g. Ringer's solution) and air is meticulously excluded from the arterial side of the circuit.

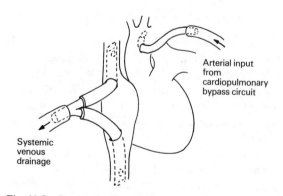

Arterial input from cardiopulmonary bypass circuit

Systemic venous drainage

Fig. 20.5   Cannulation for cardiopulmonary bypass

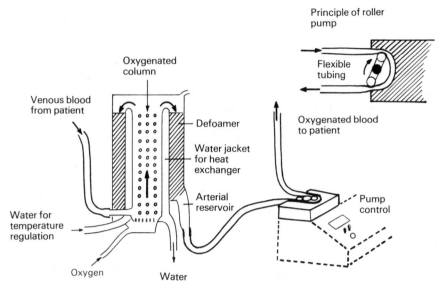

Fig. 20.6 Diagram of cardiopulmonary bypass circuit using a bubble oxygenator

Heparin

Before inserting the cannulas for cardiopulmonary bypass, heparin 3 mg/kg body weight is injected into the patient's circulation to prevent blood from clotting in the extracorporeal circuit. Additional heparin is given during long operations and is neutralized with protamine once the bypass procedure is completed.

Hazard of emboli

Care is taken to avoid introduction of air into the systemic arterial system and to remove air from the heart chambers before allowing ejection into the aorta. Intracardiac thrombosis and calcified fragments from calcific heart valves can act as emboli. The most profound effects follow cerebral emboli, as severe cerebral damage can result.

Sterility

All parts of the extracorporeal circuit with which blood comes into contact must be sterile. The commercially produced oxygenators are pre-sterilized. It is usual practice to give a broad spectrum antibiotic during the operation to reduce the risk of bacteraemia.

Myocardial protection

During most cardiac operations the ascending aorta is cross-clamped once cardiopulmonary bypass has been established. This interrupts flow into the coronary arteries and renders the myocardium ischaemic. Aortic cross-clamping is essential before opening the aortic roof for access to the aortic valve. It is also of great help in providing a bloodless, immobile, relaxed heart for most cardiac operations.

Interruption of coronary flow is followed by ischaemic cardiac arrest within a few minutes, changes in mitochondria within 15 minutes, and increasing myocardial damage after about 30–45 minutes. Where cross-clamping of the aorta beyond about 30 minutes is required (as for valve replacement), some form of myocardial protection is necessary. In the past this was achieved by directly cannulating and perfusing the coronary arteries with oxygenated blood via their ostia, or by perfusing the aortic root.

Myocardial protection is now usually achieved by cooling and arresting the heart (cardioplegia) with infusion of cold (4–10°C) isotonic crystalloid solution with a high potassium content (14–30 mmol/l) or with chilled blood containing added potassium, the aim being to produce prompt potassium-induced cardiac arrest (thus minimizing loss of high-energy phosphate stores in the myocardial mitochondria) and to reduce metabolic requirements by induction of local myocardial hypothermia. Topical irrigation of the heart within the pericardial sac with large volumes of cold saline (about 4°C) is commonly used to supplement the hypothermic effect of the cardioplegic fluid.

Cardioplegic myocardial protection is generally used in combination with systemic cooling of the patient (using the heat exchanger within the extra-corporeal circuit). Cooling to 28–30°C decreases the general metabolic requirements and provides a safety margin in the event of cardiopulmonary bypass being relatively inadequate. More profound hypothermia (20°C) is often considered necessary to reduce the rewarming effects of the non-coronary collateral flow on the myocardium. This is particularly important in coronary disease where non-coronary collateral flow may be increased. With careful technique, and reinfusion of cardio-plegic solution if myocardial temperature rises or electrocardiographic activity returns, it is possible to achieve safe cardiac arrest for 2 hours or more — sufficient for most cardiac operations to be completed. Myocardial rewarming and activity occur rapidly once coronary blood flow is restored.

Ventricular fibrillation is common after rewarming and is sometimes induced deliberately to prevent ejection of blood from the heart while air is removed. Direct application of defibrillating paddles and a countershock to the ventricles restores an effective beat.

Incisions in ventricular muscle impair contractility and are kept to a minimum. Right ventriculotomy is used for repair of Fallot's tetralogy, and sometimes for repair of an isolated ventricular septal defect. Most other cardiac lesions can be approached via incisions in the atria or major vessels, rather than in ventricular myocardium, to allow access to intracardiac structures (Fig. 20.7). Incisions are closed with continuous non-absorbable sutures.

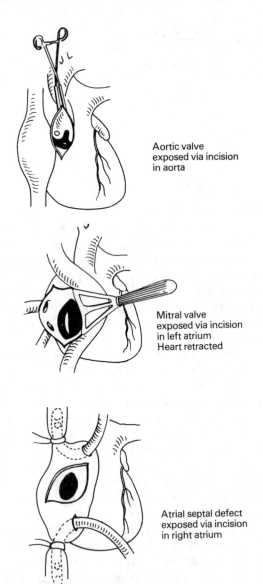

Aortic valve exposed via incision in aorta

Mitral valve exposed via incision in left atrium Heart retracted

Atrial septal defect exposed via incision in right atrium

Fig. 20.7 Surgical exploration of intracardiac structures with cardiopulmonary bypass

VALVULAR HEART DISEASE

Types of valvular disease

Mitral valve disease is usually due to rheumatic fever, although a history of rheumatic fever is not always obtained. The valve may become regurgitant due to annular dilatation during the acute episode and the condition is associated with pancarditis. Surgery is usually required for the late results of chronic inflammation which may cause (1) predominant *mitral stenosis* due to commissural fusion and leaflet thickening; (2) predominant *mitral regurgitation* due to annular dilatation and retraction of leaflet tissue; or (3) a *mixed lesion* due to combination of commissural fusion, leaflet thickening and chordal shortening. Valve calcification is common after long-standing inflammation.

Less commonly, mitral regurgitation is due to chordal rupture, leaflet degeneration, infarction or rupture of papillary muscle as a result of ischaemic heart disease, or left ventricular dilatation in severe cardiac failure.

Infective endocarditis may affect any diseased heart valve and cause rapid deterioration in valve function.

Aortic valve disease may be due to rheumatic fever with resultant predominant stenosis, predominant regurgitation, or a 'mixed' lesion. Calcification occurs in long-standing disease. A congenitally bicuspid aortic valve may be stenotic early in life, but stenosis is more commonly a late manifestation of calcification developing in such valves.

Syphilitic and dissecting aortic aneurysm are less common causes of aortic regurgitation.

Tricuspid valve disease may be due to rheumatic involvement or to 'functional' annular dilatation in patients with mitral valve disease complicated by severe pulmonary hypertension. The tricuspid valve may also be congenitally abnormal.

Pulmonary valve disease is usually a congenital stenosis with varying degrees of commissural fusion or hypoplasia of the valve annulus.

Conservative surgical measures for abnormal valves

Reasonably satisfactory haemodynamic function of the patient's own valve is preferable to that of any prosthetic valve. Conservation of valves is the aim wherever feasible.

The stenosed mitral valve may be opened by *mitral valvotomy*. This applies to a mobile abnormality, evidence for which is a loud first heart sound and opening snap, with absence of radiological calcification. With a finger inserted through a small incision in the left atrial appendage, a dilator is passed through the left ventricular apex and guided into the stenosed mitral orifice. Rapid opening of the dilator breaks down commissural fusion. The operation does not severely impede cardiac action and does not require cardiopulmonary bypass.

Pulmonary and *aortic valvotomy* are performed using cardiopulmonary bypass. The valve is visualized and the fused commissures are divided.

Regurgitant valves are less easy to conserve, particularly the aortic and pulmonary valves. Mitral or tricuspid regurgitation due primarily to dilatation of the annulus may be dealt with by reduction in the size of the annulus to restore competence — frequently by sewing a rigid or semirigid ring to the annulus to maintain normal annular dimensions (annuloplasty). Elongated chordae can be shortened, and limited areas of flail leaflets due to chordal rupture can be resected with restoration of satisfactory valve competence.

Valve replacement

Cardiopulmonary bypass is required with exposure of the valve. A diseased valve which cannot be conserved is excised, leaving a rim of valve tissue to facilitate suturing in a prosthesis. It is often necessary to remove calcium from the valve annulus.

The surgeon has a large choice of different valve prostheses for valve replacement (Fig. 20.8). This reflects the continuing problems with prosthetic valves, although many earlier problems have been largely overcome. In general there are two categories of prosthetic valve.

1. *Mechanical valves*. These are made of non-biological materials such as pyrolytic carbon and metal alloys, and do not mimic natural valves. The Starr-Edwards caged ball valve and the Bjork-Shiley tilting disc valve are perhaps the best known. All mechanical valves are subject to thrombosis on the valve, with resultant embolism or interference with valve function. Indefinite oral anticoagulation (with warfarin) is used to reduce this hazard and is started as soon as post-operative blood loss ceases. With well controlled anticoagulation the risk of thromboembolism with current mechanical valves is low. Such valves are very durable.

2. *Bioprosthetic valves*. These have moving parts made of biological tissue, usually glutaraldehyde-treated porcine aortic valves or

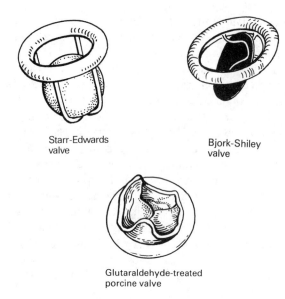

Starr-Edwards
valve

Bjork-Shiley
valve

Glutaraldehyde-treated
porcine valve

Fig. 20.8   Types of artificial heart valve

glutaraldehyde-treated bovine pericardium fashioned and mounted on a supportive frame to mimic the natural aortic valve. They can be used to replace the aortic or mitral valves.

Bioprosthetic valves have less tendency to thromboembolism and can often be used without the need for anticoagulation (usually only patients with residual atrial fibrillation need anticoagulation). Their major drawback is their limited or uncertain durability — calcification or tissue disruption is seen in many of these valves after 5–10 years, and accelerated calcification is unfortunately common in young adults and children (just the group where mechanical valves with their need for lifelong anticoagulation are least desirable).

Prosthetic valves are produced in a range of sizes, and the appropriate size is selected at operation. Postoperatively, all prosthetic valves carry a small risk of infective endocarditis on the valve, and prophylactic antibiotics are advised at times of potential bacteraemia, such as dental manipulations or whenever the patient has a septic condition.

Valve replacement surgery carries a risk of operative mortality, which is higher in the elderly, in those with coronary artery disease, and in patients with impaired liver function or severe pulmonary vascular disease. Overall, the operative mortality is in the region of 5%. Symptomatic relief is usually marked and the natural history considerably improved.

ISCHAEMIC HEART DISEASE

Surgery for coronary artery disease has become extremely common in most Western countries — indeed, in the United States the number of coronary operations now exceeds 1000 per million of population each year. *Angina pectoris* is the usual indication for surgery, and most surgeons now agree that surgery should be offered where symptoms persist or interfere with activities in spite of adequate medical therapy with beta-blocking drugs, calcium-channel blockers or nitrates. It is now widely accepted that triple vessel disease and left main coronary artery disease, particularly when associated with impaired left ventricular function, have a better long-term prognosis with surgical treatment than with medical therapy alone. For this reason, detailed investigation of all patients with angina, frequently with coronary arteriography, is required before making a decision about management. Increasingly, younger patients and those with a poor family history of ischaemic heart disease, are being investigated with a view to possible surgery (and anticipated improvement in the natural history) when a 'coronary event' such as myocardial infarction or sudden angina first occurs.

Coronary artery bypass grafting

In principle the technique of coronary surgery consists of inserting a conduit carrying a high-pressure source of arterial blood into relatively normal segments of coronary arteries distal to the angiographically demonstrated obstruction(s) (Fig. 20.9). In the past the commonest source for the conduit was the patient's own saphenous vein, which was removed at the time of operation and inserted between the ascending aorta and the distal coronary arteries jeopardized by stenosis. Increasing recognition of the late changes in saphenous vein when used in this fashion (about one-half of such grafts become occluded by thrombosis or intimal hyperplasia within the first 10 years after

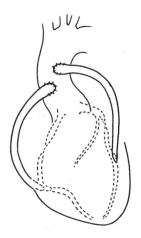

Fig. 20.9 Bypass grafts for right and left anterior descending coronary obstruction

operation), together with evidence of excellent long-term patency of internal mammary arteries when used as a coronary conduit have led to more widespread use of the patient's own internal mammary arteries.

Cardiopulmonary bypass is used to allow cardioplegic arrest of the heart and thus provide an immobile, bloodless operative field. The coronary arteries are opened beyond known obstructions which have been angiographically demonstrated prior to surgery. Typically, grafts will be needed for the anterior descending artery (see Fig. 20.9), the obtuse marginal branch of the circumflex and the distal right or posterior descending arteries. Vessels with a lumen diameter greater than 1.5 mm are large enough to permit satisfactory grafting, and most grafts are placed to vessels in their epicardial course. Fine instruments and sutures, and magnification, are needed to suture the distal end of the mobilized internal mammary artery (or the end of the saphenous vein) to the coronary arteriotomy. Where a vein is used, the other end of the vein is sewn to a small opening made in the ascending aorta. Vein grafts, and often internal mammary artery grafts, can be used as sequential grafts to allow flow into more than one distal coronary artery.

Endarterectomy, the removal of an atheromatous core, will often clear a totally blocked distal coronary artery, allowing a graft to be inserted. Revascularization of poorly functioning myocardium due to ischaemic fibrosis is unrewarding. Thus, surgery is indicated primarily in those patients with angina pectoris in whom coronary angiography has demonstrated proximal severe obstruction (loss of 50% or more of coronary lumen) in a major coronary artery. Provided that angina is present (indicating the presence of viable, ischaemic muscle), the state of left ventricular function is rarely so poor as to preclude surgery.

Result of surgery

The risk of surgery is low: in males under 70 years of age the mortality rate is about 1–2%. It is a little higher in females, in the very elderly and in those with widespread arterial disease. Relief from angina is complete in 60–80%, and much improved in most of the remainder. There is a gradual return of angina in the subsequent years, and only about 30–50% are free from angina 10 years after the operation. Recurrence is usually due to progression of disease in the coronary arteries or occlusion of vein grafts. Effects on natural history are difficult to assess. The combination of spontaneous changes in disease manifestations, improvements in both surgical and medical management, and the wide variability in coronary pathology and its frequently unpredictable correlation with clinical manifestations makes interpretation of the outcome of the relatively small number of randomized prospective trials of medical and surgical management very difficult. There is, however, general agreement that surgery improves prognosis to a greater extent than medical management in those with left main and triple vessel disease, particularly when left ventricular function is impaired.

Percutaneous transluminal coronary balloon angioplasty

Since its introduction for coronary surgery in the late 1970s, the technique of inflating a small balloon which has been introduced through a peripheral artery and positioned under radiological control across a stenosis in a coronary artery has become increasingly popular. Impressive reduction in the degree of stenosis can be achieved, and multiple vessels can be treated. The risk is low, but there is a 'learning curve' for the technique, i.e. results improve with experience. This form of treatment is generally reserved for short, subtotal stenoses located away from major bifurcations or branching. Some lesions cannot be dilated. Approximately one-third recur within 6 months. However, the relatively brief hospital stay and less invasive nature of the procedure make it a potentially attractive alternative to surgery in many patients. Its precise role is not yet defined.

Surgery for complications of coronary artery disease

Myocardial infarction is the usual complication of coronary artery disease. A few centres have adopted a policy of undertaking prompt coronary angiography, followed by immediate bypass grafting of the infarct-related artery, as well as any other stenosed vessels, provided that surgery can be undertaken within 4–6 hours of the onset of chest pain. Such surgery naturally creates logistic problems because of time constraints. Low operative mortality is reported, although salvage of significant amounts of jeopardized myocardium is difficult to prove.

Of greater practical application is the more recent development of techniques for coronary thrombolysis, either by intracoronary infusion of streptokinase or by systemic administration of specific fibrin-targetted lytic agents. This makes restoration of blood flow in the infarct-related artery a practical possibility within the first few hours of the onset of chest pain and diagnosis of evolving myocardial infarction, and leaves the option of subsequent management of any coronary stenosis by percutaneous balloon angioplasty or coronary bypass surgery. The role of such intervention in the early phase of acute myocardial infarction is not yet established. Uncertainty persists about the period of time in which intervention is worthwhile, although generally it is thought to be within the first 4–6 hours of the onset of chest pain. As with early intervention surgery, it is difficult to prove that early thrombolysis does indeed salvage myocardium otherwise doomed to infarction.

Ventricular aneurysm is a late complication of myocardial infarction. Healing of transmural infarction may leave a large fibrous scar which bulges to form an aneurysm, thus compromising left ventricular function and causing breathlessness on exertion. The aneurysm can be resected using cardiopulmonary bypass, taking care to avoid dissemination of mural thrombus, which is frequently present. The rim of the aneurysm is pulled together and sewn to a small patch to restore a more normal ventricular shape. Teflon felt buttresses and strong non-absorbable sutures are used for the sewing. The operation improves overall left ventricular function, although it leaves a significant akinetic area. Operation is indicated only for large aneurysms where exertional dyspnoea is a major symptom. It may be combined with coronary grafting if coronary angiography demonstrates stenosis of major coronary arteries.

Less commonly, where acute myocardial infarction involves the interventricular septum or a papillary muscle of mitral valve, *muscle rupture* may occur. This results in either a ventricular septal defect or mitral regurgitation, and places a major, and often rapidly fatal haemodynamic load on an already compromised heart. Urgent surgery to close the ventricular septal defect or replace the mitral valve may be life-saving.

CONGENITAL HEART DISEASE

Congenital heart disease occurs in about 6–8 of every 1000 live births. There are many different types and only the common defects are mentioned here. Although symptoms may not appear until late in life (e.g. congenital bicuspid aortic valve), the problem usually presents in childhood. The severe lesions which present in the first few months of life have a high surgical mortality. Cardiopulmonary bypass is commonly used in neonates for corrective cardiac surgery, although it is technically more difficult than in larger children.

Palliative surgery

Palliative surgery most frequently involves construction of a shunt between the systemic and pulmonary circulations to increase pulmonary blood flow and improve oxygenation in patients with poor pulmonary blood flow and cyanosis. The commonest application is in Fallot's tetralogy (see later), where anastomosis of the subclavian artery to the pulmonary artery (Blalock-Taussig shunt) is a relatively simple operation giving good palliation and allowing definitive repair to be deferred for 2 or 3 years, when the larger size may make surgery safer. However, improving techniques mean that definitive repair is now often undertaken in younger patients and palliative surgery is avoided. Palliative surgery may still be the only course open for complex anomalies.

Patent ductus arteriosus

The ductus arteriosus allows pulmonary artery blood to bypass the airless lungs during intra-uterine life. Failure of normal closure results in left-to-right shunting of systemic blood into the pulmonary circulation as pulmonary vascular resistance falls after birth. This may produce cardiac failure in infancy, requiring urgent surgery. More commonly, the shunt is well tolerated and the characteristic 'machinery' murmur in the second left interspace is the reason for referral. Cardiac failure may occur in later life if the condition is not remedied. Surgery carries little risk and is always advised. The ductus is exposed through a left lateral incision and is either divided and sutured between vascular clamps or ligated with thick non-absorbable sutures.

Coarctation of the aorta

Narrowing of the aorta usually occurs just beyond the left subclavian artery. The diagnosis is suggested by absent or delayed femoral pulses; in older patients rib notching is often seen on radiological examination. About 50% of patients die within the first year of life from cardiac failure, and complications from proximal hypertension frequently lead to death in early adult life. Operation is always advised and is undertaken through a left lateral thoracotomy incision. The aorta is temporarily cross-clamped above and below the coarctation. The narrowed segment is resected and the aortic ends are sutured together with non-absorbable sutures. In infants it may be preferable to enlarge the narrowed area, using the left sub-clavian artery as a patch (patch angioplasty). Occasionally, with a long narrowing in an inelastic aorta, an intervening graft may be needed.

Atrial septal defect

Atrial septal defects result in shunting of blood from left to right atrium because of the greater distensibility of the right ventricle and pulmonary arterial tree than of the left ventricle and systemic arterial system. The typical clinical findings are increased pulmonary blood flow, a delayed pulmonary second sound and radiological evidence of pulmonary plethora. If untreated, the defect causes breathlessness on exertion and eventually cardiac failure in middle life.

Surgical repair is advised when the diagnosis is made and carries little risk. Cardiopulmonary bypass is used and the defect is closed through an incision in the right atrium. It is usually possible to approximate the edges of the defect with a continuous suture, but a patch of pericardium or Dacron may be required for large defects in an inflexible atrial septum.

Although most atrial septal defects are of a simple nature (secundum defects), there are others which are more complex. These are the sinus venosus defect, which occurs near the orifice of the superior vena cava, and the primum defect, which occurs close to the mitral and tricuspid valves, which may have associated clefts. These more complex types can usually be diagnosed preoperatively, and require greater experience and care in closure to avoid compromising related anatomical structures.

Ventricular septal defects

Defects in the ventricular septum result in left-to-right shunting of blood because left ventricular pressure is higher than right ventricular pressure during systole. This results in excessive pulmonary blood flow, which carries the risk of pulmonary vascular obstruction developing, with consequent pulmonary hypertension, and eventually cessation and then reversal of the shunting of blood through the ventricular septal defect (Eisenmenger syndrome). This results in cyanosis and is inoperable. Surgery for ventricular septal defect may be required in infancy for cardiac failure refractory to medical treatment, but is usually advised before school age for defects of significant size. There is a possibility of spontaneous closure, but the risk of an untreated defect leading to pulmonary vascular disease must be borne in mind. Evidence of raised pulmonary vascular resistance in childhood is an indication for early surgery. Severe pulmonary vascular disease or reversal of the shunt is a contraindication to surgery.

Closure of the defect requires the use of cardiopulmonary bypass. The ventricular septal defect is exposed through an incision in the right ventricle or through a right atrial incision with retraction of the tricuspid valve. A patch of Dacron or similar material is sutured into the defect. Tricuspid valve tissue and conducting tissue are closely related to the defect and injury must be avoided.

Tetralogy of Fallot

This condition consists of (1) obstruction to right ventricular outflow due to pulmonary valve stenosis, right ventricular outflow tract muscle hypertrophy, or pulmonary artery hypoplasia; and (2) a large ventricular septal defect due to malalignment of the aorta and pulmonary artery over the interventricular septum. Both ventricles are at systemic pressure and the right ventricle is hypertrophic. Right-to-left shunting of blood across the ventricular septal defect results in cyanosis. Compensatory polycythaemia occurs and carries a risk of spontaneous intravascular thrombosis with consequences dependent on the site of the arterial tree affected.

Palliative shunting between the systemic and pulmonary circulation (Blalock-Taussig shunt; see earlier) may be undertaken in the first year or two of life if there is severe cyanosis with polycythaemia or the child has repeated cyanotic spells. Total correction is usually advised before school age. Cardiopulmonary bypass is required. If a palliative shunt is present, this must first be closed. The outflow obstruction is then removed (this may require patch enlargement) and the ventricular septal defect is closed. The operation carries a mortality of about 5% and results are good. Cyanosis is abolished, return to full activity

is possible, and there is an undoubted improvement in life expectancy. There are more severe forms of the condition in which the pulmonary arteries are hypoplastic or even missing (pulmonary atresia). These increase the complexity and mortality of surgical repair, and some are amenable only to palliation.

PERICARDIAL DISEASE

Chronic constrictive pericarditis has many causes. The commonest is tuberculous pericarditis, which is usually inactive by the time the disease is seen by the surgeon. Systemic venous congestion occurs because the heart cannot expand fully in diastole to accept normal venous return.

Resection of the dense constrictive fibrous tissue surrounding the heart can be achieved through a vertical sternotomy incision with careful dissection of the beating heart. Some surgeons prefer to use cardiopulmonary bypass.

CARDIAC TRAUMA

Cardiac injuries are not commonly seen by the surgeon. Stab wounds of the heart usually cause rapidly increasing tamponade. Urgent thoracotomy on the side of the stab wound with opening of the pericardium immediately relieves tamponade, allowing time for blood transfusion and suture of the cardiac injury.

Rupture of the first part of the descending thoracic aorta may occur with rapid deceleration injuries, usually as a result of road traffic accidents. Suspicion should be aroused by a bruise over the sternum which carries an imprint of the source of trauma, e.g. a steering wheel hub. If the injury is not immediately fatal due to intrapleural rupture and exsanguination, the diagnosis is suggested by the finding of a widened mediastinum on chest radiography, and is confirmed by urgent aortography which shows irregularity at the rupture site. Overlying aortic adventitia and mediastinal tissues may temporarily prevent total rupture of the aorta into the pleural space and give time for rapid left thoracotomy. The aorta is rapidly clamped above and below the ruptured area and aortic continuity is restored by sewing in a short Dacron tube.

POSTOPERATIVE CARDIAC SURGICAL CARE

Before closure of the chest after any cardiac operation, tubes are placed for drainage of blood and connected to underwater seal bottles. These tubes prevent tamponade by allowing escape of blood from around the heart, and permit measurement of postoperative blood loss. Postoperative observation in an intensive care area is required for the first 24 hours after surgery with cardiopulmonary bypass to pre-empt complications and ensure stable haemodynamic function.

Cardiac output

Adequate cardiac output is reflected by normal tissue perfusion as assessed by peripheral skin temperature (palpation or skin temperature probe), mental responsiveness, urine flow (measured from bladder catheter; 0.5/ml/kg per hour is adequate) and maintenance of normal acid-base balance.

Continuous monitoring of *pulse rate* (from oscilloscope display of electrocardiogram), *blood pressure* (recorded from peripheral arterial cannula used for peroperative monitoring) and *atrial pressure* is essential. The latter is usually right atrial or central venous pressure, but left atrial or pulmonary arterial wedge pressure is more useful and informative though not routine.

Low cardiac output is shown by a fall in peripheral skin temperature, mental unresponsiveness, oliguria and developing metabolic acidosis. This may be due to oligaemia, heart failure or cardiac tamponade.

1. *Oligaemia* is caused by inadequate replacement of blood loss, or vasodilatation in a patient previously vasoconstricted due to systemic hypothermia. Tachycardia, hypotension and low atrial pressure are the typical signs. Rapid blood transfusion is necessary to restore normal parameters.

2. *Heart failure* may be due to surgical trauma, ischaemia complicating perioperative myocardial infarction or dysrhythmia. The pulse rate may be normal, rapid or very slow, and there may be hypotension and high atrial pressure. Treatment includes administration of inotropic drugs such as isoprenaline, adrenaline or dopamine, and correction of electrolyte or acid-base abnormalities.

3. *Cardiac tamponade* is due to accumulation of blood around the heart, usually as a result of clot blocking the drainage tubes. Tachycardia, hypotension and high atrial pressure usually develop rapidly. Tamponade can be difficult to distinguish from heart failure, but the sudden onset of these signs, particularly when blood loss has been heavy, makes tamponade the likely diagnosis. Once the diagnosis is suspected, the chest should be re-opened immediately for evacuation of clot and control of bleeding.

Blood loss

Blood loss in excess of 200 ml/hour in an adult is usually best treated by re-opening of the chest. This may reveal an active bleeding site, but more often there is generalized oozing. Haematological studies may reveal the cause (e.g. free heparin or a low platelet count) and suggest specific therapy.

Ventilation

It is common practice to control ventilation with a mechanical ventilator for several hours after cardiopulmonary bypass. This is to ensure adequate return of spontaneous ventilatory effort and allow aspiration of bronchial secretions until cardiovascular function is stable.

Patients with poor preoperative lung function may require prolonged ventilation with gradual weaning from the ventilator, regular removal of retained bronchial secretions and treatment of pulmonary infection.

COMPLICATIONS OF CARDIAC SURGERY

Excessive bleeding and low cardiac output may complicate cardiac surgery, and have been discussed above.

Cerebral injury is often directly attributable to events occurring during cardiac surgery and ranges in severity from minor disturbances of concentration and mood to severe cerebral lesions resulting in failure to regain consciousness, hemiplegia or other serious disturbances. The more minor disturbances may be due to consequences of extracorporeal circulation (e.g. microemboli or inadequate cerebral perfusion). Major cerebral injury may complicate 1–5% of operations, depending on the type of patients in the practice, and is usually due to air embolism, arterial thromboembolism or cerebrovascular accident occurring during the altered perfusion of cardiopulmonary bypass. Treatment is supportive and the prognosis is variable.

Cardiac arrest may be due to ventricular fibrillation which can occur as a result of myocardial irritability due to falling serum potassium levels or to asystole. Treatment consists of prompt external cardiac massage, maintenance of ventilation, defibrillation, correction of any abnormality of serum potassium and acid-base balance, and inotropic support if required.

Renal failure is an occasional complication. If more than transient, it requires peritoneal dialysis or haemodialysis.

Repeat cardiac surgery

In recent years an increasing number of patients have undergone cardiac surgery for a second or even third time after the initial operation. In many cases this is for correction of congenital cardiac abnormalities following initial palliative surgery. In others it may be required for replacement of previously repaired heart valves or malfunctioning or degenerating valve prostheses. Repeat coronary artery surgery may be needed in patients who develop recurrent symptoms due to progression of coronary disease to previously normal arteries, or due to occlusion of saphenous vein conduits. There is generally an increased operative risk for repeat surgery. This is largely due to the hazard of surgical injury to the heart (which is usually adherent to surrounding pericardium or overlying sternum as a consequence of previous postoperative adhesions) at the time of re-opening of the chest and preparation for cardiopulmonary bypass.

CARDIAC TRANSPLANTATION

Although still applicable to only a relatively small number of patients with cardiac disease, cardiac transplantation for end-stage cardiac disease now offers remarkably good survival where there are no prospects for improvement with medical or surgical measures. Cardiopulmonary bypass is used to maintain the circulation during excision of the heart and replacement with a heart from a donor — excised promptly after death, using cardioplegic myocardial protective techniques and short ischaemic time. Advances in monitoring and treating rejection episodes, notably with cyclosporin, have contributed greatly to the improved survival, which is now in the region of 70% at 3 years.

21. Peripheral vascular disease

Vascular disease is the commonest cause of disability and death in the Western World. There are striking variations in geographical distribution. Venous disorders are commoner, but arterial diseases are more serious and more likely to require urgent surgical intervention.

ARTERIAL DISEASE

Large vessel disease, affecting the aorta and its branches down to 1–2 mm in diameter, behaves differently from small vessel disease, affecting small arteries and capillaries. Large vessel disease can threaten life or limb, often presents acutely but can usually be treated successfully by repair or reconstruction. Small vessel disease causes chronic disability and surgery has little to offer. Most arterial disorders are due to atherosclerosis. Morphologically this takes the form of (1) obliterative or (2) ectatic or aneurysmal disease.

ATHEROSCLEROTIC OBLITERATIVE ARTERIAL DISEASE

This disease can affect the circulation to the heart, causing angina or myocardial infarction; to the brain, causing chronic ischaemia or stroke; to the kidneys, causing hypertension or renal infarction; to the gut, causing mesenteric angina or intestinal infarction; or to the limbs, causing claudication, rest pain, gangrene or acute ischaemia. These various manifestations arise from what is essentially the same disease.

Obliterative arterial disease is partly familial. Other important aetiological factors are smoking, hypercholesterolaemia, hypertension and diet. Diabetics are prone not only to atheroma but also to neuropathy which, together with elevated sugar levels in the tissues, makes them vulnerable to sepsis.

Atherosclerosis encompasses a spectrum ranging from pure atheroma, a metabolic lesion affecting large arteries (aorta, iliac, carotid, renal, etc.), to arteriosclerosis, 'hardening of the arteries', which affects the media of the whole arterial tree.

Atheroma has a clear association with smoking and with metabolic disorders, notably hyperlipidaemia and diabetes. It may cause symptoms in young adults. The basic lesion is a subintimal deposit of lipid laid down at points of haemodynamic stress such as vessel bifurcations

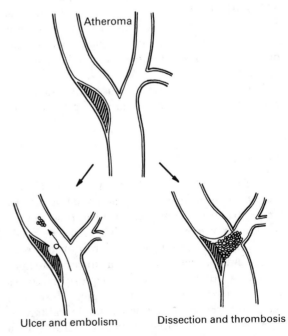

Fig. 21.1 Vascular problems caused by atheroma

and branches (Fig. 21.1). In experimental animals and possibly in man these plaques can be made to regress by altering the diet. *Arteriosclerosis* is a disease of older patients. It affects the arterial tree diffusely, including the small arteries, resulting in degeneration of muscle and elastic tissue of the media, these being replaced by fibrous tissue and calcification. These two facets of atherosclerosis usually coexist, but awareness that the patterns may differ explains some of the variable clinical features.

Serious complications arise from enlargement or extension of the atheromatous plaque by subendothelial build-up of lipid. Flow may be obstructed or ulceration may in turn lead to thrombosis, embolism or dissection of the vessel wall. Extension of the disease to involve the media and elastic lamina weakens the wall, which may result in aneurysm formation, particularly if the patient is hypertensive.

Thrombosis

The platelet aggregation which starts a thrombus is triggered by several factors, including turbulence and irregularity of the vessel wall. These effects are produced by the developing plaque which, when it obstructs the lumen by about 70%, reduces blood flow. The liability to thrombosis may be further enhanced by ulceration of the plaque to expose thrombogenic subendothelial elements.

Thrombosis of an artery causes infarction only when collateral channels are affected by the disease.

Embolism

Before a plaque and/or thrombus completely occludes a vessel, fragments of atheroma or platelet aggregates may become detached and pass into the distal arterial tree as emboli. These can be single or multiple and may give rise to pain or necrosis.

An embolus may arise from an atheromatous plaque or from an aneurysm but usually comes from the heart. The patient may give a history of recent myocardial infarction (with a mural thrombosis) or the thrombus may have formed in a fibrillating atrium. Less often the source may be

an artificial heart valve, a cusp vegetation or, very rarely, an atrial myxoma. The severity of the effects of embolism depends on the site and the adequacy of collateral compensatory flow.

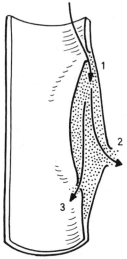

Fig. 21.2 Dissecting aneurysm of aorta. (1) Initial intimal tear; (2) adventitial rupture; (3) intimal rupture

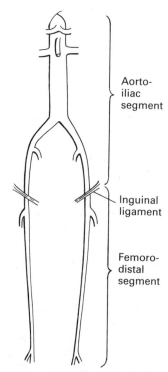

Fig. 21.3 Diagram showing aorto-iliac and femoro-distal segments

Dissection

Ulceration of the arterial wall allows blood to drive a haemodynamic wedge under the endothelium. A flap may be raised which obstructs flow and exposes subendothelial tissues so that thrombosis is promoted. Dissection may also result from the insertion of an arterial catheter. In the aorta, particularly if there is associated hypertension, the split may extend into the media and down the wall of the vessel over a distance of many centimetres (Fig. 21.2). Then it may rupture outside the vessel or track back into the lumen, creating a false channel carrying blood within the wall of the artery. Such a process will obstruct the orifices of any branches in its path. Thus, a dissection of the abdominal aorta may cause acute occlusion of the renal, mesenteric or iliac arteries.

The natural history and clinical features

Occlusion of femoro-distal and aorto-iliac segments (Fig. 21.3) causes different clinical features and requires different forms of management.

Femoro-distal obliterative disease

The femoro-distal segment includes the common femoral artery with its superficial and profunda divisions, the popliteal artery with its three divisions, the anterior and posterior tibial and the peroneal arteries. As a general rule, the older the patient the more does obliterative disease affect the small vessels and therefore the less the possibility of surgical repair. The commonest site of occlusion is the superficial femoral artery, but serious effects are limited by the relatively good anastomoses between the profunda and the popliteal via the perforating and genicular vessels. Critical ischaemia ensues when there is obstruction of collateral (profunda) channels or of the inflow or 'run-off' vessels.

Although obliterative arterial disease is a steadily progressive pathological process, the symptoms follow a pattern of relapse and remission (Fig. 21.4). The earliest lesion to cause symptoms is usually a stenosis in the femoral artery in the region of the adductor canal (A). The patient reports tightness in the calf muscle (claudication)

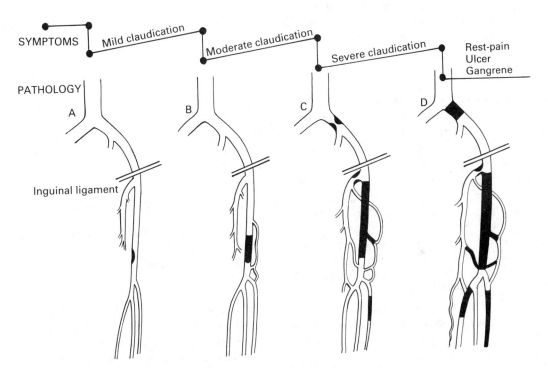

Fig. 21.4 Pattern of symptoms and pathology in obliterative arterial disease (see text)

after walking continuously for about a quarter of a mile (about 400 m). On examination the limb appears normal. Ankle pulses are palpable but diminished and a bruit can be heard at or below the adductor canal.

Over the next few weeks the collateral vessels of the profunda system enlarge to carry a higher proportion of the blood flow. The symptoms gradually improve or even disappear. With occlusion of the artery from thrombosis there is a sudden deterioration in symptoms. Claudication now comes on after about 300 metres (B). The limb still appears relatively healthy on inspection but ankle and popliteal pulses can no longer be palpated.

Over the following months collateral circulation again compensates for the reduced blood flow and the symptoms improve. Stopping smoking greatly facilitates this improvement. The patient may also consciously or subconsciously adapt by relaxing his pace. Thus the inconvenience may be only slight, especially if the individual is elderly or relatively inactive.

This phase of moderate claudication may remain apparently stable for several years. However, unless there is a radical change in the patient's life style, the atherosclerosis will progress in inflow, outflow or collateral channels to further compromise the blood supply (C). Claudication is now severe, forcing the patient to stop every 50 metres or so and he complains that the foot is cold. On examination the extremity may be cool and capillary refilling slow. Once again there may be a period of relative improvement but the scope for this is steadily diminishing as the disease spreads. In just a few months the occlusions increase and the symptoms deteriorate (D). Severe pain develops in the toes or forefoot at rest, typically arising about an hour after the patient has gone to bed. This 'night pain' is due to the accumulation of metabolites which occurs with the fall in blood flow as the lower limb rests in a horizontal position. It is severe but is relieved by hanging the limb out of bed, which in turn causes dependent oedema and a risk of infection. There may also be numbness and paraesthesia. Once a patient develops rest pain, gangrene is not far away. This is the stage of 'critical ischaemia'.

By now chronic loss of nutrition will have caused changes in muscles, skin and nails. Necrotic areas (dry gangrene) appear over pressure points such as the knuckles, metatarsal heads and heel (decubitus ulcer) and sepsis supervenes. This is more common if there is dependent oedema or diabetes, when it may lead to a spreading moist gangrene requiring amputation.

An understanding of this cyclical pattern of exacerbation and resolution is important. Medical treatment with drugs is usually prescribed when symptoms occur but improvement is more likely to be due to the natural history than to the medicine. Drug treatment has a very limited place in the treatment of obliterative arterial disease.

Aorto-iliac occlusion

Even when the blockage is above the inguinal ligament, claudication is most commonly felt in the calf. It may also be felt in the buttock and thigh. The commonest sites for occlusion are the lower aorta and the common iliac arteries. If the internal iliac arteries are blocked in a male, the patient may also complain of impotence (Leriche syndrome). Relatively young women who are heavy smokers and of small stature, with narrow-calibre vessels, are particularly prone to develop atheroma in the lower aorta.

Femoral pulses are diminished or absent and bruits may be heard. In 'pure' aorto-iliac disease the signs of ischaemia in the lower limb may be minimal, as, at rest, collaterals carry an ample blood supply. When there are blocks in both the aorto-iliac and femoro-distal segments the symptoms are severe.

Assessment of obliterative arterial disease

Particular attention is paid to a history of disease of the cardiorespiratory system, diabetes and smoking and a family history is obtained. Claudication is the cardinal symptom of early and moderate disease. It is predominantly felt in the calf, occasionally in the thigh and buttock and rarely in the foot. The discomfort, usually described as a 'tightness' rather than a pain, comes on with exercise and goes away within 1–2 minutes of rest. This rapid relief distinguishes it from other causes of exercise-related calf pain, such as spinal cord compression, which takes 5–10 minutes to settle with rest. Pain caused by osteoarthritis of the hip or knee is likely to be present when walking first commences, and that from venous insufficiency obliges the patient to sit down; it is also associated with leg swelling. Ischaemic rest pain or night pain (see above) is felt in the forefoot or toes and is worse when the leg is elevated. It disturbs sleep and is poorly controlled by analgesics.

In a chronically ischaemic limb the skin is thin and dry. On elevation of the leg there is marked pallor, and on hanging it down the foot becomes bright red; this is known as dependent rubor or 'sunset foot'. In the horizontal position the superficial veins fill sluggishly. The nails are brittle and crumbly and there is muscle wasting. Temperature differences are important. Mottling and extreme pallor are particularly serious signs.

The pulses should be carefully palpated, beginning with the femoral pulses. The strength and regularity of the impulse, the texture of the vessel wall and the presence of any thrill are noted. Auscultation over the common femoral arteries may reveal bruits. To feel the popliteal pulses, the knee should be slightly flexed to relax the muscles and popliteal fascia before palpating deeply between the condyles with the fingers of both hands. The posterior tibial artery is felt midway between the medial malleolus and the tendo-achilles, and the dorsalis pedis just proximal to where it dips down between the bases of the first and second metatarsals. The patient must be carefully examined for other evidence of arterial disease.

Doppler ultrasound is used to measure the systolic blood pressure at the ankle. If there is any doubt about the diagnosis or the severity of claudication, pressures are measured before and after a treadmill exercise test. Exercise causes a fall in systolic pressure proportional to the severity of the disease. The speed of recovery is quicker with aorto-iliac than with femoro-distal disease. There are a variety of non-invasive radiological or laboratory tests in current use of which the most valuable is Duplex B-mode ultrasound imaging. This offers the possibility of visualizing the vessel and making a simultaneous blood flow measure-

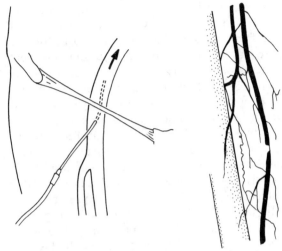

Fig. 21.5 Femoral arteriography showing stenosis in the femoro-distal segment

ment at the point of insonation. Arteriography (Fig. 21.5) remains the most important investigation but is only used if active treatment such as angioplasty or operation is being seriously considered.

Treatment of obliterative arterial disease of the lower limb

Conservative care

Most patients with claudication simply need reassurance and advice. If smoking can be stopped, the prognosis greatly improves. Patients are encouraged to undertake a programme of graded exercise such as walking but pausing momentarily *before* being forced to stop by their claudication, and gradually increasing their distance over a period of time. If combined with stopping of smoking, this will result in a progressive increase of the claudication distance. Patients are advised to take plenty of cereal, fruit and vegetables and to reduce intake of animal fats. Hyperlipidaemia and obesity are corrected as far as possible. Associated diseases such as diabetes, cardiac failure and hypertension should be controlled. Hygiene, care of the skin and chiropody are important to avoid septic complications and the onset of gangrene. Extremes of temperature and all forms of trauma should be avoided.

Vasodilator drugs are of no benefit. Drugs with more complex vasoactive actions such as naftidrofuryl oxalate (Praxilene) and oxpentifylline (Trental) may be worth a trial but only in elderly patients with severe claudication for whom no more active intervention is possible. Antiplatelet therapy (one 300 mg aspirin tablet per day) is advised; long-term anticoagulants are not.

When possible, rest pain is controlled with sufficiently strong analgesics to obviate the patient's need to hang the leg out of bed. The head of the bed is elevated. Pressure on the heel must be avoided. Sepsis should be treated promptly with antibiotics. Skin lesions are kept as dry as possible with a spirit-based antiseptic. Should gangrene occur, the limb is kept cool and dry. Reflex heating is of no value.

Sympathectomy

Where there is normal autonomic control, sympathectomy results in a warm, dry limb. It does not increase the blood flow to muscles.

The principal place for sympathectomy in obliterative arterial disease is in critical ischaemia before any tissue necrosis has developed. In some patients it will relieve coldness and rest pain. Some surgeons believe it enhances the benefits of reconstructive surgery.

Chemical sympathectomy is the usual method since it avoids operation. This is done by paravertebral injection of phenol in the region of the lumbar sympathetic chain under radiological control (Fig. 21.6).

Percutaneous angioplasty

Balloon angioplasty has added a new dimension to the management of obliterative arterial disease. Its main indication is in the treatment of stenotic lesions in the aorto-iliac segment, but it has also been used successfully lower down the leg and in other arteries. The balloon catheter is introduced into the femoral artery over a guide wire (Seldinger technique) under local anaesthesia and advanced through the stenosis (Fig. 21.7). Inflation of the balloon splits the atheromatous plaque, thereby enlarging the lumen. In some centres a laser-heated probe is used to open up a channel through blocked segments and so facilitate passage of the balloon. The treatment can be repeated after an interval if necessary. Angioplasty may avoid the need for a major operation or it can be effectively combined with surgery. It should only be undertaken by a radiologist in collaboration with a vascular surgeon since complications such as dissection and thrombosis may require emergency surgical repair.

Arterial reconstruction

For the patient with claudication, surgery is considered only if the occlusion is in the aorto-iliac segment or if the patient's way of life or livelihood

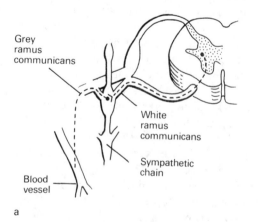
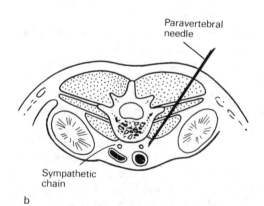

Fig. 21.6 Sympathectomy for occlusive arterial disease. Diagram showing (a) vascular sympathetic supply and (b) direction of insertion of paravertebral needle for phenol block

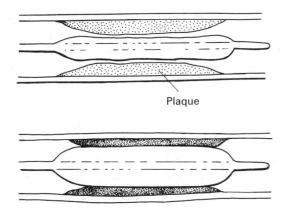

Fig. 21.7 Balloon angioplasty

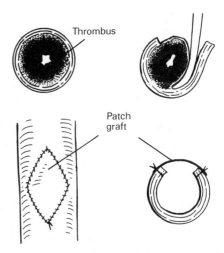

Fig. 21.8 Thrombo-endarterectomy and patch grafting

is seriously affected. A failed graft may not only leave the patient worse off than before but makes any subsequent reconstruction for critical ischaemia more difficult. Surgery is usually reserved for a limb whose viability is under threat.

In such patients, most of whom have been lifelong smokers, the risks of operation must always be considered carefully. Impaired respiratory function is very common. Since atherosclerosis is a multifocal disease, there is a much greater risk than average of cardiac complications and of stroke. Indeed, myocardial infarction is the commonest cause of death both in the perioperative period and during long-term follow-up.

Surgical techniques involve either removal of atherosclerotic plaques and thrombus (thrombo-endarterectomy) or bypass grafting. Synthetic (Dacron) grafts are used to replace large vessels. Vein is preferred for small ones. Fundamental requirements for non-thrombosis of a graft are good cardiac output and patent inflow and run-off vessels.

Aorto-iliac segment. If the occluding lesion is relatively localized, it can be treated by opening the artery and removing it (thrombo-endarterectomy) and then closing the artery with a patch of vein or Dacron to ensure patency (Fig. 21.8). Most aorto-iliac lesions are treated by aorto-iliac or aorto-femoral Dacron graft which bypasses the diseased sections (Fig. 21.9).

If the iliac artery is blocked only on one side and the patient is unfit for abdominal surgery, a femoro-femoral graft can be crossed over

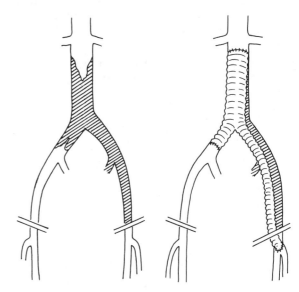

Fig. 21.9 Arterial reconstruction of the aorto-iliac segment by bypass grafting

suprapubically from the patent side to bypass the iliac block. This is one example of an 'extra-anatomic' bypass, i.e. one which does not follow a normal anatomical path. Another, which is also used in aorto-iliac disease in patients unfit for abdominal surgery, is the axillo-femoral graft. This is taken from one axillary artery down the side of the chest and flank to one or both femoral arteries. The results are less satisfactory than direct aorto-iliac reconstruction.

Patency rates are around 80% at 5 years. Graft occlusion may occur for the reasons given above. Other graft complications such as graft infection or pseudoaneurysms are rare. Infection in the graft necessitates its removal and an alternative reconstruction. Pseudoaneurysm can usually be repaired locally as long as there is no sepsis.

Femoro-popliteal segment. Saphenous vein is the preferred material for grafts of all arteries smaller than the iliacs. Other commonly used materials are polytetrafluorethylene (PTFE) or human umbilical vein (Dardik biograft). The latter is glutaraldehyde-treated to prevent graft-host reaction. These materials are very expensive. Further, patency rates are poor and sepsis is more likely than with autogenous vein.

An isolated stenosis or a short occlusion can be successfully treated by a vein patch graft with, if necessary, an endarterectomy. A good example is the narrowed orifice of the profunda which can

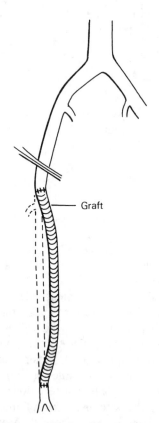

Fig. 21.10 Femoro-popliteal graft inserted to bypass an occlusion in the femoral artery.

Graft

thus be widened (profundoplasty). However, since atheroma is never confined to one area and most femoral blocks are many centimetres in length, the preferred option is to take a bypass from the common femoral artery to a point on the popliteal, tibial or peroneal artery beyond the blocked portion (Fig. 21.10).

Saphenous vein is available in 70% of cases requiring femoro-distal bypass. To eliminate the effect of the valves the vein either has to be removed and inserted upside down (reversed vein bypass) or it can be left in position and the valves disrupted by the passage of a valvulotome. This is the 'in-situ' technique which is now preferred in many centres. All the tributaries of the vein have to be individually ligated or clipped. Intravenous heparin is given before arteries are clamped. Grafts are anastomosed to arteries with fine non-absorbable sutures.

Patency rates with femoro-distal bypass are not as good as with the large-bore reconstructions, being around 50% at 5 years with vein and 30% with synthetics. The prognosis is better if the patient can stop smoking. When a graft blocks, amputation is usually inevitable, although some grafts can be cleared or replaced if the patient is referred very promptly.

Diabetes and arterial disease

About 10% of patients with arterial disease are diabetics; conversely, the proportion of patients with critical ischaemia who are diabetic is around 40%. The extent to which microvascular disease plays a part in this is debated but it is quite clear that there are two other very important factors which frequently bring diabetics under the care of surgeons. These are: (1) the high sugar content of tissues which favours bacterial growth and spread, and (2) the anaesthesia from diabetic neuropathy which allows the patient to be unaware of the minor traumas that allow ingress of bacteria. Skin care, avoidance of pressure or trauma, hygiene and chiropody are therefore doubly important in the diabetic. Good control of the diabetes and early antibiotic treatment of infections are essential. Large vessel atherosclerotic disease should be treated in the same way as in non-diabetic patients. Sympathectomy may be tried but usually has little effect. Drainage of pus and debridement of dead tissue are particularly important in patients with diabetes. Amputations can usually be more conservative than in non-diabetic ischaemia.

Amputation

Vascular disease is responsible for more than 90% of all amputations carried out in western countries. Amputation is indicated only after arterial reconstruction for 'limb salvage' has failed or if it is impractical. Fortunately the majority of patients with atherosclerosis do not reach this end stage and it is important to reassure those with early claudication that if they follow medical advice, especially concerning smoking, amputation can be avoided.

The level of amputation is determined by local blood supply and by the state of the joints, general health and age. The broad principle is to amputate at the lowest level consistent with healing. It is particularly important, from the point of view of rehabilitation, to conserve the knee joint since the energy required for walking with a below-knee prosthesis is only a fraction of that required for one above the knee. However, if the patient has other disabilities which will make walking with a prosthesis impossible, there is no point in attempting to conserve the knee joint at the expense of healing.

Thermography, percutaneous oxygen measurements and other techniques can be used to assess the local blood supply in order to determine the correct level for amputation, but clinical judgement and meticulous technique remain the most important factors.

Some 50% or more of major vascular amputations are performed below the knee, the remainder being mostly mid-thigh (Fig. 21.11). A few are performed through the knee or foot (transmetatarsal). Normally the stump is closed by primary suture. In severe septic conditions the stump may be left open with a dressing, to be closed or revised to a higher level later, when infection has been controlled.

Haemostasis is important. The end of the bone is carefully smoothed, nerves are cut cleanly as high as possible to avoid neuroma formation, muscles and fascia are approximated with fine ab-

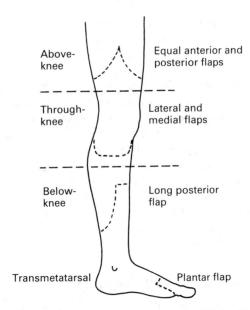

Fig.21.11 Levels of amputation and types of flap used to close the resultant defect

sorbable sutures, and the skin is closed over a drain. Inadequate blood supply, haematoma, infection and tension on the stitch line are the main causes of failure to heal. Antibiotic cover with penicillin is routine. A firm but not tight bandage is applied to an above-knee stump. A light plaster is preferred for below-knee stumps. An early return to active exercise helps to avoid contracture at the hip and/or knee. At about one week the patient should begin to bear weight on the other limb between parallel bars and at 10 days to walk with a pneumatic walking aid. If healing is progressing well, a temporary prosthesis can be fitted at about 3 weeks. Final fitting of the artificial limb must await shaping and firming of the stump. Approximately 70% of below-knee amputees and 30% of above-knee amputees eventually walk independently or with a stick or Zimmer support.

'Phantom limb' pain can be a late and troublesome complication, especially if pain has not been well controlled before and after operation. With analgesia, reassurance and time this usually settles.

Even patients who are unable to manage an artificial limb can achieve a considerable degree of independence in a wheel chair, especially if they can transfer from chair to toilet or bed and if the appropriate modifications such as ramps, wide doors and bathroom handles are made to the home.

Patients who undergo amputation for critical ischaemia are usually elderly, frail and disabled in other ways. Amputation then presents a huge psychological and physical burden. Such patients need strong support and their care is a matter of team work, with surgeon, nursing staff, physiotherapist, occupational therapist, prosthetist and social worker all playing vital parts. Amputation for vascular disease has a high morbidity and mortality rate and only a few patients remain alive for 5 years.

Occlusive disease of the upper limb

Obliterative arterial disease is much less of a problem in the upper limb than in the lower. Muscular activity is less, collateral circulation is good and atheroma does not occur to the same extent. The commonest site of occlusion is the first part of the subclavian artery proximal to the origin of the vertebral artery (Fig. 21.12). Occlusion at this level has two effects: (1) a reduced blood pressure in the arm and (2) compensatory reversal of flow down the vertebral artery to supply the limb. This effect, known as 'subclavian steal', can give rise to symptoms of vertebrobasilar ischaemia such as dizziness, classically occurring during muscular activity of the arm. More often the patient presents with weakness, tiredness or claudication in the upper limb, with subclavian steal as a radiological finding on arteriography.

Subclavian occlusion is easily corrected by inserting a bypass graft between the subclavian and one of the other arteries in the neck, usually the common carotid.

Occlusive disease of the carotid and vertebral arteries

Stroke

Stroke is an episode of focal neurological dysfunction whose symptoms last more than 24 hours and which is caused by a vascular disturbance in the brain. When such symptoms last for less than 24

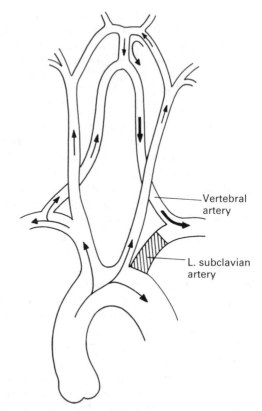

Fig. 21.12   Occlusion of subclavian artery causing 'subclavian steal'

hours, the episode is described as a transient ischaemic attack (TIA). Most TIAs last only a few minutes.

In the UK about 100 000 people per year suffer their first stroke. As a cause of death, stroke is exceeded only by heart disease and malignant neoplasm. It is the most important cause of severe disability. Four-fifths of strokes are caused by thrombosis and the majority of these are due to occlusive disease in the *extracranial* vessels, i.e. the carotid and vertebral arteries. Occlusions in these vessels give rise to two distinct syndromes: carotid ischaemia with effects in the related cerebral hemisphere, and vertebrobasilar ischaemia with effects referrable to the hind brain. TIA, especially if clearly in the carotid territory, may be an indication for carotid endarterectomy (see below).

Carotid distribution events

The origin of the internal carotid artery is particularly prone to atheroma. Following the formation of a plaque, emboli of aggregated platelets, fibrin or fragments of atheroma may pass into the carotid territory. If they enter the retinal artery, they cause transient ipsilateral blindness (amaurosis fugax) or sometimes permanent blindness. These emboli can be seen in the retina with an ophthalmoscope. If they enter the territory of the middle cerebral artery, they may cause dysphasia, dysarthria, hemiparesis, hemisensory loss, deviation of the head and eyes towards the side of the lesion, or disorientation. A TIA is a precursor of major stroke, the risk of which lies between 5 and 10% per year. Investigation and treatment should not be delayed.

Vertebrobasilar distribution events

These are more varied but frequently produce dizziness, diplopia, cortical blindness, dysarthria, 'drop attacks' and unilateral or bilateral motor and sensory deficits.

Examination and investigation

It is important to exclude other causes of cerebral ischaemia, especially cardiac arrhythmias. The carotid pulse may be diminished or absent and a bruit may be audible over the affected carotid or vertebral artery. However, the absence of a bruit does not rule out significant disease. Cerebral CT scanning is an important investigation which can quickly exclude haemorrhage and detect infarcts of more than 0.5 cm in diameter.

Useful screening tests of the vessels include Duplex B-mode ultrasound imaging and digital subtraction angiography but perfemoral arch and selective carotid arteriography are the critical investigations on which decisions regarding surgery depend.

Treatment

There is evidence that antiplatelet therapy with aspirin in small doses, e.g. 300 mg on alternate days, reduces arterial thrombotic events. Surgery, since it carries a 1–5% risk of stroke or death, is not justified unless there have been unequivocal transient ischaemic attacks or minor stroke with good recovery. The aim of surgery is to remove the source of embolism and protect the patient from major stroke. To achieve this, carotid disease must be detected before it proceeds to complete occlusion. A completely blocked internal carotid

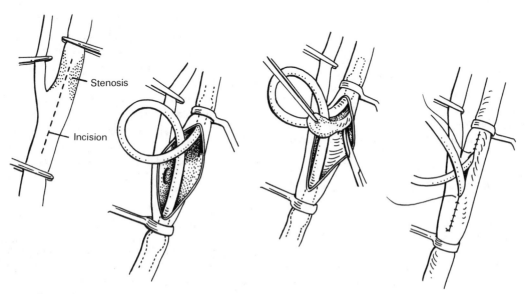

Fig. 21.13 Carotid endarterectomy using an internal Javid shunt to bypass the site of operation and thus protect cerebral blood flow

artery cannot be re-opened and operation is not indicated in the presence of a stroke with substantial residual deficit.

At *carotid endarterectomy* heparin is given and the arteries are clamped and opened. Cerebral blood flow is usually quite adequately maintained via collaterals but can be further protected by means of a shunt (Fig. 21.13). The stenosing plaque is shelled out and the artery repaired with direct suture or with a patch graft.

Stenosing plaque at the origin of the vertebral artery is removed through an incision in the subclavian artery. This operation is rarely performed.

Occlusive disease of the renal artery

Stenoses of the renal arteries can be caused by fibromuscular hyperplasia, particularly in young females, or by congenital lesions but the great majority are due to atherosclerosis. Such narrowing reduces perfusion of the juxtaglomerular apparatus, which in turn leads to increased release of renin and angiotensin, and hypertension.

Hypertension of renal origin should be suspected if the patient is relatively young or resistant to antihypertensive therapy. There may be an audible bruit on auscultation of the abdomen. Investigations include renin estimations on selective venous catheter samples, renal isotope perfusion scanning and renal angiography.

There are two indications for active intervention in cases of renal artery stenosis: (1) control of hypertension and (2) preservation of renal tissue. Perfemoral balloon angioplasty has proved to be effective in some types of stenosis. Operative reconstruction may be carried out by means of a vein graft. In technically difficult cases, especially where there are multiple renal arteries, the kidney can be removed from the body and preserved by perfusion with cooled electrolyte solution while the arteries are repaired under magnification. The kidney is then returned to its previous position or autotransplanted to the iliac fossa as in renal transplantation.

When the operation is performed for hypertension, about two-thirds of patients are either cured or the hypertension becomes easier to control.

Acute arterial occlusion

The commonest vascular emergency is sudden arterial occlusion. The causes are thrombosis, embolism, trauma or dissecting aneurysm. The severity of the effect on distal tissues depends on the level of the block and the adequacy of collateral circulation. Trauma and dissection of aneurysm aside, about one-third of acute occlusions are due to embolism and one-third to thrombosis. In the remaining third it is not possible to distinguish between the two.

Thrombosis usually occurs as the end stage of chronic obliterative disease, so the patient is likely to have a history of previous chronic ischaemia such as claudication. Aneurysms are also prone to thrombosis, especially popliteal aneurysms. The onset may be dramatic with severe pain or, because collaterals have had an opportunity to develop over a period of time, may simply consist of sudden numbness and coldness. Thrombosis is often precipitated by a fall in blood pressure due to cardiac failure, myocardial infarction or shock from any cause.

Embolism is most commonly associated with ischaemic heart disease with atrial fibrillation, cardiac failure or a recent myocardial infarction. Sometimes there is a history of previous embolism. Subacute bacterial endocarditis and prosthetic heart valves can produce multiple emboli which may be infected. Emboli may also originate from mural thrombus associated with atherosclerosis in proximal main arteries. Trauma to a vessel during arterial catheterization may dispatch emboli to distal arteries.

A typical embolus consists of partially organized thrombus and lodges at the bifurcation of an artery. Occlusion is aggravated by thrombosis spreading proximally and distally from the embolus, and occluded collaterals can lead to gangrene.

Clinical features

A typical site for an acute occlusion is the bifurcation of the common femoral artery. Coldness and pain in the foot and calf are the first symptoms. This is followed by paraesthesia, loss of sensation and loss of power. The loss of sensation is of the 'glove and stocking' variety, i.e. maximal distally and not following any segmental nerve distribution. At first the limb is pale with poor venous filling but later it becomes mottled with cyanotic patches. Muscle tenderness is a sign of ischaemic damage, and is first evident in the anterior tibial compartment. Embolism generally is more dramatic than thrombosis but either can be insidious.

Acute arterial occlusion has to be distinguished from deep venous thrombosis and venous gangrene, in which swelling is marked. A careful history and examination, supported by chest X-ray and electrocardiography, will usually define the cause. Arteriography is necessary only if there is doubt whether the occlusion is embolic or thrombotic, i.e. when there is acute-on-chronic ischaemia. A full blood count, and blood sugar, urea and electrolyte estimations are obtained routinely.

Management

Acute embolic ischaemia can be reversed completely if treated promptly. A main-stem arterial occlusion will cause permanent tissue damage only if more than 6 hours elapse without treatment. Thrombosis is not as easy to correct as embolus because of the underlying disease in the arterial wall but, owing to its more insidious nature, a little more time may be available to investigate and plan treatment.

The first step is to correct any precipitating condition such as hypotension. There is no point in clearing thrombus from an artery if flow cannot be sustained. Volume replacement, digoxin, diuretics, anti-arrhythmics and inotropic agents are used as indicated.

Systemic heparin is started immediately to minimize further spread of thrombus. All embolic occlusions and any thrombotic occlusion with signs of severe ischaemia (loss of sensation, loss of power, muscle tenderness) require urgent operation. For thromboses with less compelling clinical features, initial medical treatment with thrombolytic agents or heparin may be considered but the patient must be very carefully observed for

signs of deterioration. Expert advice must be sought.

Emergency embolectomy/thrombectomy can be performed under local anaesthesia but an anaesthetist should be available in case of difficulties or in case arterial reconstruction has to be undertaken. Most lower limb thrombi can be removed by passing a Fogarty balloon catheter through an incision in the femoral artery (Fig. 21.14). Embolectomy/thrombectomy is contraindicated in the presence of gangrene, when amputation is the only possible treatment.

Early operation has dramatically improved limb salvage rates but mortality remains around 20%. The degree of ischaemia on presentation gives a good indication of the likely outcome. Lack of motor activity with tender hard muscles suggests that amputation is likely to be necessary. In such cases embolectomy/thrombectomy has to be accompanied by fasciotomy in the compartments of the calf to relieve the tension from swelling which follows restoration of blood flow to ischaemic muscles. Restoration of blood flow may cause cardiac or renal complications (arrhythmias, hypotension, oliguria) due to release of breakdown products of myoglobin and haemoglobin.

Femoral embolectomy/thrombectomy. Thrombi in the iliac, femoral, popliteal or more distal arteries can be removed through an opening in the

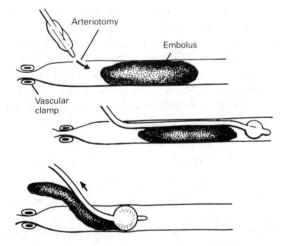

Fig. 21.14 Removal of embolus with a Fogarty balloon catheter

common femoral artery. The artery is incised longitudinally and a Fogarty catheter passed proximally or distally through the thrombus; the balloon is then inflated and the catheter gently withdrawn, extracting the thrombus (see Fig. 21.14). Several passages may be necessary to clear the vessel. The result should be checked by operative angiography. A *saddle embolus of the aorta* is dealt with by removal of the thrombus through bilateral groin incisions.

Acute arterial occlusion of the upper limb is less common. Thrombosis may form on an atheromatous patch in the subclavian artery, in a subclavian aneurysm or in an artery mechanically compressed at the thoracic outlet. Thrombosis also occurs in the axillary artery affected by previous radiotherapy for breast carcinoma. Emboli may lodge at any level. Clinical features are similar to those in acute occlusion of the lower limb although, as the collateral supply is better, the symptoms are generally less severe. Exposure of the brachial artery at the elbow gives access to the origins of the radial and ulnar as well as proximal vessels. Patency should be confirmed by operative angiography.

Postoperative care

The colour, temperature and peripheral pulses of the leg are closely monitored in case re-thrombosis should occur. If fasciotomies were not performed at the initial procedure, the muscles must be carefully checked for swelling or tenderness during the first 12–24 hours. A decompression fasciotomy may be indicated. If the occlusion was due to embolism, heparin is continued for one week and oral anticoagulants for 6 months or more. Patients with atrial fibrillation will require to remain on anticoagulants permanently.

Mesenteric embolism

The sudden onset of abdominal pain and diarrhoea in a patient known to be at risk of embolism should suggest the diagnosis of mesenteric embolism. This is based on clinical findings alone; angiography would only cause delays which cannot be afforded. Early abdominal signs are non-specific: there may be lower or mid-abdominal tenderness and increased bowel sounds. Urgent laparotomy and balloon embolectomy may prevent intestinal ischaemia, but only 2–4 hours are available before damage becomes irreversible. By the time the diarrhoea becomes bloody and there are signs of peritonitis, the bowel has infarcted and survival of the patient is unlikely.

ANEURYSM

An aneurysm is an abnormal dilatation of an artery (or occasionally a vein or a heart chamber). This may be congenital but is more commonly acquired. Aneurysms have three principal complications: rupture, thrombosis or embolism. An arterial aneurysm may be 'true' or 'false' (Fig 21.15).

True aneurysms

A true aneurysm is enclosed by all three layers of the arterial wall. Acquired aneurysms result from degeneration of the media and elastic lamina due to atheroma or arteritis (including syphilis), with expansion of the affected part of the vessel. Though not strictly an aneurysm, *dissection* of the arterial wall, usually secondary to atherosclerotic destruction of the media, is also considered (see later).

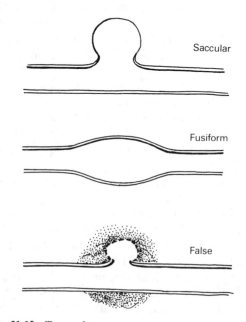

Fig. 21.15 Types of aneurysm

In subacute bacterial endocarditis or in bacteraemia, septic emboli may lodge within the vasa vasorum and form an intramural abscess. This may give rise to an infective or (as it is often wrongly termed) a 'mycotic' aneurysm.

Turbulence of the blood stream within an aneurysm leads to the laying down of thrombus. As it enlarges, it may erode adjacent structures. Since the tension in the wall of a viscus increases with its radius of curvature (Laplace's law), the liability to rupture increases as it expands.

Congenital aneurysms occur in the cerebral arteries and may be saccular or fusiform, depending on whether part of the whole of the circumference of the wall is weakened (see Fig. 21.15).

False aneurysms

If the wall of an artery is pierced, the resulting haematoma sometimes remains in continuity with the lumen. A pulsatile swelling then forms whose wall consists of compacted thrombus. If small (2–3 cm diameter), they usually thrombose and resolve but if larger they tend to expand and leak.

Abdominal aortic aneurysm

An aneurysm of the abdominal aorta is found in 2–4% of autopsies. Such aneurysms appear to be increasing in western countries and are more common in males. Fortunately 95% occur below the level of the origins of the renal arteries and can be treated surgically.

Aneurysms are often multiple. An abdominal aneurysm may be in continuity with a thoracic one or there may be associated iliac, femoral or popliteal aneurysms. Most patients are over 70 years of age. Many have hypertension, which increases the risk of rupture. This risk varies with aneurysm size. An aneurysm larger than 6 cm in diameter has at least a 50% risk of rupture within 2 years; however, the risk of dying of myocardial infarction or stroke during that period is almost as great.

Clinical features

An abdominal aortic aneurysm may present in the following ways.

1. An asymptomatic pulsatile swelling may be found on routine physical examination, X-ray or abdominal scan.

2. Pain may be felt in the central abdomen or more commonly referred to the back, loin, iliac fossa or groin; this may simulate renal colic.

3. Leakage or rupture may cause severe abdominal or back pain and hypovolaemic shock. An episode of lesser pain (a 'herald bleed') may precede catastrophic rupture by several days or even weeks. Rarely an aneurysm may form a fistula into the bowel or vena cava.

Unless the patient is exceptionally obese, a pulsating mass can be felt. Tenderness is a sign of impending rupture or of an infective aneurysm. Guarding and distension suggests rupture. Femoral pulses may be diminished.

A plain abdominal X-ray will show a rim of calcification especially on a lateral view. Ultrasound or CT scanning are useful investigations to determine the size and wall thickness and may demonstrate extravascular haematoma. Arteriography is only indicated if there is a history of claudication or if involvement of the renal arteries is suspected. The diagnosis of a ruptured aneurysm is based on history and physical examination; other investigations are contraindicated.

Management

The treatment of choice is replacement of the aneurysm with a Dacron graft. The aneurysmal sac is opened between clamps, partly excised and replaced either by a straight tube or a 'trouser' bifurcation graft whose legs are anastomosed to the iliac or femoral arteries (Fig. 21.16).

All aneurysms over 5 cm in diameter should be repaired electively unless there are general contraindications to surgery. Its progress must then be monitored by ultrasound.

A leaking or ruptured aneurysm requires immediate operation. Overenthusiastic resuscitation should be avoided; a systolic blood pressure of 80–90 mmHg is sufficient to sustain renal perfusion. Blood is immediately sent for rapid cross-matching and a urinary catheter and wide-bore venous cannula are inserted. Operative mortality depends on the experience of the surgeon and his team and

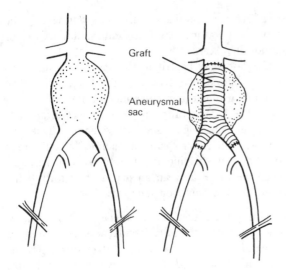

Fig. 21.16 Repair of aortic aneurysm by insertion of a 'trouser' bifurcation graft

transfer to a specialist centre is recommended. If the patient is hypotensive, and particularly if he or she has to be transported any distance, a pneumatic 'G-suit' applied to the lower limbs and abdomen will help to maintain blood pressure. The G-suit is removed in the operating theatre when the surgeon is ready to start the operation. Postoperative intensive care is essential. Myocardial infarction and renal failure are the main immediate complications.

Dissection of the aorta

Aortic dissection (see Fig. 21.2) generally begins in the ascending aorta or proximal descending aorta and extends distally. It may cause aortic valve incompetence and/or coronary artery occlusion and has a high mortality. The patients are usually hypertensive but dissection may also occur in pregnancy, as a result of trauma or in Marfan's syndrome. The onset of dissection is accompanied by excruciating central chest pain which spreads to the back and abdomen. If the ascending aorta is involved, upper limb ischaemia is noted; dissections of the descending aorta affect the lower limbs. Severe chest or back pain with diminution of arm or leg pulses should always raise the suspicion of dissection. Paraplegia, renal failure and mesenteric ischaemia may signal involvement

of aortic branches. Pulmonary oedema is often present. External rupture results in hypovolaemic shock.

Management

Pain control, antihypertensive treatment (e.g. with sodium nitroprusside) and stabilization of the circulation are the first steps. The diagnosis is confirmed by aortography.

Dissection of the ascending aorta is treated by resection of the affected part and replacement with a Dacron graft, combined if necessary with aortic valve replacement. Uncomplicated dissection of the descending aorta can be treated conservatively with antihypertensive drugs, but grafting is indicated if pain is uncontrolled, if the circulation cannot be stabilized or if rupture occurs. About 50% of untreated patients die within 48 hours; 60% of treated patients survive 5 years.

Peripheral aneurysms

Aneurysms in peripheral vessels form pulsatile swellings in the course of the vessel. The liability to complications varies according to site. For example, in subclavian aneurysm, often associated with mechanical compression at the thoracic outlet (e.g. cervical rib), emboli are carried to the fingers and hand. Popliteal aneurysm frequently presents as acute arterial occlusion. The possibilities for reconstruction are often poor because of silting of tibial and peroneal branches by previous small emboli. Aneurysms may also cause symptoms by pressure on adjacent veins or nerves. It is preferable to operate on large aneurysms electively rather than wait for complications to arise.

Arteriography defines the site and extent of the aneurysm and the state of the distal arteries. Treatment consists of bypassing the affected segment with a vein or synthetic graft, the aneurysm being resected or simply tied off.

ARTERIOVENOUS FISTULA

An arteriovenous (A-V) fistula is an abnormal communication between artery and vein which may be congenital or acquired.

Congenital A-V fistula

Congenital A-V fistulas result from persistence of fetal arteriovenous communications. They are usually multiple and affect the small vessels. They usually present in childhood and are commonest in the lower limb or pelvis. There is overgrowth of bone and soft tissues so that the limb is bigger, longer and warmer than normal. Extensive varicose veins cover the posterolateral aspect of the limb and there are areas of purple skin haemangioma (Fig. 21.17). Superficial venous hypertension may cause skin ulceration. Venous thrombosis is common.

Treatment. Surgery tends to be unrewarding and is best avoided. Venous hypertension is controlled with accurately fitted graduated compression stockings. In certain cases selective catheterization and obliteration of feeding arteries by injected sclerosants is successful, and preferable to surgical ligation. The correction of limb overgrowth by bone shortening is deferred until the epiphyses have fused after puberty.

Acquired A-V fistula

Acquired A-V fistulas are generally traumatic in origin and thus tend to be single. A penetrating injury (including a surgical mishap) of adjacent artery and vein results in the formation of a channel between the two either directly or with an intervening false aneurysm (Fig. 21.18). Blood is shunted under high pressure into the vein, which becomes thickened and arterialized. The deliberate construction of such a fistula in the forearm is used as a means of providing ready vascular access in patients requiring dialysis for chronic renal failure.

A large communication between an artery and vein gives rise to a number of serious consequences. First the blood flow to tissues beyond the fistula may be reduced, causing ischaemia in the extremity. Second the shunt places strain on the heart, leading to valve damage and high-output failure. Fistulas near the heart are more likely to cause cardiac failure, while those situated distally in the extremities tend to cause ischaemia. The clinical features are warmth and venous distension in the region of the fistula, and coldness and signs of atrophy distally. A palpable thrill and a loud to-and-fro 'machinery' murmur at the site of the fistula is characteristic. Occlusion of the fistula by pressure leads to slowing of the heart. Arteriography confirms the diagnosis and outlines the anatomy of the involved vessels.

Treatment. Where access is straightforward, the best treatment is operative closure of the fistula and repair or ligation of the vessels. In certain situations a fistula can be blocked by placement of a balloon inserted by percutaneous selective catheter technique.

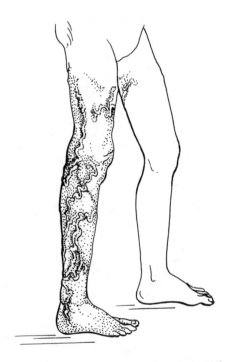

Fig. 21.17 Congenital arteriovenous fistula

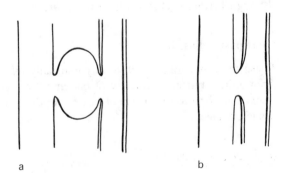

a

b

Fig. 21.18 Acquired (traumatic) arteriovenous fistula with (a) intervening false aneurysm and (b) direct communication

ARTERITIS

Buerger's disease (thromboangiitis obliterans)

This form of obliterative arterial disease is rare in the UK but common in Mediterranean countries. It usually occurs in young males who are heavy smokers and characteristically affects the peripheral arteries, giving rise to claudication in the feet or rest pain in the fingers or toes. There is often a previous history of superficial phlebitis. Wrist and ankle pulses are usually absent, but brachial and popliteal pulses are palpable. Arteriography shows narrowing or occlusion of small peripheral arteries but relatively healthy main vessels. The condition often remits if the patient stops smoking, and sympathectomy is helpful. If required, amputation can often be limited to the digits.

Giant cell arteritis

Giant cell arteritis is a rare condition involving major limb arteries, particularly the subclavian and axillary. Patients present with claudication and polymyalgia (i.e. pain and weakness) of shoulders and arms. The condition is treated with steroids; surgery has no place. Diagnosis is by temporal artery biopsy.

Takayasu's arteritis

This is a rare inflammatory disease affecting mainly the aortic arch vessels in young Asian women. Progressive ischaemia of the arms and brain may occur. Steroids may help. Surgical bypass of the affected arteries may be feasible, although further occlusions tend to occur.

Vasospastic disorders

These are very common. Disability is usually relatively minor but in a minority of patients there is associated thrombosis of small vessels leading to tissue damage.

Raynaud's phenomenon

Exposure to cold causes digital artery constriction so that the fingers become white, numb and painful. Primary and secondary types are recognized.

Primary Raynaud's phenomenon affects 5–10% of young women in temperate climates. It usually appears between the ages of 15 and 30 years; a family history is common. It does not progress to ulceration or infarction. No investigation is necessary and treatment consists of reassurance and advice on avoidance of exposure to cold.

Secondary Raynaud's phenomenon tends to occur in older people as a manifestation of underlying disease such as scleroderma or systemic lupus. It may also be caused by working with vibrating tools or by treatment with beta-blocking drugs. There is thrombosis of small vessels leading to atrophy and necrosis of the finger-tips (Fig. 21.19). Management is often unsatisfactory, particularly when no underlying disease can be found. The fingers must be protected from cold and trauma, and infection treated with antibiotics. Vasoactive drugs have no clear benefit. Sympathectomy helps for a year or two. Limited debridement of infected or necrotic digits may be necessary.

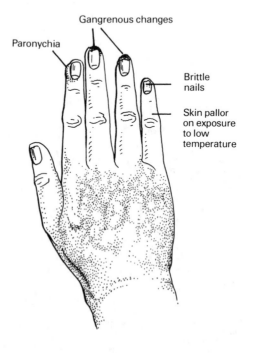

Fig. 21.19 Clinical appearance of long-standing Raynaud's phenomenon

Acrocyanosis

Acrocyanosis is characterized by red-blue discoloration of the skin on exposure to cold. When warm the extremities become bright pink. It is distinct from, but often coexists with, Raynaud's phenomenon.

Chilblains is one form of this condition. It is also seen in elderly patients with cardiac disease and in limbs affected by neurological disorders such as stroke. Reassurance and protection from cold are usually all that is needed. If symptoms are severe, sympathectomy may be indicated. Vasodilators are ineffective.

Cold injury

Although frostbite is particularly associated with mountaineering, it is also frequently seen in temperate climates in neglected elderly patients or vagrants, particularly alcoholics. At first there is swelling, redness and blistering, followed by infection and superficial gangrene. Treatment consists of reflex heating, analgesics, antibiotics and dextran infusions. Surgery is delayed until the area of dead tissue has become clearly demarcated, when debridement can be carried out.

VASCULAR TRAUMA

Arterial damage may occur as a result of blunt or penetrating trauma. Iatrogenic damage during the course of investigations (e.g. cardiac catheterization, arteriography) is becoming increasingly common and inadvertent intra-arterial injection of anaesthetic agents or sclerosants can also cause arterial injury. Compression of an artery may follow swelling of tissues within an osteofascial compartment or the application of rigid dressings, or it may be caused by direct pressure from splints or plasters.

Secondary thrombosis at the site of injury occludes the vessel. The degree of ischaemia depends on the state of the collateral circulation. While arterial spasm can occur at or beyond the site of injury, it should never be assumed to be the cause of ischaemia.

Arterial injuries can be divided into three categories: (1) complete severance or transection;

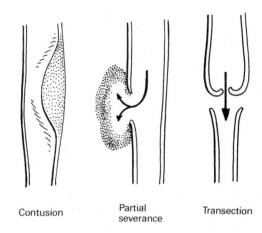

Contusion   Partial severance   Transection

Fig. 21.20 Types of arterial injury

(2) incomplete or partial severance; and (3) contusion (Fig. 21.20).

Complete severance (transection)

If the vessel is completely divided, for example by a knife, its ends retract and constrict. Thrombosis occurs rapidly at the cut end and blood loss may be surprisingly small. In patients with severe atherosclerosis there is less capacity for constriction and retraction so that serious haemorrhage is more likely.

Distal pulses in the limbs are lost immediately, and pallor, paraesthesia, pain, paralysis and poikilothermia (coldness) — the five Ps of acute ischaemia — quickly develop.

Incomplete severance

Partial division of an artery may result from penetrating injuries (including those from surgical knives, drills or needles) or from closed injury, e.g. when the vessel is lacerated by a fragment of fractured bone.

Partial continuity of the vessel prevents retraction, and contraction of the circular muscle at the site of injury tends to hold the laceration open. Haemorrhage is severe. If the overlying tissues are intact, this leads to the formation of a pulsating haematoma (see earlier). Diminution of distal pulses and signs of distal ischaemia are less pronounced than after complete severance of a vessel. If there is coincident damage to an adjacent vein, an arteriovenous fistula is likely to develop (see earlier in this chapter).

Arterial contusion

Contusion results from blunt injury or stretching and is not uncommon in fractures. An intramural haematoma may develop and occlude the vessel. Usually, however, on exploring the vessel the surgeon finds that although the adventitia is intact the intima has been split, often completely circumferentially, with resultant thrombosis.

External bleeding is absent. Pulses disappear and signs of ischaemia develop.

Management

In an open wound, severe haemorrhage indicates the likelihood of arterial damage. In closed injuries, the existence of arterial damage should always be considered if limbs and lives are to be saved. Even then some arterial injuries are not apparent at first but become obvious only when complications arise.

Control of haemorrhage is the first concern. The limb is elevated and pressure applied. Tourniquets are seldom required and are potentially dangerous. Blood volume is restored by transfusion. If the peripheral circulation does not improve despite adequate replacement, surgery is indicated. Arteriography may help to define the site and extent of the injury but is often unnecessary and should not delay definitive surgical treatment.

Surgical treatment

Early reconstruction is advised for injuries of large arteries; small ones may be ligated. Direct closure is sometimes possible but generally a vein patch or tube graft is preferred. Synthetic grafts should be avoided because of their liability to infection, thrombosis and secondary haemorrhage.

Fractures should be stabilized first by external or internal fixation. Antibiotic cover is advisable. Heparin or dextran therapy should be used postoperatively to maintain patency in the early stages.

Intra-arterial injection of noxious material is treated conservatively in the first instance. The artery is flushed with heparinized saline and irrigated with reserpine. Full systemic doses of heparin, opiates and antibiotics are given.

DISORDERS OF THE VEINS

Venous drainage of the lower limb

The superficial veins of the lower limb are the long and short saphenous veins and their tributaries (Fig. 21.21). The vessels lie outside the deep fascia and carry only 10% of the venous return from the limb. The long saphenous vein begins at the

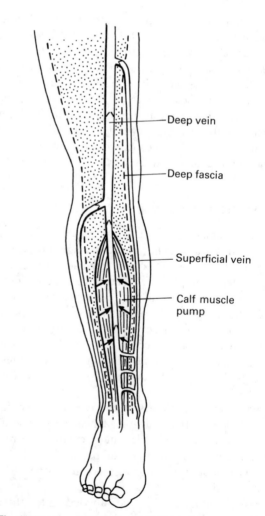

Fig. 21.21 Venous drainage of the lower limb

medial end of the dorsal venous arch, crosses the medial malleolus and ascends the medial side of the leg. It penetrates the deep fascia (cribriform fascia) at the saphenous opening 4 cm below and lateral to the pubic tubercle to enter the femoral vein. The short saphenous vein starts at the lateral end of the dorsal venous arch, passes round posteriorly to the median line of the calf, in which it ascends to join the popliteal vein behind the knee. Anatomical variations are common.

The deep venous system comprises intramuscular veins and the veins, usually paired in the calf, which accompany the main arteries. There is also liberal venous flow in the medullary cavities of the bones.

The superficial and deep systems are connected by communicating veins which perforate the deep fascia (see Fig. 21.21). The largest perforators are on the medial side of the lower calf opposite the medial border of the soleus muscle, but some also occur on the lateral side of the calf and the medial side of the thigh. It is important to remember that in the calf the perforators do not connect directly with the long saphenous vein but join its tributaries.

Venous return is an active process. There is a 'foot pump' as veins of the sole are emptied by weightbearing and a 'calf pump' comprising veins within the soleus muscle which is activated by muscle contraction within the cylinder of fascia lata. Blood flow is directed inwards and upwards by valves, and during muscle relaxation is sucked in from the superficial veins. Reflux into the superficial system is prevented by valves in the perforators and at the terminations of the saphenous veins. The venous pressure at the ankle is approximately 100 cmH$_2$O (zero in the right atrium) and, provided that valves are intact, falls to 20–30 cmH$_2$O during exercise. It is because of its exposure to this relatively high pressure that the saphenous vein is thick-walled and suitable for arterial grafting.

VARICOSE VEINS

Varicose veins of the leg are particularly common in women (female-to-male ratio 5:1). Incompetence of valves and reflux of blood from the deep system subjects the superficial veins to exces-

sive pressure not only when standing or sitting at rest but also during exercise. The veins become elongated, dilated and tortuous. It is the thin-walled tributaries that undergo these changes; the saphenous veins themselves are relatively little altered (Fig. 21.22).

Primary varicose veins are common and often show a familial tendency. There is debate as to whether the basic fault is in the valves or in the elasticity of the vein wall. The valves at the sapheno-femoral and/or sapheno-popliteal junctions are incompetent and the distension and varicosity spreads progressively through the system. The deep veins are usually normal. Aggravating factors include obesity, pregnancy, constipation and prolonged standing.

Secondary varicose veins develop after valve function has been damaged by disease (thrombosis) or occasionally trauma. The deep veins are either rendered incompetent or are occluded. The high pressure from posture and from the calf muscle

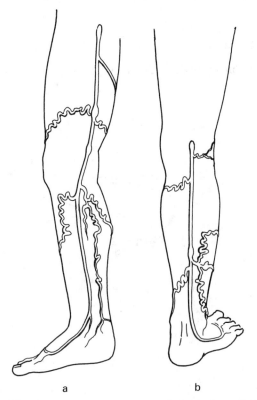

Fig. 21.22 Distribution of varicose veins in the lower limb. (a) Long saphenous system. (b) Short saphenous system

pump is transmitted to the superficial veins predominantly via calf perforators, which also become incompetent. Another cause of secondary varicose veins is arteriovenous fistula (see above).

Sustained high pressure in the superficial veins, known as chronic venous insufficiency, results in changes in the skin and subcutaneous tissues of the 'gaiter' area collectively termed lipodermato-sclerosis. They consist of oedema, inflammation, fibrosis, pigmentation, eczema and ulceration. Chronic venous insufficiency causes a disturbance in the balance between haemodynamic and osmotic pressures (the Starling equation) in the capillaries. The mechanism of the skin changes is not fully understood but it is known that increased capillary permeability permits escape of protein and red cells into the extravascular compartment. Breakdown of the red cells leads to haemosiderin deposition. Fibrin is precipitated outside the vessels and forms a barrier to nutrition. It is unusual for primary varices to lead to these changes, but they are very common in the secondary variety.

Clinical features

The main anxiety for many patients is that their varices are unsightly, but discomfort in a distended vein and general ache, tiredness and swelling in the limb are common complaints, especially after long periods of standing. The skin changes described above begin with pigmentation or eczema. Minor trauma to such an area often fails to heal and progresses to chronic ulceration.

Rupture of a varix is uncommon but can lead to severe haemorrhage. It is easily controlled by elevation of the limb and local application of pressure.

Varicose veins are prone to thrombosis (superficial phlebitis), which is discussed in more detail later in this chapter.

Examination

The aim is to identify the sites of incompetent connections between the deep and superficial systems. The patient is examined standing, preferably on a raised platform in a warm room. The experienced examiner will know the likely sites of incompetence from the anatomical pattern of the varices. *Percussion* over a varix while palpating with the other hand at a higher or lower level will help trace the pattern.

The level at which deep-to-superficial reflux is

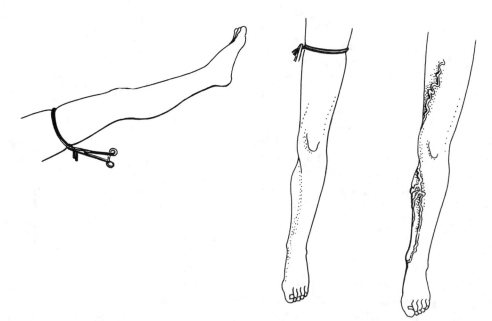

Fig. 21.23 Trendelenberg test demonstrating sapheno-femoral incompetence

occurring can be checked by the *Trendelenberg test* (Fig. 21.23). The leg is elevated and a rubber tourniquet applied just at or below the saphenofemoral junction. The patient is then asked to stand. Veins fill slowly from arterial inflow but quickly from venous reflux. If venous distension below the tourniquet is controlled, the site of reflux must be above it. By moving the tourniquet to different levels in the limb the pattern of incompetence can be mapped out.

A more effective way to demonstrate reflux is to insonate over the site of incompetence and reflux with a portable directional *Doppler ultrasound flowmeter* (Fig. 21.24). This is particularly valuable in obese patients or those with recurrent varicose veins in whom the anatomy may be obscure.

If it is suspected that the varicose veins are secondary to previous deep vein thrombosis (on account of the history or the presence of stigmata of chronic venous insufficiency), *ascending phlebography* of the deep veins may be indicated. This is performed by injecting contrast medium into a foot vein while occluding the superficial system with a tourniquet around the ankle, and then taking serial X-rays as the dye ascends the limb. Before operating on difficult cases of varicose veins, particularly recurrent ones, *varicography* is used, i.e. the direct injection of contrast material into varices to demonstrate deep connections.

Severe varicose veins, especially if in children, of atypical distribution, or associated with cutaneous haemangioma, should raise the suspicion of congenital arteriovenous fistulas (see Fig. 21.17).

Management

Conservative treatment

Elderly patients or those with mild disease can be treated conservatively. Elastic support hoses, weight reduction, regular exercise and avoidance of constricting garments all help to relieve tiredness and reduce swelling.

Sclerotherapy

Injection treatment is used for small varices below the knee which are due to incompetence of local perforators or for recurrent varices after surgery. It is not satisfactory for the majority associated with sapheno-femoral or sapheno-popliteal incompetence since recurrence is inevitable. Sclerotherapy also makes subsequent surgery more difficult.

The injection sites are marked with a pencil while the patient stands. He or she then sits with the leg hanging over the side of the couch and an elastic self-adhesive bandage is applied, starting at the base of the toes, and wound up to the first injection site. The needle is inserted at the lowest mark and the leg elevated to empty the veins; 0.5 ml of 3% sodium tetradecyl sulphate is then injected while the vein is compressed proximally to keep the segment empty (Fig. 21.25). A cotton wool ball is placed over the injection site and the bandage advanced up to the next point where the injection is repeated — and so on. Compression is maintained for 3 weeks. As the bandage is self-adhesive it stays in place undisturbed. The patient is instructed to walk several miles each day in order to redevelop an efficient muscle pump.

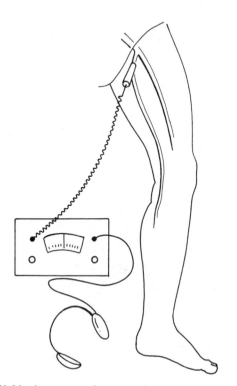

Fig. 21.24 Assessment of venous reflux using a Doppler ultrasonic flowmeter

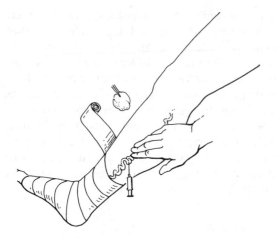

Fig. 21.25 Sclerotherapy for small varices below the knee

Surgery

When there is sapheno-femoral or sapheno-popliteal incompetence, surgery is the only effective treatment. Varicose vein surgery has three aims:

1. to intercept incompetent connections between deep and superficial veins;
2. to remove (strip) the main saphenous channels from which pressure is distributed among the superficial veins; and
3. to eradicate varices.

Sapheno-femoral ligation. General anaesthesia is preferred. The sapheno-femoral junction is displayed and all its tributaries are carefully dissected out, ligated and divided (Fig. 21.26). The saphenous vein is ligated flush with the femoral vein. In patients with sapheno-popliteal incompetence the upper end of the incompetent short saphenous vein is dealt with in similar fashion.

There is less probability of recurrence if the long saphenous vein is stripped out from knee to groin. However, this part of the operation is omitted if there is any prospect that the patient might later need the saphenous vein as an arterial bypass, e.g. if he has arterial symptoms, a strong family history of obliterative disease, is a smoker or if he has angina or a history of myocardial disease.

Varices are eradicated by dissection and ligation or by the avulsion technique, in which the varices are 'winkled out' through many tiny incisions. Bleeding is controlled by tourniquet or local pressure.

CHRONIC LEG ULCER

Ulceration of the leg is a common cause of disability, especially in the elderly. It affects approximately 4% of individuals over 60 years of age. Some two-thirds are directly attributable to chronic venous insufficiency, diabetes or rheumatoid disease.

Added to these causes are many aggravating factors such as old age, obesity, recurrent trauma, immobility, joint problems (including osteoarthritis and arthrodesis) and neurological deficits following stroke or polio.

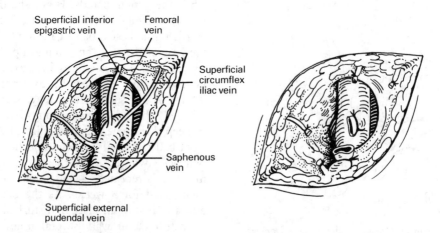

Fig. 21.26 Sapheno-femoral disconnection with ligation of the tributaries of the long saphenous vein

Clinical features

Chronic venous ulcer (Fig. 21.27) is the end-stage of lipodermatosclerosis. It is typically situated in the retromalleolar region on the medial side of the gaiter area, just below the calf perforators. Varicose veins are usually obvious. The ulcer is usually single, large and shallow with a base of unhealthy granulation tissue and is surrounded by the signs of chronic venous insufficiency, i.e. pigmentation, induration and eczema. Contact dermatitis is a very common complication because of the chronicity of the condition and the injudicious treatments, such as local antibiotics, which are often applied.

If an ulcer does not have these characteristics, an alternative aetiology should be considered. For example, if it is deep and painful and/or extends onto the foot, an arterial element is suspected. If ulcers are multiple and situated higher up on the front or lateral side of the calf, arteritis or hypertension are the likely cause. An ulcer on the front

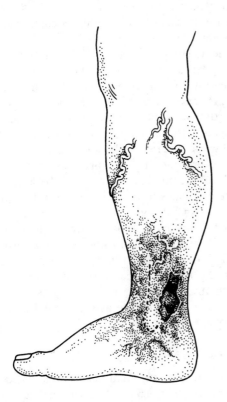

Fig. 21.27 Chronic venous leg ulcer

of the shin or foot may be traumatic. Some ulcers, for psychological reasons, are self-inflicted.

Management

A careful history should be taken, particularly noting thrombotic episodes, previous vein surgery, arterial symptoms, diabetes, locomotor problems and allergies. Examination and investigation should concentrate particularly on predisposing conditions and should include pedal pulses and Doppler pressures, ankle mobility, gait, full blood count, blood glucose determination and rheumatoid serology. If surgery is contemplated, phlebography is advisable to assess the state of the deep veins. The treatment of chronic leg ulcers depends on the aetiology. Arterial insufficiency is treated by reconstruction or sympathectomy, locomotor disabilities by physiotherapy. Mobility is encouraged, diabetes controlled and obesity, if possible, reduced. If self-infliction is suspected, covering the ulcer with a dressing incorporating tin-foil may uncover the cause, e.g. a needle prick.

The great majority of ulcers, however, are venous and are treated as described below.

Conservative treatment. Many venous ulcers can be cured while the patient remains fully active. An absorbent, non-adherent, mild antiseptic dressing is applied. Local antibiotics are contraindicated.

Dressing is of secondary importance to careful bandaging designed to counteract the venous hypertension and swelling. This is achieved by *graduated elastic compression* combined with high elevation of the limb at rest. Graduated elastic compression achieves a pressure gradient maximal in the gaiter area and diminishing as it ascends the leg (Fig. 21.28). This has been shown to have the optimal effect on flow in the deep veins. For a patient of average build a pressure of around 30 mmHg at the ankle is appropriate. While the ulcer is still present, compression is achieved by bandaging and after healing by elastic stocking. The application of effective compression bandages requires skill and experience. It is important to exclude arterial disease before compression is applied.

For the inflamed or intractable ulcer a period of bed rest is required with high elevation of the leg

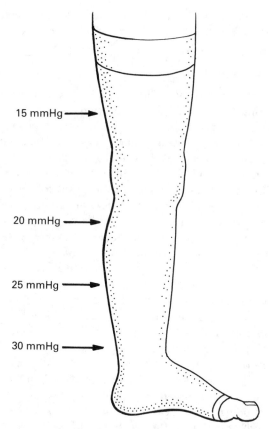

15 mmHg

20 mmHg

25 mmHg

30 mmHg

Fig. 21.28   Graduated elastic compression for venous ulcer

to counteract venous hypertension. Once the ulcer is clean, healing can be hastened with skin grafts. When the ulcer has healed, venous hypertension must be controlled. This can be achieved either by long-term wearing of high-quality elastic stockings or by surgery. Superficial varices are dealt with as described earlier and incompetent perforators in the lower calf are ligated. This is best done by incising the skin and deep fascia vertically and ligating the perforating vessels under the deep fascia.

VENOUS THROMBOSIS AND PULMONARY EMBOLISM

Superficial thrombophlebitis

Inflammation and thrombosis of a previously normal superficial vein may result from trauma, irritation from an intravenous infusion or from the injection of noxious agents. With the exception of septic puncture sites, it is usually non-bacterial. When superficial phlebitis occurs spontaneously, it almost invariably arises in a varicose vein. Redness and tenderness follow the line of the vein. Thrombosis may spread through communicating channels into the deep veins and give rise to pulmonary embolism. It resolves over 2–3 weeks, leaving a track of pigmentation and fibrosed nodular veins.

Treatment consists of analgesics, support stockings and active exercise. Rapid propagation with deep vein involvement may require heparin therapy and occasionally thrombectomy or vein ligation.

A recurrent, migrating type of superficial phlebitis is occasionally seen in association with malignant disease.

Deep vein thrombosis (DVT)

This condition is very common. It is present in some 30% of legs after major operations. It is usually asymptomatic, particularly in the first few days, which is unfortunate because it is the early thrombus which most readily becomes detached and embolizes to the lungs.

The starting point for DVT is usually a valve sinus in the deep veins of the calf (Fig. 21.29). Primary thrombus consists of adherent laminae of platelets and fibrin. When it has accumulated sufficiently to impede flow it is augmented by secondary thrombus which consists of a looser meshwork of red cells and fibrin and which propagates rapidly. It may extend into the popliteal, femoral or iliac veins. In a few cases DVT originates in the veins of the pelvis and fills the ilio-femoral segment.

Pulmonary embolism is a serious complication. Life-threatening embolism rarely occurs from calf DVT but the risk is very real when the ilio-femoral segment is involved. Since DVT commonly produces no symptoms, the first evidence of its presence may be a fatal pulmonary embolism.

Aetiology

Three factors are traditionally associated with thrombogenesis: venous stasis, intimal damage and hypercoagulability of the blood.

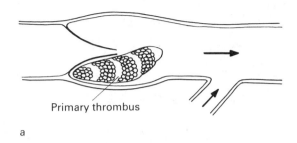

Primary thrombus

a

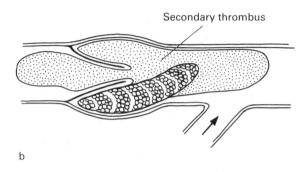

Secondary thrombus

b

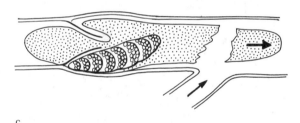

c

Fig. 21.29 Mechanism of embolus formation from thrombus in a deep vein

Venous stasis. Many of the factors we recognize as increasing the risk of thrombosis, such as immobility, obesity, pregnancy, paralysis, operation and trauma, imply an element of venous obstruction or stasis. However, stasis alone does not cause thrombosis; other factors must be present.

Intimal damage. In most instances of DVT no evidence of intimal damage can be detected, but external trauma to a vein, for example during a hip replacement operation, can provide a starting point for thrombogenesis.

Hypercoagulability. Primary hypercoagulable states are those in which an identifiable abnormality of haemostasis is present. These include deficiencies of antithrombin III, protein C, protein S and plasminogen activators. One of these should

be suspected if there are recurrent thrombotic episodes, especially if they occur in a young person or there is a strong family history. Polycythaemia rubra is also associated with a tendency to thrombosis.

Secondary hypercoagulable states are conditions known to be associated with thrombosis but the cause is not identified. These include pregnancy and the puerperium, malignancy, Behcet's disease, homocystinuria and paroxysmal nocturnal haemoglobinuria.

It is important to identify patients who are at potential risk of developing venous thromboembolism during or after operation. The most important risk factors are:

> a history of previous DVT or embolism
> advanced age
> malignant disease
> varicose veins
> obesity
> oestrogen-containing contraceptives
> polycythaemia

Curiously enough, for reasons which are not clear, smokers have a lower risk of postoperative DVT than non-smokers.

Diagnosis

Early DVT sometimes gives rise to a warm patch and dilated superficial veins over the affected area. The principal symptoms are pain and swelling. These, if present at all, are late symptoms which do not develop until the thrombus has begun to organize or has extended to obstruct venous outflow or collaterals. Swelling at the ankle or lower calf indicates that the thrombus is at least at popliteal level; swelling up to the level of the knee means femoral vein thrombosis; thigh swelling indicates iliac vein thrombosis.

Arterial spasm may accompany extensive DVT and cause a swollen white leg (phlegmasia caerulea dolens). If the limb is both swollen and cyanosed, not only are the main stem veins occluded but also the collateral channels. This may go on to venous gangrene and usually indicates a sinister underlying cause such as advanced malignant disease.

The differential diagnosis of DVT includes lymphoedema, dependent oedema, mechanical or

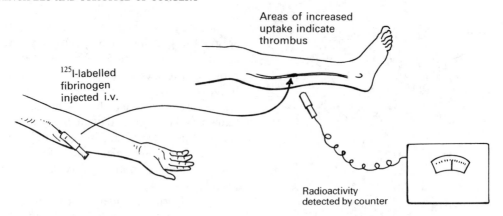

Fig. 21.30   Principles of radiofibrinogen uptake test

tumour obstruction, cellulitis, a ruptured Baker's cyst, haematoma, muscle strain and arterial occlusion.

Because of the inaccuracy of the clinical diagnosis of DVT, anticoagulant treatment (which is potentially dangerous) should not be started until the diagnosis has been properly confirmed.

The *radiofibrinogen uptake test* (Fig. 21.30) is an excellent perioperative screening test. The thyroid is first blocked with 100 mg potassium iodide. An intravenous injection of ^{125}I-labelled fibrinogen is then given and the legs are serially scanned on successive days for 'hot spots' with a portable radiation counter. A hot spot which persists on successive readings indicates that fibrinogen has accumulated in a thrombus.

When DVT is suspected clinically, a variety of non-invasive confirmatory tests may be used, including directional Doppler ultrasound, thermography, impedance or strain gauge plethysmography and Duplex B-mode scanning. Each of these improves the accuracy of diagnosis, each has its limitations and none provides as much information as phlebography, which is the 'gold standard'.

Phlebography for DVT is performed by the ascending method unless swelling of the thigh indicates occlusive ilio-femoral thrombus. Ascending phlebography (Fig. 21.31) involves injection of approximately 40 ml of non-ionic (non-irritant) contrast material into a vein on the dorsum of each foot, flow being directed into the deep veins by superficial tourniquets applied above the ankle. For suspected DVT, phlebography should always

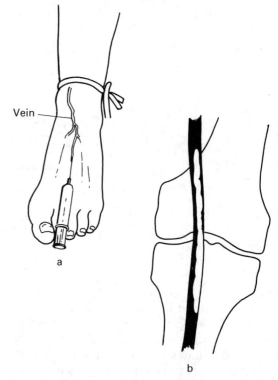

Fig. 21.31   Ascending phlebography showing (a) tourniquet around ankle to direct radio-opaque material into deep veins and (b) thrombus in popliteal vein with partial adhesion to vessel wall

be bilateral. The aim is to delineate fully any thrombus, especially its upper end since this is the dangerous portion. Should ascending phlebography fail to achieve this, perfemoral phlebography with direct injection of contrast into the femoral veins may be necessary. The appearances of the thrombus will indicate how recent it is, how extensive and how liable to embolize. These are the parameters which influence treatment.

An integral part of the investigation of DVT is to find out whether the thrombus is actively embolizing. A lung scan should be obtained at an early stage. This also provides a baseline for comparison with repeat scans should subsequent embolism be suspected.

Prevention

Pulmonary embolism is still a common cause of postoperative death. Because of our inability to diagnose DVT in its early and dangerous phase, prophylaxis is very important. Many aspects of modern surgical care help to reduce the likelihood of postoperative venous thromboembolism. These include regional anaesthesia, accurate fluid replacement, effective pain control and early ambulation. Sometimes these measures are not enough, especially in high-risk patients or high-risk operations. As mentioned earlier, previous DVT or embolism, advancing age, malignancy, varicose veins, obesity, oestrogen-containing contraceptives and polycythaemia all increase the risk. High-risk operations include hip reconstructions, spinal operations, major abdominal or pelvic procedures and others associated with severe illness, malignancy, sepsis or trauma.

Physical methods. Flow in the deep veins can be accelerated and thrombus prevented by the application of graduated compression (antiembolism) stockings. These exert a pressure of about 20 mmHg at the ankle. To avoid pressure damage it is vital to check that the patient has readily palpable pedal pulses before applying elastic stockings. If in doubt, the arterial pressure should be measured with a Doppler ultrasonic flowmeter (see earlier).

Intermittent pneumatic compression can be applied to the legs by of means of plastic sleeves connected to a pump during and after operation and is of proven benefit. So is intermittent electrical stimulation of the calf muscles.

Active exercises and early mobilization should be encouraged.

Pharmacological methods. Low-dose subcutaneous calcium or sodium heparin, 5000 units 8- or 12-hourly, has been shown in many controlled trials to protect against DVT and pulmonary embolism. The first dose is given with the premedication and treatment is continued until the patient is fully ambulant. There is a slightly increased risk of bleeding and wound haematoma, and for this reason low molecular weight heparin fractions are undergoing trials as alternatives. Heparin is not effective in major orthopaedic surgery and some surgeons combine it with dihydroergotamine, which increases venous tone and enhances the effect of heparin.

Dextran-70 is a starch solution which reduces blood viscosity and coagulability; the protection given is equivalent to that of heparin. It is administered by intravenous infusion of 500 ml perioperatively and then daily for 2–3 days. Dextran-70 tends to encourage capillary oozing at operation. Anaphylaxis is a rare but occasionally severe complication.

Oral anticoagulants are effective prophylactic agents but they require laboratory control, react unfavourably with many drugs and their effects are not easily reversed should bleeding occur. Antiplatelet agents do not provide effective prophylaxis against venous thrombosis.

For patients at particular risk of thromboembolism, physical and pharmacological methods can be combined. The surgeon has to balance the potential benefit against the inconvenience, side effects and costs of the methods available.

Treatment of acute DVT

The plan of treatment assumes that the DVT has been reliably diagnosed by an objective method, preferably phlebography. The aims of treatment are: (1) to relieve acute symptoms; (2) to protect against pulmonary embolism; and (3) to facilitate resolution and thereby reduce the likelihood of long-term post-thrombotic damage to the limb.

If thrombus is confined to the calf and the patient is fully mobile, an elastic stocking and physical exercise may be all that is required. This is a rare situation.

Usually the patient has some underlying cause for the DVT which prevents full activity and there is a risk of thrombus extension. Specific treatment is therefore essential. The foot of the bed is elevated. If there is marked swelling, additional elevation is provided with extra pillows or a foam wedge. Active movement of toes and ankle is encouraged. Elastic compression is not necessary during this phase. Once the patient starts to be mobile, graduated compression stockings are fitted. Mobilization is started as soon as swelling has resolved.

Heparin therapy is started with an intravenous injection of 5000 units and followed by continuous infusion of 1500–3000 units/hour by syringe pump. Calcium heparin can also be given by deep subcutaneous injection in full therapeutic doses of 2500 units per 10 kg bodyweight 12-hourly, which makes it easier for the patient to become mobile. Subsequent doses of heparin are adjusted to keep the activated partial thromboplastin time or thrombin clotting time at two to three times the normal value. Heparin is continued for 1–2 weeks (depending on the severity of the episode) and overlapped with oral anticoagulants by 3 days. Oral anticoagulants are continued for at least 3 months and patients with a history of recurrent episodes may have to continue treatment indefinitely.

Thrombolytic therapy with streptokinase and urokinase has proved disappointing in DVT of the lower limbs largely because of the difficulty of making the diagnosis early enough for the thrombus to be readily lysable. New thrombolytic agents such as tissue plasminogen activator and pro-urokinase are being evaluated.

In some centres venous thrombectomy is practised for ilio-femoral thrombosis but re-occlusion may occur and post-thrombotic syndrome is not necessarily prevented.

Pulmonary embolism

Pulmonary embolism is found in approximately 50% of all autopsies. It is the commonest acute lung disorder in hospital patients and an important cause of postoperative death.

Like DVT the majority of pulmonary emboli are silent and many of those which give rise to symptoms are not diagnosed. Their features are protean and non-specific.

Approximately 90% of pulmonary emboli arise from the veins of the lower limbs or pelvis. A few come from the right heart. The recent increase in the use of central venous lines for monitoring and parenteral nutrition has caused an increase in emboli from the subclavian veins.

Major embolism

Massive embolism with occlusion of two-thirds or more of the pulmonary arterial flow causes acute central chest pain, followed by severe dyspnoea, cyanosis, hypotension and collapse.

Early resuscitation is essential and includes cardiac massage, administration of oxygen (at a rate of 6 litre/min) and immediate injection of heparin 15 000 units intravenously to prevent extension of thrombus. Intravenous fluid is given to support right ventricular filling and a pressor agent (i.e. 1 in 1000 noradrenaline made up as 2 mg in 500 ml of isotonic saline) given via a paediatric burette at a rate titrated to maintain blood pressure at a minimum of 80 mmHg systolic.

An urgent pulmonary angiogram is obtained and, if the diagnosis is confirmed and the patient's condition is still serious, thrombolytic therapy is commenced with a loading dose of 250 000 units of streptokinase intravenously, followed by 100 000 units per hour by infusion pump for 24 hours. Hydrocortisone 100 mg intravenously is given before the streptokinase. New thrombolytic agents (tissue plasminogen activator; plasminogen-streptokinase complex; pro-urokinase) may prove to be equally effective but with fewer bleeding complications.

The patient's vital signs are carefully monitored. Thrombolytic therapy is followed by heparin and later by oral anticoagulants.

Rarely pulmonary embolectomy may have to be considered, but few pulmonary emboli occur in circumstances which permit immediate cardiopulmonary bypass. A new technique under trial allows extraction of the embolus from the pulmonary artery under radiological control by means of a catheter introduced through the femoral vein.

Minor embolism

This includes any embolism which does not immediately threaten life. Most emboli are multiple and many do not cause infarction. The symptoms may therefore be insidious and a high level of suspicion is essential.

Dyspnoea may be sudden or gradual. Infarction results in pleuritic chest pain, tachycardia and pyrexia. Haemoptysis is relatively uncommon. Auscultation reveals diminished air entry, moist rales and a friction rub. Some pulmonary emboli cause bronchospasm and are mistaken for asthmatic attacks. Others, by reducing cerebral oxygenation, may present as confusion, impaired consciousness or syncopal attacks. Recurrent pulmonary emboli may over a period of months or years lead to the development of pulmonary hypertension.

Blood gas analysis shows a low Po_2. ECG may show signs of right heart strain with right axis deviation, a prolonged PR interval, depressed ST segments in leads I and II and an inverted T wave in leads II and III. The chest X-ray may be unremarkable or may show diminished lung markings, a prominent pulmonary artery and enlarged cardiac shadow. Linear atelectasis may be noted. Later there may be pleural effusion, elevation of the diaphragm and wedge-shaped areas of consolidation.

Lung scanning and phlebography are the principal investigations. A perfusion scan is performed with a gamma-camera after intravenous injection of macroaggregates of albumin which have been labelled with technetium-99m. To distinguish perfusion defects from those caused by emphysematous bullae a ventilation scan may be added. This will reveal areas of increased uptake following the inhalation of xenon-133. If there is doubt about the diagnosis or if thrombolytic therapy is being considered, a pulmonary angiogram is obtained.

At least one-third of the patients who die of pulmonary embolism have had previous episodes of 'herald' embolism. In patients suspected of minor pulmonary embolism, attention must be focused on the lower limbs and residual life-threatening DVT excluded by bilateral phlebography.

Management

It is important, as the term 'thromboembolism' implies, to consider pulmonary embolism and DVT as one disease. The main objective of management is to prevent further embolism. Systemic heparin therapy is started at once, followed by an oral anticoagulant. Antibiotics and analgesics are indicated for pulmonary infarction. If phlebography reveals loose thrombus in femoral or iliac veins, embolism can be prevented by insertion of a filter into the inferior vena cava (Fig. 21.32). The filter is introduced percutaneously under radiological control through a femoral or a jugular vein. A further indication for insertion of a caval filter is the recurrence of embolism despite anticoagulation. Surgical removal of the thrombus is associated with a high thrombosis rate and is seldom indicated. Oral anticoagulants are continued for at least 6 months.

Other forms of venous thrombosis

Inferior vena caval thrombosis

Thrombosis of the inferior vena cava may result from extension of an iliofemoral thrombosis, but more often complicates abdominal malignant disease. The typical signs are bilateral leg and scrotal oedema, distended collateral veins on the abdominal wall and possibly ascites. Management is

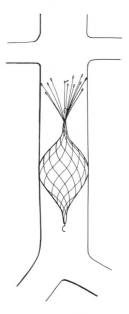

Fig. 21.32 Filter placed in inferior vena cava to prevent pulmonary embolism

symptomatic with diuretics and elastic compression stockings for the legs. Anticoagulation is indicated only in non-malignant cases.

Superior vena caval thrombosis

Mediastinal tumours or enlarged lymph nodes (e.g. from breast or bronchial carcinoma) may obstruct the superior vena cava and induce thrombosis. Central venous catheters for parenteral nutrition or pressure monitoring may cause thrombosis of the vena cava, or the subclavian or axillary veins. The patient experiences an unpleasant bursting feeling in the head, neck and upper limbs. There is oedema, cyanosis and venous distension.

The obstruction is defined by upper limb phlebography. If the cause is not malignant gratifying relief may be obtained from thrombolytic therapy followed by heparin and oral anticoagulants. Radiotherapy or chemotherapy may relieve malignant obstruction, but the outlook is poor.

Subclavian and axillary vein thrombosis

Catheter-induced thrombosis has been discussed above. Malignant disease or irradiation of axillary lymph nodes are other causes of axillary thrombosis. Spontaneous axillary thrombosis occasionally occurs in healthy young adults. Sometimes it follows exercise and is then termed 'effort thrombosis'. There may be a previous history of intermittent venous obstruction in the limb due to a mechanical cause at the thoracic outlet. A cervical rib, abnormal muscle or ligamentous bands at the inner border of the first rib, or a narrow interval between the clavicle and the first rib may constrict the vein and eventually lead to thrombosis.

The patient complains of an uncomfortable, heavy, cyanosed arm with venous engorgement. Venous collaterals develop over the shoulder and anterior chest wall.

Upper limb phlebography defines the occlusion. The arm should be elevated, e.g. in a towel suspended from a drip stand. Heparin therapy followed by oral anticoagulants is standard treatment. Thrombolytic therapy can be very effective in early cases. Many surgeons believe that after the axillary thrombosis has been cleared the thoracic outlet should be explored and the first rib or other obstructing element removed.

22. The lymphatic system

Function of lymphatics

The lymphatic system drains fluid from the interstitial spaces into the venous system. The lymphatic capillaries differ from those of the blood stream by having little, if any, basement membrane and no tight junctions between endothelial cells, an arrangement which allows macromolecules such as protein to pass through the lymphatic wall. The protein content of lymph varies from 5 g/l in the periphery to 40–60 g/l in the thoracic duct and liver.

Flow in the lymphatics is directed centrally by endothelial valves and is increased by muscle contraction. The lymphatics do not remove large amounts of fluid from the tissues. The total daily flow into the venous system is only 2–4 litres.

The lymphatics of the limbs form a plexus within the dermis and within the muscle-fascial compartments. Solitary lymph nodes occur along the course of the major lymphatic trunks which then pass through regional nodes at the root of the limb. Lymph nodes consist of a supporting framework of reticuloendothelial tissue and contain aggregates of lymphoid tissue. They have filtering, phagocytic and immunological functions (Fig. 22.1).

Lymphangiography

The subcutaneous lymphatics on the dorsum of the hand or foot are first visualized by injecting 0.5 ml of 2.5% Patent Blue dye into a web space. After 5–10 minutes of exercise, the lymphatics show clearly through the skin as blue lines. A transverse skin incision is then made over one of the lymphatics, which is dissected out and cannu-

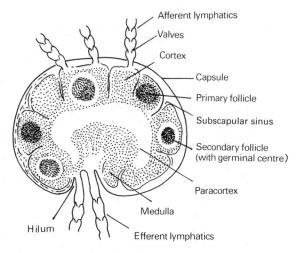

Fig. 22.1 Lymph node

lated (Fig. 22.2). Following injection of a small amount of water-soluble contrast medium, the position of the cannula is checked by image intensification and, if correct, 10 ml oily lipiodol is infused slowly from a pump. The dye can be followed by image intensification and permanent records obtained by radiography. The contrast medium remains in normal nodes for 6 months, and in pathological nodes for 2 years. Serial radiographs can therefore be used to monitor the progress of node metastases.

The examination takes 2 hours to perform. The patient should be warned that he will pass blue urine for up to 48 hours. Complications are infrequent but include skin sepsis, thrombophlebitis, oily embolus to the lung, and hypersensitivity to the oily medium.

Lymphangiography is used to display the lymphatic vessels in lymphoedema and the nodes in

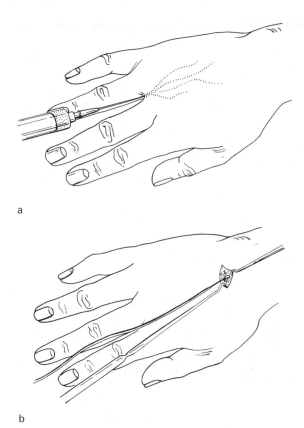

a

b

Fig. 22.2 Technique of lymphangiography. (a) Injection of Patent Blue dye into web space between fingers to demonstrate subcutaneous lymphatic vessels. (b) Dissection and cannulation of lymphatic vessel

patients with melanoma, seminoma, lymphoma and renal carcinoma. It is used occasionally to investigate obscure abdominal masses and to confirm operative clearance of lymph nodes in cancer surgery.

Normal lymph nodes are oval or reniform, and the oily medium is distributed diffusely in a granular fashion. Central translucencies are frequently due to nodules of fat. When invaded by tumour, a node becomes enlarged and has central and round or peripheral and crescent-shaped discrete filling defects. Lymphoma and seminoma may cause a foamy 'soap-bubble' appearance due to diffuse infiltration. Alternatively, a node which is invaded by tumour may fail to opacify and so give rise to a false negative interpretation.

ABNORMALITIES OF THE LYMPHATIC VESSELS

Lymphangitis

Acute lymphangitis

Inflammation of the dermal lymphatics (superficial lymphangitis) is most commonly due to streptococcal infection. The primary site of infection is often a minor wound or puncture with associated cellulitis. The inflamed lymph trunks cause linear red streaks in the skin and may be palpable and tender. There is usually associated tender enlargement of regional lymph nodes (lymphadenitis).

The affected part should be rested and elevated if there is marked swelling. Antibiotic therapy is indicated and large doses of penicillin are prescribed in the first instance. Surgery is required only if there is suppuration or a retained foreign body at the primary site of infection.

Chronic lymphangitis

This condition is uncommon. Mondor's disease is a form of chronic lymphangitis which gives rise to tense tender 'strings' in the skin or subcutaneous tissues, particularly over the female breast or in the cubital fossa.

Lymphoedema

Blockage of lymphatic flow upsets the normal balance of forces controlling the passage of fluid across capillary membranes of the blood stream. Accumulation of protein molecules in the tissue spaces increases the osmotic pressure and hence the volume of interstitial fluid (Fig. 22.3). This increase in protein-rich fluid (protein content 10–50 g/l) is known as lymphoedema. Fluid rich in protein can also accumulate without lymphatic blockage, as for example after burns, when increased capillary permeability allows more protein to accumulate in the tissue spaces than can be removed by the lymphatics.

Lymphoedema should also be differentiated from 'low-protein' or 'filtration' oedema, in which the protein content of the fluid is only 1–9 g/l. Examples are the oedema of hypoproteinaemia and

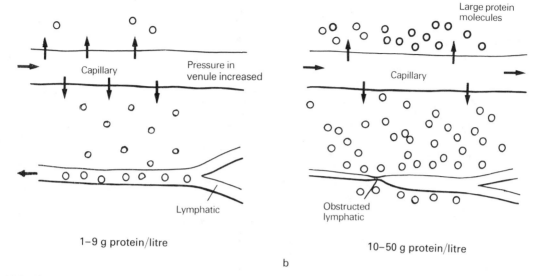

Fig. 22.3 Types of oedema. (a) Low-protein oedema due to abnormally high net fluid filtration. (b) High-protein oedema due to failure of lymphatics to remove interstitial proteins

that which accompanies the raised venous pressure of congestive cardiac failure or venous obstruction.

Lymphoedema is usually subdivided into primary and secondary forms.

Primary lymphoedema

This is a familial condition caused by developmental abnormalities of the lymphatics. The vessels are hypoplastic and reduced in number, but may show varicose dilatation or even fail to appear. Lymphoedema may be present at birth (congenital lymphoedema or Milroy's disease) but more commonly develops during adolescence and early adult life (lymphoedema praecox). A few cases develop after the age of 35 years (lymphoedema tarda).

Lymphoedema praecox affects predominantly females and may be unilateral or bilateral. It affects upper or lower limbs and begins insidiously as a painless swelling which progresses slowly up the limb. It is often more noticeable after exercise or exposure to warmth, and in the premenstrual period. The swelling is initially soft and pitting, but the high protein content of the retained fluid gradually leads to fibrosis. The limb then becomes permanently enlarged and 'woody'. As with all forms of lymphoedema, there is a constant threat

of cellulitis and lymphangitis, and a long-term risk of lymphangiosarcoma of the skin.

Lymphoedema is easily distinguished from the soft pitting oedema of congestive heart failure and systemic diseases causing hypoproteinaemia. These are bilateral conditions and, as the oedema fluid has a low protein content, fibrosis is rare.

Chronic venous insufficiency gives rise to soft pitting oedema at first. Later this may become firm, rubbery and non-pitting; secondary pigmentation, dermatitis and ulceration may then develop.

Diagnosis. Lymphangiography is the key to diagnosis (Fig. 22.4). In primary lymphoedema this may reveal (1) complete absence of lymphatics (15%); (2) widespread hypoplasia of lymphatics with small and infrequent channels below the knee or in the whole leg (55%); or (3) varicose, dilated and tortuous lymph trunks (30%).

Treatment. In the early stages, primary lymphoedema responds to treatment by elevation of the leg at night or to intermittent compression by an inflated cuff to drive fluid out from the swollen limb. A tailored elastic stocking should be worn during the day. Diuretics given in regular cycles are recommended by some.

It is important to guard against infection by

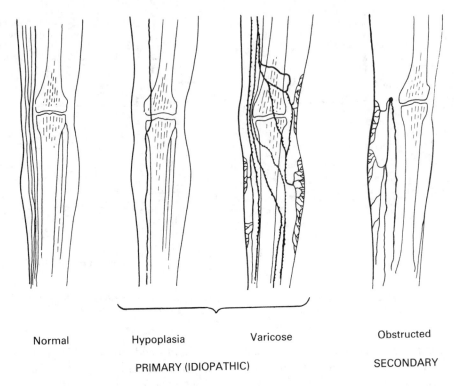

Normal	Hypoplasia	Varicose	Obstructed
	PRIMARY (IDIOPATHIC)		SECONDARY

Fig. 22.4 Lymphangiographic appearance of primary and secondary lymphoedema

adequate hygiene, to prevent trauma, and to treat minor infections such as athlete's foot promptly. In some patients who have repeated bouts of streptococcal infection, long-term prophylactic penicillin may be required.

Because of the absence of pain many patients delay seeking medical aid until faced with the cosmetic problem of a permanently enlarged limb. At this stage the lymphoedema no longer pits and is usually subject to repeated infection. Elevation and mechanical compression are no longer of value. As the failure of lymphatic development is widespread, there is little point in attempting to construct a 'lymphatic bridge' between limb and trunk. Relief demands complete excision of skin, subcutaneous tissue and deep fascia from the affected limb. Split-skin grafts of skin removed from the excised tissue are then placed directly on the exposed muscle (Fig. 22.5). The limb has a grotesque appearance after this procedure, which is used only when the swollen limb prevents ambulation or is subject to recurrent infection, or when proliferative nodular changes occur in the skin.

Secondary lymphoedema

Secondary lymphoedema develops if the lymph trunks and nodes become obstructed by tumour, recurrent infection, or infestation with filariasis, or if they are obliterated by surgery or radiotherapy. Swelling develops more rapidly than in primary lymphoedema, and is accompanied by dragging discomfort, erythema and a high risk of recurrent lymphangitis. Lymphangiography demonstrates dilated lymphatics up to the point of the obstruction (see Fig. 22.4). A characteristic feature is dermal back-flow, a fine reticular pattern extending from the subcutaneous tissue to the dermis.

Conservative measures such as elevation and compression are of value in the majority of patients. Surgery is seldom indicated and then only if a distinct local lesion has been demonstrated by lymphangiography.

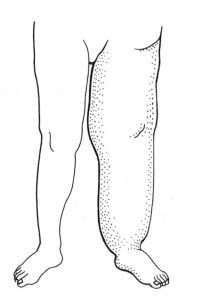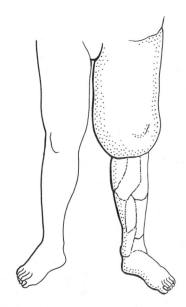

Fig. 22.5   Treatment of lymphoedema by excision of subcutaneous tissue

A number of procedures are available to bypass the lymphatic obstruction. These include burying longitudinal strips of dermis within the muscles to promote access to the deep lymphatics, pedicled omental transplants, and direct anastomosis between dilated lymphatics or transected lymph nodes and the venous system. None of these methods are wholly reliable, although the development of microsurgical techniques for vascular anastomoses has been a definite advance. Lymphaticovenous anastomoses at several sites in the limb, performed as soon as secondary lymphoedema is diagnosed, are reported to give good results. In all other cases, continued elastic support for the limb is an essential part of treatment.

As the upper limb is frequently affected, the patient must be warned to avoid even minor injuries to the hands. For gardening or any similar occupation gloves must be worn.

ABNORMALITIES OF LYMPH NODES
(Table 22.1)

The superficial lymph nodes lie subcutaneously and are readily palpable. The skin moves freely over the nodes, which are normally oval or kidney-shaped and have a smooth outline. Enlarged nodes retain their shape when involved by infec-

Table 22.1   Causes of lymph node enlargement

Infection	Acute lymphadenitis
	Chronic lymphadenitis
	Tuberculosis
	Granulomatous lymphadenitis
	HIV infection
Neoplasia	Primary (lymphoreticular neoplasia)
	Hodgkin's lymphoma
	Non-Hodgkin's lymphoma
	Secondary (metastatic cancer)

tion or lymphoreticular neoplasia, but become large, lobulated or nodular and matted when involved by metastatic cancer.

Deep-seated nodes cannot be palpated readily. Enlargement can be detected by soft tissue X-rays (mediastinal nodes), lymphangiography (retroperitoneal nodes) and CT scans. With the exception of lymphangiography, these methods indicate only whether a node is normal in size and shape. None of them defines the cause of pathological enlargement.

Acute lymphadenitis

Pyogenic infection of lymph nodes is most often due to streptococcal or staphylococcal infection. A typical example is the cervical lymph node enlargement (lymphadenopathy) which accompanies acute tonsillitis. The primary infection may be so trivial as to go unnoticed. For example, it may consist only of a tiny puncture wound of the hand or foot sustained while gardening or walking without shoes. The intervening lymphadenitis may also escape detection.

The affected node or nodes are enlarged, painful and tender, restricting movement of the limb. Fever and leucocytosis are common. Untreated infections may resolve spontaneously, progress to suppuration and abscess formation, or become chronic.

Spontaneous resolution is common. Although the nodes diminish in size, they may never completely return to normal and may remain palpably enlarged for the remainder of the patient's life. There are few normal individuals who do not have palpable nodes in some site or other. The superficial inguinal nodes of the groin are almost invariably enlarged and palpable.

Suppuration often leads to neighbouring nodes forming an adherent mass and breaking down to form a large abscess cavity. The abscess may rupture through the overlying fascia and spread into the subcutaneous tissues to form the superficial loculus of a collar-stud abscess (Fig. 22.6). The overlying skin becomes red, hot and shiny, and fluctuation can be elicited. Unless the skin is incised, it will rupture with discharge of the contained pus.

Chronic infection is heralded by the nodes becoming smaller and less tender, but they still remain larger and firmer than normal. Systemic signs gradually abate, although it is common for chronic lymphadenitis to run a 'grumbling' course with intermittent episodes of tenderness, node enlargement, and leucocytosis.

Treatment

If lymphadenitis is suspected, a careful search should be made for a primary site of infection within the catchment area of the affected nodes. The largest and most involved node is usually the first to have been infected. In many cases, the primary site cannot be found or is so trivial that it need not be treated.

In the acute phase, antibiotics are prescribed. Penicillin is usually appropriate, as most infections

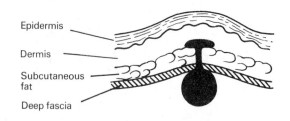

Fig. 22.6   Collar-stud abscess

occur outwith hospital. If systemic upset is not marked, oral phenoxymethyl penicillin (penicillin V) is given; otherwise parenteral benzylpenicillin (penicillin G) is preferred.

If improvement has not occurred within 48 hours, a broad spectrum antibiotic should be given. In children with acute cervical lymphadenitis this should not be ampicillin. Abnormal reactions to this antibiotic occur regularly in infective mononucleosis, a condition which frequently presents with acute lymphadenitis.

Dry heat is sometimes of value in relieving pain over the inflamed nodes. Fluctuation or other local signs of abscess formation indicate the need for incision and drainage of pus. This is best performed under general anaesthesia so that the opening in the fascia can be dilated, the deep loculus evacuated and necrotic material curetted from the node. The incision should be placed to allow dependent drainage and a small corrugated drain is inserted to maintain it.

A sample of pus should be sent for culture and determination of sensitivity to antibiotics. A biopsy from the wall of the abscess cavity is obtained if there is any doubt as to the nature of the condition.

Chronic lymphadenitis

Tuberculous lymphadenitis

At one time this was an extremely common cause of neck swellings in children. The deep cervical nodes were painlessly enlarged, and the distribution of node involvement pointed to the likely primary focus of infection. Infection entering through the teeth, tonsils or adenoids involved the upper cervical (jugulodigastric) nodes, whereas involvement of the lower cervical (supraclavicular) nodes indicated infection coming from the apex of the lung. Generalized lymphadenopathy suggested miliary tuberculosis.

Tuberculous lymphadenitis is now rare in children but is occasionally seen in adults. The nodes enlarge painlessly, become matted together and fixed to adjacent structures. Caseation leads to the formation of a 'cold' abscess which lacks the local and systemic signs of acute inflammation. When a cold abscess ruptures through the deep fascia, the skin becomes red and thin, takes on a blue tinge and then gives way to establish an indolent tuberculous sinus.

Not all nodes involved by tuberculosis undergo caseation. In some cases the capsule remains unbroken and the nodes remain discrete. With healing, tuberculous lymph nodes become calcified and thus visible radiologically.

Confirmation of tuberculous infection depends on culture of the organism from aspirated material (if the nodes have softened) or from an excised node.

Antituberculous therapy leads to resolution in the majority of cases. If the nodes remain grossly enlarged after a few weeks of treatment, or if a cold abscess has formed, surgery is indicated. The enlarged nodes may be excised, but more commonly caseous material is evacuated. A tuberculous abscess is never left with a drain, or secondary infection is inevitable. Primary skin closure is the rule for all surgery performed for tuberculous lesions.

Viral infections

Acute and chronic lymphadenitis result frequently from infections such as infectious mononucleosis and HIV infection. Occasionally lymph node biopsy may be required if the diagnosis is in doubt.

Granulomatous lymphadenitis

This includes a number of forms of chronic non-tuberculous lymphadenitis. Occipital and posterior cervical lymphadenopathy are common in the early stages of rubella; enlargement of the epitrochlear, suboccipital and posterior cervical nodes is a feature of secondary syphilis; and lymphadenitis

simulating caseating tuberculosis occurs in cat-scratch fever.

THE LYMPHOMAS

The lymphomas are a group of neoplastic disorders which originate in the primitive reticular cells of the reticuloendothelial system or their histiocytic or lymphocytic derivatives. The commonest and most important is Hodgkin's disease which is characterized by progressive painless enlargement of lymphoid tissue throughout the body.

Hodgkin's lymphoma

This disease is most frequently encountered by the surgeon when patients are referred for diagnosis or for surgical staging of the extent of the disease.

Most patients present with enlarged nodes in the anterior or posterior triangle of the neck or in the axilla. The nodes are painless, rubbery and discrete. Rarely the patient presents as an abdominal emergency due to deposits of Hodgkin's tissue causing adhesions or intestinal obstruction. The diagnosis of Hodgkin's disease is confirmed by excision biopsy of an involved node. A full haematological examination and chest X-ray are essential preoperative investigations. Lymph node dissections in the neck and axilla are more difficult than might be imagined, and good exposure and unhurried dissection are essential. For this reason, general anaesthesia is usually preferred.

Staging

The staging of Hodgkin's disease has undergone considerable revision over the past few years. The classification now used most commonly is shown in Table 22.2. The surgeon is occasionally asked to undertake staging laparotomy to supplement clinical and radiological determination of the extent of the disease.

Staging laparotomy involves splenectomy, wedge biopsy of the right and left lobes of the liver, biopsy of the para-aortic nodes at the level of the coeliac axis and duodenojejunal flexure, and removal of those nodes which appear abnormal on lymphangiography. Radio-opaque clips are placed at the site of node biopsy and on the vascular

Table 22.2 Staging of Hodgkin's disease

Stage*	Definition
I	Single involved lymph node group (or one extranodal primary site)
II	Two or more involved lymph node groups limited to one side of the diaphragm
III	Involvement on both sides of the diaphragm with or without splenic involvement
IV	Extralymphatic spread (including liver involvement)

* All stages are further subdivided into either A (no systemic symptoms) or B (to denote the presence of systemic symptoms, defined as weight loss of more than 10% in 6 months; fever; and night sweats).

pedicle of the spleen so that these regions can subsequently be localized on X-ray. In females, the ovaries and ovarian tubes may be sutured together in the midline behind the uterus to protect them from abdominal radiotherapy. A bone biopsy is performed.

All of the removed material is examined by the pathologist for the presence of Hodgkin's lymphoma tissue. As with all lymph node biopsies, the pathologist should be forewarned in case he wishes to have fresh samples of tissue for electron microscopy or for immunohistochemical evaluation.

Improved methods of diagnostic imaging, notably CT scanning, have altered the indications for staging laparotomy, which is now less commonly performed.

Treatment

The treatment of Hodgkin's disease depends on its stage, and now consists of radiotherapy and/or chemotherapy, usually with multiple cytotoxic agents given cyclically. Surgery has no place in therapy except to remove the spleen in order to reduce the field of radiation required in patients with abdominal involvement. As a result, radiation damage to the left lung and kidney is avoided.

Non-Hodgkin's lymphomas

These are lymphomas other than Hodgkin's disease which were classified previously as lymphosarcoma, reticulosarcoma and follicular lymphoma. All are now grouped together as non-Hodgkin's lymphomas but are classified according to cell type. Predominantly lymphocytic, predominantly reticulocytic, and mixed types are recognized.

All forms of lymphoma (including Hodgkin's disease) can also be classified according to whether the changes are diffuse or nodular; the diffuse forms have a more benign course. Extranodal disease is more common in non-Hodgkin's than in Hodgkin's lymphoma. The intestine and bone are most commonly involved in young children, the skin and adenoids in young adults.

Certain types of lymphoma are now known to be more common in patients with immune deficiency, lupus erythematosus and Sjögren's disease. Reticulocytic lymphoma of the brain is a long-term hazard in patients undergoing immunosuppressive therapy after organ transplantation. The surgeon is seldom required to establish the diagnosis of non-Hodgkin's lymphoma. Barium studies, lymphangiography and bone marrow examination usually suffice, although lymph node biopsy is sometimes required for confirmation.

Involvement of the stomach and intestine by tumour deposits can give rise to abdominal pain, a mass, fever, anorexia, malabsorption and weight loss. Some patients develop multiple 'punched-out' perforations of the gut at the site of tumour deposits, and then present as an acute abdominal emergency. At laparotomy the perforations are excised with a rim of surrounding bowel wall to allow histopathological diagnosis. Excision of a length of bowel may be required.

Tissue must always be removed for histological examination when an inoperable tumour of the stomach or intestine is found at laparotomy. Lymphoma can stimulate adenocarcinoma at operation but is very much more amenable to treatment by radiotherapy and chemotherapy.

The majority of lymphomas of the non-Hodgkin's type are treated by a combination of chemotherapy and radiotherapy. The MOPP regimen of nitrogen mustard (mustine), vincristine (Oncovin), procarbazine and prednisone is one of several frequently used. The prognosis of this condition is poorer than that of Hodgkin's disease.

Burkitt's lymphoma

This is a poorly differentiated lymphocytic lymphoma first described in East African children.

The disease occurs in the tropics and has a similar distribution to malaria. It is spread by an insect vector and thought to be virus-induced.

Males are predominantly affected. The area surrounding the jaw is most commonly involved, resulting in an enormous unsightly facial swelling. Most patients have multiple tumour deposits in the kidney, retroperitoneal tissues, ovaries, long bones and central nervous system.

Initially it was believed that one or two injections of cyclophosphamide induced long-term if not permanent remission. A high relapse rate has now been reported and current therapy demands full clinical and pathological staging, and combination chemotherapy with cytosine arabinoside (cytarabine) and cyclophosphamide. An immediate remission is induced in the majority of patients, and this can be maintained by further courses of combination chemotherapy.

METASTATIC TUMOURS

All forms of cancer can disseminate by lymphatic spread and via the blood stream. The concept that lymphatic invasion takes place first and that entrapment of tumour cells by the regional nodes can delay systemic involvement is no longer tenable. Although some cells are retained by the regional nodes and give rise to lymph node metastases, others pass through the nodes without being retained, bypass the nodes through lymphaticovenous communications, or enter the blood stream at the site of the primary disease.

Lymph node deposits are now taken as an indication that the tumour has invaded both lymphatic and blood channels and that there are likely to be systemic deposits elsewhere. Cancer associated with lymph node involvement is incurable by local means alone. Nevertheless, surgical removal of regional lymph nodes may be practised as part of the local control of the disease. This is discussed in Chapter 16.

Myelomatosis

This disease is characterized by a proliferation of plasma cells in the spleen and bone marrow. These cells secrete an abnormal gammaglobulin. The patient is usually over 60 years of age and may present at a surgical clinic because of intermittent bone pain, fractures or nerve pain. There may be anaemia and an abnormal bleeding tendency, and abnormal protein (Bence-Jones protein) may be found in the urine.

The most striking feature of the disease is the radiological appearance of punched-out areas in all bones due to deposits of myelomatous tissue (Fig. 22.7). Occasionally there are obvious swellings along the ribs.

It is important to differentiate these changes from those caused by multiple osteolytic metastases. X-ray of the skull is helpful as this is invariably affected by myelomatosis (see Fig. 22.7). The diagnosis is confirmed by demonstration of myeloma cells in the bone marrow and the typical paraproteinaemia.

The treatment of myelomatosis consists of combination chemotherapy. Surgical treatment is required only for stabilization of pathological fractures.

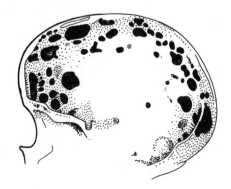

Fig. 22.7 Radiological appearance of myelomatosis showing characteristic lytic lesions in the skull

23. Endocrine disorders

THE THYROID

Anatomy and development

The thyroid gland is situated anteriorly and laterally in the lower part of the neck, opposite the 5–7th cervical vertebrae (Fig. 23.1). It develops from a diverticulum of the primitive pharynx containing epithelial elements. This thyroglossal duct grows downwards through the developing hyoid bone and in front of the larynx to bifurcate and fuse with elements from the 4th branchial arch. These form the parafollicular cells.

The 'thyroglossal duct' (see Ch. 24, Fig. 3a & b) is normally obliterated and marked only at its upper and lower ends by the foramen caecum at the back of the tongue and the pyramidal lobe of the thyroid. It may persist in part or in whole, giving rise to thyroglossal cysts or fistulas. Arrest of the process of descent may result in an ectopic thyroid.

Two pairs of parathyroid glands arise from the 3rd and 4th branchial arches. The superior parathyroids, which come from the 4th arch, are closely related to the posterior aspect of the thyroid. The inferior parathyroids arise from the 3rd arch and are more closely related to the developing thymus gland. Although usually situated behind the inferior poles of the thyroid lobes, they may be found between them and the thymus or within the thymus gland.

The developed thyroid gland consists of right and left lobes. These lie on the anterior and lateral aspects of the trachea and larynx and are connected by a narrow isthmus, which lies over the 2nd and 3rd tracheal rings. The gland weighs approximately 15–30 g.

The thyroid is bound down to the larynx, cricoid and trachea by the pretracheal fascia (Fig. 23.2). It is contained within a compartment which is bounded laterally by the carotid sheath and posteriorly by the prevertebral fascia. Anterior to the pretracheal fascia are the sternohyoid and sternothyroid muscles, which must be separated or divided to gain access to the gland. The lateral border of the sternoleidomastoid muscle overlaps the gland.

The gland derives its blood supply from the superior and inferior thyroid arteries. The superior artery arises from the external carotid artery at the level of the hyoid and runs downwards and forwards to enter the gland at its superior pole. The

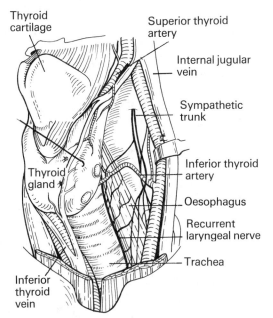

Thyroid cartilage

Superior thyroid artery

Internal jugular vein

Sympathetic trunk

Thyroid gland

Inferior thyroid artery

Oesophagus

Recurrent laryngeal nerve

Trachea

Inferior thyroid vein

Fig. 23.1 Anatomy of the thyroid gland. (Note: the middle thyroid vein has been divided to allow forward rotation of the left lobe.)

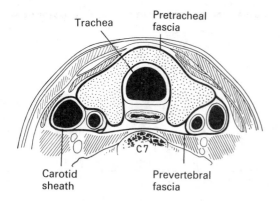

Fig. 23.2 Transverse section of the neck at the level of the seventh cervical vertebra to show the arrangement of the deep cervical fascia

inferior thyroid artery arises from the thyrocervical trunk (of subclavian origin) and runs upwards and medially behind the carotid sheath to the posterior aspect of the lower third of the gland. A short distance from the gland the artery passes behind or in front of the recurrent laryngeal nerve, or it may branch around it. The two recurrent laryngeal nerves course upwards in the groove between the oesophagus and the trachea to enter the larynx. Their inadvertent division can have serious consequences. For this reason many surgeons expose them in the neck as a preliminary step to thyroidectomy (see p. 335).

Blood from the thyroid drains through a series of veins which run upwards (superior thyroid veins) and laterally (middle thyroid veins) to the internal jugular vein, and downwards (inferior thyroid veins) to the innominate vein (see Fig. 23.1). Lymphatic drainage is laterally to the deep cervical chain and inferiorly to the pretracheal and mediastinal nodes.

Thyroid function

The follicles of the thyroid gland secrete two hormones: tri-iodothyronine (T3) and thyroxine (T4). Quantitatively T4 is the main hormone but the active hormone is T3. T4 is converted to T3 peripherally. The first step in the synthesis of thyroid hormones is the combination of iodine with tyrosyl groups to form mono- and di-iodotyrosine. These are coupled to form two active iodothyronines, T3 and T4. These hormones are stored within the follicles in the gland bound to thyroglobulin and, when released, circulate either in free form or bound to plasma proteins. The proportion of T3 which circulates in free rather than bound form is greater than that of T4.

The secretion of thyroid hormones is controlled by the thyroid stimulating hormone (TSH), a polypeptide of pituitary origin whose secretion is in turn controlled by thyrotropin releasing hormone (TRH), a tripeptide secreted by the hypothalamus (Fig. 23.3). The thyroid hormones (T3 and T4) exert negative 'feed back' on the hypothalamus and pituitary gland by suppressing secretion of TSH. Conversely, when there is deficiency in thyroid hormone production, TSH levels in the circulating blood are high.

Assessment of thyroid function

The assessment of thyroid function has been revolutionized by the development of sensitive and

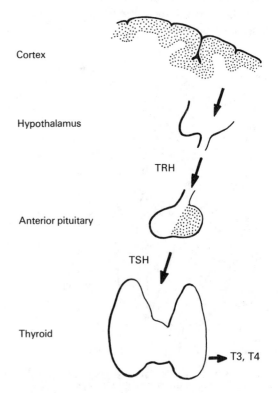

Fig. 23.3 Control of thyroid hormone secretion

precise assays for T3, T4 and TSH. As plasma levels of thyroid-binding globulin are increased in pregnancy and by the administration of oestrogens (including oestrogen-containing contraceptives), estimation of the ratio of unbound (free) to bound hormones may be necessary. TRH and TSH stimulation tests can be used to determine the site of failure to secrete thyroid hormones.

Methods of imaging the thyroid include plain X-rays, ultrasonography and radioisotope scanning using ^{99m}Tc-labelled sodium pertechnetate. This behaves like iodine and is 'trapped' by the thyroid. Its main value is to differentiate 'hot' (actively functioning) from 'cool' (normally functioning) and 'cold' (non-functioning) thyroid nodules.

Fine-needle aspiration (FNA) and FNA-cytology are now used for the preoperative diagnosis of thyroid nodules. Tests for thyroid antibodies are carried out by red-cell agglutination techniques and are used for the diagnosis of autoimmune thyroiditis.

ENLARGEMENT OF THE THYROID
(Goitre)

A goitre is a visible or palpable enlargement of the thyroid. Enlargement of the gland may occur during puberty or pregnancy. This is termed 'physiological goitre' and is a temporary phenomenon.

Lack of iodine in the diet also causes thyroid enlargement; at one time such 'endemic goitres' were common in some parts of Britain, e.g. Derbyshire and Wales.

The gland initially becomes diffusely enlarged, the follicles being filled with colloid (colloid goitre). Later multiple nodular areas develop, some of which contain abundant colloid. Others show degenerative changes with cyst formation, recent or old haemorrhage and calcification. This is the typical 'multinodular goitre'. Multinodular goitre is not restricted to iodine-deficient regions, which, with the addition of iodine to table salt, are now of only historical interest in this country.

Diffuse enlargement of the thyroid may also be due to overstimulation of the gland by TSH or TSH-like proteins, resulting in increased production of T3 and T4 and thus thyrotoxicosis. Diffuse

enlargement may also reflect an autoimmune reaction (Hashimoto's disease) or occur as part of an infective process (subacute thyroiditis).

Goitres are not always diffuse but may result from a single nodule, e.g. a cyst or a benign or malignant tumour which arises from the thyroid cells, the parafollicular cells or lymphatic elements. Although both thyrotoxicosis and myxoedema can occur in association with thyroid enlargement, most goitres occur in euthyroid individuals.

Clinically, thyroid enlargement appears as a swelling in the lower neck which takes up the shape of the thyroid gland and lies anteriorly and laterally. It characteristically moves upwards on swallowing. The patient should be asked to hold a drink of water in his closed mouth and then swallow, while the examiner observes the lower neck from in front.

Non-toxic nodular goitre

As indicated above, this common disease of the thyroid occurs endemically in areas of iodine deficiency, but may also be sporadic or occur as a reaction to drugs. It is more common in females. Multinodular goitres vary greatly in size, from little more than that of the normal thyroid to swellings weighing several hundred grams. Usually the whole gland is involved, but the changes may be confined to one lobe. On section there are multiple nodules of varied appearance, some hyperplastic with or without colloid formation, others degenerative with cysts, haemorrhage, fibrosis and even calcification. Microscopically, the glandular tissue within some nodules consists of acini which are greatly distended with colloid and lined by flattened epithelium. In others there are areas of hyperplasia, fibrosis or degenerative change.

Clinical features

Most multinodular goitres are asymptomatic. Some cause tracheal compression and dyspnoea particularly when the goitre extends downwards behind the sternum (retrosternal goitre). Dysphagia due to oesophageal compression rarely occurs. Haemorrhage into a nodule may cause pain and

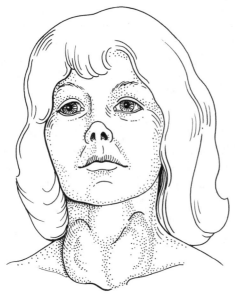

Fig. 23.4 Multinodular goitre

rapid enlargement and, if the goitre is retrosternal, respiratory distress. The thyroid is visibly enlarged (Fig. 23.4) and multiple nodules usually are palpable. However, sometimes only one nodule may be felt, giving rise to the erroneous impression that one is dealing with a solitary nodule.

X-rays of the thoracic inlet are taken to detect any retrosternal extension or tracheal compression. If there is dysphagia, a barium swallow is indicated. Tests of thyroid function (T3, T4, TSH estimations) are normally performed, but radioactive isotope scans are rarely helpful, as a 'cold' nodule is likely only to represent degenerate thyroid tissue.

Treatment

The administration of thyroxine will occasionally prevent further enlargement of the gland by suppressing TSH secretion. Regression of the goitre is unusual. Large multinodular goitres and those causing symptoms of compression require subtotal thyroidectomy (see later). As the gland is not functioning well, the risk of hypothyroidism following operation is greater than after resection for thyrotoxicosis. Thyroxine therapy is advised postoperatively to suppress TSH stimulation and prevent enlargement of residual glandular tissue.

Thyroiditis

Subacute thyroiditis (De Quervain's disease)

This rare condition is associated with a flu-like illness during which there is a painful diffuse swelling of the thyroid gland. Thyroid antibodies may appear in the serum. It is believed to be due to a viral infection and usually resolves, although in some patients it has an intermittent course.

Autoimmune thyroiditis (Hashimoto's disease)

This condition is believed to be due to destruction of thyroid follicles by immunocompetent lymphocytes. Thyroid antibodies can be detected in the serum, and are active against thyroglobulin, thyroid-cell cytosol and microsomes. The gland is diffusely enlarged, and histologically there is marked lymphocytic infiltration around destroyed follicles, hence the term 'lymphadenoid goitre'. Failure of thyroid function and myxoedema follow.

Postmenopausal females are most commonly affected (female-to-male ratio 10 : 1). The thyroid is diffusely enlarged and firm. The enlargement includes the isthmus and pyramidal lobe, giving a 'butterfly' appearance. A nodular form, which may be confused with multinodular goitre, also occurs.

The patient is usually euthyroid, but thyrotoxicosis may occur. In time the patient becomes myxoedematous.

The diagnosis depends on the demonstration of high titres of circulating antithyroid antibodies, particularly to microsomal components of the follicular cells. Biopsy of the gland is indicated only if findings such as nodularity or asymmetical enlargement raise the suspicion of malignancy.

Thyroxine replacement leads to regression of small goitres. If the goitre is large or associated with symptoms of compression, subtotal thyroidectomy may be required.

Riedel's thyroiditis

This is a very rare condition in which the thyroid is replaced by dense fibrous tissue, resulting in a firm, painless swelling and tracheal compression. The cause is unknown. Surgical decompression of the trachea may be required.

Solitary thyroid nodule

Slow-growing and painless 'solitary nodules' are common in the thyroid gland. About 50% are not true solitary lesions but a conspicuous and palpable nodule in a gland affected by multinodular goitre. Of true solitary nodules, half are benign adenomas and the remainder cysts or a differentiated cancer.

It is important to have a 'decision tree' for the diagnosis of solitary nodules based on full clinical and biochemical assessment of thyroid function; isotope scanning to determine if the nodule is 'hot' or 'cold'; ultrasonography to differentiate cystic from solid lesions; and FNA-cytology (or Tru-cut biopsy) should they prove to be solid.

Cysts can be treated by aspiration, and, provided they do not refill and the cytology of the fluid is negative, they need not be removed.

FNA-cytology and Tru-cut biopsy are not fully diagnostic, as they cannot accurately differentiate a follicular adenoma from a follicular carcinoma. All other lesions can be confidently diagnosed.

While some surgeons are prepared to treat follicular adenomas believed to be benign with thyroxine (a proportion of them undergo regression), the risk of cancer makes it preferable to excise all follicular lesions by total or subtotal lobectomy. Immediate frozen section examination is carried out so that more radical surgery can be performed should a carcinoma be present.

HYPERTHYROIDISM

Thyrotoxicosis results from overproduction of the thyroid hormones T3 and T4. Circulating levels of these hormones are increased, while, through the feedback mechanism, TSH levels in the serum are reduced or undetectable. Three well-defined conditions of the thyroid gland share, to a varying extent, the clinical features of this disease: Grave's disease (primary thyrotoxicosis), and toxic multinodular goitre and toxic adenoma (secondary thyrotoxicosis).

Primary thyrotoxicosis (Grave's disease)

This accounts for 75–80% of cases of thyrotoxicosis. It is an autoimmune disease in which the TSH receptors in the thyroid gland are stimulated by circulating immunoglobulins called thyroid-stimulating immunoglobulins (TSI). The gland is uniformly hyperactive, very vascular and has a firm, meaty appearance on section. It is usually, but not always, symmetrically enlarged. Histologically, there is marked epithelial proliferation with papillary projections into the follicles which are devoid of colloid.

As TSI can cross the placental barrier, neonatal thyrotoxicosis may develop in children born to previously thyrotoxic mothers.

Clinical features

The patient is usually female (male-to-female ratio 1:8) and young. There is a strong genetic predisposition. The main effects of increased levels of circulating T3 and T4 are to increase the basal metabolic rate and potentiate the actions of the sympathetic nervous system. Other effects (due probably to TSI) are also described.

Metabolic effects. Due to the increased rate of metabolism the patient feels hot at rest and is intolerant of warmth. The skin is moist and warm because of the peripheral vasodilatation and excess sweating. Weight loss is the rule despite increased appetite. Cardiac output is increased to meet metabolic demands.

Sympathetic activity. Tachycardia is invariably present, even during sleep. Palpitations may be troublesome and cardiac irregularities and arrhythmias occur in older patients. There is a fine tremor, the upper eyelids are retracted, gastrointestinal motility is increased and there is general hyperkinesia. Anxiety and psychiatric disturbance may be evident.

Other features. Exophthalmos is a classical feature of primary thyrotoxicosis but is not always present. Ophthalmoplegia, pretibial myxoedema, myopathy (affecting proximal muscles) and finger clubbing also are variable. Menstrual irregularities and relative infertility are common.

The *thyroid gland* is usually moderately and diffusely enlarged and soft. Because of its increased vascularity a bruit is often audible.

Diagnosis

In most patients the diagnosis can readily be made,

but in those with anxiety, distinction from other neuroses can be difficult. It should be remembered that thyrotoxicosis may be a cause of unexplained diarrhoea.

The demonstration of raised circulating levels of T3 and T4 and a low level of TSH in the serum is diagnostic. The TSH response to intravenous injection of 200 μg TRH is absent owing to atrophy of the TSH-producing cells of the pituitary.

Treatment

Thyrotoxicosis can be treated by antithyroid drugs, radioactive iodine or surgery.

Antithyroid drugs. These drugs, of which carbimazole is the most widely used, block the incorporation of iodine into the tyrosine molecule and thus prevent the synthesis of T3 and T4. Following the administration of carbimazole in full blocking doses (30–60 mg daily), symptoms improve within a few weeks and the patient can be expected to be euthyroid by 4–6 weeks. Once this has been achieved, the dose can be reduced to maintenance levels (5–15 mg daily). Alternatively the drug may be continued in full thyroid-blocking doses, in which case T3 (as liothyronine sodium) is added to provide hormone replacement. This should be given in an initial dose of 10–20 μg daily, increasing at weekly intervals to 60 μg daily in divided doses. As primary thyrotoxicosis is a disease likely to remit, carbimazole is normally stopped after 12–18 months although 60–70% of patients will have a relapse within 2 years of stopping treatment.

Carbimazole treatment is not free from problems. The drug must be taken regularly (at 6-hourly intervals) and sensitivity reactions such as skin rashes, gastrointestinal upsets and occasionally agranulocytosis have been reported. For this reason early definitive treatment with radioactive iodine or by surgery has much to recommend it.

Radioactive iodine. The risk of possible radiation damage to developing gametes from therapeutic doses of radioiodine has restricted the use of this form of treatment to patients over 40 years of age. Many consider radioiodine to be the treatment of choice for most patients over that age although, because of the difficulty in calculating the dose, progressive hypothyroidism almost invariably occurs, and affects 80% of patients after 15 years. Thyroid replacement therapy will be necessary.

Radioiodine is the treatment of choice for primary thyrotoxicosis in the USA but in the UK it is more commonly reserved for patients whose disease recurs after surgical treatment.

Surgery. Surgery by subtotal thyroidectomy is the best treatment for many patients and certainly those under 40 years of age. In experienced hands mortality is low, complications are rare and the disease is cured in 95% of cases. Recurrence is usually due to inadequate removal of glandular tissue. The aim is to leave a remnant of about 3 g. Postoperative hypothyroidism occurs in 20–25% of patients. Low levels of T3 and T4 and elevated levels of TSH persisting beyond 6 months, or signs of frank hypothyroidism, are indications for lifelong thyroid hormone replacement.

The patient should be rendered euthyroid before operation. This is usually done with antithyroid drugs, which are continued up to the evening before the operation. The previously common practice of substituting or adding iodine therapy 10 days before the operation in order to reduce the vascularity of the gland has now been largely discontinued.

Alternatively, beta-adrenergic blocking agents can be used to prepare the patient for operation. These abolish the increased sympathetic activity, but only slightly reduce T3 and T4 levels so that the metabolic effects of hyperthyroidism are not counteracted. They are contraindicated in patients with cardiac failure and best avoided in diabetics as they mask hypoglycaemic symptoms.

The usual dose of propranolol is 40–80 mg 6-hourly. This results in an improvement of symptoms within a few days. A pulse rate of 80/min or less is desirable.

With this method of preparation, the patient is admitted to hospital 3 days before operation in case minor adjustments of dose are required. The drug is given on the morning of operation and continued for 7 days postoperatively. Excessive sweating in the postoperative period indicates a need to increase the dose.

Secondary thyrotoxicosis (toxic multinodular goitre and toxic adenomas)

Toxic multinodular goitre accounts for 20–25% of cases of thyrotoxicosis and tends to occur in older patients. It usually develops in association with a non-toxic multinodular goitre of long standing. One or more nodules become hyperactive and function independently of TSH stimulation. The remainder of the gland is inactive.

A rare cause of thyrotoxicosis (1–2%) is a single functioning adenoma which autonomously secretes thyroid hormones. As TSH secretion is completely suppressed, the remaining gland is non-functional.

Clinical features and diagnosis

The disease is much more common in women than in men. Patients with toxic multinodular goitre are more prone to cardiac complications such as arrhythmias. Exophthalmos is rare. In those with a functioning solitary adenoma, exophthalmos, ophthalmoplegia and myopathies are invariably absent.

In both instances an isotope scan of the thyroid is advised. In multinodular goitre it will demonstrate one or several areas of increased uptake. In toxic adenoma the nodule is hot and the remainder of the gland suppressed.

Treatment

Treatment consists of removal of hyperfunctioning glandular tissue. This is achieved by subtotal thyroidectomy for multinodular goitre and by lobectomy for a toxic adenoma.

MALIGNANT TUMOURS OF THE THYROID

Malignant tumours of the thyroid are rare, accounting for less than 1% of all forms of malignancy. As with other thyroid disease, females are predominantly affected (male-to-female ratio 1:3). There are three main types of thyroid carcinoma: papillary (45–55%), follicular (10–25%) and anaplastic (25–40%). The remainder are medullary carcinomas and lymphomas. The incidence of thyroid cancer is increased in patients who have been exposed to radiation in childhood (as used to be accepted treatment in children thought to have 'thymic disease'). Medullary carcinoma may be familial.

Papillary carcinoma

This is a tumour of early life and is rare after the age of 40 years. It presents as a solitary lump in the thyroid and is relatively slow-growing. Rarely it presents as a so-called 'lateral aberrant thyroid'. This is due to metastatic enlargement of deep cervical lymph nodes from a microscopic primary lesion in the ipsilateral thyroid lobe.

Papillary cancers of the thyroid are not particularly hard. Enlarged cervical lymph nodes are palpable in 30% of patients but distant metastases are rare. Occasionally a papillary carcinoma is discovered incidentally during microscopic examination of a thyroid removed for other reasons. Histologically, there are complex masses of papillary folds which are lined by several layers of cuboidal cells and which project into what appear to be cystic spaces.

Treatment

As the disease is commonly multifocal, most or all of the gland should be removed by total or near-total thyroidectomy. Any involved lymph nodes are also removed, but radical neck dissection is no longer recommended. Hormone replacement therapy with T3 (20 μg four times a day) is instituted and monitored by TSH estimations. Some surgeons routinely obtain a radioiodine body scan and, if this shows increased uptake at any site, administer a therapeutic dose of radioiodine. This is not general practice.

The tumour has an excellent prognosis, with 10-year survival rates approaching 90%.

Follicular carcinoma

Follicular carcinoma usually presents as a solitary nodule in the thyroid. It tends to occur in older patients (30–50 years) than papillary carcinoma (15–40 years) and is more aggressive, with a 10-

year survival rate of 50%. Lymph node metastases are rare. The tumour spreads mainly via the blood stream, and 15–20% of patients have metastatic deposits in the lungs, bone or liver. Histologically the malignant cells are arranged in solid masses with only rudimentary formation of acini. Venous invasion is common.

Mixed follicular tumours with evidence of papillary neoplasia have a better prognosis, with a natural history similar to that of papillary carcinoma.

Treatment

Treatment consists of thyroidectomy with preservation of the parathyroids. All palpable lymph nodes should be removed and biopsied. If this shows metastatic involvement, a modified radical neck dissection is carried out.

A postoperative radioisotope scan is routinely obtained, and if this reveals areas of increased uptake in the skeleton, therapeutic doses of radio-iodine are given. Uptake in the neck region indicates residual thyroid tissue, which must first be ablated with radio-iodine. T3 is administered routinely to suppress TSH secretion.

Anaplastic carcinoma

These are rapidly growing, highly malignant tumours which tend to occur in older patients than papillary or follicular carcinoma. The prognosis is poor, with 70% of patients dying within one year.

Local invasion may involve the recurrent laryngeal nerve(s) and cause hoarseness and compression of the trachea and oesophagus. Respiratory obstruction, dyspnoea, stridor and dysphagia can occur. Invasion of the cervical sympathetic nerves gives rise to Horner's syndrome. Pulmonary metastases are common.

Resection is rarely possible but surgical decompression of the trachea may relieve symptoms. Radiotherapy is usually given.

Medullary carcinoma

This tumour arises from the parafollicular C-cells which secrete thyrocalcitonin. It occurs sporadically or may be part of the multiple endocrine neoplasia (MEN) syndrome type II (Sipple's syndrome). Associated abnormalities include phaeochromocytoma, hyperparathyroidism and mucosal neuromas.

The disease presents as a hard enlargement of one or both lobes of the thyroid. Cervical lymph node metastases are present in 50% of patients. Multiple mucosal neuromas may mark the presence of MEN II.

Thyrocalcitonin levels are elevated although the serum calcium is normal. Calcitonin assays can be used to monitor progress and also to screen relatives in familial cases.

Treatment consists of total thyroidectomy. Palpable nodes are biopsied and, if positive, a modified radical neck dissection is performed.

Other tumours

Lymphoid tumours

Primary lymphoma of the thyroid is a rare complication of autoimmune thyroiditis. It is radiosensitive and therefore amenable to treatment by radiotherapy and chemotherapy.

Thyroid metastases

Metastatic tumours of the thyroid are unusual but may be seen in cancer of the breast and bronchus.

THYROIDECTOMY

Technique

The thyroid gland is exposed through a transverse skin-crease incision placed midway between the suprasternal notch and the thyroid cartilage. Laterally the incision extends to the external jugular veins.

The incision is deepened through the subcutaneous fat and platysma muscle, and superior and inferior flaps of skin together with platysma are elevated from the cervical fascia to the level of the notch of the thyroid cartilage above and the suprasternal notch below. The deep cervical fascia is then divided longitudinally in the midline, and the strap muscles are separated and retracted to expose the gland and its investing pretracheal fascia, which is separated from the surface of the gland. Some surgeons prefer to divide the strap muscles transversely.

Each lobe of the thyroid is then mobilized in turn, ligating and dividing first the vessels at the superior pole of the gland, then the middle and inferior thyroid veins, and finally the inferior thyroid arteries. This should be done with great care so as not to damage the recurrent laryngeal nerves. Many surgeons expose the recurrent nerves routinely to define their course.

A varying amount of each lobe is removed, taking care to preserve the parathyroid glands. Drains are inserted into the thyroid space and the layers of the neck are reconstituted.

Complications of thyroidectomy

Haemorrhage

The most important early complication of thyroidectomy is haemorrhage into the confined space deep to the deep cervical fascia leading to tracheal compression and asphyxia. This is a particular risk in patients in whom pressure from a long-standing large goitre has led to softening of the tracheal rings. The patient must be intubated if necessary and returned to theatre immediately so that the wound can be reopened and any bleeding vessels ligated.

Nerve damage

Inadvertent damage to the external branch of the superior laryngeal nerve may occur during ligation of the vascular pedicle of the upper pole of the thyroid. As this nerve supplies the cricothyroid muscle, which tenses the vocal cord, temporary weakness of the voice will result.

Recurrent laryngeal nerve damage is more serious. Traction during resection results in temporary paralysis of the vocal cord in 5% of cases, but recovery within 3 months is the rule. Accidental division results in permanent paralysis.

If the injury is unilateral, the voice becomes hoarse and 'bovine'. With time, the unaffected cord compensates by increased adduction while the paralysed cord is drawn nearer to the midline. The voice becomes normal but easily tired.

Bilateral injury results in stridor and ineffective coughing in the immediate postoperative period. If this occurs, an endotracheal tube must be inserted. If there is no improvement within 10 days, a tracheostomy is required. As both cords gradually come together in the midline, there is increasing dyspnoea on exertion, which can be particularly troublesome in patients whose job involves heavy physical work. If surgical methods of repositioning the attachments of the cords are not successful, a permanent tracheostomy may be required.

It is essential to examine the vocal cords both before and immediately after thyroid surgery, not only to detect any recurrent laryngeal nerve damage but also to document their pre- and postoperative position for medicolegal reasons.

Occasionally the sympathetic chain is injured at the time of ligation of the inferior thyroid artery, causing Horner's syndrome.

Thyroid malfunction

With modern methods of preparation for surgery, postoperative 'thyrotoxic crises' with hyperpyrexia and increased sympathetic activity should not occur. Immediate treatment with iodide and beta-blockers is advised.

The risk of postoperative hypothyroidism depends on the nature of the disease and the extent of thyroid removal (see earlier).

Hypoparathyroidism

Damage to the parathyroid glands leads to a decrease in serum calcium concentration over a few days with a risk of subsequent tetany (see p. 338). Careful postoperative monitoring of serum calcium levels and motor nerve function is therefore required in all patients who have undergone total lobectomy or thyroidectomy, and in those treated by bilateral subtotal thyroidectomy for thyrotoxicosis associated with a large goitre, in whom one wishes to leave only a small remnant.

Treatment consists of calcium and vitamin D (alfacalcidol, calcitriol) administration and, if necessary, correction of magnesium deficiency.

Scar complications

Some patients develop a hypertrophic scar or keloid, particularly when the wound has been placed too low in the neck. Excision of the scar with steroid infiltration of the new wound during healing may improve the result but recurrence is common.

THE PARATHYROID GLANDS

Anatomy and function

As indicated above, there are two pairs of parathyroid glands. The right and left superior parathyroids are applied closely to the posterior aspect of the upper lateral lobes of the thyroid, at the level of the cricoid cartilage. They are constant in position, unlike the inferior pair of glands, which may be found closely applied to the posterior surface of the lower portion of the thyroid lobes, within their fascial sheath, or even within the gland. Occasionally they are found some distance below the thyroid, in the upper mediastinum or within the thymus gland. The inconstancy of the position of the inferior parathyroids is due to their development from the third branchial arch in association with the thymus, with which they descend.

The parathyroid glands receive a rich blood supply from the inferior thyroid artery, the branches of which are a valuable marker to their position.

The parathyroids secrete parathormone (PTH), a polypeptide with 84 amino acids which maintains the level of calcium in plasma and tissue fluids between 2.25 and 2.60 mmol/l. The ionized fraction of calcium (50%) is particularly relevant to body function; the remainder is protein-bound and not directly available. There is a dynamic equilibrium between the levels of calcium and phosphate.

Parathormone acts in three ways to restore a falling serum calcium.

1. It mobilizes calcium from bone by stimulating osteoclastic activity.

2. It stimulates phosphate excretion by the renal tubules, which, by lowering phosphate concentrations in plasma, increases the dissociation of calcium phosphate, so allowing calcium to be freed. (A secondary effect on the kidney is to promote the conversion of less active forms of vitamin D to the more active 1,25-dihydroxycholecalciferol.)

3. It increases intestinal absorption of calcium.

PTH secretion is in turn controlled by the level of ionized calcium in blood circulating through the parathyroid glands.

Thyrocalcitonin (secreted by the parafollicular or C-cells of the thyroid gland) has an opposite effect to PTH. It is not important in man and total thyroidectomy does not affect calcium balance.

Calcium metabolism

Hypercalcaemia is commonly due to factors other than parathyroid disease. These are:

1. excessive absorption of calcium due to vitamin D excess, the milk-alkali syndrome, sarcoidosis or drugs;

2. excessive breakdown of bone (e.g. in metastatic bone disease or myeloma);

3. ectopic secretion of a PTH-like substance (e.g. in malignant disease of bronchus or breast).

It is occasionally associated with disease or the thyroid or adrenal glands.

Hypocalcaemia is also often due to disease remote from the parathyroids. Examples are:

1. hypoproteinaemia, which may be due to nephrosis (excessive loss of protein), malnutrition (inadequate intake), or cirrhosis (deficient synthesis). This reduces the amount of protein available for calcium binding. Loss of albumin probably accounts for the hypocalcaemia of acute pancreatitis;

2. vitamin D deficiency (e.g. in rickets);

3. excess secretion of thyrocalcitonin (e.g. in medullary cancer of the thyroid); and

4. pseudohypoparathyroidism, a genetic disorder of children in which there is end-organ resistance to the action of PTH.

PARATHYROID DISEASE

Primary, secondary and tertiary forms of hyperparathyoidism are recognized. That of greatest surgical importance is the primary type.

Primary hyperparathyroidism

This is usually (in about 90% of cases) due to a secreting adenoma of the parathyoid glands affecting one gland only (Fig. 23.5a). In the remaining 10% there is hyperplasia, usually of all four glands (Fig. 23.5b). Parathyroid carcinoma is a very rare cause of the syndrome.

Adenomas of the parathyroids are benign, spherical tumours. Although usually small, they occasionally reach a size 10 times that of a normal parathyroid. Most are single but one-fifth affect more than one gland.

Macroscopically the lesion appears as a rounded

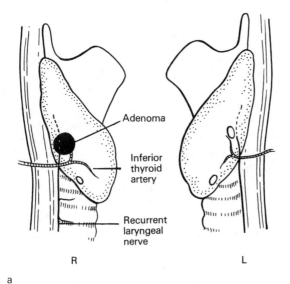

a

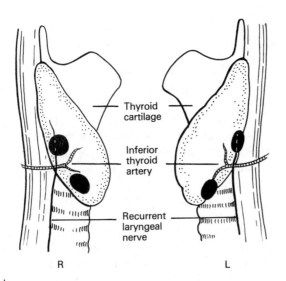

b

Fig. 23.5 Causes of primary hyperparathyroidism. (a) Parathyroid adenoma. (b) Parathyroid hyperplasia

nodular brown mass. On microscopy there is a varying proportion of chief and water-clear cells, an appearance not easy to distinguish from that of primary hyperplasia.

Primary hyperplasia is due to an increase in the number of chief cells. Before this diagnosis can be accepted, the gland must be at least twice the upper limit of normal size (i.e. 70 mg or more in weight).

Clinical features

Primary hyperparathyroidism affects women twice as often as men. It is usually found in middle age. Increasingly it is detected in asymptomatic patients during routine biochemical screening for some other reason, when an abnormally high level of serum calcium is noted.

Clinical manifestations, if they do occur, affect kidneys and bones, and rarely the nervous system, giving rise to neurological or psychiatric symptoms. Acute pancreatitis is reported to be more common in this disease.

Renal effects include formation of urinary calculi and nephrocalcinosis (speckled renal calcification). Recurrent urinary calculi are particularly significant. All such patients must be investigated by repeated estimations of serum calcium concentration. If the syndrome is untreated renal failure can result. Polyuria is an early feature of renal damage.

Bone damage used to be a common clinical presentation but is now rarely seen. Gross demineralization, subperiosteal bone resorption (typically seen in middle and distal phalanges of the fingers), cysts in long bones and jaw, and the moth-eaten appearance of the skull gave the syndrome its name 'osteitis fibrosa cystica'. Multiple fractures were common.

Diagnosis

The key investigations are biochemical. As serum calcium levels may fluctuate, they must be determined on at least three separate occasions. It is routine practice not to use a tourniquet when taking blood although this is now known to be irrelevant. Serum phosphate concentrations are abnormally low.

If hyperparathyoidism is suspected, serum PTH levels should be measured sequentially. If they are raised, other forms of hyperparathyroidism must be excluded before the parathyroid glands are explored.

Treatment

Treatment is surgical. The aim is to identify and remove all overactive parathyroid tissue. The surgical approach is similar to that for a thyroidectomy, each lobe of the thyroid being mobilized in turn. All four glands must be identified and inspected. Normal parathyroids are smooth and brownish, the surface resembling the capsule of the liver. Enlarged glands are nodular. Immediate frozen section examination is required to establish the diagnosis and exclude thyroid nodules, thymic tissue or fat.

In the majority of cases only one gland is enlarged, and this is removed. In 7–10% of cases two or more glands are enlarged, and these should be removed unless all four glands are enlarged, in which case all but a portion of one gland should be removed. In all cases the recurrent laryngeal nerves must be identified and preserved.

If neither a parathyroid adenoma nor hyperplasia can be identified at operation, it is wisest to close the incision and reoperate following additional investigations such as gallium radioisotope scans and selective venous catheterization with PTH estimations to help define the source of abnormal hormone secretion. Similar investigations are performed prior to reoperation in patients with recurrent hyperparathyroidism.

Secondary and tertiary hyperparathyroidism

In secondary hyperparathyroidism there is oversecretion of PTH in response to low plasma concentrations of ionized calcium, usually due to renal disease or malabsorption. This is an increasing clinical problem in patients on long-term haemodialysis for chronic renal failure.

Treatment is medical and consists of administration of 1α-hydroxyvitamin D_3 (alfacalcidol) to increase calcium absorption and provide a negative feedback effect on the parathyroids.

The excessive secretion of PTH in some patients with secondary hyperparathyroidism may become autonomous, and is then termed tertiary hyperparathyroidism. This may occur after renal transplantation. Total parathyroidectomy may be required with autotransplantation of a parathyroid fragment equivalent in size to a normal parathyroid gland into an arm muscle (where it is readily located if problems persist). Postoperatively, treatment is continued with alfacalcidol and calcium to heal bone disease and reduce the risk of recurrent hyperparathyroidism.

Hypoparathyroidism

A fall in ionized serum calcium below the normal level may give rise to tetany. This is a condition of neuromuscular instability in which the patient experiences 'pins and needles' in hands and feet, and muscle cramps and spasms cause flexion and bunching of fingers and toes. Respiratory obstruction with stridor due to spasm of laryngeal muscles may prove fatal.

The patient is lethargic and depressed. Clinical signs include Chvostek's sign (twitching of facial muscles in response to tapping of the facial nerve), Trousseau's sign (spasm of the hand and forearm muscles following application of a tourniquet to obliterate the pulse) and Erb's sign (hyperexcitability of muscles on electrical stimulation).

The ECG shows a lengthened Q-T interval and X-ray of the skull may reveal calcification of basal ganglia. Blood levels of ionized calcium and PTH are low.

Acute hypoparathyroidism is treated by intravenous injection of calcium gluconate (20 ml of a 10% solution given every 4 hours until calcium levels begin to rise). Oral calcium (effervescent calcium gluconate) and vitamin D (cholecalciferol 20 000 units daily) are required for maintenance. Calcium levels must be monitored regularly.

THE PITUITARY GLAND

The pituitary gland is small, weighing only 500 mg. It is enclosed within a bony shell, the sella turcica, which is sealed superiorly by a fold of dura mater, the diaphragma sellae. Through this passes the pituitary stalk which connects the pituitary to the hypothalamus.

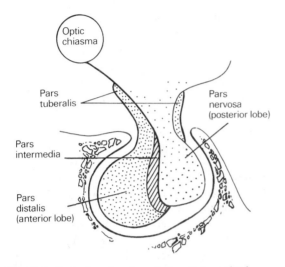

Fig. 23.6 Sagittal section through the pituitary gland

The pituitary consists of two main parts: the adenohypophysis, or anterior pituitary, and the neurohypophysis, or posterior pituitary (Fig. 23.6). These two parts have different functions and different connections with the hypothalamus.

THE ANTERIOR PITUITARY

This is part of the endocrine system, secreting hormones which act on distant targets. It contains solid cords of secreting cells which on conventional staining with haematoxylin and eosin are of three main types: acidophil, basophil and chromophobe.

Using immunofluorescent and other specific stains these cells can be further divided according to the nature of their secretion. Thus particular cell types can be shown to secrete growth hormone, prolactin, adrenocorticotropin (ACTH), gonadotropins and TSH (Fig. 23.7).

The anterior pituitary develops embryologically from the epithelium of Rathke's pouch, an outgrowth from the pharynx. Some cells are believed to be of neural crest origin and to belong to the APUD system (see p. 353).

The anterior pituitary is connected to the hypothalamus by the hypophysial stalk carrying the portal venous system, a group of veins which run down the pituitary stalk to connect capillaries in the median eminence of the hypothalamus with capillaries and sinusoids of the anterior pituitary (Fig. 23.8). This portal system carries a series of neurosecretory hormones from the hypothalamus to the pituitary where they stimulate or inhibit specific endocrine cells. The most important messengers are growth hormone releasing and inhibiting factors, corticotropin releasing factor (CRF), gonadotropin releasing hormone (Gn-RH), thyrotropin releasing hormone (TRH) and prolactin-inhibiting factor (PIF). If the hypophysial-portal tract is divided, the anterior pituitary is disconnected from these hypothalamic influences so that the secretion of all hormones but prolactin is suppressed. Prolactin-secreting cells, being released from the inhibitory effect of PIF, oversecrete.

A complex system of long, short and ultrashort

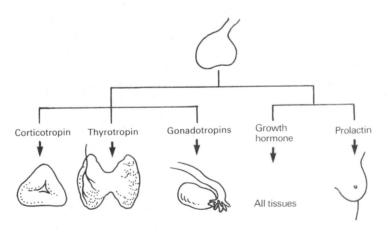

Fig. 23.7 The anterior pituitary hormones and their target organs

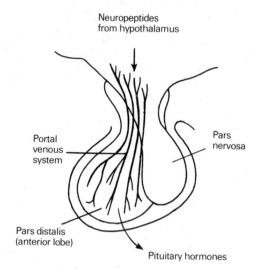

Fig. 23.8   The hypophysial-hypothalamic system

loops form a delicate feedback system by which the secretion of pituitary hormones can be adjusted according to need (Fig. 23.9).

Functions of pituitary hormones

1. *Growth hormone* is a long-chain polypeptide which has a wide variety of functions, including regulation of growth. Its metabolic effects include increased uptake of amino acids and promotion of

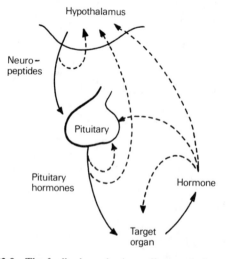

Fig. 23.9   The feedback mechanisms affecting pituitary hormone secretion

protein synthesis with increase in the size of muscles, viscera and glands. It also increases lipolysis and enhances utilization of fatty acids, causing ketosis. Growth hormone has an anti-insulin effect: it increases gluconeogenesis and decreases peripheral utilization of glucose. In large amounts it augments milk secretion.

Release of growth hormone is stimulated by stress, fasting and hypoglycaemia. It can be inhibited by bromocriptine or chlorpromazine. It stimulates secretion of somatomedin from liver and kidney, and this is responsible for some of its growth-promoting effects. Growth hormone excess causes gigantism in children and acromegaly in adults, while inadequate secretion in childhood causes dwarfism. Genetically prepared human growth hormone is now available for therapeutic use.

2. *Prolactin* is a long-chain polypeptide of similar molecular weight to growth hormone. Normally only small amounts are secreted, but these increase markedly during the night. Secretion is greatly increased during pregnancy, as prolactin, is an essential hormone for lobulo-alveolar development of the breast and the initiation of lactation.

Prolactin release is increased by oestradiol, phenothiazines (e.g. chlorpromazine) and meto-clopramide. Its release is inhibited by L-dopa and bromocriptine.

3. *Human corticotropin* is a polypeptide containing 39 amino acids. The first 23 amino acids are common to all species. Synthetic ACTH, as used in clinical practice (tetracosactrin) contains 24 amino acids. The 4–10 amino acid sequence is similar to that found in melanocyte-stimulating hormone and accounts for the pigmentation associated with excess secretion of ACTH.

ACTH is secreted as part of a larger molecule which consists of three constituent polypeptides: pro-gamma ACTH, ACTH and beta-lipoprotein (LPH). Pro-gamma ACTH is believed to act on the adrenal by sensitizing the cells to the action of ACTH. LPH mobilizes fat, but also contains the amino acid sequences of metencephalin and beta-endorphin which bind to opiate receptors and have analgesic properties.

ACTH itself acts on the inner zones of the adrenal cortex, where it stimulates secretion of cortisol and adrenal androgens. Its secretion is in turn stimulated by corticotropin-releasing factor (CRF), which is secreted in response to all forms of stress.

4. *Three glycoprotein hormones* are secreted by the pituitary: Luteinizing hormone (LH), follicle-stimulating hormone (FSH) and thyroid-stimulating hormone (TSH). Each has alpha- and beta-subunits. While the alpha-subunit is common to all three and shared with human chorionic gonadotropin, the beta-subunit is specific to each hormone and endows it with its appropriate actions. FSH stimulates follicle development towards the end of the menstrual cycle and the secretion of oestrogen from the thecal cells. LH triggers ovulation and promotes the formation of the corpus luteum and secretion of oestrogens and progesterone. In the male, FSH stimulates spermatogenesis and LH (which in the male is known as interstitial cell stimulating hormone), the secretion of testosterone by the Leydig cells (Fig. 23.10).

TSH promotes the growth of the thyroid and regulates the secretion of thyroid hormones.

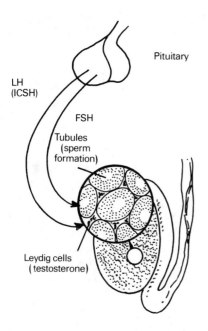

Fig. 23.10 The role of pituitary hormones in the control of male sexual function. ICSH = interstitial cell stimulating hormone

Tumours of the anterior pituitary

Functioning adenomas of the pituitary result from overstimulation by hypothalamic factors. Initially small and confined within the gland (micro-adenomas), they slowly increase in size and may ultimately expand the sella turcica. Eccentric enlargement is common and produces asymmetry of the pituitary fossa. This can be detected radiologically by lateral tomograms.

Upward extension of an adenoma may stretch the diaphragm or herniate through it as a suprasellar extension. This will compress the optic chiasma and cause visual defects. A CT scan with contrast enhancement will reveal the tumour and delineate its extent.

It is important that pituitary adenomas are detected before they enlarge the fossa or extend above it. Three endocrine syndromes are of surgical relevance.

Acromegaly

This syndrome of 'large extremities' is due to excess secretion of growth hormone, usually starting in early adult life. The resultant overgrowth of the soft tissues of hands, feet and face gives the patient a characteristic grotesque appearance with a coarse face, bulging supraorbital ridges and protruding jaw. Endochondral ossification and periosteal new bone formation account for some of these changes. All viscera are enlarged and there is muscular hypertrophy. However, muscle weakness and cardiac failure develop later. The skin is coarse and greasy and acne is common. Headaches, sweating and the carpal tunnel syndrome are common. Glucose tolerance is impaired and galactorrhoea may occur in females.

Growth hormone levels are increased and secretion is not suppressed by glucose or a meal. Increased levels of circulating somatomedin are also described.

Treatment is aimed at restoring growth hormone levels to normal. External radiation will achieve this in 70% of patients but only after 10 years. Radioactive implants give a quicker response. For small adenomas, transphenoidal surgical removal is now the treatment of choice.

Bromocriptine has also been used but normal

levels of growth hormone are achieved in only 20% of patients.

Hyperprolactinaemia

Prolactin is the commonest hormone secreted by pituitary tumours of all types. Hypersecretion causes galactorrhoea and amenorrhoea, which results from suppression of gonadotropin secretion. Young women are mostly affected.

Basal levels of serum prolactin are high, the normal nocturnal increase is absent and the response to TRH and metoclopramide is diminished. Other causes of hyperprolactinaemia, such as drug ingestion, must be excluded.

In view of the importance of preserving pituitary function in this age group, small adenomas are treated by enucleation. Larger tumours are treated by administration of bromocriptine, which inhibits prolactin release and is also reported to reduce the size of the tumour.

Careful and frequent observation is mandatory during pregnancy, as tumour expansion may threaten visual integrity.

Cushing's disease

This may be due to a functioning adenoma of ACTH-secreting cells. Only 15% of cases are associated with expansion of the pituitary fossa. Removal of the microadenoma or its irradiation relieves the syndrome (see p. 349).

Pituitary surgery and radiation

Tumours of the pituitary gland may be removed surgically or destroyed by radiation. Until recently the normal pituitary used to be removed or destroyed in the treatment of advanced breast cancer, but oestrogen-suppressing drugs are now preferred.

Surgical hypophysectomy

The pituitary can be approached transcranially (Fig. 23.11) but this is a major neurosurgical procedure involving removal of a bony flap and retraction or resection of the frontal lobes, which is now only used to remove the whole pituitary or

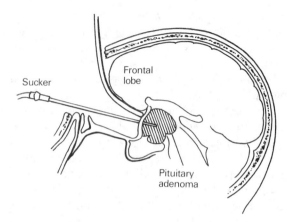

Fig. 23.11   Transcranial hypophysectomy

a large tumour with suprasellar extension. Loss of smell is a constant complication, and if the pituitary stalk is divided high, diabetes insipidus is permanent and severe.

The preferred approach for removal of a normal sized gland or enucleation of a small adenoma is transphenoidal. This is performed by an otolaryngologist who approaches the gland through the ethmoidal or sphenoidal sinuses using an operating microscope (Fig. 23.12). As the pituitary stalk is divided low down within the fossa, diabetes insipidus is rare. CSF rhinorrhoea may occur, but is usually prevented by placing a free flap of muscle into the fossa.

Occasionally a combined transcranial and transphenoidal approach is required for very large tumours.

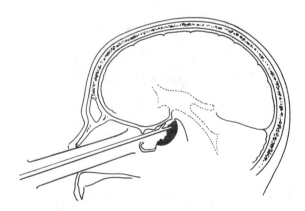

Fig. 23.12   Transphenoidal removal of a pituitary adenoma

External radiation

The pituitary gland is radio-resistant and a dose of at least 100 Gy is required to affect the function of the normal gland. Smaller doses (40–50 Gy) are used to treat acromegaly and Cushing's disease. A rotational technique avoids excessive irradiation of surrounding nervous tissue.

Larger doses of radiation can be delivered by beams of heavy particles (protons, alpha-particles or neutrons) generated by a cyclotron. These beams are narrow, with little scatter and allow high doses of radiation to be focused on small areas.

Internal irradiation

Implantation of radioactive sources by trans-ethmoidal or transphenoidal cannulation can be readily accomplished under radiological control (Fig. 23.13). The isotope most commonly used is yttrium-90, a beta-particle emitter of high energy but short half-life (64 hours). The activity of the source can be adjusted so as to achieve a complete or partial hypophysectomy.

Diabetes insipidus follows internal radiation only if the hypothalamic nuclei have been irradiated. CSF rhinorrhoea is an occasional complication. This technique has now been largely superseded by transphenoidal surgery.

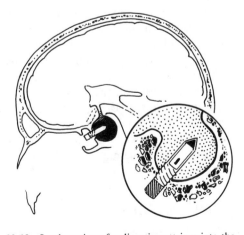

Fig. 23.13 Implantation of radioactive yttrium into the pituitary fossa

Maintenance therapy

Following total hypophysectomy, cortisol or cortisone replacement therapy is required in a dose of 37.5 mg daily. As aldosterone secretion is unaffected, there is no need for mineralocorticoid replacement.

TSH secretion is suppressed and hypothyroidism will develop over a period of some months. This is controlled by giving L-thyroxine in a dose of 0.1–0.2 mg daily.

Diabetes insipidus is a common immediate complication of hypophysectomy or insertion of radioactive implants, but is usually transient unless the pituitary stalk or hypothalamus has been damaged. Polyuria can be relieved by the vasopressin analogue desmopressin (DDAVP) given either by intranasal instillation or intramuscular injection.

Immediately following hypophysectomy additional cortisol or cortisone therapy is given to cover the normal metabolic response to surgery. During periods of further stress or trauma, protection by additional cortisone is necessary.

THE POSTERIOR PITUITARY

The neurohypophysis is a secretory and storage unit which includes the nerve cells of the supraoptic and paraventricular hypothalamic nuclei (Fig. 23.14). Fibres pass from these nuclei by the hypothalamo-hypophysial tract to the median eminence of the hypothalamus and the posterior lobe of the pituitary. The nerve cells secrete arginine vasopressin (antidiuretic hormone, ADH) and oxytocin; both of these octapeptides pass down the nerve fibres to be stored in vesicles within the pituitary.

Only vasopressin is of surgical importance. It increases the permeability of the distal renal tubule, facilitating the reabsorption of water and reducing plasma osmolality. Release of vasopressin is governed by osmoreceptors in the hypothalamus which react to slight changes (2%) in osmolality in the internal carotid circulation and by baroreceptors (both high and low pressure) in the heart and great vessels which react to changes in arterial and venous pressure.

Failure of secretion of vasopressin results in

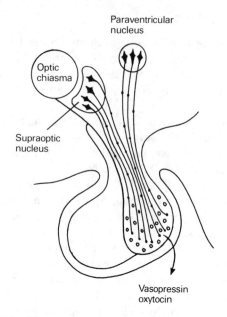

Fig. 23.14   The neurohypophysial system

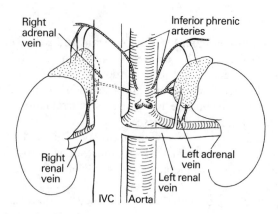

Fig. 23.15   Blood supply and venous drainage of the adrenal glands. IVC = inferior vena cava

diabetes insipidus. This may be due to trauma, inflammatory lesions, or primary or metastatic tumours. Following surgical hypophysectomy permanent diabetes insipidus occurs only if the hypothalamic nuclei have been irreparably damaged by pulling on the pituitary stalk or by its high division. Irradiation, particularly from internal sources, may cause severe diabetes insipidus.

The symptoms of diabetes insipidus are thirst and polyuria. The patient usually passes 5 to 12 litres of urine in 24 hours. The urine is dilute, with a specific gravity of 1.001–1.005 and an osmolality of 50–200 mmol/l. The osmolality of the plasma is normal (270–290 mmol/l) or slightly increased.

Inappropriate secretion of vasopressin occasionally occurs from a bronchial carcinoma or other paraendocrine tumour, leading to hyponatraemia, increased extracellular volume and renal loss of sodium. Inappropriate secretion also complicates positive pressure ventilation following surgery.

THE ADRENAL GLANDS

The adrenal glands are small, each weighing approximately 4 g. More than 90% of normal glands weigh less than 6 g. They lie immediately above and medial to the kidneys. The right adrenal lies in close contact with the inferior vena cava into which the short wide adrenal vein drains. On the left, the adrenal vein is joined by the inferior phrenic vein before running downwards to enter the renal vein (Fig. 23.15).

Knowledge of the venous drainage of the adrenals is of importance to both surgeon and radiologist. For example, in patients with suspected adrenal disorders, the radiologist may be required to cannulate the adrenal veins in order to collect blood for hormone assays.

The arterial supply arises from the aorta, the renal and the phrenic arteries. A leash of small vessels run in the periadrenal fat to reach the capsule of the gland.

Each gland consists of an outer cortex and an inner medulla which differ in origin as well as in function. The adrenal cortex is unique in that it contains highly specialized cells which secrete steroid hormones. Some steroids are also secreted by the ovary, the testis and the placenta, but only those synthesized in the adrenal cortex are termed corticosteroids. The medulla is part of the sympathetic system. It contains chromaffin cells which secrete the catecholamines adrenaline and noradrenaline.

THE ADRENAL CORTEX

Microscopically, the adrenal cortex consists of three zones of cells. Starting from the outside,

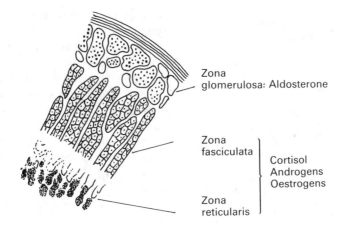

Zona
glomerulosa: Aldosterone

Zona
fasciculata

Cortisol
Androgens
Oestrogens

Zona
reticularis

Fig. 23.16 The functional zones of the adrenal cortex

these are (1) the *zona glomerulosa*, containing small cells arranged in whorls and hoops, (2) the *zona fasciculata*, with radial cords and bundles of clear fat-laden cells, and (3) the *zona reticularis*, containing small compact cells arranged indiscriminately (Fig. 23.16). These three zones form two functional layers: an outer layer, the zona glomerulosa, which secretes the mineralocorticoid aldosterone, and an inner layer, the fasciculata-reticularis, which secretes the glucocorticoids cortisol (hydrocortisone) and corticosterone, the androgenic steroids androstenedione (A), 11-hydroxy-A and testosterone, and their inactive precursor dehydroepiandrosterone sulphate (DHA-S). Precursor steroids for the synthesis of aldosterone are also synthesized. Only small amounts of progesterone and oestrogens are formed.

Control of adrenal cortical secretion

The adrenal cortex stores only a fraction of the daily requirements of hormones. They are secreted 'to order' and circulate either bound to an alpha-globulin (95%) or as free steroids (5%).

Approximately 15–20 mg of cortisol are secreted daily under the control of pituitary ACTH, which in turn is governed by the negative feedback effect of circulating cortisol (Fig. 23.17).

ACTH also stimulates the secretion of androgenic steroids. If excessive, this can cause virilization. The output of androstenedione and

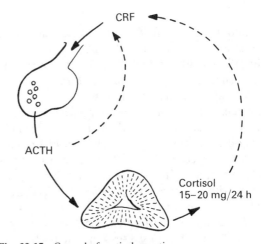

CRF

ACTH

Cortisol
15–20 mg/24 h

Fig. 23.17 Control of cortisol secretion. CRF = corticotropin releasing factor

testosterone is normally low while that of DHA-S is high (25 mg daily).

The mineralocorticoid aldosterone is secreted in small amounts of 100–200 μg daily. Circulating levels are low (0.05–0.06 μg/l). Although the secretion of aldosterone is increased by large amounts of ACTH, it is normally controlled by angiotensin (Fig. 23.18). Angiotensin is formed by the action of renin, which is secreted by the juxtaglomerular apparatus of the kidney in response to diminished perfusion. Aldosterone secretion is also sensitive to the concentrations of sodium and potassium in the circulating adrenal blood.

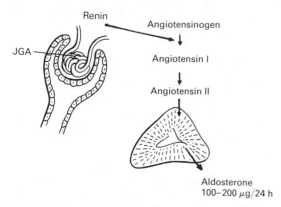

Fig. 23.18 Control of aldosterone secretion. JGA = juxtaglomerular apparatus

Functions of adrenocortical hormones

Cortisol

Maintenance of life. Cortisol is essential to life. The nature of its action is obscure, but it appears to have a vital intracellular function. It protects the body against stress, aids recovery from injury and shock, and maintains blood pressure.

Protein and carbohydrate metabolism. Cortisol has an important role in carbohydrate and protein metabolism. It encourages breakdown of proteins (catabolic effect) and stimulates gluconeogenesis while inhibiting glucose utilization (diabetogenic effect), with a consequent increase in blood sugar levels and deposition of glycogen.

Fat and water distribution. Cortisol mobilizes body stores of fat and causes hyperlipidaemia. It governs the distribution of water and fat, and has a slight mineralocorticoid effect, promoting retention of sodium and excretion of potassium, but this is of clinical relevance only when circulating cortisol levels are excessive. Renal excretion of water is enhanced.

Other actions. Excess cortisol secretion causes psychosis and mental instability. Cortisol also has an anti-inflammatory effect, reducing the number of lymphocytes and eosinophils in the blood, inhibiting fibroblastic activity and depressing antibody formation.

Aldosterone

The main action of aldosterone is to facilitate the renal exchange of potassium and hydrogen ions for sodium. It has a similar action on intestinal mucosa, sweat glands and, to some extent, on all cells. Whether potassium or hydrogen ions are exchanged depends on their availability. In low potassium states, the urine may be acid due to obligatory secretion of hydrogen rather than potassium ions despite extracellular alkalosis. Sodium retention increases plasma volume but this is limited by an escape mechanism which overrides the effect of aldosterone and permits sodium excretion.

Androgens

DHA-S is biologically inactive but is converted in fat, liver and other tissues to testosterone, its 5α-reduced products and oestrogen. Peripheral aromatization of this steroid provides the main source of oestrogen in postmenopausal women.

Adrenalectomy

Indications

Removal of normal adrenal glands was once used as palliative treatment in postmenopausal women with metastatic breast cancer. The aim was to remove the source of DHA-S and thus prevent its peripheral conversion to oestrogen. Aromatase-inhibiting drugs (aminoglutethimide and 4-hydroxyandrostenedione) have made this operation obsolete. Adrenalectomy is now only indicated for disorders due to adrenal hyperplasia (as a result of overstimulation) or adrenal tumours. This includes a wide variety of syndromes, depending on which hormone is excreted to excess.

The adrenals may be approached surgically from in front (transabdominally), from the side, or from behind (through the bed of the twelfth rib). If both glands are to be explored, a frontal approach is best.

Postoperative replacement therapy

Following bilateral total adrenalectomy, lifelong replacement therapy with corticosteroids is needed. This is best achieved with a combination of oral hydrocortisone (30 mg daily in divided doses) and the synthetic mineralocorticoid fludrocortisone acetate (0.1 mg daily). The adequacy of treatment can be assessed by estimations of blood pressure in both the erect and the supine position and by serum electrolyte determinations. Replacement therapy is not permanently required following unilateral adrenalectomy but may be necessary temporarily in Cushing's syndrome (see below). If both adrenals are removed, or the remaining adrenal is non-functional, the metabolic response to surgery must be covered by steroids during the immediate postoperative period.

Hydrocortisone sodium succinate is water-soluble and can be given by intravenous infusion during the first 24 hours. Further doses may be given intramuscularly until the patient can take cortisone by mouth. An alternative preparation for intramuscular injection is cortisone acetate in a slow-release medium. Oral cortisone is started on day 3–4 and the dose is gradually reduced to maintenance levels.

Blood pressure is the best guide to the adequacy of therapy. Should hypotension occur, 100 mg hydrocortisone sodium succinate is given immediately by intravenous injection and an intravenous infusion of saline with added cortisol (200 mg) is commenced.

Totally adrenalectomized patients must be warned to increase the dose of cortisone should stress or infection occur. They should carry a 'steroid card' giving details of their dosage and possible complications, and should be able to recognize the symptoms of steroid insufficiency (i.e. loss of appetite, nausea, cramps, muscle pains and a general feeling of malaise). If such symptoms develop, the patient should take an extra two tablets of cortisone and report to his doctor.

Failure to anticipate the need for additional steroid may precipitate an 'adrenal crisis' with acute hypotension and collapse.

Should this occur, hydrocortisone sodium succinate (100 mg) is administered intravenously and the patient admitted to hospital. An intravenous infusion with 200 mg hydrocortisone sodium succinate in 500 ml saline is set up and a regimen similar to that used in the post-adrenalectomy patient is instituted.

Cushing's syndrome

The signs and symptoms of Cushing's syndrome are due to prolonged and inappropriate secretion of cortisol. The severity and rate of progression of the disease depend on the amount of hormone secreted.

Excess secretion of cortisol may be due to a functioning tumour of the adrenal cortex (20%) or to overstimulation of normal glands by excess ACTH (80%) either of pituitary origin or from an ectopic source (Fig. 23.19).

Adrenal tumours. A benign adenoma is the commonest adrenal tumour causing Cushing's syndrome. It is almost invariably unilateral and more common in females. Histologically the tumour cells appear clear (resembling those of the zona fasciculata) or compact (resembling those of the zona reticularis).

Adrenal carcinoma is a rare cause of Cushing's syndrome. It is more common in children and young adults, grows to a large size, is highly malignant and metastasizes to liver and lungs.

The autonomous secretion of cortisol from an adrenal tumour inhibits ACTH secretion so that the contralateral gland becomes atrophic and ceases to function (Fig. 23.20).

Pituitary disease. Pituitary tumours are the commonest cause of Cushing's syndrome, accounting for almost 80% of all cases. They are usually basophil but sometimes chromophobe adenomas of ACTH-secreting cells. They may be

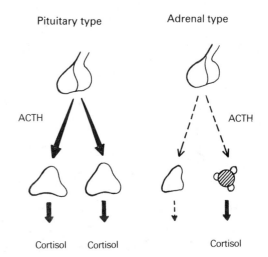

Fig. 23.19 Types of Cushing's syndrome.
(a) Overstimulation of normal gland by excess ACTH.
(b) Oversecretion by functioning tumour of the adrenal cortex.

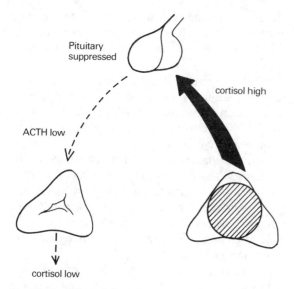

Fig. 23.20 Effect of cortisol-secreting adrenal adenoma on the opposite gland

tiny (microadenomas), large and even invasive. Both adrenals become hyperplastic. This pituitary form of the syndrome is called Cushing's *disease*.

Ectopic ACTH production. In a few cases Cushing's syndrome is caused by inappropriate secretion of an ACTH-like peptide by a tumour of

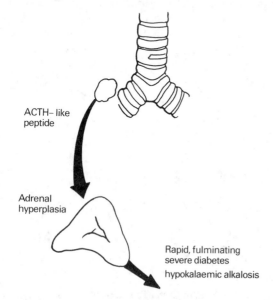

Fig. 23.21 Effects of ectopic ACTH production, in this example from a bronchial carcinoma

non-pituitary origin. This may arise in the pancreas, bronchus, thymus or other sites and is usually malignant (Fig. 23.21).

Clinical features

Cushing's syndrome occurs most frequently in young adult women. The most striking feature is truncal obesity due to redistribution of body water and fat. This may also produce the classical feature of a 'buffalo hump'. 'Mooning' of the face occurs early. As a result of protein loss, the skin becomes thin, with purple striae, dusky cyanosis and visible dermal vessels. Muscle weakness is a prominent feature. Increased capillary fragility, purpura, osteoporosis, acne, loss of libido, hirsutism, diabetes and hypertension are other common features. Amenorrhoea, hypertension and obesity tend to occur early.

These clinical signs usually develop gradually over several years and can best be recognized by reviewing old photographs. In some cases the disease runs a fulminant course, particularly when it is due to an adrenal carcinoma or ectopic secretion of ACTH. Electrolyte disturbances, pigmentation, severe diabetes and psychosis are common in these patients. Cachexia is prominent and may overshadow other features.

Investigation

Before carrying out adrenalectomy on a patient with Cushing's syndrome, it is essential to establish the source of hypersecretion of cortisol. The surgeon should assure himself of the following:

1. That cortisol hypersecretion is outwith normal control. In patients with Cushing's syndrome plasma cortisol levels are increased, its diurnal variation is lost and its secretion is not suppressed by low-dose dexamethasone or increased by insulin-hypoglycaemia.

2. That the cortisol excess is of adrenal origin. In patients with a functioning adrenal tumour, ACTH cannot be detected in the plasma and urinary secretion of cortisol is not suppressed by high-dose dexamethasone (Fig. 23.22).

3. That pituitary causes and ectopic sources of excess secretion can be excluded. In Cushing's syndrome due to a pituitary adenoma, plasma

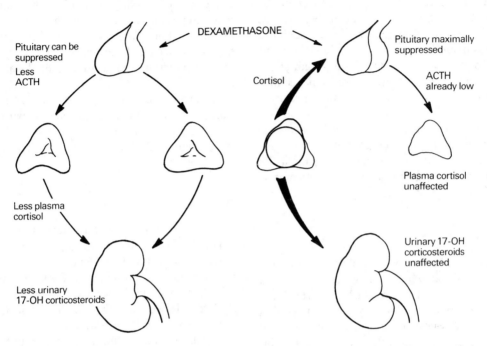

Fig. 23.22 The dexamethasone suppression test to distinguish between adrenal and pituitary causes of excess cortisol secretion

ACTH levels are inappropriately high and urinary cortisol excretion is suppressed by dexamethasone. (see Fig. 23.22).

4. That attempts have been made to localize the lesion, e.g. by CT scanning or isotope scanning using radio-labelled iodocholesterol. The source of excess cortisol secretion can be defined by selective adrenal vein catheterization with determination of cortisol levels in venous blood and injection of contrast medium to outline the tumour.

Treatment

Adrenal tumours. Adrenal adenomas are rarely bilateral, and unilateral adrenalectomy is the usual treatment. Only the affected adrenal need be explored. As the other adrenal gland is atrophic, steroid replacement therapy with cortisone is required postoperatively. Once the patient is maintained on small doses, cortisone can gradually be withdrawn, allowing the remaining adrenal a resume normal function.

Carcinomas of the adrenal causing Cushing's syndrome should also be removed if possible, but this may prove difficult. Recurrence of tumour, both locally and systemically, is common and adjuvant systemic therapy with an adrenal cytotoxin such as *o,p'*-DDD is advised. Unfortunately this drug has unpleasant gastrointestinal side effects and may not be tolerated.

Pituitary disease. The symptoms of bilateral adrenal hyperplasia due to pituitary hyperfunction (Cushing's disease) can be relieved permanently by bilateral adrenalectomy, and in some centres this is still standard practice. There are, however, two major disadvantages: (1) the patient will require lifelong steroid replacement and (2) the removal of the source of cortisol means that the pituitary is no longer suppressed by the normal feedback mechanism so that large amounts of ACTH and MSH are secreted, leading to characteristic pigmentation of the skin. Moreover, an untreated pituitary adenoma may continue to grow and cause pressure on the optic chiasma.

Irradiation of the pituitary may prevent these effects of adrenalectomy, but a direct attack on the pituitary, leaving the adrenal undisturbed, is now preferred. Microsurgical removal of the adenoma is the treatment of choice, as this preserves the function of the normal gland, thus avoiding the need for replacement therapy. In some centres implantation of yttrium-90 is the preferred treatment.

In fulminating cases with severe metabolic upset, metyrapone, aminoglutethimide or trilostane can be used to prepare the patient for operation. Some surgeons advise such preparation in all cases.

Aldosteronism

Hyperaldosteronism most commonly occurs as a secondary phenomenon in chronic liver, renal or cardiac disease. Activation of the juxtaglomerular apparatus by diminution in plasma volume, renal ischaemia or excessive use of diuretics causes hypersecretion of renin and increased stimulation of the zona glomerulosa by angiotensin.

Primary hyperaldosteronism (Conn's syndrome) is usually due to a benign adenoma and most commonly occurs in young or middle-aged women. The lesion is small (1–3 g), single, canary yellow and composed of cells of glomerulosa type. Occasionally an adrenal cortical carcinoma causes primary hyperaldosteronism. Bilateral adrenal hyperplasia and multiple adrenal microadenomas are other possible causes.

Clinical features

The classical clinical features are due to the metabolic effects of aldosterone excess, i.e. sodium retention and potassium loss. Most patients are now discovered in the course of investigation at a hypertension clinic.

Sodium retention. Retention of sodium expands plasma volume and causes hypertension. This may give rise to severe headache and visual disturbance but serious retinopathy is uncommon. Oedema is rare.

Potassium loss. In the early stages, the only evidence of potassium loss may be a moderate depression of serum potassium levels. Later there may be episodes of muscle weakness and nocturnal polyuria, the latter due to the effect of hypokalaemia on the kidneys. This is associated with vacuolation and distortion of distal tubular cells.

If unrecognized, the syndrome progresses to a state of severe hypokalaemic alkalosis with attacks of periodic muscle paralysis, tetany and paraesthesia. This full-blown picture is now rare.

Diagnosis

The finding of a low serum potassium in a hypertensive patient should alert the clinician to the possibility of primary hyperaldosteronism. Further investigations are designed to confirm hypokalaemia, demonstrate hypersecretion of aldosterone and exclude secondary hyperaldosteronism.

1. *Confirm hypokalaemia*. The demonstration of hypokalaemia may require repeated estimations on venous blood samples taken without an occluding cuff.

2. *Demonstrate hypersecretion*. Plasma aldosterone levels are measured by radioimmunoassay at 4-hourly intervals to compensate for the diurnal variation in secretion. Administration of spironolactone (an aldosterone antagonist) should result in a reduction in blood pressure and reversal of hypokalaemia.

3. *Exclude secondary hyperaldosteronism*. Measurement of plasma renin concentration is the critical investigation in the differential diagnosis. It is increased in secondary hyperaldosteronism but undetectable in the primary form. Spironolactone will increase renin levels in secondary hyperaldosteronism.

If primary hyperaldosteronism is confirmed, an attempt should be made to localize the adenoma by CT or isotope scanning using radio-labelled iodocholesterol. Blood samples are collected from both right and left adrenal and from the inferior vena cava for aldosterone estimations.

Plasma cortisol levels should always be estimated to exclude the possibility of atypical Cushing's syndrome.

Treatment

Primary hyperaldosteronism due to an adenoma is treated by removal of the adrenal with its contained tumour. It is important that hypokalaemia is first corrected. This can be done with oral potassium supplements and spironolactone or triamterene.

Primary hyperaldosteronism due to adrenal hyperplasia can be cured by bilateral adrenalectomy, but at too great a price. Chemotherapy with triamterene and amiloride is preferable to long-term administration of spironolactone.

Adrenogenital syndrome (Adrenal virilism)

This syndrome is due to a genetically determined enzyme defect which impairs cortisol synthesis. The resultant deficiency in this hormone stimulates the pituitary to increase production of ACTH. This causes adrenal hyperplasia and inappropriate secretion of adrenal androgens.

The effect depends on the sex and age at which the disease become manifest. Female infants show enlargment of the clitoris and varying degrees of fusion of the genital folds. Later, other signs of virilism appear, leading to precocious heterosexual puberty. Young boys have isosexual precocious puberty.

In both sexes there are striking abnormalities of growth. Bone growth is rapid at first, but the epiphyses fuse early so that the final height is stunted. Excess muscle growth produces the 'Infant Hercules' appearance. Milder forms of the disease may affect older girls and cause hirsutism and acne. Associated metabolic abnormalities depend on the type of enzyme block. Thus, 21-hydroxylase deficiency may lead to excessive loss of salt due to aldosterone deficiency, while 11-hydroxylase deficiency commonly gives rise to hypertension as a result of the accumulation of 11-deoxycortisol.

The syndrome is effectively treated by glucocorticoid administration which both supplies the patient's needs for cortisol and suppresses ACTH overproduction. Surgical correction of the genital abnormality may be required.

Rarely virilism may be due to an adrenal tumour, which is usually large and malignant.

Adrenal feminization

Exceptionally, a tumour of the adrenal cortex may secrete oestrogens. Such tumours are usually large and malignant. In the female there is isosexual precocity; in the male feminization with gynaecomastia, decreased libido and testicular atrophy. Treatment consists of removal of the tumour but recurrence and metastatic spread are invariable.

THE ADRENAL MEDULLA

The adrenal medulla contains chromaffin cells which are derived from the neural crest and secrete catecholamines into the circulation. The cells belong to the APUD series (see below) and are supplied by preganglionic sympathetic nerves. The adrenal medulla is not essential to life. There are other collections of chromaffin cells in paraganglia in the retroperitoneum, mediastinum and neck. The normal adrenal medulla produces catecholamines in the ratio 80% adrenaline to 20% noradrenaline. It also secretes dopamine which acts as a precursor to noradrenaline.

Adrenaline

Adrenaline acts on both alpha- and beta-adrenergic receptors to redistribute blood flow by constricting skin and splanchnic vessels and dilating those of the heart, skeletal muscles and brain. It causes tachycardia, induces a sense of anxiety and has a number of metabolic effects. These include the conversion of glycogen to glucose in the liver, and an increase in the concentration of free circulating fatty acids.

Noradrenaline

Noradrenaline acts on alpha-receptors to constrict all blood vessels and raise the systolic and diastolic blood pressure. It has little effect on the central nervous system or metabolism.

Small amounts of catecholamines are excreted in the urine in free and conjugated form. Larger amounts are excreted as metabolites such as meta-derivatives (e.g. metnoradrenaline); 3-methoxy-4-hydroxymandelic acid (VMA); and 3-methoxy-4-hydroxyphenylglycol.

Phaeochromocytoma

Phaeochromocytomas are tumours of the adrenal medulla which secrete large amounts of adrenaline and noradrenaline. They may also occur in extra-adrenal paraganglionic tissue, most often in the retroperitoneum near the kidneys and occasionally in more distant locations such as the posterior mediastinum or neck, pelvis or urinary bladder. Extra-adrenal phaeochromocytomas secrete only noradrenaline. Virtually all tumours (99%) arise within the abdomen, 90% in the adrenals. One-tenth of patients have multiple tumours which may affect both adrenals.

A phaeochromocytoma is usually benign, about 5 cm in diameter, highly vascular and chocolate-brown in colour. Histologically the cells resemble those of the normal adrenal medulla and stain with chromate. Approximately 5% are malignant and metastasize.

Associated conditions are neurofibromatosis, medullary carcinoma of the thyroid (as part of multiple endocrine neoplasia type II), duodenal ulcer and renal artery stenosis.

Clinical features

Phaeochromocytomas present before the age of 50 years. Their clinical features depend on the proportions of adrenaline and noradrenaline secreted by the tumour. Noradrenaline excess causes hypertension, while excess secretion of adrenaline has metabolic effects (e.g. thyrotoxicosis) and may give rise to hypotension.

Paroxysmal hypertension is the most characteristic symptom and is due to the sudden release of catecholamines from the tumour. This may be precipitated by abdominal pressure, exercise or postural change. During an attack, the blood pressure rises to above 200/100 mmHg and there is headache, palpitations, sweating, extreme anxiety and chest and abdominal pain. Pallor, dilated pupils and tachycardia are notable.

In some patients persistent hypertension may develop at the age of 30–40 years. In this case the clinical features are those of severe hypertension associated with moderate or severe retinopathy. Fundal changes include vascular spasm, optic atrophy and blindness. Glycosuria is common.

There is mottling of the skin and tingling of the extremities. Extra-adrenal phaeochromocytomas are always associated with persistent hypertension. If the tumour in the bladder, micturition may precipitate a syncopal attack.

A few patients present in other ways. In some, metabolic effects predominate and the patient may present with thyrotoxicosis. In others the presenting feature may be paroxysmal hypotension.

An unsuspected phaeochromocytoma may cause sudden unexplained death after trauma or an operation. The possibility that a patient may have a phaeochromocytoma and thus need further investigations must therefore never be ignored.

Investigation

All young hypertensives should be screened for a catecholamine-secreting tumour. The most reliable test is urinary determination of the catecholamine metabolite vanillylmandelic acid (VMA) following a paroxysm.

A CT or iodobenzylguanidine scan may visualize the tumour. As the tumour is highly vascular, it may be demonstrated by arteriography. Selective adrenal venous sampling may help to define the site of excess catecholamine secretion. These invasive techniques should be performed only under full adrenergic blockade.

Treatment

Surgical removal of the tumour is the treatment of choice. The introduction of alpha- and beta-adrenergic blocking drugs has greatly reduced the risks of this operation. The potential for hypertensive attacks during induction of anaesthesia or handling of the tumour is reduced and tachycardia and arrhythmias are prevented.

The patient should come to operation with both blood pressure and pulse rate controlled (see below). As preoperative adrenergic blockade also restores blood volume, troublesome hypotension following removal of the tumour is now unusual but must be borne in mind. Maintenance of blood volume during operation is important.

Long-acting preparations are preferred. The alpha-receptor blocker phenoxybenzamine is started 7–10 days preoperatively to control blood pressure. The beta-blocker propanolol may then be added to reduce tachycardia. A combined preparation may be used, but beta-blocking agents should never be given first, as this may precipitate cardiac failure.

Atropine should not be used for premedication and thiopentone is best avoided. Enflurane is the preferred anaesthetic. Pulse and blood pressure are monitored. Phentolamine and propranolol (short-acting alpha- and beta-blocking agents), sodium nitroprusside (which acts directly on vessels independent of adrenergic receptors and allows additional control of hypertension) and blood should be available. Because of the frequency of multiple tumours, both adrenals are examined.

Non-endocrine tumours

Neuroblastoma

This is a highly malignant tumour of the adrenal medulla arising from primitive sympathetic nervous tissue of neural crest origin. It is one of the commonest malignant tumours of infants and young children, and metastasizes widely to lymph nodes, liver, bones and lung. Skeletal metastases may be confused with bone sarcoma. About 75% of these tumours secrete catecholamines.

Treatment by radical surgical excision, radiotherapy and chemotherapy offers the only hope of benefit.

Ganglioneuroma

These are benign, firm, well encapsulated tumours arising from ganglion cells. They grow slowly, do not metastasize and may reach a large size. Severe diarrhoea may be a feature. Treatment by surgical excision gives excellent results.

APUDOMAS AND MULTIPLE ENDOCRINE NEOPLASIA

Cells which secrete amines and polypeptide hormones have certain characteristics in common. These are a capacity to store amines (e.g. catecholamines), the ability to take up amine precursors (such as dopamine), and the possession of the decarboxylating enzyme which is necessary

for amine synthesis. The acronym APUD (amine precursor uptake and decarboxylation) reflects the common properties of these cells, which can be demonstrated by specific histochemical and immunofluorescent techniques.

Derived from neural ectoderm, they are believed to migrate from the neural crest to various endocrine tissues, where they serve specific functions. For example, APUD cells in the anterior pituitary secrete ACTH; those in the carotid body and adrenal medulla secrete catecholamines; while those in the thyroid secrete calcitonin. APUD cells abound in the intestinal tract, both singly and in conglomerates, as in the pancreatic islets. In the gut they are responsible for the secretion of the 5-hydroxytryptamine and histamine, and a large series of polypeptide hormones (including secretin, cholecystokinin, gastrin, enteroglucagon, somatostatin, vasoactive intestinal peptide) which regulate gastrointestinal secretion and motor function. Some believe the origin of the gut APUD cells to be endodermal.

Tumours and hyperplasia of APUD cells account for many of the endocrine syndromes described in this chapter as well as those which affect the pancreatic islets (see Ch. 37). They are also believed to be responsible for ectopic hormone secretion from non-endocrine sites, e.g. secretion of ACTH or serotinin by bronchial carcinomas.

Multiple endocrine neoplasia

Tumour formation by APUD cells is not limited to single sites. For example, in multiple endocrine neoplasia (MEN) a number of endocrine glands are affected. The commonest syndromes are due to abnormal production of hormones by the anterior pituitary, adrenal medulla, pancreas and C-cells of the thyroid. However, parathyroid hyperplasia is also a feature although, as APUD cells do not contribute to the formation of parathormone, the mechanism is obscure. The MEN syndromes are very rare. They are inherited as autosomal dominant traits with varied penetrance. The tumours may be benign or malignant.

MEN I is characterized by hormone-producing lesions (hyperplasia and/or tumours) of the parathyroid, pancreatic islets and anterior pituitary. A variety of non-endocrine tumours may also occur, e.g. in the thyroid, pituitary, adrenal gland and soft tissues (lipomas), and carcinoid tumours have been described.

There is a disparity between the clinical presentation and the endocrine abnormality. Thus, while most cases present with peptic ulceration or its complications, the most common (90–95%) endocrine abnormality is hyperparathyroidism. Excess secretion of gastrin from pancreatic islet cells occurs in 20–40% and hypersecretion of insulin in 10%. Pituitary syndromes (acromegaly) are rare; chromophobe adenomas of the pituitary are more common.

Treatment is directed at the dominant feature. As hyperplasia of the parathyroid inevitably affects all four glands, these should be removed and a remnant implanted into an accessible site from which it can later be removed if recurrence develops. As the disease is familial, screening of other family members is important.

MEN II is an inherited syndrome characterized by the triad of medullary carcinoma of the thyroid, phaeochromocytoma and parathyroid hyperplasia. Two main subgroups are described.

In MEN type IIa medullary carcinoma of the thyroid is predominant. One-third of cases also have a phaeochromocytoma or parathyroid hyperplasia or both.

In MEN type IIb medullary carcinoma of the thyroid and phaeochromocytoma occur without parathyroid abnormality. However, there is overgrowth of nervous tissue causing multiple mucosal neuromas, thickened nerves and ganglioneuromatosis of the gut. The patient develops a typical facies with thick nodular lips, Marfan-like habitus, lax ligaments and a tendency to joint subluxation.

Both these syndromes are diagnosed by the demonstration of increased levels of plasma calcitonin reflecting hypersecretion from neoplastic parafollicular cells in the thyroid. This test is also used to screen other family members for occult lesions. Patients with asymptomatic MEN II syndrome show a rapid rise of calcitonin following bolus intravenous injection of pentagastrin.

The surgical treatment of MEN II is directed primarily at the medullary carcinoma of the thyroid, which is treated by total thyroidectomy. In all cases, urinary catacholamines and VMA must be determined. If this points to a phaeochromocytoma, this should be treated first. In patients with metastatic carcinoma, doxorubicin is the chemotherapeutic agent of choice. The success of treatment can be monitored by regular plasma calcitonin estimations.

Carcinoid syndrome

This syndrome is caused by excessive circulating levels of 5-hydroxytryptamine (serotonin). The carcinoid tumour responsible consists of argen taffin APUD cells.

Carcinoid tumours arise most commonly in the appendix and small bowel but can develop anywhere in the gastrointestinal tract. Only about 10% of such tumours give rise to the carcinoid syndrome, which consists of flushing attacks, abdominal colic with diarrhoea, and bronchospasm. The flushing is characteristically patchy and of variable duration and, like diarrhoea, it is sometimes precipitated by food or exercise. Heart rate and cardiac output may increase and lesions of the valves of the right side of the heart may develop.

The carcinoid syndrome occurs only when the humoral products of the tumour are not inactivated by the liver. In the case of carcinoids arising from the gut this usually implies that there are extensive liver metastases, and hepatomegaly is often detected in such patients. Occasionally the syndrome develops in association with cancer of the thyroid or testis.

The diagnosis is confirmed by finding high urinary concentrations of the serotonin metabolite 5-hydroxyindoleacetic acid (5-HIAA). Resection of the primary tumour should be undertaken wherever possible and resection of liver metastases can give worthwhile palliation. Somatostatin analogues can also relieve symptoms but at present they can only be given parenterally.

Carcinoid tumours of the small bowel and appendix are described in Chapters 31 and 33 respectively.

24. Head, neck and salivary glands

DISEASES OF THE HEAD AND NECK

The majority of head and neck conditions present as swellings. From the anatomical position of the swelling it is usually possible to diagnose which structure is affected (Fig. 24.1). The clinician's next task is to decide which pathological process is involved, and this decision is based initially on the history and findings on clinical examination. Clinical examination entails inspection followed by systematic palpation of all areas of the head and neck, and not just the area giving rise to symptoms. Classification of neck swellings into midline or lateral swellings is of great help in diagnosis (Table 24.1). Inflammatory conditions give rise to tenderness, whereas neoplastic swellings can usually be palpated without causing distress. Cysts in the head and neck may be too deep-seated or

Table 24.1 Classification of neck swellings (other than skin, subcutaneous tissues and lipomas)

Midline swellings
  Sublingual dermoid
  Thyroglossal cyst
  Pretracheal lymph node
  Subhyoid bursa
  Nodule in thyroid isthmus

Lateral swellings
1. *Anterior triangle*
  Lymph nodes
  Enlargement of submandibular salivary gland
  Pharyngeal diverticulum
  Laryngocoele
  Branchial cyst
  Lesion of the lower pole of the parotid
2. *Posterior triangle*
  Lymph nodes
  Carotid body tumour
  Cystic hygroma
  Cervical rib

tense to allow fluctuation to be elicited. If a mass is hard and indurated, it is likely to be neoplastic (although some neoplasms can feel surprisingly cystic).

On completion of history taking and clinical examination the site and nature of the disease process are often so clear that detailed laboratory and radiological examination is unnecessary. Diagnostic difficulty may be encountered if the swelling is only present intermittently, as in the case of intermittent blockage of the duct draining a salivary gland. Radiology can then be of value. If a swelling is considered to be neoplastic, spread into structures such as bone can also be assessed radiologically. If it is thought to be a secondary neoplastic deposit in a lymph node, the primary site has to be sought, and detailed examination of the upper alimentary and respiratory tracts,

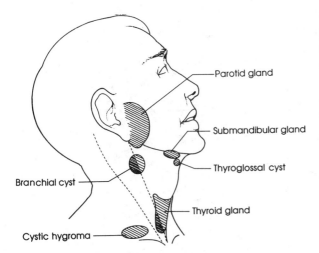

Fig. 24.1 Location of common swellings in the head and neck shown relative to the sternocleidomastoid muscle. Thyroglossal cysts are located in the midline of the neck

355

including endoscopy under general anaesthesia if need be, is essential.

In most cases a definitive diagnosis can be obtained by excising the lesion and examining it histologically. It is important that this is done by total *excision* of the lesion and not by incision biopsy. Excision is curative in many instances, whereas incision biopsy of a neoplasm increases the risk of tumour cell spillage and local recurrence even if the tumour is subsequently excised.

Congenital abnormalities

The mandibular region and neck are thought to develop from five branchial arches, each consisting of a mesenchymal core covered by ectoderm and lined by endoderm. The arches are separated externally by four branchial clefts matched internally by the pharyngeal pouches (Fig. 24.2).

Thyroglossal cyst

The thyroid gland develops from a midline tubular outgrowth of cells from the foramen caecum at the base of the tongue (Fig. 24.3a). This thyroglossal duct tracks through the body of the developing hyoid bone and then bifurcates to give rise to solid masses of cells which form the isthmus and lobes of the thyroid gland. The duct normally disappears in early fetal life; persistence of any part of it may give rise to midline thyroglossal cysts (Fig. 24.3b) and on extremely rare occasions to aberrant masses of thyroid tissue.

Thyroglossal cysts are the commonest congenital neck swelling. Although they may be present at birth, they more often present in adolescence or early adult life as a painless, smooth, rounded midline swelling. The swelling is usually located between the thyroid isthmus and hyoid bone and is non-tender and of a rubbery consistency. The cyst sometimes transilluminates but fluctuation is rarely elicited. Characteristically, the cyst moves upwards when the patient protrudes his tongue or swallows. Rarely the patient presents with a discharging sinus (if the cyst has become infected).

Thyroglossal cysts are normally excised for cosmetic reasons and to avoid recurrent infection. General anaesthesia is required and the body of the hyoid may have to be removed so that all of the

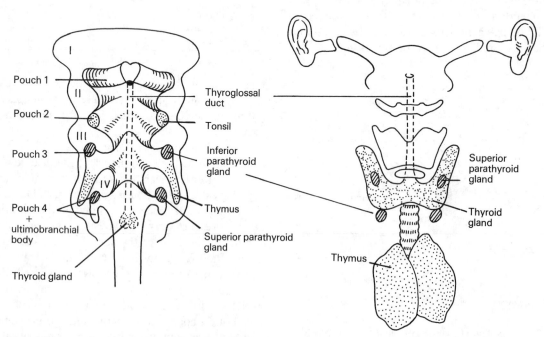

Fig. 24.2 Diagrammatic representation of the embryonic development of the floor of the mouth and neck. Roman numerals refer to the branchial arches

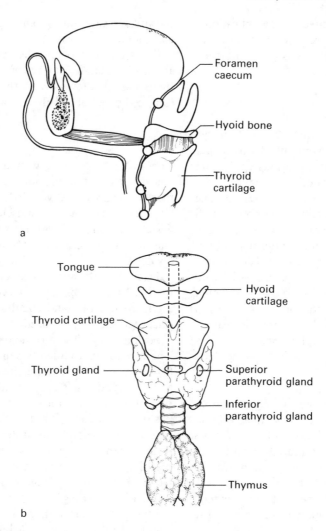

Fig. 24.3 Development of thyroglossal cyst. (a) Course of the thyroglossal duct in the midline of the neck. (b) Potential sites for the development of thyroglossal cysts

thyroglossal duct remnant can be cored out as far as the base of the tongue.

Branchial cyst

Branchial cysts rarely present before adolescence, calling into question the belief that they arise from congenital failure of fusion of the second and third branchial arches. The cyst presents as a deep-seated painless swelling bulging forwards from the anterior border of the sternocleidomastoid muscle at the level of the hyoid bone (see Fig. 24.1). The cyst has an epithelial lining and contains opaque watery or milky fluid in which cholesterol crystals are suspended. As they contain lymphoid tissue in their walls, branchial cysts are prone to infection, which tends to be recurrent. Rarely, infection is followed by the appearance of a discharging sinus. Even more unusual is the development of a branchial fistula in which there is an internal opening into the tonsillar fossa. Such fistulas are present at birth and are frequently associated with a mucopurulent discharge from the external opening at the anterior border of the lower third of the sternocleidomastoid muscle.

Branchial cysts should be excised for cosmetic

reasons and to prevent infective complications. General anaesthesia is required, and in the case of a branchial fistula, complete excision of the tract is essential.

Dermoid cyst

Dermoid cysts result from sequestration of epidermis during fusion of embryonic blocks of tissue. They are lined by stratified squamous epithelium and contain cheesy material produced by desquamation. They present as painless mobile swellings of the forehead, eyebrow region (external angular dermoid), at the base of the nose, and in the midline of the neck (submental dermoid). Sublingual dermoids may protrude from beneath the tongue, while submental dermoids are easily confused with thyroglossal cysts although they do not move on protrusion of the tongue.

Dermoid cysts are excised for cosmetic reasons and to prevent infective complications.

Cystic hygroma

Cystic hygroma is a rare type of benign lymphangioma which is usually present at birth and causes problems during delivery. The multilocular cysts contain clear lymphatic fluid and are lined by endothelium. They form a soft and readily transilluminable swelling just lateral to the sternocleidomastoid muscle and the cysts may extend into the axilla or mediastinum to cause pressure symptoms.

Surgical removal under general anaesthesia is indicated and may have to be undertaken urgently if there is airway obstruction or any evidence of infection.

Sternocleidomastoid tumour

This hard fusiform swelling of the lower third of the sternocleidomastoid muscle is thought to result from ischaemic fibrosis during birth injury. The swelling may resolve spontaneously, or fibrosis of the muscle may pull down the mastoid process on the affected side so that the head is tilted to look to the opposite side (congenital torticollis). If uncorrected, the deformity becomes permanent and the child compensates by lifting the shoulder on the affected side, thus producing secondary cervical and thoracic scoliosis.

Deformity can be avoided by rotating the head and neck through a full range of movement several times daily. Alternatively, the shortened muscle can be divided above the clavicle.

Cut throat

The majority of such wounds are self-inflicted. The neck is often extended during wounding so that the main blood vessels are protected by the taut sternocleidomastoid muscles. However, major vessels within the carotid sheath may be cut and the upper alimentary and respiratory tracts opened.

Damage to the airway poses an immediate threat to life. Inhaled blood and secretions should be aspirated urgently and endotracheal intubation or tracheostomy may be needed.

Haemorrhage is the commonest cause of death. The bleeding is frequently venous and usually follows damage to the external jugular vein. Straining and struggling increase venous bleeding and the patient should be nursed in a slightly head-up position to reduce venous pressure. Air embolus may follow the sucking of air into the open vein if the patient is allowed to sit up or stand. Internal bleeding after a stab injury can produce subfascial haematomas, compression of neck structures, and sudden haemorrhage into a pleural space.

Emergency surgical exploration is obviously mandatory if the airway has been opened, a major vessel continues to bleed or a haematoma has developed. It is also necessary if there is any suspicion that the pharynx or oesophagus has been opened, as leakage of food and fluids into the neck with resultant infection must be prevented. Otherwise it is unnecessary to explore the wound; the risk of infection is low and surgery itself can damage important structures.

Acute infections in the neck

Applied anatomy

Spread in cervical fascial planes is a dangerous complication of acute infections involving the neck. The superficial cervical fascia has no surgical importance. The deep cervical fascia, however, which lies beneath the platysma and invests the neck muscles, has considerable surgical importance (Fig. 24.4).

The investing layer of the deep fascia passes from the ligamentum nuchae and the spine of the seventh cervical vertebra to invest the sterno-cleidomastoid, and then continues across the anterior triangle to merge with the corresponding layer from the other side.

The carotid sheath is a condensation of the deep cervical fascia which encloses the common and internal carotid arteries, the internal jugular vein, the vagus nerve and the ansa cervicalis. The prevertebral lamina of the cervical fascia covers the prevertebral muscles, then extends laterally to cover the scalene muscles as a floor for the posterior triangle. The nerves of the brachial plexus carry this fascia down behind the clavicle as the axillary sheath.

Anteriorly the vertebral fascia is separated from the pharynx by the retropharyngeal space, which contains loose areolar tissue. The pretracheal lamina of the cervical fascia forms a thin fascial sheath which encloses the thyroid gland and attaches it superiorly to the arch of the cricoid cartilage.

The investing layer of the cervical fascia opposes the spread of infection superficially and enclosed pus tends to spread within these fascial planes. Pus in the anterior triangle may spread down into the mediastinum in front of the pretracheal lamina, but the investing layer is relatively thin over this

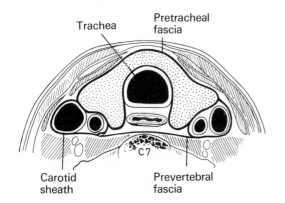

Fig. 24.4 Diagrammatic transerve section of the neck at the level of the seventh cervical vertebra to show the arrangement of the deep cervical fascia

area and abscesses may point to the surface above the sternum. Pus behind the prevertebral lamina may track laterally from the spine to point in the posterior triangle, or penetrate anteriorly to occupy the retropharyngeal space and bulge into the pharynx.

Superficial infection

1. *Furuncles* (superficial boils) are common in the back of the neck and pinna. Infection begins in a hair follicle and the overlying skin becomes reddened before it turns white and necrotic. Induration, pain and tenderness are common, but lymphadenitis and systemic upset are rare. Most boils discharge spontaneously but incision and drainage may be required. Diabetes must be excluded if the problem is recurrent.

2. *Carbuncles* develop if hair follicle infection spreads to involve the dermis and subcutaneous tissues. Many of the infected extensions open to the surface as multiple discharging sinuses. There is death of the central portion of the carbuncle and a black necrotic core develops. Carbuncles are usually more extensive than their surface appearance suggests and wide excision is needed to remove all infected sinus tracts. The patient is often febrile and toxic, may prove to be diabetic, and requires antibiotics in addition to surgery.

Deep infection

Deep cervical infections arise from a primary focus in the mouth, salivary glands, pharynx, oesophagus or larynx. Cellulitis can spread rapidly and widely beneath the investing layer of the deep cervical fascia to involve the mediastinum or compress the trachea and larynx.

Ludwig's angina denotes infection involving the floor of the mouth and often arising from a sub-mandibular lymph gland. Faulty oral hygiene is common. The patient presents with swelling in the floor of the mouth or suprahyoid region, protrusion of the tongue, trismus, difficulty in speech, dysphagia and dyspnoea. Treatment consists of antibiotic therapy, bearing in mind that the organism responsible is usually a haemolytic streptococcus. Surgical incision and drainage may be needed if there is compression of respiratory or vascular structures, or if oedema and fever persist for more than a few days despite energetic antibiotic therapy. Tracheostomy is required if there is airway obstruction. Future problems are avoided by attention to dental and oral hygiene and eradication of any focus of infection.

Other swellings within the skin and subcutaneous tissues

These are the commonest swellings in the head and neck, and the fact that swellings originate in the skin is relatively easy to determine because they can be picked up in a skinfold.

Sebaceous cysts

These cysts (see Ch. 18) are common in the sebum-producing areas of the skin and are particularly common in the scalp and neck. The presence of a punctum on the swelling is the key to diagnosis. The cyst can be excised under local anaesthesia using an elliptical incision which contains the punctum. Frequently the cysts become infected and then have to be distinguished from furuncles. Incision and drainage allows resolution and if the cyst recurs it can be excised while uninfected.

Lipomas

Lipomas in the head and neck are similar to those found elsewhere in the body and their diagnosis and management are identical (see Ch. 18).

Skin carcinoma

Apart from the hands, the head and neck are the areas most exposed to sunlight and hence are a common site for basal cell carcinomas, squamous carcinomas and malignant melanomas (see Ch. 18). These lesions are all commoner in fair, freckly, non-tanning individuals and should be suspected if any skin lesion increases rapidly in size. Excision biopsy is then indicated for histological diagnosis and is curative in most cases. Excision is best done under general anaesthesia so that adequate margins can be included and a satisfactory cosmetic result can be achieved by direct closure, local skin flaps or full thickness grafts, depending on the site and size of the lesion. Histological examination will then determine which type of malignancy, if any, was present and whether excision has been complete.

SALIVARY GLAND SWELLINGS AND DISEASE

There are three paired major salivary glands (the parotid, the submandibular and the sublingual) in addition to multiple small unnamed glands scattered throughout the mucosa of the mouth, cheeks, lips and palate. Inflammatory disease and tumours generally involve a single gland, the main exceptions being viral parotitis (mumps) and autoimmune diseases.

Surgical anatomy

Parotid gland

The parotid gland lies below the external acoustic meatus in a recess bounded by the ramus of the mandible and the sternocleidomastoid muscle. It projects forwards on the surface of the masseter. Its upper pole extends to just below the zygoma, its lower pole into the neck (Fig. 24.5). The gland is enclosed in a sheath of deep cervical fascia,

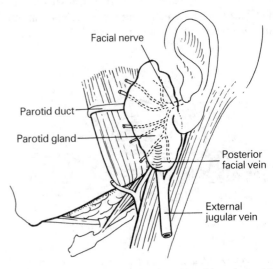

Fig. 24.5 Anatomy of the parotid gland and its relationship to the facial nerve

which makes palpation difficult and means that any acute swelling is extremely painful. Normally the only palpable part is that which overlies the ramus of the mandible. The parotid duct system combines within the gland to form a common duct which runs over the edge of the masseter muscle to enter the mouth opposite the second upper molar tooth. The anterior part of this duct can be palpated bimanually and is readily cannulated. The facial nerve runs through the superficial part of the parotid gland after leaving the stylomastoid foramen, and divides within the parotid into its main branches, which emerge to supply the muscles of facial expression. Though the gland is often described as having a superficial and a deep lobe, this division is created surgically when the gland superficial to the facial nerve is removed while preserving the nerve.

The main diagnostic difficulty with parotid lesions is usually to distinguish them from enlarged upper cervical lymph nodes when the parotid swelling is in the neck. Less commonly an enlarged preauricular lymph node may be thought to be a parotid swelling. Rarely, retrotonsillar enlargement in the oropharynx may be the result of an infiltrating parotid neoplasm.

Submandibular gland

The larger superficial portion of the submandibular gland fills most of the digastric triangle, extending upwards beneath the body of the mandible (Fig. 24.6). It rests on the mylohyoid muscle, hyoglossus and posterior pharyngeal wall. The smaller deep portion of the gland extends between the mylohyoid and hyoglossus muscles, and from it the submandibular duct runs forward to open on the floor of the mouth at the side of the frenulum of the tongue (Fig. 24.7). The normal gland is palpable bimanually with one finger on the floor of the mouth and the other in the submandibular region. The facial artery and vein and the cervical branch of the facial nerve run over the lateral border of the gland, and the lingual and hypoglossal nerves are deep to it. All of these structures can be easily damaged during surgery. The commonest cause of swellings in the digastric triangle is disease in the submandibular gland.

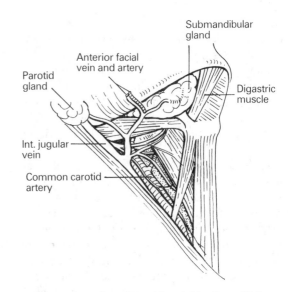

Fig. 24.6 Anatomical relationships of the submandibular gland

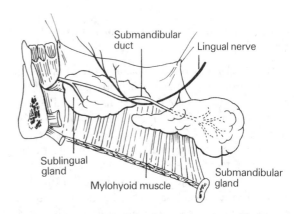

Fig. 24.7 Anatomical relationships of the submandibular duct as seen from within the floor of the mouth

Sublingual gland

The sublingual gland is the smallest of the named paired salivary glands. It lies submucosally in the floor of the mouth. It is adjacent to the submandibular duct, into which it secretes, as well as having several other separate openings. It is rarely affected by disease.

Surgical physiology

Saliva has several important functions. It lubricates food to enable swallowing, cleanses the mouth, digests starch, mediates taste and provides an immunological defence system. The composition of saliva secreted by each gland varies, the submandibular gland providing large volumes of high-viscosity calcium-enriched fluid, whereas the parotid gland secretes smaller volumes of serous fluid. Secretion is continuous throughout the day, but is highest during eating and lowest during sleep.

In diseases where the secretory cells are damaged, such as sialadenitis and autoimmune disease, the volume and composition of saliva changes, although it is not usual to analyse the secretions for diagnostic purposes. The commonest result of altered saliva composition is stone formation — sialolithiasis. This most frequently occurs in the submandibular duct because submandibular secretions are mucinous and high in calcium content. Calculi consist of concentric lamina of calcareous and organic material.

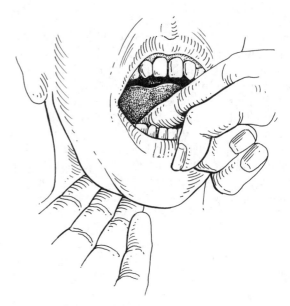

Fig. 24.8 Bimanual palpation of the submandibular gland and duct

Examination and investigation of salivary gland disease

Salivary gland disease usually presents as a unilateral or bilateral glandular enlargement which may be painful. These distinctions are of diagnostic value (Table 24.2). The affected gland must be carefully palpated for any enlargement and tenderness. Frequently the enlargement is diffuse rather than discrete because the fascia covering the gland is tight. With parotid disease, a change in the contour of the face may be the only sign of enlargement. Bimanual palpation of the submandibular and sublingual glands and ducts (Fig. 24.8) and of the parotid duct should always be carried out. Stones within the ducts can be palpated and the orifices should be inspected to

identify any exudate following massage of the gland.

Plain transoral X-ray of the submandibular region is used to detect stones, and sialography can be used to outline any of the duct systems if a secretion abnormality is suspected. In a normal sialogram the arborizations of the duct are fine, regular and symmetrical. Abnormalities include displacement, distortion, stricture, dilation and sacculation (sialectasis). Radiology is usually of little value in distinguishing benign from malignant tumours, but fine needle aspiration cytology can be valuable if an experienced pathologist is available. Antinuclear antibody determinations and lip biopsy to examine the minor salivary glands histologically can provide the diagnosis in autoimmune disease.

Infective conditions

Mumps

After a prodromal period, patients with viral parotitis (mumps) usually develop bilateral, diffusely enlarged and tender parotid glands. These changes subside spontaneously, and symptomatic treatment is all that is needed. Less commonly the

Table 24.2 Symptomatology and laterality of parotid gland disease

| | Pain | Swelling | |
		Unilateral	Bilateral
Mumps (viral parotitis)	+		+
Acute parotitis	+	+	
Sialadenitis	+	+	
Autoimmune disease	+		+
Neoplasia	−	+	

condition involves other salivary glands or is associated with sensorineural hearing impairment or orchitis (in adults). The incidence of mumps should gradually fall in countries where immunization programmes are active.

Acute parotitis

The parotid duct is normally flushed continuously by the flow of secretions. Ascending infection is likely if flow becomes depressed in elderly, debilitated and dehydrated patients with poor oral hygiene. The gland is particularly vulnerable in the postoperative period, and if infection occurs, staphylococcal organisms are usually responsible. With improved standards of care the condition has now become extremely uncommon.

Because the gland cannot expand, pain is severe. Systemic upset is marked and the patient has a swinging temperature. The parotid is tender and diffusely enlarged, forming a smooth convex swelling in front of the ear and overlying the angle of the jaw. The skin becomes stretched, shiny and reddened, and trismus is marked. The duct orifice is red and patulous and there may be a purulent discharge. Gentle 'milking' of the gland may evoke a gush of pus from the duct. A bacteriological swab should be taken.

Treatment of acute parotitis. Prophylaxis is vital. All elderly and debilitated patients who require surgery must be adequately hydrated. In addition they should have frequent mouthwashes and have their gums painted with a viscous antiseptic (bromoglycerol). They are encouraged to masticate, and acid drops or chewing gum are helpful stimulants to salivation.

As soon as acute parotitis is suspected, the patient is given full doses of a broad spectrum antibiotic and is fully rehydrated. If there is no marked improvement within the next 48 hours, the gland should be surgically decompressed.

Inflammatory conditions

Sialectasis

Sialectasis, or chronic dialation of the duct system, usually affects the parotid, and leads to episodes of pain and distension due to stasis and infection.

Sialography is diagnostic and shows a dilated, distended duct system. An autoimmune basis should be excluded. Management is symptomatic, superficial parotidectomy being reserved for patients with severe problems.

Sjögren's syndrome

This is the commonest form of autoimmune disease affecting both the major and the minor salivary glands and comprises the triad of dry mouth (xerostomia), dry eye (keratoconjunctivitis sicca) and other evidence of collagen disease, most frequently rheumatoid arthritis or Raynaud's phenomenon. Clinically, there is chronic enlargement of any or all of the major salivary glands and the mouth is dry. If the patient is still dentulous, there may be gross caries. Dryness of the eye can be confirmed by Schirmer's test (measuring the rate of secretion by hooking a strip of filter paper over the lower lid). The diagnosis is best confirmed by biopsy of the minor salivary glands in the lip, and organ-specific and non-organ specific antibodies can be sought serologically. Management is symptomatic with attention to oral hygiene and eye drops. Rarely, lymphoma can develop secondarily.

Sialolithiasis

Salivary calculi are most common in the submandibular gland or duct and the patient usually presents with intermittent painful enlargement of the gland associated with eating. In the chronic condition, the gland becomes fibrosed, enlarged and palpable. If the stone cannot be felt within the duct on bimanual palpation, the duct can be probed, but the final diagnosis is usually made by transoral radiology. The calculi are composed of calcium carbonate and phosphate and are therefore radio-opaque. Sialography may be helpful early in the condition.

The treatment of a submandibular calculus depends on its site and whether the gland is chronically enlarged. A stone in the intra-oral portion of the duct is removed through the floor of the mouth (Fig. 24.9). However, when the stone is impacted within the gland or when the gland is chronically enlarged, the whole gland must be

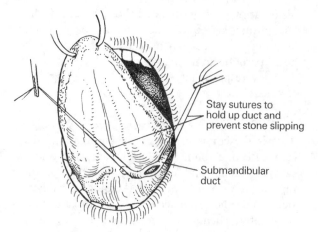

Fig. 24.9 Removal of a calculus from the submandibular duct within the floor of the mouth

removed. This is performed through an external approach, taking care to avoid the cervical branch of the facial nerve, and the lingual and hypoglossal nerves.

Salivary gland neoplasia

Neoplasms, benign and malignant, can arise from the secretory tissue, the duct system and from the myoepithelial or lymphoid tissue in the salivary glands. Thus, many different histological types of tumour can occur. Their classification is controversial but in the majority of patients the clinical distinction between them does not influence management, although it may have an important bearing on prognosis. Approximately 80% of all neoplasms of the major salivary glands are found in the parotid. The great majority of parotid tumours (roughly 85%) are benign. About half of the tumours arising in the submandibular gland are benign, and the majority of tumours of the minor salivary glands are malignant. The great majority of benign tumours are pleomorphic adenomas. Adenolymphomas are much rarer but also benign.

Pleomorphic salivary adenoma

A pleomorphic adenoma has a wide variety of histological features. It is composed primarily of epithelial glandular tissue which contains irregular

spaces. In the mucoepidermoid type, epidermoid characteristics predominate and there is stratification and prickle cell formation. The epithelial elements form a mucous matrix thought originally to be cartilage and responsible for the term 'mixed salivary tumour'. There is a dense collagenous stroma which may enclose tubules of epithelium (the so-called cylindroma) and form a dense capsule. The capsule is incomplete and portions of neoplastic epithelial tissue project into the surrounding salivary tissue.

Pleomorphic adenoma of the parotid gland

The superficial portion of the parotid gland is predominantly affected but no salivary tissue is immune. The tumour is found most frequently in middle-aged adults of either sex. Mixed salivary tumours are extraordinarily slow-growing and may reach a large size without causing symptoms. They are not frankly malignant and do not invade or metastasize. However, there is a high incidence of recurrence if the lesion is incompletely excised.

Usually the patient presents with a firm swelling in the lower part of the parotid gland (Fig. 24.10). A tumour arising from the lower pole of the gland often feels surprisingly superficial and may be mistaken for a simple dermoid or sebaceous

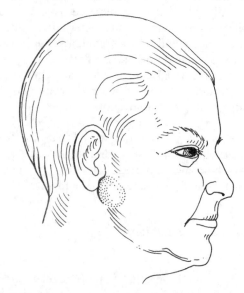

Fig. 24.10 Common appearance of a patient presenting with a pleomorphic adenoma of the parotid gland

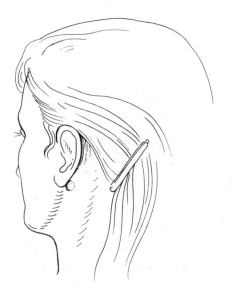

Fig. 24.11 A diagnostic trap — a 'sebaceous cyst' at the angle of the jaw which is in reality a pleomorphic adenoma of the parotid gland

cyst, or more frequently a cervical lymph gland (Fig. 24.11).

Most surgeons now consider that it is better to remove the tumour together with that portion of the parotid which lies superficial to the facial nerve (superficial parotidectomy). The key to successful completion of this operation is early definition of the facial nerve where it enters the gland and careful preservation of its branches. In expert hands the operation gives excellent results and is preferable to enucleation with its high recurrence rate (Fig. 24.12). Post-gustatory sweating (Frey's

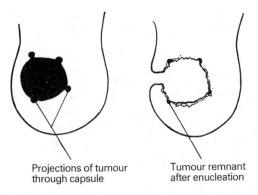

Projections of tumour
through capsule

Tumour remnant
after enucleation

Fig. 24.12 The reason for tumour recurrence after enucleation of a pleomorphic adenoma of the parotid gland (projections of tumour tissue remain after enucleation)

syndrome) is an unusual complication of surgery in which there is sweating and flushing in the distribution of the auriculotemporal nerve with aberrant regrowth of parotid parasympathetic secretomotor fibres to innervate the sympathetic end-organs of the skin.

Plemorphic adenomas in other salivary glands

Pleomorphic adenomas affecting the submandibular gland form a hard nodular swelling. The entire gland should be removed. Tumours of minor salivary glands can occur within the mouth and form lobular firm submucous swellings. They are commonly of cylindromatous type and particularly prone to recur. They should be excised widely and adjuvant radiotherapy may be considered.

Salivary adeonolymphomas

This is a rare benign solid or cystic tumour of the parotid which may affect males late in life. It is slow-growing and characteristically soft when cystic. Such tumours contain creamy material and epithelial elements associated with a mixed lymphoid stroma. The tumour feels superficial and is freely mobile. Some believe that it arises from heterotopic salivary tissue in lymph nodes.

Anaplastic carcinoma

Frankly malignant tumours of the parotid occur at a later age than pleomorphic adenomas, grow faster and invade surrounding tissues. They form a stony-hard fixed mass which may be associated with pain in the temple and scalp corresponding to the distribution of the auriculotemporal nerve. Facial palsy due to invasion of the facial nerve is uncommon but diagnostic of malignancy. Complete surgical removal, combined with radiotherapy, offers the only possible hope of cure.

THYROID GLAND SWELLINGS AND DISEASE

These are discussed separately in Chapter 23.

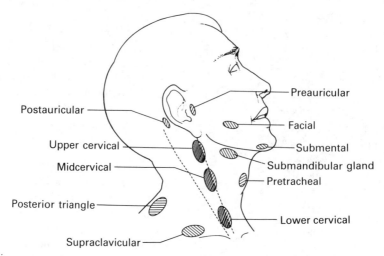

Fig. 24.13 Important lymph node groups in the head and neck shown relative to the sternocleidomastoid muscle

LYMPH NODE SWELLINGS AND DISEASE

Several hundred lymph nodes are scattered throughout the head and neck but the majority fall into well-recognized superficial groups (Fig. 24.13). In addition, there is a deep retropharyngeal chain which cannot be palpated. Drainage to lymph nodes follows a well-defined pattern (Fig. 24.14), so it is usually possible to determine the primary site of the disease by knowing which nodes are involved. Unfortunately, nodes along a drainage pathway can be bypassed; for example, dissemination of oral malignancy may skip the submental or submandibular nodes and involve the upper cervical lymph nodes. Nodes have to be at least 1 cm in diameter to be palpable and can be histologically involved by tumour while impalpable. Whether a node is fixed by tumour can be difficult to determine given that the nodes lie adjacent to muscles and within fascial sheaths. Consequently they should not to considered unresectable unless surgery proves them to be so.

Most children have several non-tender palpable nodes in the cervical chain because they are prone to recurrent upper respiratory tract infections. This should not cause concern, but by adolescence and the early twenties, these nodes should have regressed. In contrast, palpable nodes in older patients should always be investigated. In general, tender nodes are inflammatory and non-tender nodes are neoplastic. In all instances, the entire

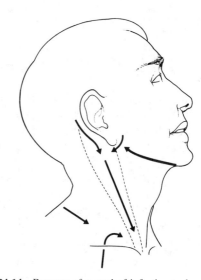

Fig. 24.14 Patterns of spread of infection and neoplasms to involve lymph nodes in the head and neck

head and neck, and in particular the oral cavity, the nose, the pharynx and the larynx, should be examined endoscopically (under general anaesthesia if necessary) to identify a primary cause.

Disorders affecting the cervical lymph nodes can be classified as follows.

1. Infective
   a. acute (pyogenic) lymphadenitis
   b. chronic (granulomatous) lymphadenitis

2. Neoplastic
   a. primary lymphoreticular neoplasia
   b. secondary carcinoma

Infective disorders

Acute lymphadenitis

Acutely tender lymph nodes are common in association with infections, particularly of the teeth, tonsils and pharynx. In most instances the cause is evident on examination and management is directed at the primary cause. Rarely the node may suppurate with spread to local tissues so that incision and drainage may be indicated.

Chronic infective lymphadenitis

In adults, chronically enlarged nodes secondary to infection are relatively uncommon but may be difficult to distinguish from neoplastic nodes as they are often not painful or tender. If no obvious cause can be identified after a thorough examination of the head and neck, including endoscopy, the nodes should be excised and sent for histological examination. This excision should be carried out by an experienced surgeon for two reasons. Firstly, as the node might be neoplastic, it has to be excised without being incised. Secondly, there are many anatomical structures that can be damaged, notably the facial and hypoglossal nerves.

Histologically the nodes often show non-specific inflammatory changes. In developed countries, diagnoses such as syphilis, actinomycosis, brucellosis, toxoplasmosis and cat scratch fever are exceptionally rare.

Tuberculous lymphadenitis is now uncommon in developed countries but should be suspected in any patient with chronically enlarged lymph nodes, particularly when there is an associated sinus, if there are several matted nodes, or when calcification is seen on X-ray. The primary route of infection is through the tonsil and involves bovine bacilli in milk. It is rare therefore for there to be associated lung tuberculosis. The final diagnosis is made by histological indentification of acid-fast bacilli; culture for *M. tuberculosis* is more time-consuming. Treatment consists of antituberculous chemotherapy.

Infectious mononucleosis (glandular fever) produces bilateral multiple enlarged lymph nodes in association with a sore throat. This combination of symptoms and signs in adolescents and young adults requires only a mono-spot test to confirm the diagnosis. As this viral infection is spread by mouth, a history of contact with a fellow-sufferer is not unusual. Sometimes the lymph glands remain chronically enlarged for months without oropharyngeal symptoms. The differential diagnosis then includes lymphoma, but a mono-spot test is again diagnostic. Treatment is symptomatic.

Neoplasia

Primary lymphomas

Patients with lymphoma frequently present with bilateral, multiple rubbery firm cervical nodes. There are few other causes of bilateral, non-tender multiple neck nodes in adolescence and early adult life. Excision biopsy will determine the histological type of lymphoma and, after investigations to stage the tumour, the appropriate treatment is given (see Ch. 22).

Secondary carcinoma

There is virtually only one diagnosis to be entertained when a painless lymph node swelling develops in a patient over the age of 45, namely metastasis from a primary carcinoma which is often, but not always, located in the head or neck. Most commonly, there are also symptoms suggestive of a primary tumour but these may well be so mild (e.g. hoarseness or the sensation of 'something' at the back of the throat) that the patient does not seek advice until a lymph node appears. Even then he may not mention the other symptoms unless questioned specifically. The primary tumour is often apparent on examination of the mouth, nose, naso-oro-hypopharynx or larynx, and can then be biopsied. If a primary tumour cannot be identified, endoscopy under general anaesthesia will usually identify a lesion in one of the more difficult areas to examine. If a primary tumour is identified, there is no need to biopsy the cervical node, as the cause for its enlargement is evident. Furthermore, surgery usually consists of excision of the primary tumour and entire lymph node system in a block dissection of the neck. Biopsy of a node prior to thorough head and neck examination is not advisable, as it will not identify the primary site and may compromise subsequent surgery. If a supraclavicular node is involved, potential primary tumours, in addition to those in the head and neck, include a bronchial or gastric neoplasm.

CAROTID BODY TUMOURS

Chemodectoma (carotid body tumour) is a rare cervical tumour which arises from chemoreceptor cells within the carotid body. The tumours are not hormonally active and metastasis is exceptional.

Characteristically, these tumours present as relatively symptomless swellings in the region of the carotid bifurcation. Secondary lymph node involvement from a primary neoplasm in the head and neck is more common and will also appear to pulsate due to transmitted pulsations from the carotid. Carotid angiography is necessary if there is any doubt about the diagnosis before the neck is explored.

Detection of a chemodectoma is not necessarily an indication for surgical removal, particularly in the elderly in whom operation can compromise the cerebral circulation. In healthy younger patients the tumour should be excised.

25. Mouth, nose, throat and ear

The upper respiratory tract extends from the nares through the nasal cavities, nasopharynx, oropharynx, hypopharynx and larynx to join the trachea, the first part of the lower respiratory tract (Fig. 25.1). The upper alimentary tract starts at the lips, goes through the oral cavity, past the fauces, over the base of the tongue, into the oro- and hypopharynx and then joins the oesophagus behind the cricoid cartilage of the larynx at the level of the 6th cervical vertebra. These two tracts might initially appear distinct but the only parts that cannot be used for both eating and breathing are the nose, nasopharynx and larynx.

Because food is relatively abrasive, the alimentary tract is lined by a non-keratinized squamous epithelium which is bathed in digestive and lubricative secretions, not only from the named salivary glands but also from multiple small salivary glands scattered throughout the mouth.

Because the primary function of the upper respiratory tract is to filter, warm and humidify the air, it is mainly lined by a mucus-secreting ciliated columnar epithelium. The exceptions are the anterior nares and the glottis, which are lined by squamous epithelium; the nares bear hairs to filter larger particles, while the glottis is subjected to mechanical trauma from vibrations. The Eustachian tube opens on the lateral wall of the nasopharynx and is lined by a ciliated mucus-secreting epithelium in continuity with that of the middle ear. The middle ear can be regarded as an extension of the upper respiratory tract. The Eustachian tube aerates the middle ear space and keeps it at atmospheric pressure while allowing secretions to drain into the nasopharynx.

As potential portals of entry for infection, the two tracts have a well-developed immunological system of lymphoid tissue which is concentrated in a ring (Waldeyer's ring) around the naso- and oropharynx. The tonsils are localized aggregations and therefore excisable (Fig. 25.2). The adenoids are patches of lymphoid tissue scattered within the mucosa of the posterior wall and have to be scraped off to be removed, while the lingual tonsils are spread diffusely within the muscle of the base of the tongue and cannot be removed. Hypertrophy of this lymphoid tissue is normal in childhood, but with ageing there is a variable

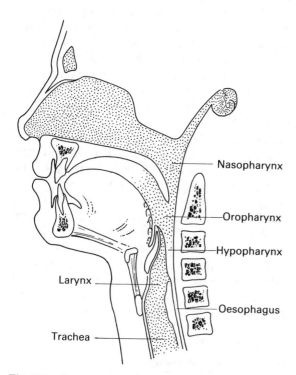

Fig. 25.1 Anatomy of nasopharynx, oropharynx and hypopharynx in relation to larynx and oesophagus

369

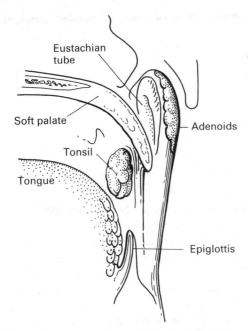

Fig. 25.2   Distribution of lymphoid tissue in pharynx

Table 25.1   Incidence of head and neck tumours

| | Incidence per 100 000 | | |
	Males	Females	Total
Larynx	4.3	0.9	2.6
Pharynx	2.1	1.5	1.8
Mouth	2.0	1.2	1.6
Salivary glands	1.4	1.6	1.5
Tongue	1.5	0.9	1.2
Nose/sinuses	0.6	0.4	0.5
Total			9.2

degree of atrophy. Localized enlargement at any age should be regarded as a possible sign of a reticuloendothelial neoplasm.

DISEASES OF THE UPPER ALIMENTARY AND RESPIRATORY TRACTS

Diseases of the upper respiratory and alimentary tracts can be classified as congenital, inflammatory, neoplastic and traumatic. Inflammatory and neoplastic conditions are seen more frequently in individuals who smoke or chew tobacco, in alcohol drinkers, those with poor dental hygiene and those in the lower socioeconomic groups.

It is not unusual for disease in one part of these tracts to be associated with similar disease in another part. For example, a viral infection may involve the epithelium of the nose, Eustachian tube and larynx. Similarly, it is not uncommon for an individual who has been successfully treated for a laryngeal tumour, for example, to develop a carcinoma of the tongue some years later.

The commonest histological type of malignant tumour in both tracts is a squamous carcinoma, which is not surprising considering that the tracts are lined mainly by squamous epithelium. Less commonly, reticuloendothelial tumours arise in the lymphoid tissue and very rarely other types of tumour occur, particularly in the nasal passages. The incidence of malignant tumours varies from country to country, depending on culture and habits, but Table 25.1 illustrates what might be expected in a Caucasian country.

Unfortunately both tracts are relatively capacious so that patients with tumours frequently present late, i.e. when the tumour finally starts to cause obstructive symptoms. The exception to this are the common glottic tumours, which often cause hoarseness early in the course of the disease, prompting the patient to seek medical attention. Another common presentation is with a secondary deposit in a neck node; as might be expected, this usually carries a bad prognosis.

In general, small (T1 and T2) head and neck squamous carcinomas respond well to radiotherapy or excisional surgery, with a 5-year survival rate of over 75%. With larger tumours (T3 and T4) which have spread to adjacent structures or lymph nodes (N1 and N2), the response to either form of therapy is considerably worse. Excisional surgery with or without secondary radiotherapy gives the best survival rates (approximately 35% at 5 years), but there are problems in repairing the defect so that the patient can eat, speak and breathe as normally as possible. Primary radiotherapy is associated with lower cure rates but may be the preferred option for patients such as the very elderly and those with poor support at home. To date chemotherapy has been reserved mainly for palliation but its benefits are marginal.

THE MOUTH
Infections and swellings

Because the oral cavity is large, lesions tend not to obstruct eating or swallowing unless they are large.

Patients often just notice that 'something is there' which can make eating difficult although the feeling is as frequently relieved by eating. Inflammatory lesions are usually painful whereas malignant ones are not. However, if there is any concern about the nature of a lesion an expert opinion should be sought and biopsy undertaken as a definitive investigation.

Mucosal disease

The mouth is the portal of the alimentary tract, and mucosal disease in the ileum or colon, notably Crohn's disease, is occasionally associated with oral ulcers. Deficiencies of vitamins (B12 or C) or minerals (such as iron) can be evident as a general dryness of the lips, cheeks and tongue, with cracking at the angles of the mouth (angular cheilitis).

Aphthous ulcers

These are recurrent painful ulcers which are usually multiple and found on mobile mucosa such as that lining the cheeks, tongue and gingival sulci. The ulcers are small, yellowish-white and punched out with a surrounding halo of erythema. Their aetiology is unknown but they are common in normal individuals and are occasionally seen in patients with Crohn's disease or ulcerative colitis. Treatment may not be necessary but some patients find that topical antiseptics or topical corticosteroid pellets are helpful.

Stomatitis and gingivitis

Inflammation of the oral mucosa (stomatitis) and gums (gingivitis) is particularly common in dehydrated, febrile and ill-nourished patients with faulty oral hygiene. Carious teeth, ill-fitting dentures and heavy smoking favour their development. The mucosa becomes reddened and dry, the tongue is swollen and furred, and halitosis (bad breath) is prominent. Pain on eating may be marked if ulceration occurs, and fever and malaise are common.

Stomatitis is largely preventable by attention to oral hygiene and adequate hydration. Established stomatitis is treated by removing causal factors, by hydration, regular mouth washes and promoting the flow of saliva. Antibiotics are rarely indicated.

Cancrum oris is a rare form of stomatitis in debilitated children in which ulceration progresses to full-thickness gangrene and destruction of the cheek. The gangrenous area is excised, penicillin is given, and the state of nutrition and oral hygiene is improved. Cancrum oris carries a poor prognosis and is often a preterminal event.

Traumatic ulcers

Trauma from broken teeth or ragged or loose dentures can cause painful ulcers on the lips, cheeks or tongue. Neglecting to remove the dentures to inspect the mouth may mean that the diagnosis is missed. If the ulcer persists after eradication of the dentition problem, it should be biopsied to exclude carcinoma.

Retention cysts

Mucus retention cysts can occur anywhere within the oral cavity or indeed in any part of the upper alimentary and respiratory tract. Those located under the tongue are ranulas. They occur if the drainage of mucous or accessory salivary glands is blocked. Many are discovered incidentally and can be disregarded. Others may have been seen by the patient or given rise to the sensation of 'something being there'. The classical appearance is that of a pearly-white, rounded swelling lying superficially in the mucosa. Excision is curative. Alternatively, the cyst may simply be deroofed. This operation is known as marsupialization.

Candida infections

In otherwise well patients, the commonest site for candida infection is underneath dentures or at the angles of the mouth. In debilitated patients and those on broad spectrum antibiotic therapy, candidiasis can be a considerable problem anywhere in the mouth but affects particularly the palate, fauces, tongue and oropharynx. The classical appearance is that of a whitish membrane which resembles milk curds and which, when scraped off, reveals a localized area of raw mucosa. The diagnosis is usually obvious but is confirmed by taking scrapings for microscopic examination.

Therapy consists of topical nystatin lozenges or suspensions (500 000 units four times a day for 4 days), stopping any unnecessary antibiotic therapy, and improving the patient's oral hygiene and general health.

Other forms of specific oral infection

Syphilitic and tuberculous ulcers are now extremely rare. *Actinomyces israeli* is a rare cause of orofacial induration in patients with faulty oral and dental hygiene. The gum becomes indurated, nodules form beneath the jaw and the overlying skin becomes hard and bluish. Pus discharges intermittently from multiple sinuses. The diagnosis is confirmed by microscopic examination and treatment consists of a 6-week course of penicillin and attention to oral and dental hygiene.

Leukoplakia

Leukoplakia denotes mucosal hyperkeratosis and is caused by long-standing irritation, notably by tobacco. It appears as white areas located most commonly on the tongue and buccal mucosa. Desquamation may expose sensitive areas resembling raw beef. Hyperkeratosis may proceed to papillomatous proliferation and fissuring, and cancer may supervene. Although premalignant, leukoplakia should regress with attention to oral hygiene and abstinence from tobacco and alcohol. Such patients should be observed regularly and any suspicious thickened areas should be biopsied.

Cancer of the tongue and oral cavity

Cancer arising in the mouth has become less common over the past 50 years but still accounts for some 5% of all malignancies. Tobacco smoking is the major aetiological factor. Other factors include heavy alcohol consumption, poor oral hygiene and betel nut chewing, although it is often difficult to dissociate these factors from the effects of coexisting tobacco consumption. Syphilitic glossitis is no longer a common predisposing factor. Oral cancer is commoner in males than in females, is uncommon before the age of 45 and half the patients are over 70 years of age.

The cancer is usually painless and patients tend to seek advice late. They frequently complain of 'something being there' and the tumour may have become quite large before diagnosis, particularly if located in 'silent' areas such as the gingivo-lingual sulcus or posterior third of the tongue. The diagnosis is usually obvious from the appearance of raised ulcerated areas with overhanging edges which sometimes bleed. The lesions are only painful if there is secondary infection. The diagnosis is confirmed by incision biopsy. The great majority (over 90%) of oral cancers are squamous carcinomas, with pleomorphic salivary adenomas accounting for most of the remainder.

Management depends primarily on the stage of the tumour. Although widespread dissemination is rare, nearly 50% of patients have involved cervical lymph nodes at the time of presentation and in some the mandible is also involved. When the tumour is small, excisional surgery and radiotherapy appear to be equally effective. When it is large and there is mandibular or nodal involvement, the primary method of curative treatment is surgery, with or without radiotherapy. To gain access it may be necessary to split the mandible temporarily. The tumour can then be excised 'en bloc' with any involved bone or cervical lymph nodes. Large defects left after excisional surgery require skilled repair using skin flaps or free grafts with microvascular anastomoses.

Approximately one-third of patients with oral cancer survive for 5 years following diagnosis.

Dental disease

Dental caries is common, and over one-third of the UK population over the age of 16 years are edentulous. Caries is due to erosion of the dental enamel by the bacterial products associated with plaque formation. In children, the commonest sites are in the cusps and in adults the areas between the teeth and at the gum margins. Caries at the gum margin is made worse by chronic gingivitis. The incidence of caries has been dramatically reduced since the introduction of fluoridation of drinking water and toothpaste. Management consists of prevention and avoidance of an oversweet diet along with regular oral hygiene and removal of debris and plaque by a combination of brushing and flossing.

Congenital abnormalities

Cleft lip and cleft palate

These are the commonest developmental abnormalities of the head and neck, with an incidence of about 1 in 700 live births. Such children pose considerable management problems involving many disciplines for periods which may exceed 20 years. Clefts are due primarily, but not solely, to abnormal fusion of the central premaxillary (nasal) process with the lateral maxillary processes to form the lip, nose, alveolus and its dentition, and the hard and soft palate (Fig. 25.3). They can occur unilaterally or bilaterally and are classified as cleft lip with or without cleft palate, and cleft palate alone (Fig. 25.4). The abnormality is considerably commoner in those with a family history, and genetic counselling should be offered.

The diagnosis is usually obvious at birth. Nasal regurgitation during suckling can usually be overcome with special teats. When the child is 3–6 months old, any cleft in the lip is usually repaired, although multiple operations to the lip and nose may be required to achieve a satisfactory cosmetic result. The next objective is to ensure that speech develops as normally as possible by closing any palatal defect surgically at about 18 months of age. Again, many operations may be necessary over the years to lengthen the palate so that the nasopharynx can be closed during phonation and eating. The next problem is to ensure good dentition and encourage maxillary growth by appropriate orthodontic splints and braces.

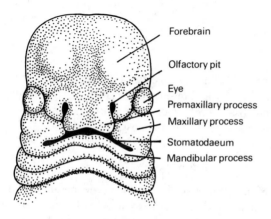

Fig. 25.3 The development of the lips and mouth

Forebrain

Olfactory pit

Eye
Premaxillary process
Maxillary process

Stomatodaeum
Mandibular process

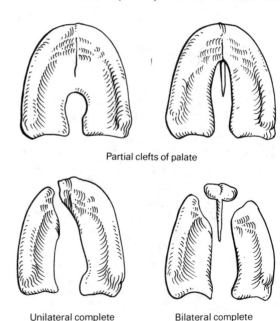

Partial clefts of palate

Unilateral complete
cleft palate

Bilateral complete
cleft palate

Fig. 25.4 Types of cleft palate

Finally, throughout the growing period, there is the problem of persistent otitis media with effusion (see later) which requires regular observation and management. Needless to say, tonsillectomy and adenoidectomy are contraindicated in children with cleft palates.

THE NOSE

Surgical anatomy

The external nose consists of the nasal bones and the paired upper and lower lateral cartilages (Fig. 25.5). Internally the nose is divided in two, anteriorly by the cartilaginous septum and posteriorly by the bony septum (Fig. 25.6). The three turbinates on the lateral wall increase the surface area of mucus-secreting mucosa which warms, humidifies and filters the inspired air. The inferior turbinate is readily seen on anterior rhinoscopy and should not be confused with a nasal polyp. Little's area is an area on the anterior septum within reach of a poking finger (Fig. 25.7) from which bleeding is common.

There are four groups of nasal sinuses: the frontal, ethmoid, maxillary and sphenoid sinuses

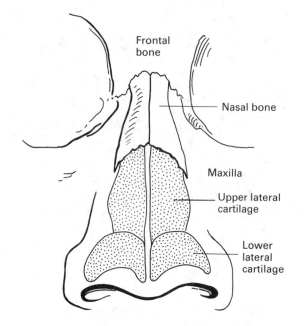

Fig. 25.5   External nasal anatomy

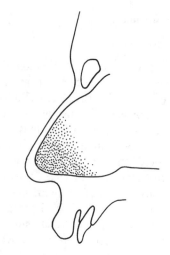

Fig. 25.7   Little's area on septum

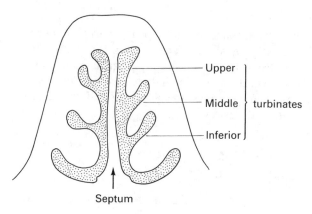

Fig. 25.6   Internal nasal anatomy

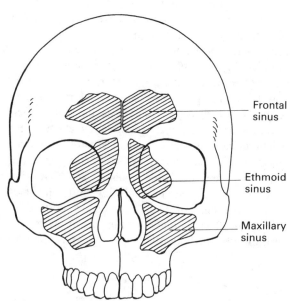

Fig. 25.8   The nasal sinuses

(Fig. 25.8). With the exception of the sphenoid sinus, they drain into the nose below the middle turbinate. Tears from the eye drain via the nasolacrimal duct, which enters below the inferior turbinate.

Nasal symptoms and diseases

Blockage

The sensation of having a blocked nose may be constant or cyclical, unilateral or bilateral. Con-stant blockage suggests deviation of the septum or a nasal tumour. Cyclical blockage suggests mucosal problems. Clinical examination will usually reveal the diagnosis.

Deviated nasal septum

Some degree of deviation of the nasal septum is normal and causes no symptoms because of com-pensatory shrinkage of the turbinates on the narrower side. In a few individuals the deviation is such that the nose feels blocked. Submucosal resection of the deviated part or repositioning the deviated parts (septoplasty; see later) will give relief.

Nasal polyps

Multiple benign nasal polyps are the commonest nasal tumour and most frequently arise bilaterally from the ethmoidal air cells. If small, they may regress with topical steroid application (e.g. beclomethasone) but otherwise management consists of surgical avulsion. Unfortunately recurrence is common, but this may be prevented by prophylactic topical steroids. If this fails, repeat avulsion or ethmoidectomy, in which the air cells are opened to clear them of disease, is indicated.

Nasal cancer

Suspicion that a nasal tumour may not be a simple polyp should be aroused if it is unilateral, does not have the classical glistening pale appearance and if it bleeds. The many different histological types of nasal tumour can only be distinguished by biopsy. Management almost invariably involves surgery; its extent depends on the degree of malignancy as assessed by biopsy, on invasion of neighbouring structures such as the paranasal sinuses and the orbit as assessed by endoscopy and radiology, and on whether there are regional or distant metastases. The tumour is removed together with any involved bone, and any resultant defect in the skull is made cosmetically more acceptable by attaching a prosthesis to a dental plate.

Rhinorrhoea

A runny nose is due to an increase in secretions (catarrh) from an inflamed nasal and/or sinus mucosa, and is usually associated with nasal blockage due to mucosal oedema. The secretions are normally clear, but may become yellow, green or brown if secondary bacterial infection occurs.

The common cold

Coryza is the commonest cause of a running nose and the diagnosis is usually obvious.

Allergic rhinitis

Allergic rhinitis is less common than non-specific rhinitis but, as the latter is diagnosed by excluding the former, allergic rhinitis is considered first. Allergic rhinitis may be seasonal or 'all-year-round' (perennial). Seasonal allergies can be due to pollens and are easy to diagnose from the typical history of a runny nose and watery eyes at a specific time of the year. Perennial rhinitis is less easy to diagnose from the history, and house dust and animal mites are the commonest allergens.

The differentiation from non-specific rhinitis rests on the identification of an allergen. Skin tests may be used but false positive reactions are common in asymptomatic individuals and a test battery can be difficult to interpret.

Management consists of avoiding the allergen and prescription of topical steroids (beclomethasone) or sodium cromoglycate. Antihistamines can be given if eye symptoms are dominant. Desensitization is contraindicated because of the dangers of anaphylactic reactions. Surgical trimming or diathermy of enlarged turbinates is an option if medical treatment fails.

Non-specific (vasomotor) rhinitis

Non-specific rhinitis is often attributed (without much evidence) to imbalance in the vasomotor system. The symptoms tend to be perennial but running eyes are infrequent in comparison to allergic rhinitis. The same medications are given as for allergic rhinitis and again turbinate surgery is an option if this fails.

Chronic sinusitis

Chronic sinusitis is akin to chronic bronchitis in that periodically the nasal and sinus mucosa becomes inflamed, resulting in the production of a mucupurulent discharge which is difficult to eradicate. It is like having frequent, mucopurulent colds. Headaches and facial pain are not common. Predisposing factors such as obstruction to the sinus ostia by a deviated nasal septum, dental caries affecting the maxillary sinus, smoking and poor general health should be excluded or dealt with. X-rays are not helpful in arriving at a diagnosis because of the poor correlation between radiological mucosal oedema and surgical findings.

Management consists of encouraging drainage with steam inhalations and topical nasal steroids. Courses of broad spectrum antibiotics may be given. In some patients, sinus washouts or more radical removal of the sinus mucosa may be indicated.

Acute sinusitis

If the ostium of a sinus becomes blocked during an upper respiratory tract infection, an abscess may form. There is acute pain and local tenderness over the affected sinus. Drainage and antibiotics are indicated.

Bleeding (epistaxis)

In younger individuals bleeding occurs most frequently from a small blood vessel in Little's area. In older patients it most frequently arises from an arteriosclerotic blood vessel located more posteriorly. Occasionally a nasal tumour bleeds.

In the acute stage the anterior septum should be compressed by pinching the cartilaginous nose. This applies pressure to Little's area (Fig. 25.9) and should stop any bleeding from this site. A pledget of cotton wool soaked in 1 in 1000 adrenaline can be inserted just inside the vestibule to encourage this. The fingernails of children with recurrent epistaxis should be kept short to prevent trauma from picking, and nasal crusts are kept soft with vaseline. Prominent blood vessels on Little's area may be cauterized.

If bleeding does not stop with anterior pinching, the epistaxis is arising further back and may be managed by nasal packing. Half-inch (1.25 cm) ribbon gauze in vaseline or BIPP (bismuth iodine paraffin paste) is inserted in a zig-zag fashion into the bleeding nasal cavity, which normally accommodates 2 feet (60 cm) of ½-inch wick (Fig. 25.10). It is usually unnecessary to pack both sides because, even if blood issues from both sides, it usually originates from only one point. Blood may be coming round the septum posteriorly and the side that initially bled is the side to pack. Hospital admission is advisable if the nose has to be packed, because of the dangers associated with any

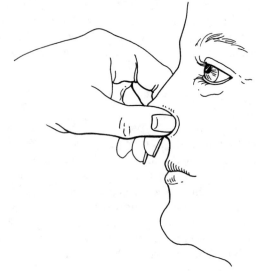

Fig. 25.9 Pressure to control haemorrhage (see text)

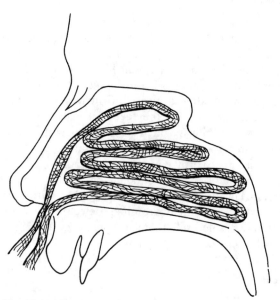

Fig. 25.10 Nasal packing

haemorrhage. Sedation and general measures to anticipate and treat shock should be instituted. If bleeding continues, the nose can be repacked more carefully with an inflatable balloon, such as a Foley catheter, to block off the nasopharynx. Surgical ligation of the arterial supply to the bleeding point is sometimes indicated if the problem persists.

Nasal trauma

Nasal fractures

Pugilistic and accidental nasal injuries are common. In the majority there is just bruising and perhaps epistaxis. In some the nasal bones and/or the septal cartilage may be fractured (Fig. 25.11). The diagnosis is a clinical one and is made by detecting local tenderness over the fracture site(s). Management depends on whether the nose is misaligned. X-rays will not help to make this distinction and even an experienced clinician may find it difficult to differentiate radiologically between an old and a newly displaced fracture. Individuals who get their nose bashed tend to do so frequently.

No treatment is necessary for undisplaced fractures apart from dealing with any epistaxis. If the bony or cartilaginous nose is displaced, manipulation under general anaesthesia has to be performed within 10 days of injury because after that time the fragments will be difficult to disimpact because of healing.

Chronic deformities

In an age of increasing personal awareness and desire to appear attractive many individuals with previously ignored nasal deformities attend some time after the incident complaining of their appearance and perhaps of increased difficulty in breathing. Other patients may present with an unsatisfactory appearance despite manipulation. Rhinoplasty with controlled chisel or saw refracturing of the nasal bones via intranasal incisions will improve the appearance. Septoplasty with repositioning of the cartilaginous and bony septum in the midline after partial removal of grossly deviated segments will clear the airway (Fig. 25.12).

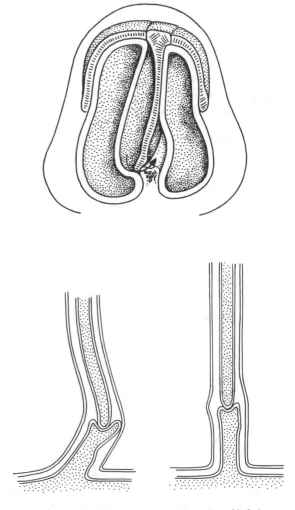

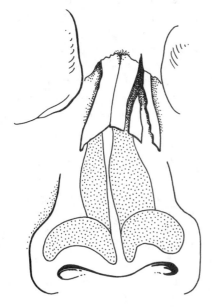

Fig. 25.11 Nasal fracture

Fig. 25.12 Septoplasty. Submucosal dissection of inferior part of septum and repositioning of the cartilaginous and bony septum in the midline

THE PHARYNX

Surgical anatomy

The pharynx is divided into three parts. The nasopharynx extends from the base of the skull to the soft palate and is part of the upper respiratory tract into which the Eustachian tubes open on the posterolateral wall. There are scattered patches of lymphoid (adenoid) tissue on the posterior wall. The oropharynx opens anteriorly to the mouth and is bounded above by the soft palate and below by the tip of the epiglottis. It contains the (palatal) tonsils, the lingual tonsils and the base of the tongue. The hypopharynx is bounded above by the tip of the epiglottis and ends at the cricoid cartilage at the level of the sixth cervical vertebra. The laryngeal inlet is bounded anteriorly on either side by the pyriform fossae, which are the main routes taken by food when it is swallowed and before it enters the oesophagus at the base of the hypopharynx.

The muscles of the pharynx are under voluntary control via the vagus nerve and mucosal sensation is subserved mainly by the glossopharyngeal nerve.

The nasopharynx

Adenoid hypertrophy and neoplasia are the two main diseases of the nasopharynx and they usually present with symptoms caused by their size. The nose may become blocked and/or the Eustachian tube may be unable to function, giving rise to otitis media with effusion. Sometimes nasopharyngeal tumours will bleed and, even when small, they may metastazise to the cervical lymph nodes.

Adenoid hypertrophy

Adenoid hypertrophy in childhood is normal and in the majority of cases causes no symptoms. However, large adenoids may be a factor in recurrent nasal infections and otitis media with effusion. The size of the adenoids can be assessed indirectly with a mirror but this is often difficult; lateral X-rays are more reliable. If hypertrophy is considered to be a factor, the adenoids can be removed by curetting. Although a simple operation, it should not be embarked upon lightly because of the dangers of haemorrhage. It is also definitely contraindicated if there is any suggestion of a cleft palate because of the subsequent development of hypernasal speech and nasal regurgitation of food.

Tumours

In children and adolescents the majority of tumours are congenital in origin, and benign. This does not mean that they can be considered trivial. They can erode bone at the base of the skull by pressure and thereby cause cranial nerve palsies. The commonest tumour is an angiofibroma and, because of the risk of bleeding from biopsy, arteriography is the initial investigation. The ideal treatment is total surgical removal but because of the danger of bleeding many lesions are now managed initially by embolization.

In adults, particularly those of Chinese extraction who have lived in the Far East, squamous cell carcinoma is the commonest tumour of the nasopharynx. It usually presents late, often with erosion of the base of the skull or with neck metastases. Many patients have otitis media with effusion due to Eustachian tube blockage, hence the importance of considering a nasopharyngeal tumour in adults with this condition. Complete surgical excision of the primary tumour is not possible because of its relationship to important neurological structures and surgical clearance of the neck can never be complete because of the almost invariable presence of retropharyngeal nodes which cannot be removed. Radiotherapy is therefore the mainstay of management and in the majority of patients is palliative rather than curative, relieving the pain associated with erosion of the skull base.

The oropharynx

As in the mouth, lesions in the oropharynx have to be large before they obstruct swallowing. However, unlike those in the mouth, oropharyngeal lesions frequently cause pain.

Acute pharyngitis

Viral infections of the pharynx are common and

present as a sore throat which is exacerbated by tobacco smoke or dust. Usually a runny nose or hoarse voice indicates that other parts of the upper respiratory tract are involved. Clinically the oropharynx can look surprisingly normal but is hypersensitive to touch. Pain relief pending resolution is obtained in children by paracetamol elixir and in adults by aspirin gargles, which are then swallowed to give both a topical and systemic effect.

Acute tonsillitis

Bacterial tonsillitis due to beta-haemolytic strepto-cocci is a condition of childhood and adolescence. Episodes of sore throat are associated with fever, malaise and cervical lymphadenopathy but without a runny nose, cough or hoarse voice. Both tonsils appear inflamed and enlarged with mucopus in the crypts. Analgesics, as in acute pharyngitis, are the mainstay of management, with prescription of parenteral penicillin for the more severely ill.

In the acute stage, differentiation from acute pharyngitis is easy. Between episodes, it is not possible to make the distinction on the appearance of the tonsils. Some tonsils which are chronically enlarged give no problems while others which are recurrently infected may be small.

If the episodes of tonsillitis are frequent and in-capacitating, tonsillectomy is the surgical option. This is done under general anaesthesia with en-dotracheal intubation to protect the airway from haemorrhage. The tonsils are dissected out and any bleeding points are controlled. Post-tonsillar haemorrhage is the major complication and can be fatal (1 in 10 000 operations). Monitoring, es-pecially of the pulse rate, for 24 hours after operation is essential. Fluid replacement, preferably with blood, is vital if bleeding occurs. Once the child is resuscitated, the bleeding point should be ligated. Secondary haemorrhage can occur several days later but is usually minor and does not require surgery.

Because of its dangers and the psychological dis-turbances associated with admission of children to hospital, tonsillectomy should not be considered a minor operation. The natural history of recurrent tonsillitis is one of spontaneous resolution over a two-year period so that all tonsillectomy does is hasten this.

Peritonsillar abscess (quinsy)

The most frequent complication of acute tonsillitis is a peritonsillar abscess, which should be suspected when there is asymmetry in the size of the tonsils in a patient with acute tonsillitis. This is due to the abscess displacing the tonsil downwards and medially. Trismus denotes dif-ficulty in opening the mouth due to reflex spasm of the masseter and buccinator muscles and also suggests an abscess.

Drainage of the abscess by stab incision under local anaesthesia or by tonsillectomy under general anaesthesia gives quick resolution. In the early stages, parenteral penicillin is an alternative.

Parapharyngeal abscess

Very occasionally infection from the tonsils or teeth may track into the parapharyngeal space lateral to the pharynx and present with gross symptoms of infection and a lateral tender neck swelling. Treatment consists of systemic anti-biotics and internal or external surgical drainage.

Infectious mononucleosis

Infectious mononucleosis (glandular fever) due to the Epstein-Barr virus should be suspected if an adolescent or young adult has grossly enlarged bilateral cervical lymph nodes in association with a sore throat and general malaise. The pharynx may be only mildly infected, there is a mononuclear leucocytosis, and the mono-spot test is positive. Symptoms are often protracted over several months and there is no specific treatment. Interestingly, if ampicillin is given for the sore throat, over 90% of patients will develop a skin rash.

Hypopharynx

Pharyngeal problems usually present as a sensation of 'something being there'. There is no difficulty in swallowing or obstruction, indeed swallowing can relieve the symptoms. In many patients, no pathology can be detected despite a thorough clinical examination with a mirror, plain lateral X-rays and barium swallow.

However, such symptoms should always be treated seriously because of the possibility of an underlying tumour. To exclude this, many patients have to be examined under general anaesthesia to allow evaluation of areas such as the pyriform fossae on either side of the larynx that are otherwise difficult to inspect.

Once pathology has been excluded, the patient can be reassured that symptoms will abate with time. It is likely that in future, many of these unexplained symptoms will increasingly be diagnosed as due to motility disorders, but the term 'globus hystericus' as a label for idiopathic symptoms is somewhat inaccurate as there is no hysteria. The term 'globus syndrome' may be more appropriate.

Gastro-oesophageal reflux

Reflux may produce the sensation of 'something being there' and is not always associated with heartburn. It is easy to understand how refluxed acid and bile can irritate the pharynx. The diagnosis and management of gastro-oesophageal reflux are described in Chapter 26.

Pharyngeal pouch

This is a midline mucosal herniation through the lower pharyngeal muscles (Killian's dehiscence) which gradually enlarges with retained food (Fig. 25.13). The condition is caused by incoordination between contraction of the pharynx and relaxation of the upper oesophageal sphincter and usually affects the elderly. It causes progressive difficulty in swallowing due to pressure on the hypopharynx and upper oesophagus from the diverticulum. Mirror examination and endoscopy frequently miss the pouch and the diagnosis is best made by barium swallow. It is unusual to palpate a swelling in the neck.

Treatment consists of excision of the pouch, repair of the defect and division of the cricopharyngeal muscle (myotomy) below the defect (Fig. 25.14).

Pharyngeal tumours

These are mainly squamous cell carcinomas and, when small, only cause the sensation of 'something being there'. In some sites, particularly the pyriform fossae, they can grow quite large before causing obstruction to swallowing and, perhaps, hoarseness due to laryngeal involvement. Enlargement of cervical lymph nodes is a common form of presentation.

As these tumours tend to be relatively large by

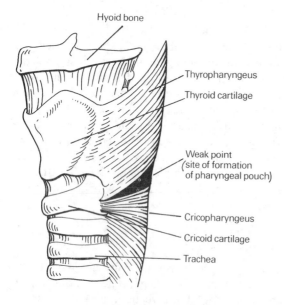

Fig. 25.13   Site of formation of pharyngeal pouch

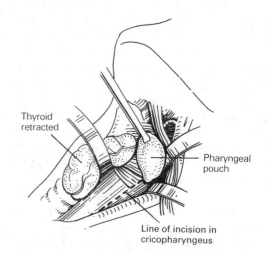

Fig. 25.14   Cricomyotomy and 'suspension' of pharyngeal pouch

the time they are diagnosed, excision with repair of the pharyngeal defect by a vascularized skin flap such as the myocutaneous deltopectoral flap is the curative method of choice. When the larynx is involved, this has to be removed as well (pharyngolaryngectomy) and repair may involve the use of a free jejunal graft (with vascular anastomosis) or consist of advancing the oesophagus upwards after freeing it in the chest and abdomen. Any involved cervical nodes are excised during block dissection of the neck and radiotherapy can be given as an adjunct.

LARYNX

Applied anatomy

The larynx is the muscular organ of speech and coughing and is enclosed within the cartilaginous framework of the thyroid and cricoid cartilages. It also has the function of preventing food and fluids from entering the lower respiratory tract. This is achieved because the tongue is attached to, and the larynx is suspended from, the hyoid bone. When a bolus of food is propelled by the tongue into the pharynx, the hyoid bone is automatically elevated and this raises and tilts the larynx backwards. Food then goes round the sides of the epiglottis via the pyriform fossae into the hypopharynx and oesophagus. If any material manages to enter the larynx, it is sensed in the supraglottis by virtue of the superior laryngeal nerves. The larynx then goes into spasm and coughing subsequently expels the inhaled material.

Sound vibrations produced by the larynx are transformed into articulate speech by movements of the tongue, lips and teeth and by the resonance of the nose. The sound vibrations come from the muscular vocal cords, which are attached to the mobile arytenoid cartilages posteriorly and fixed together anteriorly to the thyroid cartilage. By varying the tension of the vocal cords, vibrations of different pitch can be produced. The motor supply to the vocal cords comes from the recurrent laryngeal branch of the vagus nerve. On the right side of the neck the branch goes directly to the larynx but on the left it first passes intrathoracically below the arch of the aorta.

Coughing is achieved by building up intra-thoracic pressure behind a closed glottis, which is then opened, suddenly releasing the air which carries with it any secretions or inhaled particles.

Symptoms of laryngeal disease

As disease most frequently affects the glottis, hoarseness is the commonest laryngeal symptom. It needs only a minor mucosal abnormality to cause hoarseness so that in theory all glottic tumours should be detected early. Stridor or obstruction to breathing is less common but is the way in which supraglottic and subglottic disease most frequently presents. Inhalation of food and loss of the ability to cough it up is the least frequent symptom and is usually a complication of neck surgery (notably tracheostomy) or neurological disease.

Examination of the larynx

The larynx can be visualized indirectly with a mirror or fibreoptic laryngoscope and directly with a rigid laryngoscope. Laryngoscopy is not an investigation for the inexperienced clinician, especially when a tumour has to be excluded. This means referral of all patients with potential laryngeal problems to a specialist. In the majority of cases, laryngoscopy will give the diagnosis but plain radiography and tomography can be helpful in assessing the size of the airway, particularly in the subglottic region and trachea.

Acute laryngeal conditions

Acute laryngitis

Short episodes of hoarseness are common after excessive use of the voice or in association with upper respiratory tract infection. With the avoidance of further trauma, especially from tobacco smoke and voice use, the hoarseness should settle within days and certainly within three weeks. Steam inhalations can give symptomatic relief but antibiotics are not indicated.

Acute laryngo-tracheo-bronchitis and epiglottitis

Laryngo-tracheo-bronchitis (croup) and acute epiglottitis are the alternative diagnoses in a child with an upper respiratory infection who develops stridor. Both are life-threatening because of their acute onset and the relatively small size of a child's airway. In laryngo-tracheo-bronchitis the whole mucosa becomes inflamed but particularly in the subglottic region. Acute epiglottitis is a potentially more life-threatening infection which is due to *Haemophilus influenzae*. It is almost invariably painful and there is drooling of saliva. Examination of the mouth and throat is contraindicated because it may precipitate obstruction. The child is best managed in hospital, and should be accompanied there by a doctor in case acute obstruction occurs. The majority of patients will settle with aspiration of secretions, humidification and parenteral antibiotics, usually amoxycillin. Sometimes, however, it will be necessary to intubate the child or perform a tracheostomy.

Chronic laryngeal conditions

Chronic laryngitis

In chronic laryngitis the whole laryngeal mucosa is inflamed and this is frequently associated with chronic disease elsewhere in the respiratory tract, e.g. bronchitis. Excessive alcohol intake and smoking are often implicated and neoplasia can develop secondarily. Management hinges on the avoidance of predisposing factors, but it is almost impossible to get patients to comply.

Vocal nodules

Vocal nodules are hyperkeratotic patches which develop in the middle third of the cords, i.e. their main point of contact. They are caused by excessive or inappropriate use of the voice. Voice rest and speech therapy can help. Resolution may be speeded by microsurgical stripping of the cords.

Vocal cord palsy

Vocal cord palsies are commoner on the left because the intrathoracic course of the recurrent laryngeal nerve allows it to be affected by bronchial neoplasms, tuberculosis or arteriosclerosis of the aortic arch. In the neck the commonest cause of palsy is surgical trauma, for example following thyroidectomy. However, many cases are idiopathic, but this should not be assumed until a tumour has been excluded. In addition to a weak or hoarse voice, many patients have difficulty in coughing up sputum and this can be particularly disabling when palsy has been caused by a bronchial neoplasm. The natural history is one of symptomatic recovery either because the palsy recovers or because the other cord compensates. If this does not occur within 6 months, Teflon injection of the cord can be of value. This can be done endoscopically under general anaesthesia or externally under local anaesthesia with fibreoptic vision if the patient is unfit. In individuals whose main problem is coughing up sputum, Teflon injections can give considerable relief and one should not wait to see if spontaneous improvement takes place.

Laryngeal tumours

The larynx is the commonest site in the head and neck for tumours to develop. Thankfully the majority are on the glottis and in theory can be detected early by examining everybody who is hoarse for more than 3 weeks. By comparison, supra- and subglottic tumours present when they are considerably larger, giving rise to compression of the airway or hoarseness following extension to the glottis.

The majority of tumours are squamous cell carcinomas and occur in male smokers in the lower socioeconomic groups. Untreated, they spread within the larynx, immobilizing the cord and then spreading outwith the cartilaginous framework to the thyroid gland. Cervical lymph node metastases are frequent with larger tumours but distant metastases are rare.

The diagnosis is confirmed by biopsy under direct vision with a rigid laryngoscope. While the patient is under general anaesthesia, the size and extent of the tumour within the larynx are assessed. With small tumours confined to a mobile vocal cord, the 5-year survival rate after radiotherapy is in the region of 80%. However, with larger tumours or cervical lymph node involvement, the survival rate following radiotherapy falls to below 50%. For these patients, laryngectomy with block neck dissection gives superior cure rates but the patient has to develop some other form of speech. Traditionally this is achieved by regurgitation of air from the oesophagus but only about half of all laryngectomy patients manage this successfully; accordingly methods of partial laryngectomy have been developed which are suitable for some patients. Alternatively, a tracheo-oesophageal fistula may be created into which a tube with a one-way valve is inserted through the tracheostomy to prevent tracheal aspiration of food or fluids. To speak, the laryngectomy patient closes off the tube and tracheostomy with his finger, thus directing air from the trachea into the oesophagus.

MANAGEMENT OF ACUTE AIRWAY OBSTRUCTION (Stridor)

Acute difficulty in breathing (stridor) is an alarming problem which requires urgent medical attention. Its cause is usually easy to determine (Table 25.2) and in all cases the first emergency action is to clear secretions from the mouth and pharynx. The next step depends on where the emergency has occurred, its urgency and its cause. If transfer to hospital is deemed advisable, the patient must be accompanied by trained personnel.

Conservative management

Humidified oxygen will rapidly ease symptoms, give confidence and allow secretions to be more easily aspirated. Hydrocortisone 100–300 mg intravenously will often buy time until a more definitive procedure can be performed.

Table 25.2 Common causes of acute airway obstruction

Cause	Distinguishing features
Children	
Inhaled foreign bodies	Sudden stridor in previously well child
Laryngotracheal bronchitis	Increasing illness and fever
Acute epiglottitis	Drooling and painful throat
Adults	
Laryngeal trauma	History of accident
Acute epiglottitis	Ill with painful throat
Tumours	Often chronic hoarseness

Heimlich's manoeuvre

Inhaled foreign bodies in children, such as peanuts, are best expelled from the larynx or trachea by a sudden bear hug around the chest and abdomen.

Laryngotomy

A large-bore needle inserted through the cricothyroid membrane can give temporary airway relief if necessary. So will the barrel of a ballpoint pen inserted through a stab incision.

Intubation

Endotracheal intubation past an obstructing lesion can be difficult but should be attempted if the obstruction persists, and is normally carried out in a hospital environment. If it fails, emergency tracheostomy is necessary.

Emergency tracheostomy

The best site for this is between the second and third tracheal rings, which in adults is two finger-breadths above the suprasternal notch. With the head extended over a pillow, and under local anaesthesia if the patient cannot be intubated for general anaesthesia, a vertical midline incision is made to expose the tracheal rings; a transverse incision between them at the correct level then allows a tracheostomy tube to be inserted. Sometimes the thyroid isthmus has to be divided or retracted to gain access.

THE EAR

Anatomy of the ear

The ear is the organ of hearing and balance. It has three parts: the outer, the middle and the inner ear (Fig. 25.15). These parts have different physiological functions and each has its own diseases.

Outer ear

The outer ear consists of the pinna and the external auditory canal. Both are covered by keratinized

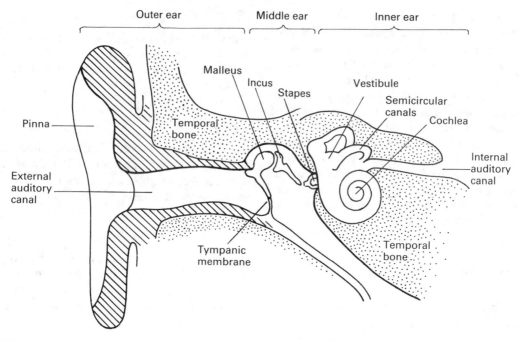

Fig. 25.15   Anatomical relationships of the external ear, middle ear and inner ear

squamous epithelium so that skin diseases are common. The substance of the pinna is fibroelastic cartilage and this extends into the outer third of the canal, the remaining two-thirds being bony. In the outer third of the canal there are, in addition, ceruminous glands which secrete wax. The canal terminates at the tympanic membrane (see Fig. 25.15), which is part of the middle ear.

Middle ear

The middle ear is an air-containing space in continuity with the nasopharynx via the Eustachian tube and with the mastoid air cells via the mastoid antrum (Fig. 25.16). The Eustachian tube is lined by a mucus-secreting, ciliated respiratory tract epithelium which extends into the middle ear. The remainder of the middle ear and the mastoid spaces are lined by a simple flat mucosa which, when inflamed, undergoes metaplasia to an upper respiratory tract mucosa. The majority of middle ear conditions are due to mucosal disease. The middle ear contains the three ossicles (malleus, incus and stapes) which transmit sounds as vibra-

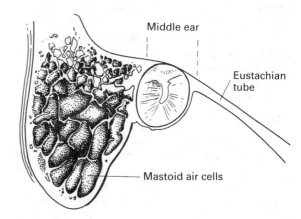

Fig. 25.16   Anatomical relationships between the mastoid air cells and the middle ear

tions from the external auditory canal to the fluids of the inner ear.

Inner ear

The inner ear is within the temporal bone and consists of the cochlea (the sense organ of hearing) and the vestibular labyrinth (the sense organ of balance) (see Fig. 25.15). These are supplied by the eighth (cochleovestibular) cranial nerve from the brain stem. The seventh (facial) cranial nerve runs alongside the eighth nerve in the internal auditory canal, then progresses through the middle ear and mastoid air cell system to exit via the stylomastoid foramen. In the inner ear, pathology most frequently affects the neurosensory elements.

Otological symptoms

Otological symptoms are common and their cause is usually easy to ascertain by taking a relevant case history, by examining the ear and by assessing the hearing. Investigations apart from audiology play a minimal role.

Hearing impairment

Hearing impairment may affect one ear, or both ears to an equal or different extent. Although impairments are common they are not always complained of, particularly at the extremes of life. In children, bilateral impairment can seriously hinder education, and screening by health visitors before the age of 1 year (by distraction testing) and again in the first school year (by pure-tone audiometry) is therefore routine in the UK.

Hearing impairments are classified according to whether the defect is in the external or middle ear conduction mechanism or in the sensory or neural parts of the inner ear. The former are called conductive and the latter sensorineural impairments. The distinction has considerable diagnostic and management implications.

Ear discharge (otorrhoea)

Wax is normally shed unnoticed but there are some who consider it to be a discharge. It should not be difficult to distinguish wax from the foul-smelling, watery or mucopurulent discharge that is often associated with inflammation of the external or middle ear. Sometimes there may be blood in the discharge but this is usually due to trauma from attempts to clean out the ear.

Pain (otalgia)

There are two distinct types of otalgia. One is the itchy, uncomfortable pain associated with inflammation of the skin of the external auditory canal which makes the patient want to 'poke' it. The other is a more deep-seated pain due to a difference in pressure across the tympanic membrane. This can be due to a malfunctioning Eustachian tube which is unable to equate pressure in the middle ear with atmospheric pressure. Alternatively, it may be due to pus under positive pressure or fluid under negative pressure.

Otalgia is by no means always otological in origin; pain from the pharynx, teeth and neck can present as referred otalgia as those areas are supplied by the same nerves as the ear.

Tinnitus

Tinnitus is the intermittent or constant hearing of sounds variously described by terms such as whistling, television interference or rushing water. Tinnitus is usually associated with hearing impairment but this can be of any type or aetiology. Its presence does not make a specific diagnosis more likely, it only determines whether management is required. The vast majority of individuals are able to adjust to their tinnitus.

The pathophysiology of tinnitus is unknown but perhaps the easiest explanation to give a patient is that there has been some damage to the ear which then sends off inappropriate nerve signals which are heard as tinnitus.

Disequilibrium

Balance upset is one of the more difficult symptoms to disentangle. Faulty or absent input from any of the organs that normally help to control balance (Fig. 25.17) can cause disequilibrium. Ophthalmic disease rarely causes disequilibrium and proprioceptor disease is relatively easy to diagnose because of the associated problems of limb control. With time and patience it is usually possible to categorize the patient's symptoms as one of the following.

Vertigo. This is the sensation of rotation, either of the patient or of the environment. Vertigo tends to be episodic, can come at any time, is made worse by shutting the eyes and is often associated with nausea but not with vomiting. The subject

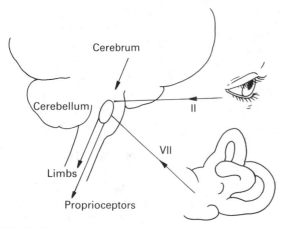

Fig. 25.17 Physiology of balance

feels off-balance but does not fall, and the episodes last at most for minutes. Vertigo is usually otological in origin but not all otological balance problems present as vertigo.

Lightheadedness. If this occurs on changing the body's position, the patient can be advised to do this more slowly. The most likely cause is postural hypotension, which occurs when the pressure receptors do not respond quickly enough to a change in posture, notably on getting up from a sitting or lying position. Drugs can cause lightheadedness, including those prescribed for hypertension and for disequilibrium.

Imbalance. This typically occurs only on movement. The patient often staggers to one side and the commonest cause is the general incoordination of ageing. Most patients with imbalance have non-otological problems but otological disease can, in the acute stage, cause imbalance. This tends to compensate with time whereas central causes do not.

Blackouts and falls. Patients will usually have no difficulty in deciding whether they temporarily lose consciousness, fall to the ground or both. A history of loss of consciousness rules out otological conditions as being responsible.

Assessment of the ear

Otoscopy

In most instances, the cause of a conductive hearing impairment will be revealed by otoscopy although this can sometimes be difficult and require a microscope. Otitis media with effusion can be particularly difficult to detect but a pneumatic otoscope, which varies the pressure in the external auditory canal, should help to detect an immobile tympanic membrane (see below).

Hearing

Hearing impairment is present if a patient cannot repeat words whispered to him at the quietest level possible from behind and at arm's length while hearing in the non-tested ear is masked by rubbing the tragus. By varying the voice level and distance, the severity of the impairment can be assessed.

Tuning-fork tests, particularly the Rinne test, have been used to identify the presence of a conduction defect. If bone conduction appears louder than air conduction there is conductive impairment, but a high proportion of ears with such impairment do not give this response. The best way to determine the type of impairment is by pure-tone audiometry.

Audiometry

Pure-tone audiometry determines the thresholds of hearing by both air and bone conduction. The air conduction thresholds reflect the severity of the impairment, while the difference (if any) between air conduction and bone conduction thresholds reflects the magnitude of any conduction defect.

Electric response audiometry measures electrically the neuronal responses to sound stimuli at various levels in the auditory pathway and allows thresholds to be determined in patients who are otherwise difficult to test, notably infants.

Management of hearing impairment

If an individual with a hearing impairment is disabled, the mainstay of management is a hearing aid; surgery may be considered if the impairment is of a conductive type.

Hearing aids

These are miniature sound amplifiers whose frequency output and gain can be modified to suit the patient's impairment. The majority are worn behind the ear and are suitable for most types of impairment. In the UK supply and servicing of these aids is free. 'In-the-ear' aids are available commercially but are only suitable for the mildly impaired and have no acoustic advantage.

Benefit from a hearing aid is not as simple to achieve as the benefit to vision given by spectacles. Many find the ear mould difficult to insert, and learning to use the aid at different settings in different listening circumstances can be difficult. Follow-up is essential to ensure that the aid can be used. It is unfortunate that extra loudness often does not make speech any clearer for those with poor frequency discrimination due to a sensorineural impairment.

Surgery

Ear surgery (see below) may be necessary to treat ear pathology but in the majority of patients surgery is undertaken to improve hearing. When successful, the results are superior to those of a hearing aid. Such surgery is usually done with the aid of an operating microscope and under local or general anaesthesia.

General management of tinnitus

The patient should be reassured that tinnitus is common and does not indicate serious brain disease or portend total loss of hearing. Background noise, for example from a radio, can be used to distract the attention when tinnitus is troublesome. The majority require little else. For those more severely troubled, a tinnitus masker, a behind-the-ear aid that produces a broad band noise, can be a psychological prop. There are no specific anti-tinnitus drugs but sedatives and tranquillizers may be used with caution in selected patients.

General management of vertigo

Thankfully otological vertigo is self-limiting, and long-term medication is seldom indicated. Indeed, drug-induced disequilibrium is common, and many individuals feel better without their medication. The drugs available for treatment are non-specific 'sedatives' and include anti-histamines, such as cinnarizine (Stugeron), phenothiazides such as prochlorperazine (Stemetil) or vasodilators such as betahistidine (Serc).

For the rare patient whose vertigo does not subside with time, various destructive surgical procedures, such as labyrinthectomy and vestibular nerve section, may be helpful.

CONDITIONS OF THE PINNA

Bat ears

Bat ears are a common developmental abnormality in which the absence of an antehelix fold causes the ears to stick out. This may cause embarrassment unless covered by long hair. Various methods of surgical correction can recreate the absent fold.

Trauma

Because of its position, the pinna is frequently injured. Minor subperichondrial haemorrhage is common and, if repeated, the cartilage will thicken and result in a deformed 'cauliflower' ear (typical of boxers). Any definite haematoma should be surgically drained to prevent cartilage necrosis. If local signs and symptoms of inflammation occur, secondary bacterial infection has occurred. Such perichondritis should be treated with antibiotics.

CONDITIONS OF THE EXTERNAL AUDITORY CANAL

Wax

Wax is secreted in the outer third of the canal and in this position, even if it obscures the view of the tympanic membrane, will not impair hearing because it does not impede sound vibrations. Only if wax becomes impacted against the tympanic membrane by misguided attempts to remove it with cotton buds will impairment result, and even then the impairment is minor. The mould of a hearing aid can also impact wax.

Wax frequently has to be removed to visualize the tympanic membrane. This is best done by syringing. Impacted wax requires softening with olive oil, almond oil or sodium bicarbonate ear drops (BP). Commercial preparations are not superior and can cause skin irritation.

Otitis externa

Otitis externa is dermatitis of the external auditory canal which sometimes involves the pinna. The ear is uncomfortable and itchy, making the patient want to clean it out. There is sometimes a watery discharge and the canal is inflamed, oedematous and weepy. The mainstay of management is to remove the debris, often by syringing. Topical low-strength steroid cream or glycerol and ichthamol ear drops can soothe the discomfort. If the canal is narrow, these medications can be applied daily on a wick. Topical antibiotics are contraindicated, as otitis externa is not normally an infective condition and they can cause allergic skin reactions.

CONDITIONS OF THE MIDDLE EAR

Acute otitis media

Acute otitis media is a bacterial infection of the middle ear which is extremely common in childhood, especially under the age of 5 years. The typical history is of a child with an upper respiratory tract infection who wakes at night crying with a painful ear. It arises because the products of secondary bacterial infection of the middle ear mucosa are unable to drain down an oedematous Eustachian tube. The differential diagnosis is from transient negative middle ear pressure or from referred pain from the teeth or upper respiratory and alimentary tracts. The distinction is made by the otoscopic finding of an inflamed, bulging tympanic membrane. The natural history is one of spontaneous resolution or drainage after rupture of the tympanic membrane. Such ruptures almost invariably heal spontaneously.

Management consists of analgesics (e.g. paracetamol elixir) and perhaps antibiotics (e.g. amoxycillin to cover upper respiratory bacteria, including *Haemophilus influenzae*) if there is gross systemic upset with fever. Drainage of pus by myringotomy is usually unnecessary. Rarely, pus

within the mastoid is unable to drain, causing mastoiditis which may spread intracranially to give rise to meningitis or an abscess. Surgical drainage and removal of infected mucosa and bone (mastoidectomy) is then mandatory.

Otitis media with effusion

Otitis media with effusion (secretory/serous otitis media, glue ear) is due to a combination of factors (adenoid enlargement, poor Eustachian tube function, inflammation of the middle ear mucosa) which initially results in negative middle ear pressure and thereafter progresses to non-infected middle ear effusion. This immobilizes the tympanic membrane, causing hearing impairment.

The classical history is of a child who previously had normal hearing, as demonstrated by the development of normal speech, becoming dull of hearing. The impairment may or may not be noticed by the parents and is often detected at school screening. Occasionally there is otalgia due to a change in middle ear pressure. The natural history is one of episodes of recurrence and resolution followed by permanent resolution unless there are severe predisposing factors such as poor Eustachian tube function from a cleft palate.

Management is expectant unless bilateral hearing impairment (as demonstrated by the inability to repeat a whispered voice at arm's length) persists for 3 months. Active management is then indicated because the child may suffer educationally. Medication is of unproven value, and surgery in any combination of adenoidectomy, myringotomy and aspiration, or insertion of ventilating tubes (grommets) is indicated (Fig. 25.18).

Chronic otitis media

Chronic otitis media is due to chronic inflammation of the middle ear and mastoid mucosa and is associated with permanent perforation of the tympanic membrane. The inflammation may be constant, intermittent or inactive. When active, there is a mucopurulent, foul-smelling discharge which may or may not be noticed by the patient. In all cases there is a conductive hearing impairment the magnitude of which depends on the size

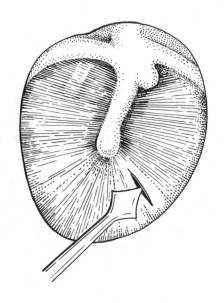

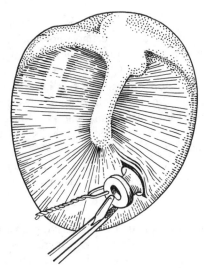

Fig. 25.18 Treatment of otitis media with effusion. (a) Myringotomy. (b) Insertion of grommet

in the attic. A cholesteatoma is a retraction pocket lined with squamous epithelium in which debris builds up because of its narrow neck.

In inactive ears, the hearing impairment may require surgical closure of the perforation to prevent future activity. Active ears require more aggressive treatment because of the risk (albeit low) of developing meningitis, intracranial abscess or facial nerve palsy due to spread of infection. The discharge is dealt with by regular aural toilet. Instillation of topical antibiotic and steroid drops improves the cyclical resolution rate but permanent cure depends on surgical eradication of the inflammation and repair of the tympanic membrane. This involves rebuilding of the tympanic membrane and/or the ossicular chain with autologous or homograft fascia and ossicles.

Otosclerosis

Otosclerosis is new bone growth in the region of the oval window which fixes the stapes. The diagnosis is assumed when a patient with a conductive hearing impairment has a normal tympanic membrane. Surgical alleviation consists of stapedectomy, in which the fixed stapes is partially removed and replaced with an artificial prosthesis.

CONDITIONS OF THE INNER EAR

Sensorineural hearing impairment

Some 20% of adults have a sensorineural hearing impairment, the majority being over the age of 50 years. In most the aetiology is unidentifiable and, in the absence of a history of noise trauma or other cause, the term presbycusis is often used to describe the syndrome in older patients.

Sensorineural impairments are usually symmetrical. It is important to investigate asymmetrical impairments because of the possibility of an acoustic neuroma, although this is rare (see below).

Noise. Industrial noise from machinery may cause hearing impairment, depending on a combination of genetic predisposition, noise level and duration of exposure. Damage can be mitigated by wearing ear defenders, but cotton wool is useless.

of the perforation and on whether the ossicular chain has been eroded. Once mucopus has been removed by mopping with a cotton bud or syringing, the defect in the tympanic membrane should be seen via an otoscope. Sometimes the middle ear mucosa becomes polypoidal and polyps can enlarge through the perforation to fill the external auditory canal. In some ears, in addition to mucosal disease, a cholesteatoma may be identified

Firing guns also causes damage, but occasional visits to discotheques will not.

Drugs. Many drugs can cause inner ear damage, particularly in patients with impaired renal function. In this respect the aminoglycosides (e.g. gentamicin) and loop diuretics can be particularly dangerous if blood levels are not monitored.

Infection. Mumps and measles can be associated with unilateral sensorineural impairment but the incidence is falling because of increasing immunization of infants. Meningitis is also fairly frequently associated with deafness.

Head injury. A temporal bone fracture, which is usually evident from the presence of blood in the middle ear and sometimes from the passage of blood or CSF from the ear, may cause sudden unilateral hearing impairment, often associated with vertigo.

Barotrauma. Sometimes, after an aeroplane flight or underwater diving, unequal pressure between the middle and inner ear ruptures the round window membrane. Sudden unilateral impairment with vertigo results and surgical repair of the rupture may be indicated.

Congenital. Genetic abnormalities, Rubella infections, prematurity, birth trauma and haemolytic crises are the main causes of sensorineural impairments in infants. These have to be recognized early so that amplification can be provided to enable speech to develop as normally as possible.

Acoustic neuroma. Acoustic neuromas are benign slow-growing neurofibromas of the eighth cranial nerve which can cause neurological problems and death by pressing on the brainstem. Early diagnosis is vital and is achieved by investigating all patients with an idiopathic unilateral or asymmetrical impairment by electric response audiometry and appropriate radiology. The tumours can be excised through the ear (translabyrinthine approach), or the middle or posterior cranial fossa, depending on their size.

Labyrinthine disorders

Acute labyrinthitis

Acute labyrinthitis produces an acute attack of vertigo which lasts for several days, is prostrating, and is associated with a sensorineural hearing impairment and sometimes tinnitus. Temporal bone fracture and ear surgery are readily identifiable causes, while viral infection or transient ischaemia are postulated as more common causes. In the absence of hearing impairment, the pathology is thought to be retrocochlear (as opposed to labyrinthine) and the syndrome is termed vestibular neuronitis. Spontaneous resolution is the rule and medication until this occurs is all that may be required.

Chronic labyrinthitis

Chronic labyrinthitis is diagnosed when there are recurrent episodes of vertigo. Fortunately, most cases resolve spontaneously. The aetiology in most patients is unknown. Chronic otitis media must be excluded because episodic vertigo in this condition implies spread of infection to the inner ear and an increased risk of intracranial complications. Surgical management in such patients is usually mandatory. If the recurrent episodes of disequilibrium are associated with transient deterioration in hearing and perhaps tinnitus or fullness in the ear, the condition is referred to as Menière's syndrome.

In the rare patient in whom symptoms do not regress with time, destructive operations such as labyrinthectomy (in which the inner ear is totally destroyed) or vestibular nerve section via the middle cranial fossa (which preserves hearing) should be considered. Various other, somewhat controversial surgical procedures have been advocated for Menière's syndrome but their value is unproven.

26. The oesophagus

Surgical anatomy

The oesophagus is a hollow muscular tube which extends from the termination of the pharynx (C6) to the oesophagogastric junction (Fig. 26.1). It has cervical, thoracic and abdominal portions and is 25 cm long, the final 2–4 cm lying within the abdomen. The muscle coat comprises an inner circular and outer longitudinal layer. The muscle fibres are striated in the upper third, with a gradual transition to smooth muscle below that level. The oesophageal lumen is lined by squamous epithelium which occasionally contains islands of ectopic gastric mucosa. The distal 1–2 cm of oesophagus are lined by columnar epithelium. The submucosa contains numerous mucous glands, a rich lymphatic network and the neural plexus of Meissner. Auerbach's neural plexus is found between the two muscle layers.

There are two oesophageal sphincters. The *upper oesophageal sphincter* is 3–4 cm long and is formed by the cricopharyngeus muscle and first few centimetres of oesophagus. It is closed at rest to prevent air from entering the oesophagus, but opens on swallowing. The *lower oesophageal sphincter* cannot be defined anatomically but is detected as a high-pressure zone on manometry. The sphincter is tonically closed at rest, is 3–5 cm long, and is located in the region of the oesophageal hiatus in the diaphragm.

Three areas of oesophageal narrowing can be demonstrated on barium swallow and are often seen during endoscopy. They are situated: (1) at the beginning of the oesophagus, (2) as it passes to the right of the aortic arch and behind the left bronchus, and (3) as it traverses the oesophageal hiatus of the diaphragm.

The oesophageal hiatus consists of an encircling noose of muscle drawn mainly from the right diaphragmatic crus, with a variable contribution from the left crus (Fig. 26.2). The lower oesophagus and oesophagogastric junction are held loosely in the hiatus by a condensation of fascia known as the phreno-oesophageal ligament.

The oesophagus receives arterial blood from the gastric and phrenic vessels below, from the aortic and bronchial vessels in the thorax, and from the

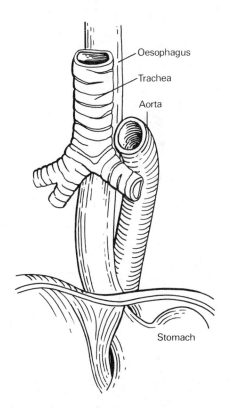

Oesophagus

Trachea

Aorta

Stomach

Fig. 26.1 Anatomical relationships of the oesophagus

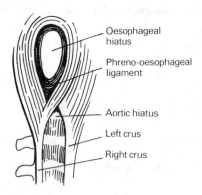

Oesophageal hiatus

Phreno-oesophageal ligament

Aortic hiatus

Left crus

Right crus

Fig. 26.2 Anatomy of the oesophageal hiatus

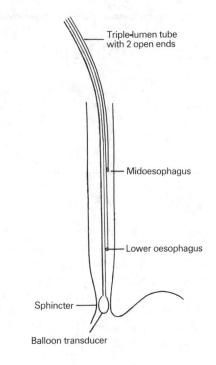

Triple-lumen tube with 2 open ends

Midoesophagus

Lower oesophagus

Sphincter

Balloon transducer

a

inferior thyroid arteries in the neck. Venous drainage corresponds to the arterial supply. The communication between the left gastric veins (portal system) and thoracic oesophageal veins (azygos and hemiazygos system) is important in the development of oesophageal varices in portal hypertension (see Ch. 36).

Lymphatic drainage does not correspond to blood supply. The lymphatics run longitudinally within the submucosa before penetrating the muscle coat to drain into regional lymph nodes. Submucosal extension of tumour is common in oesophageal carcinoma. Lymph from the upper and midoesophagus drains first to the thoracic and cervical nodes, while the lower oesophagus drains to gastric and coeliac nodes.

Surgical physiology

The upper oesophageal sphincter relaxes to allow entry of food from the pharynx. Subsequent contraction of this sphincter initiates a peristaltic wave (amplitude 50–100 cm water) which propels food distally. The lower oesophageal sphincter relaxes as the wave approaches and food passes into the stomach. Passage of the peristaltic wave can be monitored by recording luminal pressure at varying levels in the oesophagus (Fig. 26.3).

Resting pressure within the thoracic oesophagus reflects intrathoracic pressure, and mean values are subatmospheric. Intra-abdominal pressure exceeds atmospheric pressure but reflux of gastric content is normally prevented by the lower oesophageal sphincter. A number of mechanical factors may

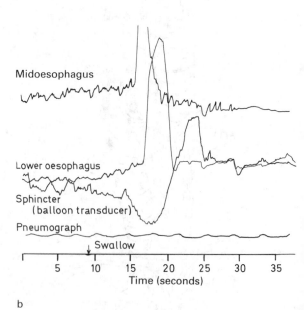

Midoesophagus

Lower oesophagus

Sphincter (balloon transducer)

Pneumograph

Swallow

5   10   15   20   25   30   35
Time (seconds)

b

Fig. 26.3 Recording of intraoesophageal pressure. (a) Balloon-covered measuring device and open-tipped tubes in place. (b) Pressure recording of deglutitive response in healty subject. Note that relaxation of the lower sphincter procedes arrival of the peristaltic wave.

contribute to gastro-oesophageal competence. They include the diaphragm, the prominent folds of gastric mucosa (mucosal rosette) at the oesophagogastric junction, and the oblique entry of the oesophagus into the stomach, which creates a flap-valve effect.

The vagus controls peristalsis in the body of the oesophagus and induces relaxation of the lower oesophageal sphincter during swallowing. However, sphincter tone is not abolished by vagal or sympathetic denervation and the sphincter continues to relax on swallowing.

Symptoms of oesophageal disease

There are three principal symptoms of oesophageal disease.

Dysphagia

Difficulty in swallowing is usually an indication of organic disease and requires urgent and careful investigation. Some patients localize the site of obstruction accurately but in many cases localization is poor. For example, the patient may indicate that food sticks at the level of the sternal angle when the lesion is located at the lower end of the oesophagus. It is important to establish the length of history, whether dysphagia is intermittent, constant or progressive, and whether liquids and solids are equally affected. Patients with oesophageal obstruction may complain of *hiccough* during eating. The mechanism responsible is uncertain but the symptom may predate the onset of dysphagia by several weeks.

Some of the main causes of dysphagia are shown in Table 26.1. Peptic oesophagitis and carcinoma are common causes of this symptom.

Globus hystericus is often confused with dysphagia. The patient feels as if there is a lump in the throat or upper oesophagus, but on close questioning the symptom is often found to be more troublesome between meals than during eating. The symptom is associated with nervous tension and has no organic cause. However, it may prove difficult to distinguish clinically between globus hystericus and dysphagia, and the former diagnosis can only be accepted after organic disease has been excluded by rigorous investigation.

Pain

Heartburn is a retrosternal burning discomfort or pain associated with gastro-oesophageal reflux. The pain may radiate up to the neck and jaws, through to the back, or down the arms. It is often

Table 26.1 Causes of dysphagia

	Intraluminal	Intramural		Extrinsic
Pharynx and upper oesophagus	Foreign body	Mucosal	Pharyngitis Tonsillitis Moniliasis Sideropenic web Corrosive poisons Carcinoma	Thyroid enlargement
		Muscular Neurological	Myasthenia gravis Bulbar palsy	Pharyngeal pouch
Body of oesophagus	Foreign body	Mucosal	Corrosive poisons Peptic oesophagitis Carcinoma	Mediastinal lymphadenopathy Aortic aneurysm Dysphagia lusoria
Lower oesophagus	Foreign body	Mucosal	Corrosive poisons Peptic oesophagitis Carcinoma	Unfolded aorta Para-oesophageal hernia
		Muscular	Oesophageal spasm Scleroderma	
		Neurological	Achalasia Post-vagotomy Gastric carcinoma	

brought on by recumbency or stooping, occurs soon after meals, and may be precipitated by hot liquids or fruit juice. The pain can usually be reproduced by instillation of 0.1-molar HCl and is usually relieved by alkali. However, acid is not essential for the production of heartburn and the symptom may occur after total gastrectomy and in patients who are achlorhydric. Alkaline bile reflux may be responsible for heartburn in such individuals. Although conditions which cause reflux oesophagitis usually produce heartburn, the symptom has an inconstant relationship with endoscopic and histological evidence of inflammation. Oesophageal motor abnormalities are also associated with production of heartburn but the exact relationship between the two is uncertain.

Oesophageal spasm is thought to produce a diffuse gripping retrosternal sensation or pain which may resemble angina pectoris or heartburn. However, the pain of spasm is not related to exercise and, in contrast to heartburn, is unaffected by posture or ingestion of alkali.

Regurgitation

Some patients with oesophageal obstruction complain of food regurgitation rather than dysphagia. The patient often states that he vomits, but careful questioning reveals that there is no associated nausea and that the 'vomiting' is effortless. The patient spits out food rather than vomits, and the 'vomitus' usually consists of undigested food uncontaminated by gastric juice or bile. Nocturnal reflux and aspiration of food may wake the patient with coughing fits, and can cause aspiration pneumonia which so dominates the clinical picture that the primary problem is easily overlooked.

Investigation of oesophageal disease

A careful history and thorough physical examination are essential when oesophageal disease is suspected. Most of the oesophagus is inaccessible, but particular attention is paid to examination of the neck, chest and upper abdomen.

A *chest X-ray* may raise suspicion of oesophageal disease by revealing enlarged mediastinal lymph nodes, evidence of aspiration pneumonia, or even pulmonary metastases. The gastric air bubble is seen within the chest in some patients with hiatus hernia, and is occasionally indented by tumour arising in the region of the cardia. Following penetrating oesophageal trauma, air may be seen in the mediastinum and root of the neck.

Barium swallow and meal are essential investigations and *cine-radiography* often assists in the assessment of motility disorders.

Endoscopy is mandatory even when the diagnosis appears certain on radiological grounds; unsuspected additional pathology may be revealed, as for example the presence of early carcinoma in a patient with long-standing hiatus hernia. The oesophagus, stomach and proximal duodenum are inspected and all suspicious lesions are biopsied. The flexible fibreoptic endoscope has largely replaced the rigid oesophagoscope because it is less uncomfortable for the patient, carries less risk of oesophageal perforation and allows inspection of the entire stomach and proximal duodenum. Fibreoptic endoscopy suffers from the limitation that only small mucosal biopsies can be obtained and submucosal extension of cancer may escape detection.

Oesophageal pressure recordings may aid in detection and assessment of abnormal motility. Pressure readings are obtained from a series of fine tubes perfused with saline and bound together so that their openings are 5 cm apart (see Fig. 26.3). The assembly can be used to detect the lower oesophageal sphincter and measure sphincter pressure, or to monitor propulsion of the peristaltic wave during swallowing. Abnormal motility patterns are a feature of achalasia, diffuse oesophageal spasm and scleroderma (see below).

Bernstein's test entails passing a narrow-bore nasogastric tube into the lower oesophagus and infusing 0.1-molar HCl or a control solution of saline. Acid reproduces the patient's symptoms if they are due to reflux oesophagitis, but false positive and false negative results are not uncommon (Fig. 26.4).

pH measurements can be made using an intraluminal electrode and are used to detect gastro-oesophageal reflux. In an extension of the Bernstein test, the electrode can also be used to determine the number of swallows needed to clear acid from the lower oesophagus. Systems are now available to monitor pH over a 24-hour period

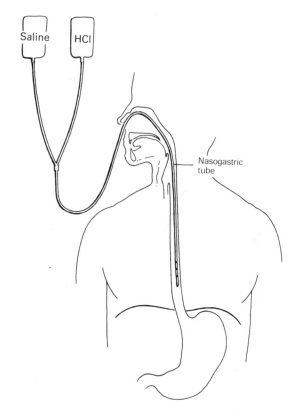

Fig. 26.4 Bernstein's test. The two bottles containing HCl and saline allow interchange of the infusion without the knowledge of the patient

while the patient goes about his normal activities.

Oesophageal scintigraphy is a quantitative test of reflux. A gamma-camera is used to scan the lower oesophagus and stomach after filling the stomach with saline to which ^{99m}Tc-labelled sulphur colloid has been added.

DISORDERS OF OESOPHAGEAL MOTILITY

Abnormalities of the upper oesophageal sphincter

Lack of coordination between pharyngeal contraction and relaxation of the upper oesophageal sphincter is implicated in dysphagia due to myasthenia gravis and bulbar palsy, and may follow extensive surgery in the oropharyngeal region. Oesophageal manometry can define those patients in whom cricopharyngeal myotomy will be of value. Abnormal motility has also been incriminated in the development of pharyngo-oesophageal diverticulum (see p. 398).

Achalasia of the cardia

Achalasia is the commonest oesophageal motility disorder although its annual incidence is less than 1 per 100 000 population. Males and females are affected with equal frequency and, while the disease occurs in all age groups, it is most common in patients between 30 and 60 years of age. The cause of achalasia is unknown but a neurogenic basis is suggested by the disintegration or absence of Auerbach's plexus. Degenerative changes have also been demonstrated in the vagal branches to the lower oesophagus, and degeneration of the myenteric plexus may be secondary to lesions in the vagus or brainstem.

Infection with *Trypanosoma cruzi* (Chagas' disease), prevalent in South America, causes degeneration of Auerbach's plexus and leads to motor changes indistinguishable from those of achalasia.

Manometric and radiological studies reveal that motility is disordered throughout the oesophagus in achalasia. Resting pressure in the body of oesophagus is high, propulsive peristalsis is absent, and the lower oesophageal sphincter fails to relax on swallowing.

Clinical features

Dysphagia is the cardinal symptom and is at first intermittent but usually becomes progressive. It may be aggravated by anxiety or fatigue, is often worse with liquids rather than solids, and may be more troublesome with cold food. Gravity rather than peristalsis is responsible for food leaving the oesophagus, and the patient may develop tricks to aid oesophageal emptying. For example, he may stand while eating or drinking, and may force food through the oesophagus by expiring forcibly against a closed glottis. Marked weight loss occurs if dysphagia is severe.

Food regurgitation is common and occurs during sleep. Repeated bouts of aspiration pneumonia may lead to pulmonary fibrosis.

Retrosternal pain occurs in about 25% of patients and is described as bursting or burning, with radiation to the neck, throat, back or arms. Hiccough may predate dysphagia.

Minor mucosal erosions of the oesophagus are common but peptic ulceration is exceptional. Carcinoma can develop in long-standing achalasia, even after successful surgical treatment. Its development is insidious and the resulting oesophageal obstruction may be attributed to the dysphagia of achalasia, leading to late diagnosis of cancer at an inoperable stage.

Diagnosis

Barium swallow reveals gross distension and/or tortuosity of the oesophagus, with a conical narrowing at the cardia leading to a string-like ('rat-tail') passage to the stomach (Fig. 26.5). Cine-radiology shows irregular disorganized contractions of the body of the oesophagus and failure of relaxation of the lower oesophageal sphincter. Despite classical radiological appearances, endoscopy is essential to exclude carcinoma or benign oesophageal stricture.

Manometry confirms the lack of propulsive peristalsis and failure of relaxation of the lower oesophageal sphincter. The denervated oesophagus is hypersensitive to subcutaneous injection of small doses of the parasympathomimetic drug methacholine, but in practice this test is rarely necessary.

Treatment

Diet and drugs are ineffective in the treatment of achalasia. Forcible dilatation by hydrostatic, pneumatic or mechanical means (Fig. 26.6) will relieve symptoms in about 80% of cases, but complications (notably oesophageal perforation) occur in 5%. Repeated dilatations may be necessary. Cardiomyotomy (Heller's operation) is employed if dilatation fails, although some surgeons now regard this operation as the primary treatment of choice. The oesophagus is usually approached through the thorax. A 10–12 cm longitudinal incision is made through the oesophageal musculature without breaching the mucosa, and taking care to preserve the vagus nerves (Fig. 26.7). The incision is extended onto the stomach for less than 1 cm. Good to excellent results are obtained in 85% of patients, but the results can be marred by gastro-oesophageal reflux with stricture formation if the incision is extended too far distally. Because of the problem of reflux some surgeons advocate combining cardiomyotomy with an antireflux procedure such as a Nissen fundoplication (see Fig. 26.11).

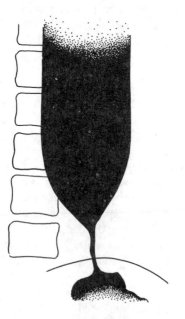

Fig. 26.5   Radiological appearance of achalasia of the cardia

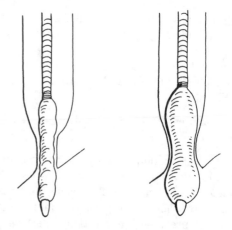

Fig. 26.6   Hydrostatic dilatation of achalasia

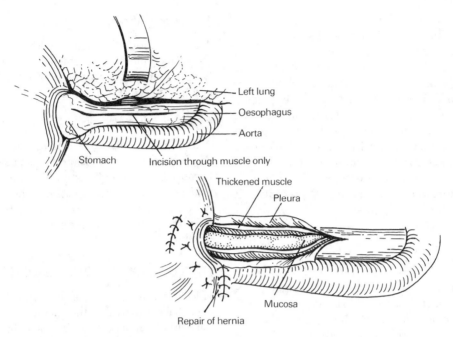

Left lung

Oesophagus

Aorta

Stomach   Incision through muscle only

Thickened muscle

Pleura

Mucosa

Repair of hernia

Fig. 26.7 Cardiomyotomy (Heller's operation) for relief of achalasia

Diffuse oesophageal spasm

This disease differs from achalasia in that the lower oesophageal sphincter is hypertensive in addition to failing to relax. Hypermotility of the body of the oesophagus leads to repeated spasmodic contractions. The cause of diffuse oesophageal spasm is unknown.

Pain is the cardinal clinical feature and varies in severity from retrosternal discomfort to severe colicky retrosternal pain which may radiate widely and mimic angina pectoris. The pain is frequently provoked by eating but sometimes occurs spontaneously and may wake the patient at night.

Barium swallow reveals a 'corkscrew' oesophagus in 50% of cases, the appearance being due to indentation of the lumen by contracted muscle bundles (Fig. 26.8). Manometry demonstrates that oesophageal peristalsis is replaced by simultaneous repetitive contractions, and may show that the lower oesophageal sphincter is hypertensive with failure to relax on swallowing.

Patients with such abnormal motility can be treated by pneumatic dilatation or by a long myotomy which may extend from the aortic arch to the cardia. The length of incision is determined

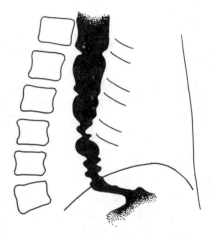

Fig. 26.8 'Corkscrew' oesophagus as seen on barium swallow

by the extent of manometric abnormality. The results of treatment are less satisfactory than those of achalasia.

Miscellaneous motility disorders

Abnormal oesophageal motility leads to dysphagia in a number of collagen diseases and neuromuscular disorders. Scleroderma is probably the commonest of these disorders, its oesophageal manifestations being fragmentation of submucosal connective tissue and smooth muscle atrophy. The lower oesophageal sphincter is incompetent, leading to reflux oesophagitis, stricture and dysphagia. Associated fibrosis leads to shortening of the oesophagus and a hiatus hernia. Motor failure can be confirmed manometrically and radiologically.

Treatment consists of medical measures to combat reflux oesophagitis, forcible dilatation if a stricture forms, and an antireflux procedure if these measures fail (see p. 400).

OESOPHAGEAL DIVERTICULA

Diverticula of the oesophagus can be classified according to their location (pharyngo-oesophageal, mid-thoracic or epiphrenic), their mode of formation (pulsion or traction), and depending on whether they contain all or only some layers of the oesophageal wall (true or false).

Pharyngo-oesophageal diverticulum (pharyngeal pouch)

This is the commonest type of diverticulum affecting the oesophagus and is dealt with in detail in chapter 25.

Mid-thoracic diverticulum

These traction diverticula used to be associated with tuberculous involvement of tracheobronchial lymph nodes. They seldom produced symptoms and are now rare.

Epiphrenic diverticulum

These diverticula are located just above the diaphragm and are pulsion diverticula which arise because of an underlying motility disorder such as achalasia or diffuse spasm. The majority of patients experience no symptoms, but dysphagia from the motility disorder may be an indication for myotomy.

HIATUS HERNIA AND OESOPHAGITIS

Herniation of a portion of the stomach through the oesophageal hiatus in the diaphragm is common, particularly in later life. It must be emphasized that hiatus hernia is not necessarily associated with symptoms; conversely, reflux oesophagitis often occurs in the absence of demonstrable gastric herniation.

There are two main types of hiatus hernia. Sliding hiatus hernia is common (95% of cases) whereas para-oesophageal (or rolling) hiatus hernia is rare (less than 5% of cases). Mixed hiatus hernia in which there is both a sliding and a rolling component is exceptional (Fig. 26.9).

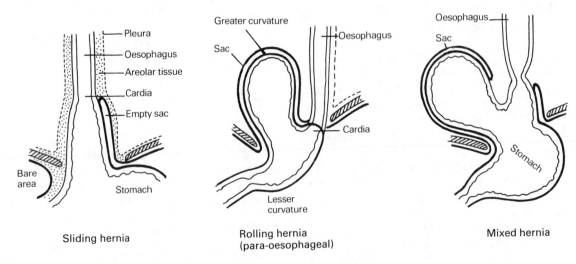

Fig. 26.9 Types of hiatus hernia

Sliding hiatus hernia

Pathological anatomy

As intra-abdominal pressure normally exceeds intrathoracic pressure, herniation of the stomach upwards is facilitated. Any additional increase in intra-abdominal pressure (as occurs during stooping, straining, coughing and in pregnancy) favours herniation. The phreno-oesophageal ligament becomes attenuated and allows the upper stomach to pass through the hiatus in a concentric fashion. Once herniation has occurred, the oesophagogastric junction slides upwards and downwards through the hiatus (hence the term 'sliding' hiatus hernia).

Provided the lower oesophageal sphincter remains competent, this does not lead to reflux of gastric contents and oesophagitis. Should reflux occur, the resulting inflammation and fibrosis may prevent further movement of the oesophagogastric junction, leading to a fixed concentric hiatus hernia with shortening of the oesophagus (Fig. 26.10).

Clinical features

The majority of patients have no symptoms referrable to their hiatus hernia and the condition is frequently discovered coincidentally during upper gastrointestinal radiology or endoscopy. It is the development of reflux oesophagitis which produces the cardinal symptom of heartburn. Heartburn occurs soon after meals, particularly large ones, is often promoted by stooping or recumbency, and is relieved by antacids. Patients may have learned to avoid tight clothing and to sleep with the head of the bed elevated to minimize symptoms.

The patient may complain of waterbrash and reflux of bitter irritating fluid into the pharynx and mouth. In waterbrash the mouth suddenly fills with clear tasteless fluid, probably from paroxysmal excessive salivation. Regurgitation of fluid and food may be associated with aspiration pneumonitis, particularly if reflux occurs during sleep.

Dysphagia is a relatively uncommon symptom and may reflect spasm of the inflamed distal oesophagus or stenosis due to long-standing oesophagitis. Stenosis may prevent further regurgitation and lead to abatement of the symptoms of reflux oesophagitis.

Acute haemorrhage is unusual, but chronic blood loss is a common cause of iron deficiency anaemia in elderly patients with reflux oesophagitis and hiatus hernia.

Diagnosis

There are two important steps in diagnosis: (1) to demonstrate the hernia and (2) to determine if reflux of gastric contents has caused oesophagitis.

The hernia may be evident on an ordinary barium swallow and meal, but in many patients it only becomes apparent when intra-abdominal pressure is increased by applying external pressure, placing the patient in the head-down position, or asking him to strain. Oesophagitis may be suspected if there is mucosal irregularity with oesophageal spasm.

Endoscopy is the key investigation for oesophagitis, the mucosa appearing red, friable and haemorrhagic. It should be biopsied. Endoscopy also allows the exclusion of carcinoma in patients with stenotic lesions, and definition of other lesions such as peptic ulceration of the oesophagus, stomach and proximal duodenum.

Oesophageal manometry and the Bernstein test (see above and Figs. 26.3 & 26.4) may aid in the

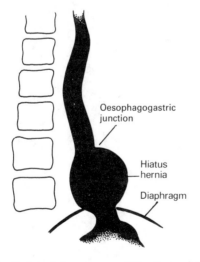

Oesophagogastric junction

Hiatus hernia

Diaphragm

Fig. 26.10 Radiological appearance of 'short' oesophagus

evaluation of patients with an atypical presentation but are not essential as routine investigations. A cholecystogram (or ultrasonic scan) should be obtained to exclude gallstones.

Management

Asymptomatic hiatus hernia does not require treatment. Reflux oesophagitis is managed in the first instance by conservative measures, which are successful in 85% of cases. These include weight reduction, avoidance of tight clothing and stooping, elevating the head of the bed at night (either by blocks or by increasing the number of pillows), stopping cigarette smoking, and pharmaceutical agents to neutralize gastric contents (antacids) or prevent the secretion of acid (e.g. cimetidine). Antacid-alginate mixtures (such as Gaviscon) or antacid-dimethicone mixtures (such as Asilone) may give more effective symptom relief. Large meals are replaced by more frequent small ones, and the patient is advised to avoid foods which induce symptoms.

Surgery is indicated if:

1. medical measures fail to control symptoms;
2. there is evidence of continuing gastrointestinal blood loss; or

3. dysphagia and stricture formation are established.

In the past, emphasis was placed on anatomical hernia repair, and a number of operations were designed to narrow the oesophageal hiatus and reconstruct the phreno-oesophageal ligament. With realization that reflux was the cause of symptoms and complications, emphasis shifted to its prevention. Modern operations combine these two principles.

Most surgeons now favour the operation of fundoplication described by Nissen. The operation can be performed through the chest or through the abdomen. The mobilized fundus of the stomach is 'wrapped around' the lower oesophagus so that the oesophagogastric junction and lower oesophagus are enclosed in a tunnel of stomach (Fig. 26.11). As pressure rises within the stomach, the enclosed segment of lower oesophagus is compressed and reflux is prevented.

The margins of the oesophageal hiatus are approximated behind the oesophagus so that the fundoplication is retained below the diaphragm. However, this is not essential in that reflux is still prevented if the fundoplication is left within the chest.

Approximately 90% of patients are rendered

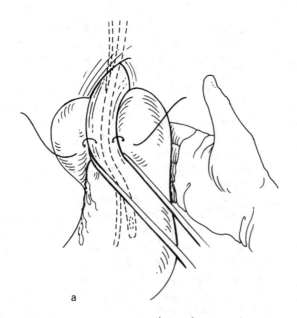
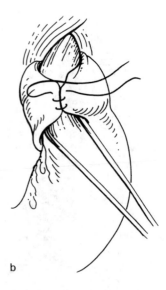

a   b

Fig. 26.11 Fundoplication. (a) Fundus wrapped around lower oesophagus. (b) Sutures in position

symptom-free and recurrence of reflux symptoms is uncommon. The 'gas-bloat' syndrome with inability to belch or vomit is experienced by about 10% of patients following fundoplication. This syndrome may improve with time and is minimized by avoiding large meals. Measures designed to reduce gastric acid-pepsin secretion (e.g. truncal vagotomy and drainage, highly selective vagotomy) are unnecessary unless the patient has associated peptic ulceration.

Para-oesophageal hernia

Pathological anatomy

There is usually a wide defect in the oesophageal hiatus lying to the left of the oesophagus. The fundus of the stomach passes upwards into a well-defined hernial sac lined by peritoneum, and the greater curve rolls upwards into the chest as the hernia enlarges. In time the entire stomach may roll into the chest so that the cardia and pylorus are approximated, the stomach appearing upside down when examined radiologically (Fig. 26.12).

Clinical features

The patient is frequently middle-aged or elderly, and herniation occurs without a recognizable precipitating cause. Symptoms of reflux are exceptional, the patient usually complaining of

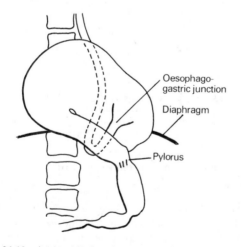

Oesophago-gastric junction

Diaphragm

Pylorus

Fig. 26.12 An 'upside-down' stomach

discomfort or pain from distension of the thoracic portion of the stomach by food. The pain is deep-seated within the chest, often described as crushing, and closely related to meals. Flatulence with belching is common and probably reflects attempts by the patient to gain relief. Weight loss and malnutrition may supervene as the patient cuts down on food intake to avoid symptoms.

Incarceration, pressure necrosis, gangrene and rupture can complicate para-oesophageal herniation and lead to an acute illness with potentially fatal rupture of gastric contents into the mediastinum. Peptic ulceration, due possibly to inadequate drainage, may occur in the incarcerated stomach and in turn can be complicated by perforation or bleeding.

Diagnosis

The diagnosis is often apparent on chest X-ray, which reveals a gas bubble and fluid level in the entrapped thoracic portion of stomach. The diagnosis is confirmed by barium meal examination. Endoscopy is not essential but may be used to exclude reflux oesophagitis.

Management

There is no medical management for para-oesophageal hiatus hernia and surgery is advised in all cases to relieve symptoms and avoid complications. The hernia can usually be reduced by an abdominal approach and the margins of the hernial defect approximated. An antireflux procedure is unnecessary but any associated gastric ulcer should be treated by vagotomy and drainage or gastric resection (see p. 455). Recurrence of herniation is uncommon but the risk can be reduced by suturing the replaced stomach to the diaphragm or abdominal wall. Symptoms are relieved promptly and nutrition improves rapidly.

Strangulation of a para-oesophageal hernia necessitates emergency thoracotomy, and gastric resection may be required if gangrene has supervened.

Reflux oesophagitis with stricture formation

This occurs as a result of long-standing reflux with oesophagitis and fibrosis. Fibrotic shortening of the oesophagus may draw the cardia up into the chest, giving rise to the so-called 'short oesophagus' (see Fig. 26.10). This was once believed to be congenital. Heartburn is the dominant clinical feature of reflux oesophagitis but is later replaced by dysphagia with stricture formation.

Treatment

Dilatation alone does not prevent continuing gastro-oesophageal reflux and stricture recurrence is common. A trial of dilatation and intensive medical therapy is used in most centres as a first-line treatment of oesophageal stricture. Dilatation followed by a surgical antireflux procedure is used when more conservative measures have failed to produce relief.

Dilatation used to be undertaken by advancing a rigid oesophagoscope to the site of narrowing and passing bougies of increasing diameter through the stricture. This was facilitated by asking the patient to swallow a piece of string on the previous evening to mark the path to be followed. A fibreoptic endoscope is now preferred to pass a fine guide wire through the stricture under vision. The endoscope is then withdrawn and a series of flexible sounds are passed over the guide wire to dilate the narrowed area.

Rigid tough strictures may fail to respond to dilatation, and operation (which should include an antireflux procedure) may then be needed. This may be either resection or repair by the fundal patch technique.

Resection. The strictured portion of oesophagus is resected and continuity is restored by anastomosis of oesophagus to the mobilized stomach or to a gastric tube fashioned from the greater curvature. Alternatively, the resected portion of oesophagus can be replaced by a pedicled length of jejunum or colon.

Fundal patch technique. Short strictures are opened longitudinally and the defect is covered by the serosal surface of the mobilized gastric fundus (Fig. 26.13). The fundus is sutured in place and its incorporated serosal surface becomes covered by stratified squamous epithelium within 3 weeks.

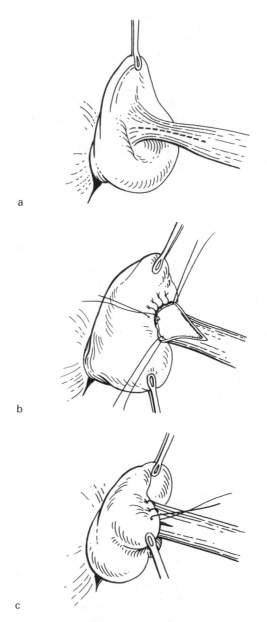

a

b

c

Fig. 26.13 Fundal patch repair. (a) Incision of strictured area. (b) Gastric fundus sutured over the defect. (c) Completion of the fundal patch.

Peptic ulceration in oesophagus lined by columnar epithelium

This condition is known as Barrett's ulcer (Fig. 26.14). It is now considered that the columnar epithelium lining the lower oesophagus represents

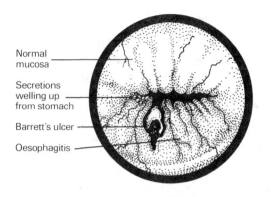

Normal mucosa

Secretions welling up from stomach

Barrett's ulcer

Oesophagitis

Fig. 26.14 Endoscopic appearance of Barrett's ulcer

a metaplastic response to persistent gastro-oesophageal reflux, and is not a congenital anomaly. Ulceration occurs at the squamocolumnar junction and may be complicated by bleeding, perforation or stricture formation. An associated hiatus hernia is common. The abnormal epithelium should be regarded as premalignant since adenocarcinoma develops in 10% of patients.

Treatment

Elective surgery is advisable and consists of dilatation of any associated stricture and an antireflux procedure. Perforation or bleeding may require an emergency oesophageal resection.

Corrosive oesophagitis

This occurs most commonly in young children who accidentally swallow household caustics, corrosives or bleaches, and is no longer a common method of suicide. Necrosis and perforation of the oesophagus or stomach may occur, and strictures form in approximately 20% of surviving patients. Strictures are frequently multiple and extensive.

Immediate management

1. Water is given to dilute the corrosive agent and effective analgesia is provided. Fluid is replaced by intravenous infusion. The passage of a tube for gastric lavage is contraindicated because of the risk of perforation.

2. Early gentle fibreoptic endoscopy is used to assess the degree and extent of damage.

3. The use of parenteral corticosteroids and antibiotics is controversial. At one time they were prescribed for 2–3 weeks while the patient was observed for signs of necrosis or perforation. Many centres no longer use these agents routinely.

4. Early feeding is encouraged if endoscopy shows only mild inflammation. If damage is severe, parenteral feeding is commenced.

5. Evidence of full thickness necrosis and perforation of oesophagus and/or stomach demands urgent surgical resection of the damaged area.

6. Barium studies or endoscopy are repeated at intervals for 12 months to detect stricture formation if the patient has been treated conservatively. The return of dysphagia is a sign of stricture and an indication for repeat radiology.

Management of strictures

Mild early stricture formation sometimes responds satisfactorily to a single dilatation. Established strictures require multiple dilatations and patients may need a feeding gastrostomy. In these patients retrograde bouginage through the gastrostomy is probably safer than bouginage by the usual route.

Patients with extensive or multiple strictures require surgical treatment. Extensive perioesophageal scarring makes resection difficult and the oesophagus is better bypassed. The right or left colon can be used, the upper anastomosis being made in the neck (Fig. 26.15). The segments are long and the blood supply may be impaired, so that potentially lethal ischaemic necrosis may develop in the upper portion of the segment.

To improve the blood supply to the segment of colon used for the bypass, a microvascular anastomosis can be made between a neck vessel (e.g. the inferior thyroid artery) and the pedicle of the segment of gut. Alternatively, a buried skin tube may be constructed to connect the pharynx and abdominal oesophagus.

Patients with corrosive strictures of the oesophagus have a high risk of developing oesophageal carcinoma and should be kept under long-term review. For this reason, many surgeons

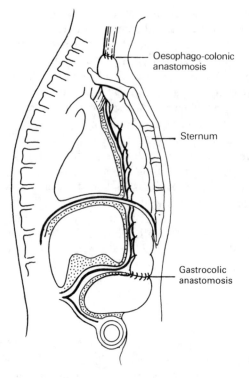

Oesophago-colonic anastomosis

Sternum

Gastrocolic anastomosis

Fig. 26.15 Bypass of the oesophagus using a loop of colon

favour resection whenever possible in patients requiring operation for corrosive stricture. Carcinoma developing in oesophageal strictures appears less aggressive than the usual oesophageal carcinoma (see later).

OESOPHAGEAL PERFORATION

Perforation of the oesophagus may be caused accidentally at endoscopy or bouginage, and during the passage of a wide-bore gastric lavage tube. Perforation is particularly liable to occur at the pharyngo-oesophageal junction (due to spasm of the cricopharyngeus muscle) or at the lower end of the oesophagus. Perforation is more common during passage of rigid oesophagoscopes but can occur during endoscopy with a flexible fibreoptic instrument. Perforation may also be caused by foreign bodies, penetrating wounds, trauma and operative mobilization of the oesophagus at vagotomy. Spontaneous rupture of the lower oesophagus can be caused by forceful retching and vomiting (Boerhaave syndrome).

Clinical features

The severity of the clinical signs is influenced by the site and size of the perforation. Perforation in the neck causes surgical emphysema, throat pain and bruising. Perforation of the thoracic oesophagus in a conscious patient causes severe substernal pain, inability to swallow, tachycardia and fever. If the perforation is above the diaphragm, escape of air will cause mediastinal emphysema which spreads upwards to the neck. Tearing of the mediastinal pleura results in pneumothorax. A perforation of the abdominal oesophagus produces acute upper abdominal pain with clinical features resembling those of perforated peptic ulcer (see p. 457).

Awareness of the diagnosis is essential and chest X-ray should always be performed after rigid endoscopy, seeking evidence of cervical and mediastinal emphysema, pleural effusion or pneumothorax.

Endoscopy is only indicated if the perforation has been caused by ingestion of a foreign body. Otherwise, the site of the perforation should be localized by a Gastrografin swallow.

Management

Conservative treatment by broad spectrum antibiotics and insertion of a nasogastric tube is indicated for perforations of the cervical oesophagus. Drainage of the retro-oesophageal space through an incision in the neck may be required. Perforation of the thoracic oesophagus demands immediate thoracotomy with repair of the perforation or, if necessary, resection of the affected segment. A patch of gastric fundus may be used to close the defect. The mediastinum and pleura should be drained. Provided operation is undertaken promptly and there is no sinister underlying cause, the prognosis is good.

OESOPHAGEAL WEB

A fibrous web at the entrance of the oesophagus causes the dysphagia which occurs in the Paterson-Kelly syndrome. Typically this occurs in middle-aged edentulous women and is associated with atrophic mucosa, anaemia and spoon-shaped fingers with brittle nails. However, all features of the syndrome are not necessarily present.

The presence of a web is confirmed by barium swallow and oesophagoscopy. Treatment consists of its disruption and correction of the anaemia, if present. As the atrophic mucosa is prone to malignancy, patients must be kept under regular supervision.

TUMOURS OF THE OESOPHAGUS

Benign tumours

Benign tumours of the oesophagus are rare, accounting for less than 1% of all oesophageal neoplasms. The majority are asymptomatic, but dysphagia and bleeding may occur. Leiomyoma is the commonest benign tumour and is detected radiologically as a filling defect covered by intact mucosa. Local resection is indicated. Other benign neoplasms include fibrovascular polyps and lipomas, for which endoscopic removal may be feasible.

Carcinoma of the oesophagus

The incidence of oesophageal carcinoma varies widely throughout the world. It is particularly common in the Far East, Iran, Africa and the West Indies. In Europe it is a relatively rare form of cancer and in Scotland accounts for just over 1% of all cases of malignancy.

Oesophageal cancer is rare before the age of 40 years. Thereafter its incidence increases progress-ively and is greatest in those over 70. Men are more commonly affected than women although hypopharyngeal cancer is more common in women.

Aetiology

The aetiology of oesophageal cancer remains unknown but chronic irritation, alcohol, tobacco chewing and smoking are risk factors. Hot spicy foods are also believed to favour development of the disease. Other dietary factors include nitrosamines and the aflatoxin of the mould *Aspergillus flavus* which can affect nuts and seeds stored in damp conditions. Nutritional and dietetic deficiency has also been implicated.

Local conditions associated with an increased risk of oesophageal cancer include the Paterson-Kelly syndrome, achalasia, hiatus hernia, Barrett's oesophagus and corrosive strictures.

Pathology

More than 90% of oesophageal cancers are of squamous type. About 80% of such tumours occur in the middle third of the oesophagus, the remainder being distributed between the upper and lower thirds. Adenocarcinomas can arise in columnar epithelium in the lower oesophagus although they usually arise from the upper stomach and extend upwards to involve the oesophagus.

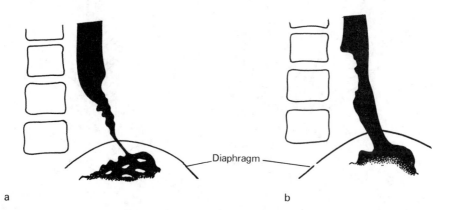

a   b

Fig. 26.16 Radiological features of oesophageal carcinoma. (a) Long irregular stricture. (b) Irregular filling defect.

Oesophageal cancer may become manifest as a polypoidal, ulcerating or hard infiltrating growth which spreads along the oesophageal mucosa and submucosa and invades adjacent structures.

Clinical features

Progressive dysphagia (first for solids and then for liquids) and weight loss are typical. Excessive

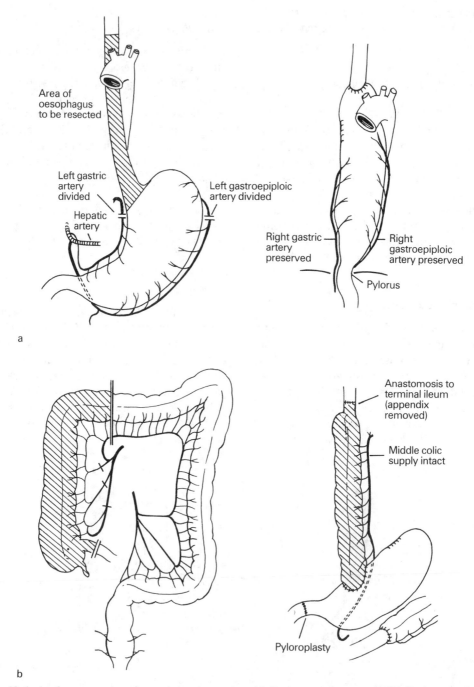

Fig. 26.17   Methods of reconstruction after total oesophagectomy. (a) Replacement by stomach. (b) Replacement by colon.

salivation, aspiration pneumonia, anaemia and lassitude are late effects. The tumour may also erode into a bronchus to establish an oesophageal bronchial fistula, perforate into the mediastinum, or infiltrate the recurrent laryngeal nerves to cause hoarseness. Distant metastases are rare.

As the oesophagus lies deeply within the thorax, clinical examination is rarely helpful. However, the lower neck and upper abdomen should be carefully palpated to detect any lymph node enlargement, tumour mass, or hepatomegaly. Barium swallow usually reveals an irregular filling defect or localized stricture of the oesophagus (Fig. 26.16). The oesophagus above the tumour does not dilate to the extent seen in achalasia. Endoscopy demonstrates an oedematous and friable oesophagus above the tumour. The cancer usually forms a hard occluding mass which prevents further advancement of the instrument. Its upper level is noted and a biopsy is taken.

Management

Oesophageal cancer can be managed by resection, by irradiation, or by a combination of both, depending on the extent and site of the lesion. Tumours of the upper third of the oesophagus are generally treated by radical radiotherapy, those of the lower third by surgery, and those in midoesophagus by either of the two. Some surgeons prefer to perform a total oesophagectomy in all cases, bringing a tube of stomach or colon up to the neck to anastomose to the pharynx (Fig. 26.17).

In patients with non-resectable cancer, dysphagia can be relieved by insertion of a Celestin tube (Fig. 26.18) to ensure that the patient can swallow and maintain nutritional intake. Such tubes can now be inserted endoscopically without the need for surgery.

Laser photocoagulation is now being assessed as

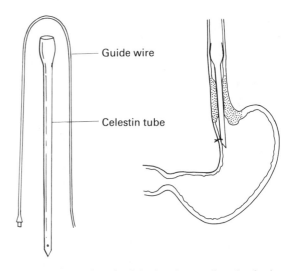

Guide wire

Celestin tube

Fig. 26.18 Insertion of a Celestin tube to relieve dysphagia in non-resectable oesophageal carcinoma. Note that following operative insertion the tube is anchored to the stomach. (This is not possible following endoscopic insertion.)

an alternative means of maintaining swallowing without the need for intubation. These methods of palliation have now virtually eliminated the need to undertake palliative surgical bypass in patients with unresectable lesions.

Resectability and prognosis are influenced by tumour size. About 50% of tumours under 5 cm in length have lymph node involvement whereas 90% of those longer than 5 cm have nodal deposits. Oesophagotracheal fistula and hoarseness are signs of inoperable disease, and resection is seldom worthwhile in patients with metastatic spread. Of 100 patients presenting with oesophageal cancer, 60 will undergo surgical exploration, and only 40 of these will undergo resection.

Resection still carries an operative mortality of 10–20%. The overall 1-year survival rate following diagnosis of oesophageal cancer is 20%, and the 5-year survival rate is less than 5%.

27. The abdominal wall and hernia

UMBILICUS

The umbilicus is the site of attachment of the umbilical cord, the 'life-line' of the developing fetus. Various congenital defects may affect the vitello-intestinal duct and urachus, which connect the umbilical cord to the intestinal and urinary tracts of the fetus.

Developmental anomalies

Vitello-intestinal duct

In the fetus the vitello-intestinal duct runs from the middle of the midgut loop to the umbilicus to connect with the yolk sac. Normally it is obliterated at birth. The duct may remain open for its whole length (vitello-intestinal fistula) causing a faecal fistula at the umbilicus at birth. A Meckel's diverticulum (see Ch. 31) is due to persistence of its intestinal extremity. Less commonly a portion of the duct may remain patent to form a cyst or mucocele which hangs from the anti-mesenteric border of the ileum (enterocystoma). Alternatively the umbilical portion of the duct may form a polypoidal raspberry-like tumour on the surface (enteroteratoma). The clinical syndromes caused by these various developmental anomalies are summarized in Figure 27.1.

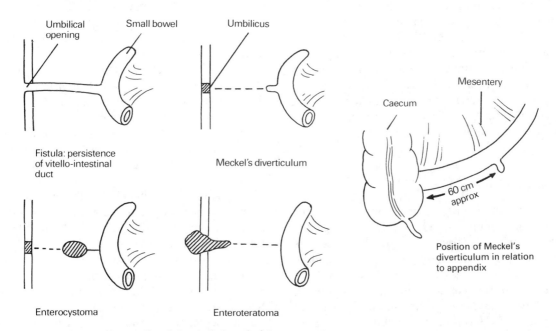

Fig. 27.1 Developmental anomalies of the vitello-intestinal duct

Symptomatic remnants, e.g. a fistula or an obvious lesion at the umbilicus, are best treated by excision. Asymptomatic remnants, e.g. enterocystoma or a Meckel's diverticulum, may be discovered as an incidental finding at laparotomy. These may be excised to prevent complications, although a Meckel's diverticulum can safely be left if broad-based.

A vitello-intestinal band (obliterated duct) may cause intestinal obstruction.

Urachus

The urachus runs from the apex of the bladder to the umbilicus. It is normally obliterated at birth but may remain patent, giving rise to a urinary fistula at the umbilicus. Cysts may form from persistent urachal remnants. Symptomatic remnants of the urachus are best treated by excision.

Umbilical sepsis

In newborn children umbilical sepsis may be the cause of portal thrombophlebitis and fatal jaundice or portal hypertension. Tetanus neonatorum due to the application of cow dung to the umbilicus to promote healing was once common. In adults, umbilical sepsis can result from retention of inspissated sebum within the folds of the umbilicus. Pilonidal sinus of the umbilicus, similar to those in the natal cleft, are also described. In infants sepsis is treated by frequent cleansing with an antiseptic and application of an antibacterial powder. Adult lesions are eradicated by excision.

Umbilical tumours

Squamous carcinoma and melanoma may occur within the umbilicus. They may only be discovered when excision of the umbilicus is performed for a persistent discharge. Secondary deposits of carcinoma at the umbilicus arise from the spread of tumour along the ligamentum teres, either from the liver or from lymph nodes in the porta hepatis. Hernias in the umbilical region are discussed later in this chapter.

AFFLICTIONS OF THE RECTUS MUSCLE

Haematoma of the rectus sheath

Rupture of the inferior epigastric artery may follow direct trauma or may arise spontaneously following sudden contraction of the rectus. It causes a painful swelling of the rectus sheath associated with muscle rigidity. This condition is rare but can arise during pregnancy. Exploration, with ligature of the ruptured artery and evacuation of clot is indicated.

Desmoid tumour

This rare fibromatous tumour arises from a fibrous intramuscular septum in the lower rectus. It is said to be commoner in women of childbearing age, and may be associated with intestinal polyposis (Gardner's syndrome). As it is prone to recur and give rise to a fibrosarcoma, it must be widely excised.

ABDOMINAL HERNIAS

A hernia or rupture is a swelling caused by the protrusion of part of an organ or other tissue through an aperture in the wall surrounding the space in which it is situated (Fig. 27.2). Such an aperture may be present normally or it may be abnormal, in which case it can be congenital or acquired (e.g. due to trauma).

A hernia can affect any viscus (e.g. brain, lung, intestine) or tissue (e.g. muscle, tendon) which lies within a cavity or constraining sheath. It may take the name of the organ involved (e.g. cerebral, small bowel hernia), the aperture through which it has occurred (e.g. hiatus hernia), or the region where it presents (e.g. lumbar or epigastric hernia).

Hernias of the abdominal wall are common. While in theory they can occur at any site, they commonly exploit natural orifices in the abdominal wall through which structures enter and leave the abdominal cavity. These are the inguinal and femoral canals, the umbilicus, the obturator canal and the oesophageal hiatus in the diaphragm. Other hernias protrude through an area of weakness in the abdominal wall, which may be due to stretching of the abdominal muscles (direct in-

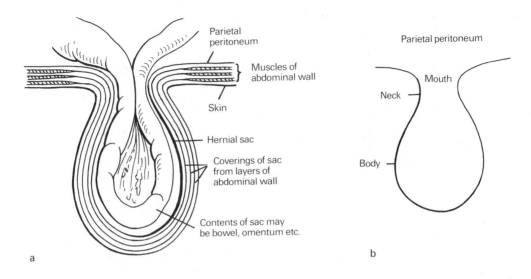

Fig. 27.2 Hernia. (a) Anatomical structure. (b) Parts of the hernial sac

guinal hernia), a gap in a fibrous layer (epigastric hernia) or a surgical incision (incisional hernia).

An abdominal hernia is immediately enclosed by the peritoneal lining of the abdominal cavity. This forms the peritoneal *sac* which is covered by those tissues stretched in front as it protrudes to the surface (the *coverings*). The neck of the sac is that part which corresponds to the orifice through which it protrudes. A hernia may contain any intra-peritoneal structure. Most commonly this is bowel or omentum. If only a segment of the circumference of the bowel wall is included, the resulting lesion is called a 'Richter's hernia' (Fig. 27.3).

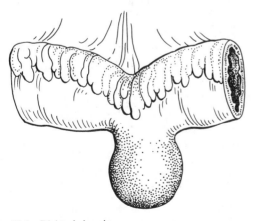

Fig. 27.3 Richter's hernia

A hernia may be reducible (i.e. it can be returned to the abdominal cavity) or irreducible. If irreducible, its contained bowel may become obstructed (if the lumen is constricted) or strangulated (if the blood supply is impaired). Omentum may also become strangulated. These effects are due to constriction at the neck of the sac.

HERNIAS OF THE GROIN

Hernias in the region of the groin account for 75–80% of all abdominal wall hernias. There are three common types: indirect inguinal (60%), direct inguinal (25%) and femoral (15%). The majority (85%) of all groin hernias occur in males.

In early life an indirect inguinal hernia is by far the commonest groin hernia. After middle age, increasing weakness of the abdominal musculature leads to an increase in the incidence of direct hernias, particularly in males. Femoral hernia is relatively more common in females, but indirect inguinal hernia is still the commonest groin hernia in women.

Anatomy of inguinal canal

The inguinal canal is formed by the descent of the testis through the abdominal wall during fetal life.

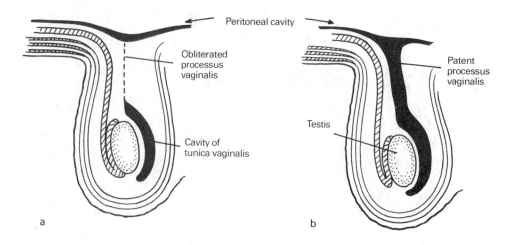

Fig. 27.4　Processus vaginalis testis. (a) Normal obliteration of processus vaginalis testis. (b) Persistence of patent processus

The testis drags with it a tube-like covering of peritoneum, the processus vaginalis. This covering of peritoneum persists as the tunica vaginalis testis in the scrotum; the processus is normally obliterated (Fig. 27.4).

The testis and its peritoneal covering pass obliquely through the three muscles of the anterior abdominal wall on their route to the scrotum. The internal opening lies 1 cm above the mid-inguinal point (internal inguinal ring), while the external opening lies just above and medial to the pubic tubercle (the external inguinal ring). The internal ring is bounded medially by the inferior epigastric artery (Fig. 27.5). At birth the inguinal canal is

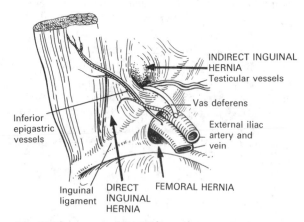

Fig. 27.5　Anatomy of the internal inguinal ring showing sites of herniation from within

short and straight so that the internal and external rings lie one on top of the other. The spermatic cord, consisting of the vas deferens and testicular vessels, lymphatics and fascial coverings, occupies the inguinal canal and runs down from the external ring into the scrotum.

As it passes through the abdominal wall, the testis and its supporting vessels receive a covering from each layer. The innermost layer is derived from the transversalis fascia (the internal spermatic fascia), the middle layer from the internal oblique muscle (cremasteric muscle and fascia) and the outer layer from the external oblique muscle (external spermatic fascia). The testis and that part of the cord which lies outside the full thickness of the abdominal wall are covered by all three layers. Within the inguinal canal the cord is covered only by the cremasteric and internal spermatic fascias.

An *indirect inguinal hernia* and its peritoneal sac descends in the line of the processus vaginalis and vas deferens. It lies within all the coverings of the spermatic cord (including the internal spermatic fascia) and may descend within them into the scrotum. A *direct hernia* enters the inguinal canal through the posterior wall of the canal medial to the internal ring. Its sac lies behind and distinct from the cord and its coverings, and is covered only by transversalis fascia. If it protrudes through the external ring, it picks up a covering of external spermatic fascia but does not normally descend into the scrotum.

Indirect inguinal hernia

The commonest cause of an indirect inguinal hernia is believed to be failure of obliteration of the processus vaginalis (see Fig. 27.4), so that the sac of peritoneum still extends for a varying distance down the inguinal canal. If persistence is complete, the sac extends into the scrotum and is continuous with the tunica vaginalis. The vas deferens is closely adherent to the medial wall of the sac.

It is uncertain whether all indirect hernias can be explained on the basis of a persistent processus and preformed sac. However, even if a peritoneal sac is acquired by descent of the hernia, it occupies the same anatomical position as the obliterated processus.

An indirect inguinal hernia usually descends through the external inguinal ring. If it remains within the inguinal canal, it forms a localized swelling or bubonocele. Alternatively, it may enlarge between the muscular layers of the abdominal wall to form an *interstitial hernia* (see later).

The contents of the hernial sac may include omentum, small intestine, the appendix, an ovary or even a Meckel's diverticulum. As these viscera lie free within the peritoneal cavity, they can descend freely within the sac.

Should large intestine form the hernia, it may be covered only partially with peritoneum and form a sliding hernia (see later).

The internal and external inguinal rings in themselves seldom constrict the contents of the hernia and an indirect hernia is usually reducible. Irreducibility is usually due to thickening of the neck of the peritoneal sac to form an unyielding fibrous ring.

Clinical features

Indirect inguinal hernia is commoner in males and on the right side. Herniation may be associated with sudden pain in the groin or it may pass unnoticed. Thereafter, there is at most a dragging discomfort in the groin, particularly during lifting or strain. Further pain *in the hernia* occurs only when it is complicated by strangulation.

An indirect hernia usually forms a swelling in the inguinal canal, at the external ring or in the upper part of the scrotum, but may occupy one entire side of the scrotum. An inguinal hernia passes through the abdominal wall above and medial to the pubic tubercle, in contrast to a femoral hernia, which emerges below and lateral to the tubercle (Fig. 27.6). A cough impulse may be visible or palpable as a thrill. Bowel sounds may be heard on auscultation of the hernia.

Adult inguinal hernias are best treated surgically. As hernia repairs can be adequately performed under local anaesthesia, there are few contraindications to operation. If the patient refuses operation or there are other contraindications, a truss may be prescribed, but this tends to be uncomfortable. As a truss causes pressure atrophy of the muscles, subsequent surgery becomes more difficult.

An indirect hernia often reduces spontaneously when the patient lies down or when gentle pressure is applied in an upward and lateral direction. The only sign of a hernia may then be thickening of the spermatic cord (due to the sac) or a cough impulse.

Once reduced, an indirect hernia can be controlled by placing a finger over the internal ring.

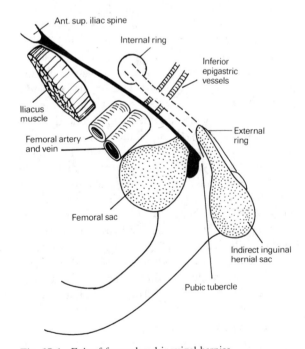

Fig. 27.6 Exit of femoral and inguinal hernias

A cough impulse may then be palpated. Alternatively the skin of the upper scrotum can be invaginated by the little finger which is run along the spermatic cord to the external ring, and the patient then asked to cough.

If a patient complains of a bulge or swelling on exercise but there is no visible or palpable hernia, the cough impulse should be sought with the patient standing up and his legs apart. If the diagnosis is still in doubt, he should be asked to exercise and report back when the hernia is down. Exploration is justifiable if the patient gives a clear history of a reducible swelling in the inguinal region.

Interstitial inguinal hernia

In this type of hernia, the sac extends between the layers of the abdominal wall to form a large diffuse bulge extending upwards and medially from the internal ring. Such extension is rarely seen in Europeans unless the inguinal canal is obstructed by an undescended testis. However, it is common in some African countries.

Direct inguinal hernia

Direct inguinal hernias account for 40% of all inguinal hernias. They are due to a weakness of the abdominal wall and may be precipitated by increased intra-abdominal tension in conditions such as obstructive airways disease, obesity, chronic constipation or prostatism. The hernia protrudes through the transversalis fascia as it forms the posterior wall of the inguinal canal. The defect is bounded above by the conjoint tendon, below by the inguinal ligament and laterally by the inferior epigastric artery. This vessel lies medial to the internal inguinal ring and separates the neck of an indirect from that of a direct hernial sac (Fig. 27.5). The hernia may protrude through the external ring but the transversalis fascia cannot stretch sufficiently to allow it to proceed down to the scrotum. As the defect is large and the neck of the sac wide, a direct hernia is seldom irreducible and rarely obstructs or strangulates.

Clinical features

A direct hernia most commonly forms a diffuse

bulge over the medial part of the inguinal canal and is easily reduced by backward pressure. Following reduction the edges of the defect in the posterior wall of the canal may be palpable. Reduction by backward pressure is in contrast to that required in an indirect hernia, which reduces obliquely by pressure directed upwards and laterally. Occasionally the sac of a direct hernia is funicular and extends down through the external ring to present just above the pubic tubercle.

Sliding direct inguinal hernias are common (see later). As they are medially placed, the urinary bladder may descend in the medial wall of the sac.

Treatment of uncomplicated inguinal hernia

Conservative treatment

In infants, an indirect inguinal hernia may disappear spontaneously due to fusion of the walls of its sac. A simple pressure pad of wool, inserted in the diaper to maintain reduction, is all that is required as a preliminary measure.

Infantile hernias seldom strangulate and little risk is incurred by leaving them alone. Operation is indicated if the hernia is still present at 2 years of age.

Adult inguinal hernias can also be controlled by

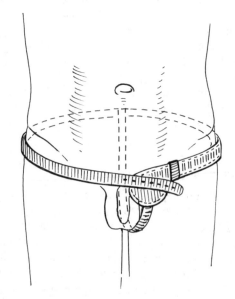

Fig. 27.7 Inguinal hernia truss

a truss but this is now seldom indicated. A truss consists of a pressure pad which is incorporated in a steel spring clipped around the waist (Fig. 27.7). The pad lies over the internal inguinal ring and the hernia must be reduced before it is applied. A patient will usually apply the truss before getting out of bed each morning and wear it throughout the day. The adequacy of control can be checked by asking the patient to stand with his legs apart and cough violently.

A truss is uncomfortable, causes pressure atrophy of the muscles and makes subsequent surgery more difficult. It should therefore be used only if operation is refused or contraindicated. It should be remembered that hernia repairs can readily be performed under local anaesthesia.

Surgical repair of direct and indirect inguinal hernias

Indirect inguinal hernia. The first principle of repair is to free the sac and remove it after transfixing its neck with a ligature (Fig. 27.8). In young children the abdominal musculature is normal, the internal ring is not dilated and simple excision of the sac (herniotomy) is all that this required.

In older children and young adults the internal ring is dilated. Provided the musculature is nor-

mal, narrowing of the ring around the cord with a few non-absorbable sutures will complete the operation. Careful suture of the transversalis fascia around the internal ring is advised.

In older patients the posterior wall of the canal is stretched and weakened, and a variety of surgical procedures are used to tighten the deep inguinal ring and strengthen the posterior wall and so prevent recurrence. The simplest method is to plicate the transversalis fascia (Fig. 27.9). More

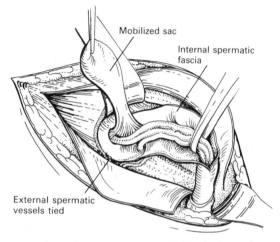

Fig. 27.8 Principle of dissection in the repair of an inguinal hernia

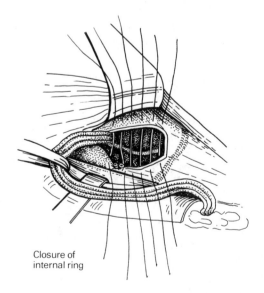

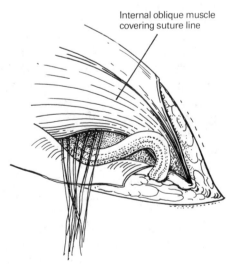

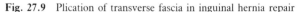

Fig. 27.9 Plication of transverse fascia in inguinal hernia repair

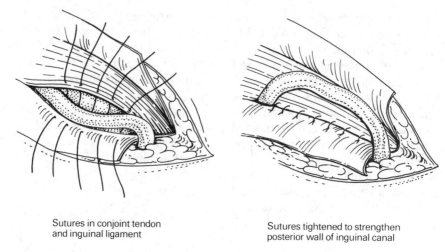

Sutures in conjoint tendon
and inguinal ligament

Sutures tightened to strengthen
posterior wall of inguinal canal

Fig. 27.10   Bassini-type of inguinal hernia repair with strengthening of the posterior wall of the canal

commonly, in the so-called Bassini repair, the conjoint tendon and internal oblique muscles are
sutured to the pubic tubercle and undersurface of
the inguinal ligament with non-absorbable interrupted sutures (herniorrhaphy) (Fig. 27.10). Some
surgeons also incise the anterior rectus sheath to
relieve tension.

Direct hernia. In a direct hernia, excision of the
diffuse sac is not usually required. The sac is
simply invaginated by a few sutures placed in the
transversalis fascia. If the sac projects through a
clearly defined defect in the posterior wall of the
canal, it can be excised. Repair of the posterior
wall of the canal can be difficult as the tissues
are stretched and thinned. In some cases it is
necessary to use a synthetic mesh (e.g. Terylene)
for reinforcement.

In all hernia repairs a tunnel must be left for the
emerging spermatic cord. This may compromise
the repair of large hernias, and in older patients
removal of the testis and cord with complete
obliteration of the inguinal canal may be the most
practical method of preventing recurrence.

Prognosis. After any form of repair of an
inguinal hernia there is a risk of recurrence. This
varies in different reported series, but can be as
high as 10%. The commonest form of recurrence
after repair of an indirect hernia is another indirect
hernia, usually due to incomplete excision of the
sac. After repair of a direct hernia, a recurrent
hernia is more likely to be direct.

Surgical repair of sliding hernia

A sliding hernia is one in which part of the circumference of the sac is formed by a viscus whose
wall is only partly covered by peritoneum, e.g.
caecum, colon or bladder. The viscus is part of the
hernial sac but lies outside the peritoneum (Fig.
27.11). A sliding hernia is usually large and occurs
most commonly in elderly patients. Repair can be
difficult, and a variety of operative procedures
have been used to re-peritonealize the bowel so
that it can be returned to the abdomen. This is
unnecessary and it is better to excise the sac distal
to the bowel, which is then gently pushed back
into its normal retroperitoneal position before
repair is carried out.

Femoral hernia

A femoral hernia projects through the femoral
canal. The canal lies medial to the femoral vein
and opens into the abdomen through the femoral
ring. The femoral ring is bounded in front by the
inguinal ligament, laterally by the femoral vein
and medially by the lacunar ligament. Posteriorly
the pubic bone has a thickened ridge of periosteum known as the pectineal ligament of Cooper
(Fig. 27.12).

A femoral hernia pushes the extraperitoneal fat
and peritoneum through the femoral ring and
down into the femoral canal. On leaving the canal

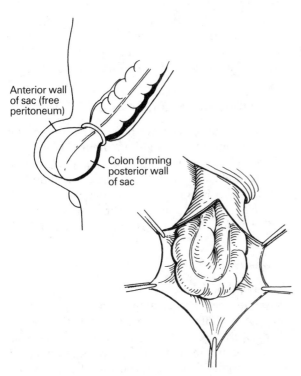

Anterior wall
of sac (free
peritoneum)

Colon forming
posterior wall
of sac

Fig. 27.11 Sliding hernia. In this example the colon forms the posterior wall of the hernial sac and cannot be reduced when the sac is opened

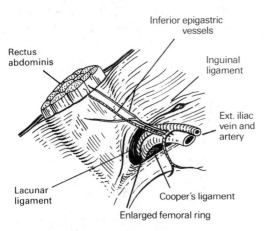

Inferior epigastric
vessels

Rectus
abdominis

Inguinal
ligament

Ext. iliac
vein and
artery

Lacunar
ligament

Cooper's ligament

Enlarged femoral ring

Fig. 27.12 Anatomy of the femoral ring as viewed from within the abdomen. The external iliac vessels become the femoral vessels as they enter the groin

the hernia turns superficially to pass through the deep fascia of the thigh at the saphenous opening. The cribriform fascia is pushed in front of it. It then turns upwards to lie over the inguinal ligament. Because of its many coverings, the size of a femoral hernia is deceptive, and only a small sac may be present in the middle of a large mass of fatty and fibrous tissue.

A femoral hernia normally contains omentum, small bowel or both. Urinary bladder may be found in the medial wall of the sac.

Femoral hernias account for 5% of groin hernias in men and 20% in women. This sex difference is attributable to the stretching of the pelvic ligaments and widening of the femoral ring during pregnancy. Nulliparous females have the same incidence of femoral hernias as males.

Clinical features

A femoral hernia typically presents as a bulge in the upper inner aspect of the thigh just beneath the inguinal ligament. Once it emerges from the saphenous opening, it forms a well-defined soft or firm swelling which is situated below and lateral to the pubic tubercle but which may extend upwards over the inguinal ligament. This type of hernia is particularly difficult to distinguish from an inguinal hernia, but the diagnosis is suggested by the absence of a cough impulse over the inguinal ring and the fact that a femoral hernia is difficult to reduce along its tortuous J-shaped course.

The relationship of the hernia to the pubic tubercle is the key to the diagnosis. The tubercle is defined by tracing the tendon of adductor longus upwards to its insertion. A femoral hernia emerges below and lateral to the pubic tubercle while inguinal hernias emerge above and medial to it. If there is doubt about the nature of a hernia in the groin it usually proves to be femoral.

A femoral hernia must also be differentiated from inguinal lymph nodes, a saphenous varix, and lipoma.

1. *Inguinal lymph nodes* are usually multiple and occupy the normal distribution of the inguinal nodes. There is no cough impulse and they cannot be reduced.

2. *A saphenous varix* is a dilated terminal portion of the saphenous vein. The soft swelling in the upper medial part of the thigh disappears when the patient lies down and the leg is elevated. There is a clearly palpable impulse on coughing

(saphenous thrill) and when the long saphenous vein lower down the leg is percussed.

3. *A lipoma* forms a soft lobulated subcutaneous swelling which is irreducible.

Surgical repair

A femoral hernia is particularly liable to strangulate. As it cannot readily be reduced and its point of emergence from the abdomen is deep-seated, a truss will not control it. Operation is indicated and, as with an inguinal hernia, may be performed under local or general anaesthesia.

The aim of operation is complete excision of the hernial sac and repair of the defect (obliteration of the femoral ring). The femoral canal can be approached (1) from below the inguinal ligament; (2) through the posterior wall of the inguinal canal; or (3) from above, by incising the anterior wall of the rectus sheath and dissecting downwards between the transversalis fascia and peritoneum to expose the inner surface of the pubis (Fig. 27.13). The third approach (McEvedy's) gives best access to the femoral ring and is generally preferred. It should be used if there is any hint of strangulation. Following reduction and excision of the hernial sac, the femoral ring is obliterated by suturing the inner surface of the conjoint tendon to the pectineal ligament of the pubis.

If reduction of the sac from above is difficult, the lower flap of the wound can be elevated from the subcutaneous tissues, allowing the sac to be exposed and freed below the inguinal ligament.

VENTRAL HERNIAS

Ventral hernias occur through areas of natural weakness in the anterior abdominal wall (Fig. 27.14). These are the linea alba (epigastric hernia), the umbilicus (umbilical and paraumbilical hernia), the lateral border of the rectus sheath (Spigelian hernia) and the scar tissue of poorly healed abdominal incisions (incisional hernias).

Epigastric hernia

Extraperitoneal fat may protrude through a small defect in the linea alba to form a soft palpable midline swelling in the epigastrium. Occasionally there is also a small sac of peritoneum. This hernia usually occurs in thin men and can cause marked local discomfort. The presence of a hernia should not be regarded as sufficient explanation for a history of dyspepsia. This complaint should always be investigated by orthodox means.

An epigastric hernia is easily repaired by closing the slit-like defect in the linea alba with a few non-absorbable sutures.

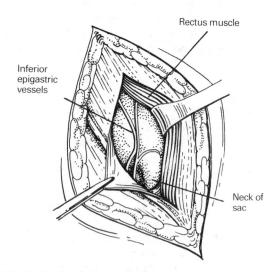

Fig. 27.13 Surgical approach to femoral hernia from above (McEvedy approach). The rectus abdominis muscle is retracted medially to reveal the neck of the hernial sac

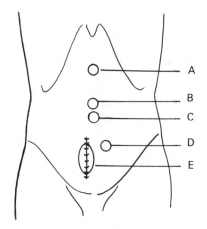

Fig. 27.14 Types of ventral hernias. A = epigastric (through the linea alba); B = umbilical (through umbilical scar); C = paraumbilical (above or below the umbilicus); D = Spigelian (adjacent to rectus sheath); E = incisional (anywhere)

Umbilical hernia

A true umbilical hernia occurs in infants. A small sac of peritoneum protrudes through the umbilicus, everting the skin when the child cries. It is easily reduced, and the edges of the ring-like defect are then clearly palpable. An umbilical pad will maintain reduction.

Although these hernias always close by puberty, persistence to the age of 2 years is usually an indication for operation. This is a simple procedure. If the neck of the sac is narrow it can be ligated by inserting a subcutaneous suture (Fig. 27.15). If larger, a formal repair may be required. Even then the umbilicus need not be excised.

Paraumbilical hernia

This arises from gradual weakening of the tissues around the umbilicus. It affects predominantly obese multiparous women. The hernia passes through the attenuated linea alba and may be situated above or below the umbilicus. It gradually increases in size. The coverings become stretched and thinned and loops of bowel may be visible under parchment-like skin. The skin may become reddened, excoriated and ulcerated, and a faecal fistula can occur.

The sac is multilocular and contains adherent omentum with loops of large and/or small bowel. These can become entrapped, and obstruction and strangulation are common. Such large hernias are invariably irreducible.

Operation is advised unless the patient is unfit. Strangulation, when it occurs, has a high mortality. The Mayo operation consists of excision of the hernia sac and its overlying skin, including the umbilicus (Fig. 27.16). An elliptical incision is made around the umbilicus and deepened to define the linea alba and anterior sheath of the rectus. The edges of the defect are defined around its outer circumference and the peritoneum is then divided around the neck of the hernia. The omentum and bowel are separated from the sac, which is then removed with its overlying skin. The aponeurotic defect in the linea alba is closed by overlapping the layers of the abdominal wall using mattress sutures of non-absorbable material. Occasionally in large defects a synthetic (e.g. Terylene) mesh implant may be required.

Incisional hernia

There is diffuse protrusion of peritoneum and abdominal contents through a weakened area in an abdominal scar. Midline vertical incisions are most frequently affected, particularly below the umbilicus. The weakened area is due to non-healing or stretching of the linea alba. Poor suture technique, wound dehiscence, chest and wound infection, and postoperative distension are precipitating factors.

The diffuse bulging of the wound is best seen when the patient is asked to lie down and then raise his head and shoulders (or straight legs) from

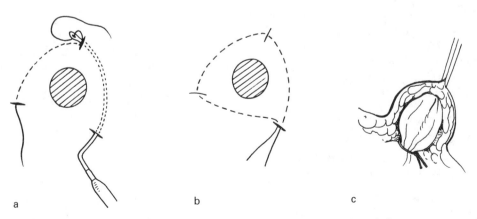

a   b   c

Fig. 27.15 Repair of infantile umbilical hernia. (a & b) Insertion of subcutaneous suture through three puncture wounds. (c) Suture tied while keeping sac taut and cut short to allow retraction into subcutaneous tissue

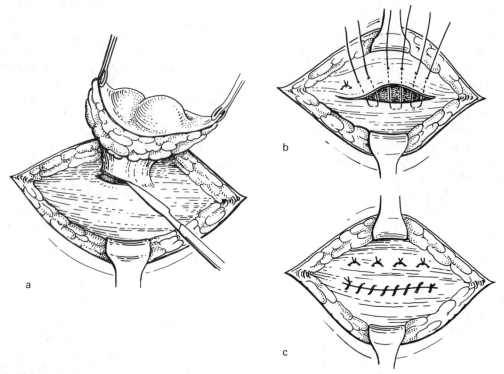

Fig. 27.16 Mayo repair of adult paraumbilical hernia. (a) Excision of sac together with overlying skin. (b) Insertion of overlapping sutures into rectus sheath. (c) Final appearance

the bed and so contract his abdominal muscles. Herniation may be associated with a sensation of weakness.

Strangulation is rare but surgical repair is usually advised. Some patients prefer to wear an abdominal belt, which may give adequate control of the hernia.

The skin wound is excised and the flaps are elevated to expose normal aponeurosis. The edges of the defect are defined and repaired either by overlapping sutures or by the insertion of a Terylene mesh. The sac is either excised or invaginated depending on its size.

COMPLICATIONS OF HERNIAS

The main complications associated with a hernia are irreducibility, obstruction and strangulation.

Irreducibility

An irreducible hernia cannot be returned to the abdominal cavity by manipulation. Most commonly this is attributable to narrowing of the neck of the sac by fibrosis, distension of the contained bowel or adhesion of contained omentum to the walls of the peritoneal sac.

Obstruction

An irreducible hernia is a common cause of intestinal obstruction. Abdominal pain, vomiting and distension may indicate the need for urgent operation. The hernial orifices *must* be inspected in all patients with suspected acute intestinal obstruction. In fact, this is an important step in *any* examination of the abdomen.

Strangulation

The vessels supplying the loop of bowel contained in the hernia are compressed by the neck of the sac or constricting ring. The veins are affected first, and the bowel becomes cyanosed and oedematous, with an exudation of blood-stained fluid. The arterial supply is then compromised and gangrene follows. Organisms and toxins pass out through the bowel wall causing local peritonitis of the hernial sac.

The patient complains of pain in the hernia which is associated with the clinical features of intestinal obstruction. The hernia is tender, the cough impulse is lost and, if the hernia is in the groin, the hip is held in a flexed position. In a Richter's hernia, where only part of the wall of the bowel is strangulated, features of intestinal obstruction may be absent.

Treatment

Provided there is no suggestion of strangulation, an attempt can be made to reduce an *irreducible hernia* by the administration of analgesics, elevation of the foot of the bed, and gentle pressure. Heavy pressure should never be used for fear of rupturing the bowel or of returning it to the abdomen 'en masse' within the sac, which would not relieve the obstruction. If reduction is not achieved within a few hours, operation is advised. In young children strangulation rarely occurs and it is reasonable to wait longer.

Except in infants, immediate operation is indicated for all cases of *obstructed hernia*. One can never be certain that the hernia is not strangulated and delay may be dangerous. The hernia is explored, the sac opened and the cause of the obstruction ascertained. In the case of an inguinal hernia, this is likely to be narrowing of the neck of the sac; in the case of a femoral hernia, constriction of the femoral ring; and in the case of an umbilical hernia, adhesions within the sac. The bowel is carefully inspected, and preserved only if there is no doubt as to its viability. Devitalized bowel is resected. The contents are returned to the abdomen, the sac is excised and the hernia is repaired.

RARE EXTERNAL HERNIAS

Lumbar hernia

This rare hernia forms a diffuse bulge above the crest of the ileum, between the posterior border of external oblique and anterior border of latissimus dorsi.

Obturator hernia

Commoner in women, this rare hernia is a protrusion of peritoneum and small bowel into the obturator canal, normally occupied by the obturator nerve and vessels. The diagnosis is normally made only when the hernia has strangulated, when it is discovered at laparotomy. The characteristic clinical feature of pain referred down the inner side of the thigh and knee (in the distribution of the geniculate branch of the obturator nerve) is very rare.

INTERNAL ABDOMINAL HERNIA

A variety of cul-de-sacs and peritoneal gaps resulting from the rotation of the bowel may be responsible for entrapment of bowel and acute intestinal obstruction.

For example, herniation may occur through the foramen of the lesser sac (epiploic foramen of Winslow) into various fossae around the duodenum (paraduodenal fossae) or through a gap at the attachment of the mesocolon of the pelvic colon (the intersigmoid fossa).

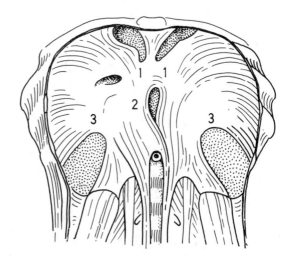

Fig. 27.17 Sites of diaphragmatic herniation.
(1) Parasternal, between the sternal and costal slips of the diaphragm, through the foramen of Morgagni.
(2) Oesophageal hiatus. (3) Pleuroperitoneal canal (foramen of Bochdalek)

Iatrogenic hernias may also occur through holes in the mesentery made at operations. Such gaps must always be carefully closed at the primary operation.

Diaphragmatic hernia

The sites of diaphragmatic herniation are shown in Figure 27.17. *Congenital* diaphragmatic hernias occur through a persistent pleuroperitoneal canal (foramen of Bochdalek) or through the foraman of Morgagni between the central and anterolateral portions of the developing diaphragm (parasternal hernia). *Acquired* diaphragmatic hernias occur through the oesophageal hiatus (see Ch. 26). *Traumatic* diaphragmatic hernia occurs following stab and gunshot wounds. Blunt abdominal trauma may also result in unrecognized diaphragmatic rupture or weakness, with immediate eventration, or later development of a large diaphragmatic hernia. Such hernias may also follow operations in which the diaphragm is divided (e.g. oesophagogastrectomy).

28. The peritoneum

Anatomy

The abdominal cavity is lined by a thin sheet of mesothelium which forms the internal layer of the abdominal wall (parietal peritoneum). During development of the abdominal viscera and organs, the peritoneal sac is invaginated to clothe these viscera with a layer of peritoneum (visceral peritoneum) and to form several pouches and compartments between them. The largest of these are the greater and lesser sacs of peritoneum connected by the epiploic foramen.

The peritoneum is smooth and glistening and secretes a small amount of fluid. In certain circumstances, abnormally increased secretion may lead to obvious free fluid in the abdominal cavity (ascites).

The visceral peritoneum is insensitive to touch, heat or chemical stimuli. In contrast, the parietal peritoneum is exquisitely sensitive to all of these.

The peritoneum is relatively resistant to infection but contamination of the peritoneal cavity, e.g. by perforation of a hollow viscus or spread of inflammation from a contained organ, may lead to peritonitis.

The omentum (Fig. 28.1) is a double fold of peritoneum connecting the liver to the stomach (lesser omentum) and the stomach to the colon (greater omentum). As the greater omentum is folded back on itself, it consists of four layers enclosing a continuation of the lesser sac of peritoneum which extends behind the stomach. The omentum contains variable amounts of fat.

PERITONITIS

Peritonitis means inflammation of the peritoneum. The process may be acute or chronic; septic (due

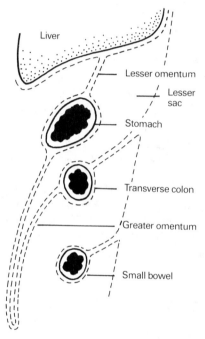

Fig. 28.1 Sagittal section through the abdomen showing the arrangement of peritoneal folds which form the lesser and greater omentum

to pyogenic organisms) or aseptic (due to chemical irritation); primary (without pre-existing visceral disease) or secondary (caused by pre-existing visceral disease). Aseptic peritonitis usually becomes secondarily infected within 6–12 hours.

Acute suppurative peritonitis

Acute septic or pyogenic peritonitis may be primary or secondary. The common surgical form of peritonitis is usually secondary to one of the following: (1) inflammatory disease of the abdominal viscera; (2) perforation of the bowel or biliary tract; (3) infection of the female genital tract; (4) penetrating injury of the abdominal wall; (5) rupture of an intra-abdominal abscess, e.g. of the liver; or (6) ischaemia of the bowel, e.g. from strangulation.

The site and extent of the inflammation depends on the origin of the infection. In acute cholecystitis or acute appendicitis, peritonitis may remain localized for some time. With perforated peptic ulcer or small bowel strangulation, it may rapidly become generalized.

Pathology

The pathological process is similar to that of acute inflammation elsewhere. Both visceral and parietal peritoneum become acutely inflamed and there is a purulent exudate. Localization of the inflammatory process may occur as the omentum 'walls off' the primary site of infection. An intra-abdominal abscess may then form.

Alternatively, the infection may remain diffuse, in which case the abdomen is filled with foul-smelling purulent material. The intestine becomes flaccid and dilated and covered with fibrinous plaques which form adhesions between bowel loops.

Clinical features

The initial symptoms of acute secondary peritonitis may be preceded by those of the primary condition, which may cause visceral pain or other symptoms. Once the parietal peritoneum is involved, the pain becomes somatic and well localized to the site of infection. As infection spreads within the peritoneal cavity the pain becomes diffuse. Pain in the shoulder indicates involvement of the diaphragmatic peritoneum. Vomiting is common but initially is not severe.

In these initial stages the patient lies still and is afraid to move. Respiration is shallow and the abdomen is scaphoid. The most important single clinical sign is tenderness on direct pressure, the extent of which depends on the area of involvement. Maximum tenderness occurs over the site of origin and may be defined by percussion or

rebound tenderness. Other local signs include muscular rigidity and guarding, which are maximal over the site of greatest tenderness. On auscultation the abdomen is silent. The pulse and temperature are usually moderately elevated.

If untreated the clinical picture gradually deteriorates. Pain becomes less prominent and vomiting more profuse. The vomitus consists first of gastric contents (which often contain bile) and then small bowel contents. With dilatation of the bowel from accumulation of fluid and lessening of rigidity from increasing toxicity, the abdomen becomes distended and the patient becomes obviously toxic and dehydrated. The pulse becomes rapid and weak and hypovolaemia, sepsis and shock supervene.

Plain abdominal X-rays may give a clue to the cause of the peritonitis, but usually they do not contribute greatly to the diagnosis. Biochemical tests are also of limited diagnostic value, although an increase in serum amylase levels suggests acute pancreatitis. Urea and electrolyte determinations are an essential aid in resuscitation, and blood gas determinations are helpful in shocked patients.

Treatment

The most important aspect of treatment of secondary peritonitis is to deal with the cause, e.g. repair a perforated viscus, resect infarcted bowel, or drain or remove an infective focus. Operation should be performed with the minimum of delay. The only time which should be spent before operation is that necessary to resuscitate an ill patient. In established pyogenic peritonitis, antibiotic cover is indicated. Peritoneal lavage, with or without added antibiotics, should be performed at operation to wash out bacteria and infected material.

Peritonitis which complicates chronic ambulatory dialysis seldom requires operation and can usually be controlled by antibiotics.

Primary peritonitis

In paediatric practice, primary acute peritonitis accounts for approximately 15% of acute abdominal emergencies.

The condition used to be most common in girls

under the age of 10 years, and was usually due to pneumococcal or haemolytic streptococcal infection spreading to the peritoneal cavity from the genital tract. Nowadays *Escherichia coli* is the predominant causative organism. It usually gains access to the peritoneal cavity through the wall of the intestine but some cases may be due to blood-borne spread from a septic focus elsewhere.

Primary peritonitis is relatively rare in adults but is a recognized complication of cirrhosis of the liver and of the nephrotic syndrome, particularly when associated with ascites.

Clinical features

The onset of primary peritonitis is abrupt. Classically, diffuse peritonitis with generalized abdominal tenderness and rigidity develops within 24 hours of onset. Fever and leucocytosis occur early. A plain abdominal X-ray shows no specific changes.

Treatment

Appropriate antibiotic therapy is the mainstay of successful treatment. An exploratory laparotomy is usually required to rule out a correctable surgical cause and a specimen of peritoneal exudate is obtained for immediate Gram stain and culture. The appendix is removed and the abdomen closed without drainage. Irrigation of the peritoneal cavity with an antibacterial solution is advised by some.

Antibiotic therapy based on the results of the Gram stain is started immediately. This is modified once the results of culture and sensitivity tests are available.

Tuberculous peritonitis

Most commonly occurring in females between the ages of 20 and 40 years, tuberculous peritonitis is now rare in this country. It is invariably secondary to tuberculosis elsewhere although the site of the primary infection is frequently unrecognized.

Two types of tuberculous peritonitis are described: ascitic (or 'moist') and plastic (or 'dry').

Ascitic tuberculous peritonitis

Fever and progressive ascites are the most common clinical features. Abdominal pain is not usually severe. Anorexia, weight loss and night sweats may occur.

Percutaneous needle biopsy of the peritoneum can be used to establish the diagnosis. Culture of the ascitic fluid is unhelpful. If laparotomy or laparoscopy is undertaken, a biopsy should be obtained from the multiple caseating tubercles which stud the peritoneum.

Plastic tuberculous peritonitis

In this condition there is a dense inflammatory exudate with adhesions which mat the coils of intestine into multiple abdominal masses (Fig. 28.2). Fistulas may follow operation, and laparotomy should be avoided unless required to relieve intestinal obstruction.

Both forms of tuberculous peritonitis are treated by a full course of antituberculous chemotherapy.

Aseptic peritonitis

Various agencies such as foreign bodies, bile, blood, gastric juice and pancreatic enzymes, can irritate the peritoneal lining and produce an exudate which is initially sterile. Secondary infection

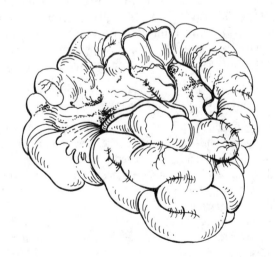

Fig. 28.2 Plastic tuberculous peritonitis

is, however, common. The management then is as for secondary peritonitis.

A foreign body may gain access to the peritoneal cavity (1) through the abdominal wall as a result of a penetrating injury, e.g. a gunshot wound; (2) from the alimentary tract, e.g. if the gut wall is penetrated by a swallowed object or one inserted per rectum; or (3) during abdominal operations, e.g. a swab, instrument or prosthetic material left behind after operation. A sterile collection or abscess may then develop with subsequent formation of a sinus or fistula.

If symptoms are severe, the abdomen should be explored and the foreign body removed. Surgical swabs and instruments must be removed as soon as their misplacement is discovered.

Although *bile* is only a mild chemical irritant, infected bile causes a virulent peritonitis with severe toxaemia. Leakage of bile may complicate acute cholecystitis but occurs most commonly following biliary surgery.

Blood is also only a mild peritoneal irritant but sudden massive haemorrhage into the peritoneal cavity can cause severe abdominal pain and signs of acute abdominal disease. Large quantities of intraperitoneal blood should be removed, as the collection may form a nidus for secondary infection.

Gastric juice is very irritating to the peritoneum. Perforation of a peptic ulcer causes acute chemical peritonitis with severe abdominal pain, rigidity and shock. Sterile *urine* from intraperitoneal rupture of the bladder behaves similarly. In both cases secondary bacterial infection is the rule. *Pancreatic enzymes* escape into the peritoneum in acute pancreatitis and are also strong irritants.

Granulomatous peritonitis

Foreign body reactions of a chronic nature occur following contamination of the peritoneum with the talc or starch once used to powder surgical gloves. Multiple granulomas form on the peritoneal surfaces, leading to the formation of fibrous adhesions.

Leakage of barium into the peritoneal cavity causes a severe plastic peritonitis with multiple dense adhesions.

Postoperative peritonitis

Peritonitis may follow any abdominal operation. It may be a residual effect of the primary disease for which the operation was carried out or occur as a direct complication of the operation, such as leakage from an anastomosis or strangulation of a trapped loop of bowel.

The diagnosis is notoriously difficult as (1) the patient is receiving postoperative sedation and may not complain of pain; (2) any pain and tenderness that *is* present may be attributed to the presence of the wound; and (3) after any abdominal operation there is normally a period (usually lasting 48 hours) when bowel sounds are absent or diminished and the abdomen is distended.

Persistence of abdominal distension for more than a few days after operation or the development of distension or vomiting after an initial return to normality should raise the suspicion of peritoneal infection. In some patients the first signs of this development are tachycardia or an altered mental state. Plain abdominal X-ray shows dilatation of the intestine. A leaking anastomosis may be demonstrated by Gastrografin studies.

Fluid and electrolyte replacement, nasogastric tube decompression and broad spectrum antibiotics are the mainstays of treatment. If major or continuing intraperitoneal infection is suspected, laparotomy is indicated.

ASCITES

Ascites is the accumulation of free fluid within the peritoneal cavity. Commonly, ascitic fluid is clear and straw-coloured and due to *transudation* across the peritoneal membrane in conditions such as cardiac failure, certain types of renal failure, and portal hypertension. In surgical wards, ascites is more often due to involvement of the parietal peritoneum by malignant deposits which irritate the peritoneum, producing an *exudate* with a higher protein content than a transudate. Occasionally free fluid accumulates in the peritoneal cavity due to blockage of lymph flow through the thoracic ducts; it is then milky in appearance because of the high content of absorbed fat in abdominal lymph (chylous ascites). Rarely the ascites is due to major pancreatic inflammation with escape of pancreatic secretions (pancreatic ascites).

Clinical features

The cardinal signs of ascites are abdominal distension and dullness on percussion of the flanks which shifts to the dependent side as the patient rolls first onto one side and then onto the other (shifting dullness). (An ovarian cyst or a full urinary bladder is dull on percussion in the suprapubic region).

A 'fluid thrill' can be elicited by placing one hand flat on one flank while tapping the other with the fingers of the other hand. If an impulse is present, transmission through the abdominal wall must be prevented by placing a third hand on the abdomen (Fig. 28.3).

A plain abdominal X-ray will demonstrate a uniform ground-glass appearance.

If ascites is present and its cause is unknown, a peritoneal tap (paracentesis) is performed by inserting a needle at a point halfway between the umbilicus and the anterior superior iliac spine.

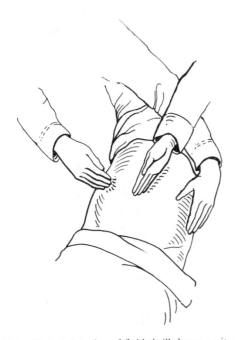

Fig. 28.3 Clinical detection of fluid thrill due to ascites

Samples of the aspirated fluid are sent for cytological examination, for bacteriological examination and culture, and to the clinical chemistry laboratory for determination of protein content.

The treatment of ascites is aimed at its cause. If it is due to malignancy, instillation of chemotherapeutic drugs into the peritoneal cavity may prevent re-accumulation of fluid. In non-malignant cases which are resistant to diuretic therapy, bed rest with restriction of fluid and salt intake and shunting of the ascitic fluid to the venous system (LeVeen shunt) has been advocated (see p. 562).

ABSCESS

An intraperitoneal abscess is a common complication of peritonitis. It may also occur postoperatively as a result of contamination of the peritoneal cavity or following a leak from an anastomosis. Intraperitoneal abscesses commonly form in the pelvis, the subphrenic and subhepatic spaces, and between loops of bowel.

The main clinical signs of an intra-abdominal abscess are continuing pyrexia, tachycardia and evidence of toxicity. Complications can occur and include erosion into a large vessel causing catastrophic haemorrhage or rupture with consequent generalized peritonitis. Septicaemia may complicate any abscess.

The site of the abscess may be suspected from clinical examination but this can prove difficult and ultrasonic, CT and isotope scans (following injection of ^{111}In-labelled leucocytes) are of great value in localization. Ultrasound may also be used to guide the percutaneous insertion of a needle into the abscess cavity so that a definitive diagnosis can be made, material can be obtained for culture and sensitivity determinations, and percutaneous drainage can be instituted should this be necessary.

Surgical drainage is still the most important method of treatment. Antibiotic therapy without drainage may confuse the picture by abolishing systemic signs and giving a false sense of security. An undrained intra-abdominal abscess is a potent source of septicaemic shock.

Subphrenic and subhepatic abscess

Approximately half of all intra-abdominal abscesses occur in the subphrenic space. Three main separate spaces are described on each side according to whether the collection is above, below and in front, or below and behind the liver (Fig. 28.4). Abscesses are frequently multiple and this classification is of little practical importance.

Because of the relative inaccessibility of these spaces, locating physical signs are often notoriously lacking in patients with subphrenic infections. Unexplained fever after a peritoneal infection or operation should always raise the suspicion of a subphrenic abscess.

In some cases, the site of the abscess can be suspected if the origin of infection is known. There may be pain and tenderness anteriorly or posteriorly on the affected side, and this may be intensified by compression of the lower ribs. Shoulder pain and oedema over the lower intercostal spaces may also occur and there may be dullness to percussion over the lower chest.

Radiographic examination by anterior, lateral and oblique views is necessary in all suspected cases. This may demonstrate a pleural effusion and/or a fluid/gas-filled space below the diaphragm. Screening of the diaphragm or X-rays taken in full inspiration and expiration may reveal relative immobility on the affected side. Ultrasonic and CT scans may be diagnostic.

Until recently, surgical drainage was the standard treatment. However, improved techniques of radiological localization now allow percutaneous drainage in some patients. For surgical drainage, the route may be anterior or posterior, intraperitoneal or extraperitoneal, depending on the site of the abscess (Fig. 28.5). Repeated operations may be necessary in some patients.

Pelvic abscess

A pelvic abscess is a common complication of any form of intraperitoneal sepsis given that the infected material gravitates into the pelvis. It is a particularly common complication of acute appendicitis and may follow appendicectomy. Fever, lower abdominal discomfort and diarrhoea are characteristic. Rectal examination discloses a tender boggy swelling anteriorly (Fig. 28.6). If large, a pelvic abscess may form a palpable mass in the suprapubic region.

Spontaneous drainage of the abscess into the rectum can occur and treatment is normally expectant, with frequent rectal examination to assess progress. If it is clear that spontaneous drainage is unlikely, or if the abscess is increasing in size and the patient becoming increasingly toxic, surgical

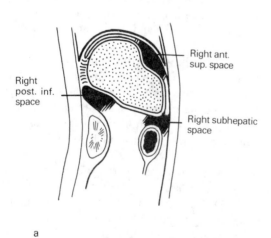

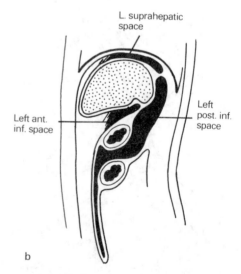

Fig. 28.4 The subphrenic and subhepatic spaces. (a) Right lateral view. (b) Left lateral view

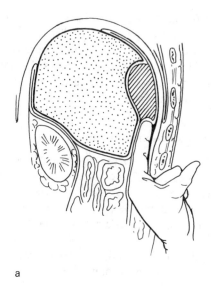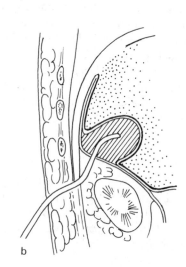

Fig. 28.5 Surgical drainage of (a) an anterior subphrenic abscess using a finger to break down loculi within the abscess, and (b) a posterior subphrenic abscess, leaving a drain within the abscess cavity

drainage is indicated. This may be done either through the rectum or by an extraperitoneal suprapubic approach. Following adequate drainage, the symptoms and signs rapidly resolve. Unfortunately, involvement of the ostia of the Fallopian tubes may be a cause of infertility in female patients.

DISORDERS OF THE MESENTERY AND OMENTUM

Mesenteric cyst

This is a rare embryonic cyst which occurs in the mesentery of the small intestine. It forms a round tense swelling in the right lower quadrant of the abdomen which is classically mobile in a vertical but not horizontal direction. Similar cysts may form in the omentum. Surgical removal is indicated.

Omental torsion

If fixed by an adhesion, the omentum may undergo torsion and give rise to acute abdominal pain associated with a tender palpable central abdominal mass. Treatment consists of laparotomy and excision of the omental mass.

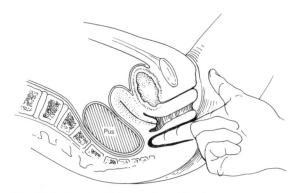

Fig. 28.6 Rectal examination for pelvic abscess

TUMOURS OF THE PERITONEUM AND RETROPERITONEUM

Primary tumours

Primary tumours of the peritoneum are rare but *mesothelioma* has been described in asbestos workers. It may present as a bulky epigastric mass or as diffuse involvement of the peritoneal surface associated with ascites.

Pseudomyxoma peritonei is a low-grade malignant tumour which spreads throughout the peritoneal cavity and is probably of ovarian origin. It may also follow rupture of a mucocele of the appendix. Lobulated deposits form on the peritoneal surfaces and there may be abundant mucus secretion causing abdominal distension. The condition is commonly associated with intermittent bouts of intestinal obstruction, and repeated operations to debulk the abdomen of tumour may be necessary. In view of its low-grade malignancy, survival may be prolonged.

Secondary tumours

The peritoneal cavity is a common site of spread of malignant disease. Seedling deposits form on the peritoneal surfaces and ascites follows. Palpable deposits of tumour may be detected in the rectovesical pouch.

In most cases, the primary site is known and and if the diagnosis is confirmed by cytological examination of the ascitic fluid there is little that can be done to alleviate symptoms. Chemotherapeutic agents may be instilled but any relief is often temporary.

Retroperitoneal tumours

A variety of retroperitoneal tumours, usually of connective tissue origin, may present as a retroperitoneal abdominal mass. Abdominal exploration and biopsy are necessary in all cases but the prognosis is usually hopeless. Occasionally, however, if the tumour is lymphomatous, radiotherapy and/or chemotherapy may cause regression and prolong life.

29. The acute abdomen

Many conditions produce acute abdominal pain. Comprehensive coverage of all of these is not feasible but the principles of assessment and management of patients with acute abdominal pain will be defined, and certain problem areas considered. Specific causes of the acute abdomen are considered in detail in other sections of this book.

Patients with acute abdominal pain may present at any time of the day or night demanding prompt assessment and treatment without recourse to many of the usual diagnostic aids. There is no substitute for experience in the management of these patients, and a full history and physical examination is fundamental to a successful outcome.

Abdominal pain

Innervation of the abdomen

The perception of abdominal pain is subserved by both autonomic (visceral pain) and somatic nervous systems (somatic pain).

Visceral afferents run from nerve endings in the muscle of the intestine and other abdominal organs along the path of the sympathetic nerves, joining the presacral and the splanchnic nerves to cross to the sensory roots through rami communicantes to enter the lumbar (L1–2) and thoracic (T6–12) regions of the spinal cord. Those viscera which have developed from the primitive gut, which embryologically is a midline structure, have a bilateral nerve supply, while that to paired organs such as the kidneys and testicles is unilateral. Visceral pain is abolished by division of the splanchnic nerves or by blocking their conduction by local anaesthesia. The vagus nerve has no role in the appreciation of abdominal pain but vagal afferents are concerned with stretch reflexes.

Somatic afferents supply the abdominal wall, including its lining of parietal peritoneum. These accompany the segmental nerves and gain access to the spinal cord through the appropriate dorsal root (T5–L2). The peritoneum under the diaphragm is an exception in that it is supplied by the phrenic nerve (C3–5) which innervates the diaphragm and descends with it from the neck (Fig. 29.1).

Perception of pain

Visceral pain. Pain arising from a hollow viscus such as the intestine, gallbladder or ureter is evoked by distension or excessive contraction. Local ischaemia may also contribute to intestinal

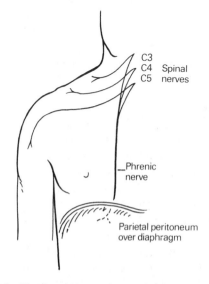

Fig. 29.1 The shared sensory innervation of the shoulder and diaphragm

pain and in some conditions, e.g. mesenteric vascular occlusion, may be the dominant component. Obstruction of a hollow viscus leads to increased muscle contractions in an attempt to overcome the blockage which are associated with bouts of excruciating cramping pain. This is called 'colic'. The frequency of the bouts of pain varies according to the viscus involved. For example, intestinal and ureteric colic are characterized by short bursts of pain lasting only 1–2 minutes, while in biliary colic the pain increases up to a plateau of intensity where it remains, with slight fluctuations, for some hours.

Handling, cutting or clamping the intestine does not cause pain unless the mesentery is dragged or stretched. The pain of peptic ulceration is due to muscular spasm and/or direct irritation of exposed nerve endings by acid.

Pain arising from a solid organ is the result of pressure and/or congestion. There are distinctive differences between organs. The liver, spleen and kidney are insensitive to pressure or incision unless inflamed, while the testes and renal pelvis are normally sensitive to pressure alone. Thus acute hepatitis is painful, as is compression injury to the testis.

Visceral pain is dull, deep-seated and cannot be precisely localized. It is appreciated in the area of the embryological position of the affected viscus so that pain arising from the intestine and its outgrowths (liver, spleen, pancreas) is felt in the midline; pain from the foregut (e.g. peptic ulcer pain) in the epigastrium; that from the midgut (e.g. from obstruction of small bowel or appendix) in the periumbilical region; and that from the hindgut (e.g. colonic obstruction) in the hypogastrium.

The unilateral pain which arises from paired organs (kidney and testis) is also perceived in the area of the embryological position of the organ. Pain from the testis (as opposed to the somatic pain from its coverings) is often felt low in the abdomen, rather than in the scrotum.

Somatic pain. While the visceral peritoneum is insensitive, the parietal peritoneum, lining the abdominal wall, is sensitive to tactile, thermal and chemical stimuli. It cannot be cut, cauterized or handled painlessly. Potent chemical irritants include bile, escaped intestinal contents, enzyme-rich exudates and blood.

Somatic pain is sharp (knife-like) and readily localized to its site of origin. The exception is pain arising from the diaphragmatic peritoneum, which is perceived in the shoulder region, the embryological position of that muscular structure (see Fig. 29.1). Painful stimulation of the parietal peritoneum is associated with reflex muscle guarding, rigidity and hyperaesthesia. Diffusion of the products of inflammation through the peritoneum into the overlying muscle may contribute to some of these effects.

Mixed pain. Some abdominal conditions cause both visceral and somatic pain. For example, an attack of acute appendicitis may start with visceral pain due to obstruction of the appendix. This pain is dull, diffuse and experienced in the region of the umbilicus. Once the inflammatory process has spread through the wall of the appendix and started to irritate the parietal peritoneum, the pain becomes somatic and is sharp and well localized.

History

Abdominal pain

The *mode of onset* of the pain is important. Explosive onset of excruciating abdominal pain suggests a vascular accident or perforation of a hollow viscus. Colic due to obstruction of the biliary tract, gut or urinary tract may also have a sudden onset, but this is not often described as explosive. Pain which starts gradually and worsens progressively is typical of peritonitis.

The *severity* of pain is difficult to define objectively as patients vary greatly in their reaction. Excruciating pain which is unrelieved by conventional doses of narcotics usually indicates a vascular catastrophe. The severe, intermittent pain of colic and the severe pain of acute pancreatitis or perforation of a peptic ulcer are usually more amenable to relief by such drugs. Pain which arises as a consequence of progressive peritonitis without initial perforation (e.g. acute appendicitis) is typically dull, gradually increases in severity, and becomes less well localized with the passage of time.

Localization is another important feature. While

visceral pain cannot be localized accurately, localization of parietal pain is precise but is complicated by the spread of peritonitis. *Referred pain* may give rise to confusion unless interpreted correctly. For example, irritation of the diaphragmatic peritoneum by blood, air or gastrointestinal content may cause pain and hyperaesthesia in the shoulder tip, while pain from the biliary tract may be referred to the right scapular region and that from ureteric colic to the groin. A *shift* in pain may also aid diagnosis. The classic example is acute appendicitis where the initial central abdominal colic of appendiceal obstruction eventually gives way to pain in the right iliac fossa as parietal peritonitis develops. Gradual spread of pain throughout the abdomen usually indicates development of diffuse peritonitis.

It is important to appreciate that a lessening of pain does not necessarily indicate that the underlying condition has resolved. The excruciating pain of mesenteric vascular occlusion may wane despite the presence of gangrenous bowel. Following perforation of a peptic ulcer there is frequently a 'period of illusion' during which pain diminishes temporarily despite progressive peritonitis. This is due to dilution of the irritant fluid by exudated serum. Diminution of pain may also occur in the terminal stages of peritonitis, regardless of cause.

Anorexia, nausea and vomiting

These are common symptoms in patients with acute abdominal pain, but are not always present. Anorexia is particularly common in acute appendicitis, while nausea, retching and vomiting are prominent features of acute pancreatitis, high intestinal obstruction and obstruction of the biliary tract. Gastroenteritis can simulate an acute surgical condition, but the nausea and vomiting frequently *precede* the onset of colic which is associated with diarrhoea.

Alteration in bowel habit

Many acute abdominal conditions develop so rapidly that there is no time for alteration in bowel habit to become apparent. With complete intestinal obstruction, inability to pass flatus or faeces eventually occurs, but in the initial stages there may be one or more bowel movements as the gut distal to the obstruction is evacuated by strong peristaltic waves passing on beyond the site of obstruction. Diarrhoea is a marked feature in gastroenteritis or colitis but can also occur as a manifestation of pelvic sepsis, as for example in acute pelvic appendicitis. Blood is present in the stool in some cases of mesenteric vascular occlusion, but repeated bloody diarrhoea is much more likely to be due to ulcerative colitis or dysentery. It must not be forgotten that bleeding from the upper gastrointestinal tract may produce massive melaena without haematemesis.

Menstrual status and gynaecological disease

The frequency of menstruation and date of the last menstrual period must be established in female patients.

The Graafian follicle normally ruptures 14 days after the start of the last menstrual period, and release of the ovum may be complicated by bleeding. This is the cause of the lower abdominal pain which occurs half-way through the menstrual cycle, notably in young girls, the so-called 'mittelschmerz' (middle-pain). The follicle then becomes a corpus luteum which degenerates before the start of the next period unless conception occurs. Bleeding from the corpus luteum is an occasional cause of pain in the late stages of the menstrual cycle.

Females of childbearing age should be asked about contraceptive practice and the likelihood of pregnancy. Rupture of an ectopic pregnancy is an acute abdominal emergency which demands prompt treatment. Lower abdominal and shoulder-tip pain (due to blood irritating the diaphragmatic peritoneum) is characteristic and 'withdrawal bleeding' due to cessation of hormone production following death of the embryo is frequent. This is scanty and dark, and follows the pain, in contrast to the profuse bright red bleeding which precedes the pain of abortion.

Low abdominal pain and tenderness can also be caused by acute salpingitis. A history of purulent vaginal discharge may provide a useful clue.

PHYSICAL EXAMINATION

Examination of the abdomen

Physical signs may be diminished in the elderly, grossly obese, gravely ill, and in patients on steroid therapy. As sedation also obscures pain and tenderness, it is best avoided until a decision on management has been made. This rule is relaxed when pain is severe or in young children in whom abdominal examination may not be practicable without sedation.

Abdominal examination is carried out with the patient lying flat and the abdomen uncovered from xiphisternum to groin. Flexing of the thighs will relax the anterior abdominal wall. The clinician sits or kneels beside the bed (traditionally on the right side) so that his arm and hand can be extended horizontally across the abdomen.

Inspection

Inspection is the essential first step. Any scars, bulging of hernias, distended loops of gut or other abnormal masses are noted. It should be ascertained whether the abdomen moves freely with respiration and the patient should be asked to 'blow out his abdomen' so that the flaccidity of the abdominal wall can be assessed. The abdominal contour is noted.

The abdomen is distended in most cases of intestinal obstruction, whereas it is indrawn and scaphoid in the early stages of perforation of a viscus. Following a perforation the patient usually lies still with the abdomen rigid for fear of exacerbating the pain by movement, whereas patients with colic are restless and may not be able to lie still during examination. Patients with acute pancreatitis sometimes find that sitting forwards relieves their pain, and are uncomfortable when lying flat. Peristalsis is occasionally visible in intestinal obstruction and can sometimes be stimulated by 'flicking' a distended loop of gut with a finger.

Palpation

Once the abdomen has been inspected, it is gently palpated to detect tenderness and muscle guard-ing. Tenderness is sought by gentle palpation with all of the fingers of one hand, holding them extended at the interphalangeal joints and gently flexing and extending the metacarpophalangeal joints. Tenderness is sought first in areas furthest from the patient's pain. Inflammation of the parietal peritoneum causes a reflex increase in overlying muscle tone which is detected on palpation as *guarding* of the muscles concerned, and in its extreme form as board-like *rigidity* of the abdominal wall.

Inflammation of the peritoneum lining the anterior abdominal wall is easy to detect. Direct tenderness and guarding are obvious on abdominal examination. Detection of peritonitis affecting other areas of the abdominal cavity may prove more difficult. Pelvic peritonitis may produce little or no tenderness or guarding on examination of the abdomen, although digital rectal examination is very painful. Inflammation of the diaphragmatic peritoneum does not cause abdominal guarding or tenderness but shoulder-tip pain (see earlier). Radiological screening is needed to reveal restricted diaphragmatic movement. Peritonitis involving the posterior parietal peritoneum may produce few signs on abdominal examination. It is for this reason that the symptoms of acute pancreatitis and retrocaecal appendicitis overshadow the abdominal signs.

Guarding and rigidity of the muscles of the anterior abdominal wall usually denotes peritonitis. However, it may also occur in renal colic, rare neurological disorders, and hysteria or malingering. In renal colic, rigidity is confined to the muscles of the affected side, while the spasm of hysteria can be overcome if the examining hand remains on the abdomen while the patient is asked to breathe deeply or when his attention is distracted by questioning.

Deep palpation. Once gentle palpation has defined areas of tenderness and guarding, deep palpation is used to detect abdominal masses. In the acute situation, these include intra-abdominal abscesses, empyema of the gallbladder, diverticulitis, aortic aneurysm, twisted ovarian cyst, and intussusception.

It is also important to palpate each organ in turn, seeking enlargement of the liver, spleen and kidneys.

Percussion

Percussion is used to delineate abdominal organs and abnormal masses, and to determine the cause of abdominal distension. The percussion note is tympanitic when distension is due to gas, as in intestinal obstruction, and dull when distension results from fluid, as in ascites or a full bladder. The site of dullness (whether in the flanks or suprapubically) and any shift in its position on change of posture are noted. Free air rises within the peritoneal cavity so that perforation of the gastrointestinal tract may be associated with diminution or absence of liver dullness as air accumulates beneath the diaphragm.

Gentle percussion may also be used to detect rebound tenderness in inflammatory disease.

Auscultation

Auscultation is an essential part of the examination. It should be carried out centrally to detect bowel sounds, and over masses and major arteries to detect vascular bruits. It should be remembered that normal heart sounds may be heard in a distended abdomen. Auscultation may have to be prolonged and repeated when there is doubt about the presence or frequency of bowel sounds (peristaltic activity). Peristalsis is increased in mechanical intestinal obstruction, in gastroenteritis, and in the presence of blood in the bowel lumen. Activity ceases in paralytic ileus but bowel sounds may still be heard in the initial stages of mesenteric vascular occlusion. The detection of a bruit during auscultation may indicate vascular disease.

Examination of the groin

Examination of the groin is important. As this step is easily forgotten, many experienced clinicians begin their examination in this area. Detection of a small inguinal or femoral hernia is particularly important in intestinal obstruction. The patient may be unaware that he had a hernia and the central localization of abdominal colic may focus attention away from the region.

Pus tracking down the psoas sheath is a rare cause of groin swelling. A colonic neoplasm may occasionally perforate retroperitoneally and cause crepitus and erythema in the groin.

The femoral pulses must be palpated routinely during examination of the groin, as diminished pulsation may point to aortic disease. In the male the testes and scrotum are also examined (see Ch. 39).

Digital rectal examination

Digital rectal examination is mandatory and should be preceded by careful inspection to reveal any pathology at the anal verge (Fig. 29.2). Tenderness on rectal examination may be the only sign of pelvic appendicitis. Tenderness of the uterine cervix may be associated with salpingitis, and abnormalities of the male prostate should be sought. Faecal impaction can be detected. Some lesions such as carcinoma of the rectum may be outwith the reach of the examiner's finger, but may become palpable when the patient is asked to strain. A specimen of stool can be tested for occult blood so that the need for proctoscopy or sigmoidoscopy can be assessed.

If disease of the uterus, Fallopian tubes or ovaries is suspected, a vaginal examination is also performed.

Miscellaneous clinical tests

Murphy's sign is associated with peritoneal tenderness in acute cholecystitis. The patient is asked to take a deep breath while the examiner palpates the region over the gallbladder. A catching of breath at the zenith of inspiration occurs as the inflamed gallbladder enters the area under the examiner's fingers.

Rovsing's sign can be elicited in some cases of acute appendicitis. Deep palpation in the left iliac fossa causes pain in the right iliac fossa. In practice the sign is inconstant and of little value.

Rebound tenderness denotes a resurgence of pain as the examiner's hand is withdrawn sharply while palpating the abdomen. It indicates parietal peritonitis but its value is controversial. Over-zealous attempts to elicit rebound tenderness inflict unnecessary pain, and light percussion of the abdominal wall is a better way to determine whether the parietal peritoneum is inflamed.

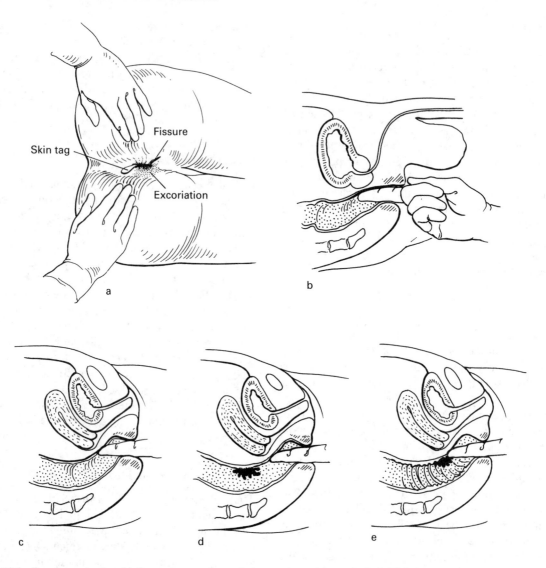

Fig. 29.2 Rectal examination. (a) Inspection revealing pathology at the anal verge. (b & c) Digital rectal examination allows palpation of the prostate in the male and of the cervix in the female. (d & e) A lesion outwith the reach of the examiner's finger may become palpable by asking the patient to strain

Cutaneous hyperaesthesia is a non-specific sign of inflammation of the peritoneum and is tested by pricking the skin. A triangle of hyperaesthesia in the right iliac fossa is strongly suggestive of appendicitis but the test is seldom employed.

The iliopsoas test is used to detect restriction of movement of the iliacus and psoas major muscles. The patient is asked to lie on his side (with the side to be tested uppermost) and the iliopsoas muscle is stretched by fully extending the thigh.

Restriction of movement may occur with retro-caecal inflammation, e.g. from appendicitis or a perinephric abscess. When inflammation is advanced the patient sometimes lies with the hip flexed on the affected side to relax the irritated psoas muscle. The iliopsoas test cannot be interpreted when there is rigidity of the abdominal wall muscles.

The obturator test is a method of detecting pelvic peritonitis irritating the obturator internus muscle.

Deep-seated pain occurs when the thigh is flexed at right angles to the trunk and the leg internally rotated.

The iliopsoas and obturator tests are now seldom used.

Vital signs

The *temperature* is often normal in the early stages of peritonitis. Elevation denotes infection but not necessarily within the abdomen. In a severely shocked patient it may be normal or below normal despite advanced infection.

Tachycardia is common in most acute abdominal conditions. The pulse rate may be increased by severe pain alone. When the pain is intermittent, as in renal colic, the pulse rate may return to normal between bouts of pain. The pulse must be monitored in all cases. A progressive increase usually indicates infection or circulatory insufficiency.

The *blood pressure* is determined routinely on admission, and then monitored at regular intervals. The frequency of recording depends on the severity of the condition and whether the patient is shocked.

The *respiration rate* is typically rapid and shallow when abdominal pain is severe. Intrathoracic disease can produce abdominal pain, but high fever, cough, flaring of the alae nasi and cyanosis are the typical signs of respiratory disease. Flaring of the alae nasi occurs in abdominal disease only when movement of the diaphragm is impeded. Hyperventilation is an early sign of septicaemic shock.

Thorough examination of the chest (including chest X-ray) is essential in all patients with acute abdominal pain. Laparotomy in a patient with basal pneumonia is a classical mistake.

ESTABLISHING A DIAGNOSIS

Once a full history has been obtained and physical examination has been completed, an attempt should be made to define the nature of the disease process responsible, and to identify the organ or organ system involved (Table 29.1). A working diagnosis and its likely alternatives are made and further investigations arranged.

Laboratory and radiological aids to diagnosis

Haematology

The haemoglobin concentration, haematocrit (packed cell volume) and white cell count are determined routinely in patients with an acute

Table 29.1 Common non-traumatic causes of acute abdomen

Pathological process	Organ commonly involved	Disease
Inflammation	Appendix	Acute appendicitis
	Gallbladder	Acute cholecystitis
	Colon	Acute diverticulitis
	Meckel's diverticulum	Acute diverticulitis
	Fallopian tube	Acute salpingitis
	Pancreas	Acute pancreatitis
Obstruction	Small intestine	Acute intestinal obstruction
	Colon	Acute intestinal obstruction
	Ureter	Ureteric colic
	Urethra	Acute retention of urine
Ischaemia	Small intestine (hernia)	Volvulus (strangulation)
	Mesenteric arteries	Intestinal infarction
	Ovary	Torsion of ovarian cyst
Perforation	Duodenum	Perforated peptic ulcer (peritonitis)
	Gallbladder	Biliary peritonitis
	Colon (diverticulum or tumour)	Faecal peritonitis
	Ectopic pregnancy	Haemoperitoneum
Arterial rupture	Abdominal aorta	Ruptured arterial aneurysm

abdomen. The white cell count is usually elevated in the presence of infection, although it may be normal in the early stages.

Urinalysis

The urine is tested routinely for sugar, acetone, protein, bile and urobilinogen. Testing for sugar is essential for the detection of undiagnosed diabetics and to assess control in those with known diabetes. Diabetic patients are just as likely to develop an acute abdomen due to intra-abdominal pathology as non-diabetics but require special care during the operative and postoperative period (see Ch. 10). Diabetic keto-acidosis may produce abdominal pain without organic pathology and in such cases unnecessary laparotomy must be avoided.

Porphyria occasionally causes abdominal pain (see below) and in those with a family trait the urine should be tested for porphobilinogen by the addition of Ehrlich's aldehyde reagent.

Microscopic examination will reveal pus cells and bacteria in urinary tract infections, and red blood cells in patients with renal colic. Measurement of urine osmolality or specific gravity may be useful in assessing dehydration or shock.

Radiology

A chest X-ray should be taken on admission. This may show primary chest pathology; secondary chest pathology (e.g. pleural effusion or pulmonary aspiration); evidence of cardiac failure; or free gas under the diaphragm. In patients with suspected obstruction or perforation of an abdominal viscus, both erect and supine abdominal films should be taken and may show distension and fluid levels or intraperitoneal gas. Otherwise, a supine film is satisfactory. For suspected aortic aneurysm a lateral decubitus film is indicated.

Radiological signs include localized ileus in inflammatory conditions such as appendicitis and pancreatitis; radio-opaque opacities in some patients with gallstones and urinary calculi; and vascular calcification in aortic aneurysms. Abnormal enlargement or displacement of abdominal organs may point to the site of disease.

Gastrointestinal perforation is not always associated with radiological evidence of free air in the peritoneum. In cases of doubt a Gastrografin meal may be indicated. As Gastrografin is water-soluble, it does not irritate the peritoneum. Gastrografin meals and enemas can also be used in the investigation of suspected intestinal obstruction.

Ultrasonography is the key investigation in the assessment of patients thought to have biliary tract disease and has been reported to increase the accuracy of diagnosis in acute appendicitis. Intravenous pyelography is invaluable in the diagnosis of urinary tract obstruction or trauma. Angiography is used occasionally to investigate severe gastrointestinal bleeding and genitourinary haemorrhage. Ultrasonography is now preferred to aortography if a ruptured aortic aneurysm cannot be excluded on clinical examination.

Peritoneal lavage

Peritoneal lavage has an established place in assessing blunt abdominal trauma (see Ch. 14). Its value is less certain in acute abdominal conditions. Lavage is contraindicated in the presence of distension or scarring. False negative (and to a lesser extent false positive) results may be misleading and most surgeons prefer to undertake laparotomy when a surgical cause for an acute abdomen cannot be excluded by conventional clinical examination.

Laparoscopy

Laparoscopy is being used increasingly to determine whether pelvic inflammatory disease or other conditions affecting the pelvic viscera (e.g. rupture of a follicle) are present. Its role in the diagnosis of other acute abdominal conditions is under review.

Clinical chemistry

Urea and electrolyte determinations are seldom of diagnostic value, but are essential in the assessment of fluid and electrolyte needs. The result of liver function tests are seldom available in time to influence initial management, but the earliest opportunity should be taken to establish a baseline, particularly in patients with liver and biliary tract disease. Serum amylase determination is valuable when acute pancreatitis is suspected, provided its limitations are borne in mind (see Ch. 37). Arterial blood gases, hydrogen ion concentration and standard bicarbonate should be measured in all shocked patients and those with respiratory problems.

Computer-assisted diagnosis

Computer-assisted diagnosis (by which the most probable diagnosis is derived from a large data base) has been shown to improve the accuracy of diagnosis of acute abdominal pain. Part of this improvement is due to the strict system used for recording the history and results of clinical examination. In the final analysis these are the most important factors in deciding the need for laparotomy, and a computer-assisted system must never be used as a substitute for careful assessment of the patient by an experienced clinician.

INITIAL TREATMENT

All patients suspected of having acute abdominal disease should be confined to bed and given nothing further by mouth. Wherever possible, analgesics are withheld until a firm decision has been taken on the likely diagnosis and proposed management. If the patient has vomited or upper gastrointestinal disease, obstruction or perforation is suspected, a nasogastric tube should be passed and the stomach kept empty by regular or continuous aspiration. Patients requiring urgent laparotomy who have eaten within the past 4–6 hours should also have a tube passed so that the stomach is empty when anaesthesia is induced.

If there is blood loss, dehydration, shock or electrolyte disturbance, or if these are anticipated, an intravenous line is inserted. A fluid balance chart is essential in all cases. In shocked patients or when urinary retention is suspected, a catheter should be inserted into the bladder. Pulse and temperature are recorded regularly in all cases, and regular recording of blood pressure, central venous pressure and hourly urine output are essential in those with shock.

Suspicion of infection is *not* an indication for antibiotic therapy. Prescription of antibiotics should await specific indications. For example, the majority of patients with acute pancreatitis or perforated peptic ulceration do not require antibiotics. Antibiotics are usually (but not invariably) prescribed in acute cholecystitis and are essential if peritonitis is thought to be due to colonic perforation. If antibiotic treatment is started before operation, blood samples for culture should be taken before the first dose is given.

Assessment of the need for laparotomy is an important aspect of the surgeon's evaluation of the acute abdomen, but must never become the sole objective. One should always construct a list of differential diagnoses first, and attempt to define the diagnosis of greatest probability. The nature of the disease process and the organ or system involved should wherever possible be recorded in writing in the case notes.

The timing of operation is determined by the nature of the underlying disease, the patient's general condition and the need for preoperative resuscitation. Considerable delay may have occurred before the patient is first seen by the surgeon, and, as a general rule, conditions requiring surgery do deteriorate with time. However, while delay may be disastrous for a patient with a ruptured aortic aneurysm, adequate preoperative resuscitation may prove life-saving for a grossly dehydrated patient with mechanical intestinal obstruction.

In many patients the diagnosis and the indications for operation are uncertain at presentation; re-examination over the next few hours will then clarify the position.

There are many instances when the surgeon must balance the risk of needless surgery against the danger of not operating promptly. For example, the penalty of not operating early in acute appendicitis far outweighs the dangers of laparotomy in mesenteric adenitis. To await signs which would make the clinical diagnosis of appendicitis certain would inevitably increase morbidity and mortality from gangrene and perforation. For this reason some surgeons accept that the appendix may be normal in up to 20% of emergency appendicectomies.

SURGICAL CAUSES OF THE ACUTE ABDOMEN

The surgical causes of the acute abdomen (see Table 29.1) include obstruction, inflammatory disease (most commonly appendicitis, cholecystitis, diverticulitis and pancreatitis), perforation and strangulation, and mesenteric ischaemia. All of these may lead to peritonitis and are considered in detail elsewhere in this volume. Gynaecological and non-surgical causes are discussed in this chapter.

GYNAECOLOGICAL CAUSES OF THE ACUTE ABDOMEN

Ruptured ectopic pregnancy

The fertilized ovum implants at an abnormal site once in every 200 pregnancies. The Fallopian tube is by far the commonest site, possibly because of delayed transit of the ovum as a result of previous tubal infection such as gonococcal salpingitis. If the erosive trophoblast penetrates the wall of the tube, it may rupture, usually after about 6 weeks of pregnancy. Alternatively, the conceptus may be extruded from the fimbrial end of the tube.

Clinical features

In many cases, bouts of cramping pain in one or other iliac fossa associated with fainting attacks and vaginal bleeding point to an abnormal pregnancy. With rupture, there is sudden, severe pain, blood loss and circulatory collapse. The abdominal pain is generalized and there is shoulder pain which may become apparent on elevating the foot of the bed. A missed period is reported by the majority of patients but the menstrual history may be confused by bleeding at the time of implantation or following death of the embryo.

Signs of pregnancy such as enlargement of the breasts and uterus are not usually present but cervical softening and tenderness are apparent on gentle pelvic examination. If a haematoma has formed between the layers of the broad ligament, a tender mass may be palpable.

Pregnancy tests are unhelpful in detecting an ectopic pregnancy prior to rupture because of inadequate placental production of chorionic gonadotrophin. Laparoscopy may be used as a diagnostic aid.

Treatment

The diagnosis of ruptured ectopic pregnancy demands urgent surgery. Following rapid resuscitation to compensate for blood loss, laparotomy is performed and the involved tube removed. Following an ectopic pregnancy, there is a 10% chance of an ectopic pregnancy occurring in the remaining tube.

Rupture of a functional ovarian cyst

Bleeding from a ruptured Graafian follicle or corpus luteum may cause abdominal pain.

Clinical features

The patient is usually between 15 and 25 years of age and complains of sudden pain in one or other iliac fossa. Nausea and vomiting may be present but there are no systemic signs and the pain usually settles within a few hours. Tenderness and guarding in the right iliac fossa can mimic acute appendicitis and a few patients bleed sufficiently to suggest rupture of an ectopic pregnancy. On rectal examination there may be tenderness in the rectovaginal pouch.

Treatment

The patient is observed and laparotomy advised only when acute appendicitis or ruptured ectopic pregnancy cannot be excluded. Laparoscopy is helpful in such cases.

Torsion of an ovarian cyst

Benign ovarian cysts are common in women under 50 years of age and may undergo torsion (Fig. 29.3). Dermoid cysts account for some 50% of torsions in young women but only for a minority of all ovarian cysts (10%). Their long pedicles make them particularly vulnerable to twisting.

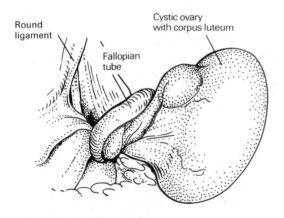

Round ligament

Cystic ovary with corpus luteum

Fallopian tube

Fig. 29.3   Torsion of an ovarian cyst

Clinical features

The patient complains of severe cramping lower abdominal pain. A smooth round mobile mass may be palpable in the abdomen. This is often higher than would be expected from an ovarian mass. There may be tenderness and guarding over the mass, particularly if there is leakage from the cyst. Rupture results in diffuse peritonism.

The Fallopian tube or a pedunculated uterine fibroid may also undergo torsion and present with a similar clinical picture.

Treatment

Laparotomy is performed. The twisted pedicle is transfixed and ligated and the cyst is removed. Care should be taken to avoid rupture of the cyst as, should it be malignant, cells may disseminate throughout the peritoneal cavity. The histology must be carefully reviewed. If the lesion is malignant, a further radical operation will be required.

Acute salpingitis

Acute salpingitis is most often due to gonococcal infection but streptococci and *M. tuberculosis* may also be responsible. Urethritis, cervicitis and a vaginal discharge occur 3–6 days following infection. At this stage, tubal involvement is unusual but after a menstrual period organisms spread to the lining of the uterus and tube. Both tubes are commonly involved and adhesions may seal the fimbriated end, leading to the formation of a pyosalpinx.

Clinical features

Bilateral pain is felt low in the abdomen, often just above the inguinal ligament. This may be associated with increased frequency of micturition. The menstrual history is often irregular and there is pyrexia (39–40°C) and leucocytosis.

On vaginal examination there is unusual vaginal warmth, the cervix is tender and there is a purulent discharge. On inspection, the cervix is red and inflamed and a swab reveals the causal organism. If the tube is sealed and distended with pus (pyosalpinx), the vaginal findings may be less marked.

Treatment

Treatment consists initially of antibiotic therapy. Laparotomy is undertaken only if acute appendicitis and ectopic pregnancy cannot be excluded or if a tubal abscess is suspected. In acute salpingitis, laparoscopy is being used increasingly to avoid unnecessary laparotomy. At laparotomy (should this be considered necessary) the inflamed tubes appear red and oedematous. On 'milking' them gently there is a purulent discharge from which a swab should be taken for bacteriological examination. The abdomen is closed without drainage. The appendix is removed only if the infection is mild.

CAUSES OF THE ACUTE ABDOMEN NOT AMENABLE TO SURGERY

Acute abdominal pain can be produced by a number of conditions for which operation is contraindicated. However, even when a non-surgical cause is suspected, it may not be possible to exclude serious abdominal disease and laparotomy may be required.

Non-specific abdominal pain

Approximately one-half of all patients sent to hospital with acute abdominal pain have no demonstrable cause or only a minor urinary tract infection of doubtful significance.

Non-specific abdominal pain is commonest in the young. Mesenteric adenitis, low-grade urinary tract infection, mild gastroenteritis, irritable bowel syndrome, cyclical ovarian problems and emotional upsets are all possible causes. Tenderness in the right iliac fossa is common and acute appendicitis is most frequently suspected.

In such cases a period of careful observation is desirable. Laparotomy is undertaken only if pain and tenderness persist or if systemic signs of an inflammatory condition develop.

Acute mesenteric adenitis

At one time acute mesenteric adenitis was believed to be viral in origin. It is now known that the majority of cases are caused by *Yersinia entercolitica* or *Y. pseudotuberculosis*. Most patients are between 5 and 15 years of age and present with a history of central or right-sided abdominal pain, anorexia, nausea and vomiting. There may have been previous attacks of pain or a recent upper respiratory tract infection.

The patient is frequently flushed and pyrexial and has an inflamed throat and cervical lymphadenopathy. Abdominal tenderness is usually higher in the abdomen and more diffuse than in appendicitis and may vary in its position on repeated examination or when the patient moves. Guarding and rebound tenderness are unusual.

Laparotomy is performed if appendicitis cannot be excluded. The lymph nodes in the mesentery of the terminal ileum are fleshy and enlarged and this may be associated with a red and thickened ileum (terminal ileitis). The appendix is normal but should be removed to avoid confusion in the future.

The diagnosis can be confirmed by culture of the responsible organisms from the stool or lymph nodes or by serological testing. However, as the condition is self-limiting and the patient usually makes an uneventful recovery, these investigations are not normally requested. There are no specific histological features on examination of lymph nodes or appendix.

Diabetes mellitus

Acute abdominal pain and tenderness occur in 25% of patients with diabetic metabolic problems. The cause of the pain is uncertain but pancreatitis, stretching of the liver capsule, gastric distension and dehydration are possible explanations. Hyperamylasaemia occurs in two-thirds of patients with diabetic keto-acidosis.

There is a history of thirst and polyuria, drowsiness, and in some instances failure to maintain stabilization on insulin therapy. The patient appears dehydrated and ill, there is acetone in the breath and he or she may become comatose. The urine contains large amounts of sugar and acetone and there is hyperglycaemia and metabolic acidosis.

If the abdominal pain is due solely to diabetes, it should disappear rapidly with treatment. Persistence of pain and tenderness suggests an underlying surgical cause. In this regard, it should be remembered that a primary surgical problem, e.g. appendicitis, can cause secondary instability of diabetic control.

If surgery is considered necessary, vigorous treatment of keto-acidosis is required before the operation.

Acute intermittent porphyria

An attack of acute porphyria is a rare cause of abdominal pain, the nature of which resembles that of small bowel colic. Vomiting is common but abdominal signs are seldom prominent. There may be a history of barbiturate ingestion, which in a susceptible person can initiate an acute attack.

The diagnosis is suggested by the finding of porphyrins in the urine. Freshly passed urine is normal in appearance but becomes red on standing or on addition of Ehrlich's aldehyde reagent. This test must be carried out on all patients with a familial trait of porphyria who are admitted with abdominal pain. Most now carry identification discs.

Porphyria and acute abdominal disease can coincide. Should it be considered advisable to operate, the anaesthetist must be informed that the patient is porphyric so that barbiturates and other sensitizing drugs can be avoided.

Haemochromatosis

Abdominal pain occurs in one-third of patients with haemochromatosis. The pain is usually dull and boring but can become severe and simulate acute cholecystitis or acute appendicitis. Other signs of haemochromatosis, e.g. slate-like pigmentation, will be present.

Lead poisoning

The clinical picture of lead poisoning resembles that of porphyria. The diagnosis is suggested by a history of exposure to lead or by associated clinical findings of muscle palsy, a blue line on the gums or punctate basophilia on examination of the blood. Severe constipation is typical.

Disease of the blood and blood vessels

Hereditary spherocytosis

Attacks of abdominal pain, nausea and vomiting associated with abdominal tenderness and icterus can coincide with episodes of haemolysis, probably as a result of minor intra-abdominal haemorrhage. Emergency laparotomy is seldom indicated. Cholelithiasis is common and cholecystitis should always be considered as a cause of abdominal pain in patients with this disease.

Haemophilia

Abdominal pain in haemophiliacs is more often due to haemorrhage than to surgical pathology. Extraperitoneal bleeding is common and haemorrhage into the psoas sheath can simulate appendicitis. Haematoma formation in the gut wall can cause intussusception.

Obviously a haemophiliac is not immune to surgical problems. If serious intra-abdominal pathology is suspected and operation advised, a haematologist must be consulted concerning factor VIII and other therapy. In view of the unfortunate infection of a proportion of haemophiliacs with human immunodeficiency virus (HIV), full precautions to protect theatre and ward staff must be instituted.

Anaphylactoid purpura (Henoch-Schönlein Purpura)

This is a rare cause of abdominal pain in children. It is usually associated with a streptococcal sore throat, abdominal colic, vomiting, bloody diarrhoea or intussusception preceding the development of skin purpura.

Sickle-cell disease

This hereditary disease is virtually confined to negroes, particularly those from West Africa. There is an abnormal form of haemoglobin S which crystallizes when oxygen tension is reduced and results in increased osmotic fragility of the red cells and haemolytic attacks. These may be associated with abdominal pain, tenderness, guarding and icterus. The abdominal pain is most commonly due to splenic infarcts.

The correct diagnosis is suggested by associated chronic anaemia, bone and joint pain, and leg ulcers. Examination of a blood film reveals the characteristic sickle shape of the red cells. Gallstones occur in one-third of patients with sickle-cell disease. Cholecystitis must always be considered as a cause of abdominal pain.

Polycythaemia vera

In this condition spontaneous thrombosis can cause splenic and mesenteric infarcts with acute abdominal pain.

Polyarteritis nodosa

Nausea, vomiting, abdominal pain and diarrhoea affect 50% of patients with this disease. Occasionally severe protracted pain with fever, leucocytosis and abdominal tenderness suggests focal infarction within the abdomen. Pancreatitis, bleeding, perforation and obstruction are also reported as complications of this disease. Steroid therapy is indicated unless perforation or infarction of the intestine is suspected. In this case operation must not be delayed.

30. Gastroduodenal disorders

SURGICAL ANATOMY

The stomach consists of three main areas: fundus, body and pyloric antrum (Fig. 30.1). The gastric lumen is lined by a row of tall columnar epithelial cells which commence abruptly at the cardia at the point of termination of the stratified squamous epithelium of the oesophagus. The gastric epithelium is pitted throughout by the opening of gastric glands. These glands are of three types.

The *cardiac glands* secrete mucus and electrolytes, and occupy a small ring around the oesophagogastric junction.

The *oxyntic glands* occupy the entire fundus and body of the stomach, taking up some 75% of gastric mucosal surface area. There are at least five types of cell lining these glands (see Fig. 30.1). *Mucous neck cells* lie in the narrow neck beneath the gastric pits. *Undifferentiated neck cells* divide throughout life to replenish the surface epithelium and oxyntic glandular cells. *Parietal cells* produce hydrogen ions and intrinsic factor and are most

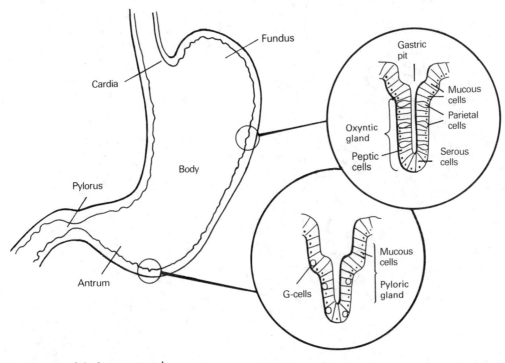

Fig. 30.1 Anatomy of the human stomach

445

numerous in the upper half of the glands. *Peptic cells* secrete pepsinogen and are most numerous in the lower half of the glands. A number of *endocrine cells* are found between the peptic cells but their physiological function is uncertain.

The *pyloric glands* occupy the antrum and are separated from the oxyntic gland area by a transitional zone. The glands are lined by cells resembling mucous neck cells which secrete mucus and electrolytes, and by G-cells which produce the hormone gastrin (see Fig. 30.1).

Nerve supply

The stomach receives its autonomic nerve supply from the vagus nerves and from the sympathetic nervous system. The left and right vagus nerves form an anterior and posterior oesophageal plexus around the lower thoracic oesophagus, each plexus containing fibres from both nerves (Fig. 30.2). Each plexus forms one or more vagal trunks just above the diaphragm, and the anterior and posterior trunks enter the abdomen by passing through the diaphragm with the oesophagus. The anterior trunk gives off hepatic branches and then descends along the lesser curvature to supply the front wall of the stomach (Fig. 30.3). The posterior trunk gives off a coeliac branch on entering the abdomen and then descends along the posterior aspect of the lesser curve supplying the back wall of the stomach. Approximately 80% of vagal fibres are afferent, and almost two-thirds of the fibres entering the abdomen innervate the stomach. The remaining one-third pass in the hepatic and coeliac branches to innervate the liver, gallbladder, pancreas, small intestine and large intestine as far as the distal transverse colon.

Sympathetic post-ganglionic fibres pass from the coeliac ganglion and reach the stomach by accompanying the gastric arteries.

SURGICAL PHYSIOLOGY

Gastric motility

After ingestion, food is stored in the stomach, where it is ground, mixed and prepared for controlled release into the duodenum. Receptive relaxation is the process by which the body and fundus of stomach relax to accommodate increasing volumes of food without major pressure

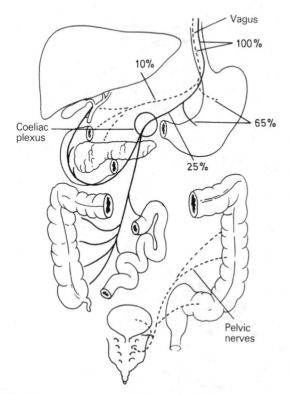

Fig. 30.2 Distribution of abdominal parasympathetic nerves

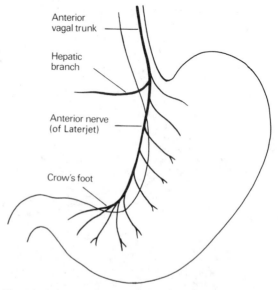

Fig. 30.3 Anatomy of the anterior vagus nerve

increase. The antrum is not concerned with receptive relaxation, but powerful antral contractions mix and grind the food, and expel it into the duodenum as the pylorus relaxes. The intrinsic neural plexuses (myenteric and submucosal) play an important role in governing gastric motility but are regulated in turn by the extrinsic nerve supply. Bilateral truncal vagotomy abolishes receptive relaxation and greatly diminishes the power of antral contraction. The sympathetic nerves inhibit gastric motility.

Gastric secretion

Mucus is secreted by all regions of the stomach and, in addition to serving as a lubricant, protects the surface epithelium against autodigestion by acid and pepsin.

Gastric acid and pepsin secretion is not essential for protein digestion, as great quantities of proteolytic enzymes are secreted by the pancreas. Four substances normally present in the body are capable of stimulating gastric secretion. *Calcium* acts as a stimulant to acid, pepsin and gastrin secretion when there is hypercalcaemia but is not a normal physiological stimulant. *Acetylcholine* and *gastrin* have established physiological roles as secretory stimulants, while *histamine* has strong claims for a physiological role. Acetylcholine acts as a neurocrine regulator and mediates vagal stimulation. Gastrin serves as a conventional endocrine regulator and is carried by the blood stream from antrum to body of stomach, while histamine is probably released from cells in the immediate vicinity of parietal and peptic cells, and acts as a *paracrine* regulator. The parietal and peptic cells possess separate receptor sites for acetylcholine, gastrin and histamine, but the action of each chemical is potentiated by a tonic effect of the other two (Fig. 30.4). This means that surgical vagotomy not only removes stimulation by acetylcholine, but also reduces the efficacy of gastrin and histamine as stimulants.

Control of gastric secretion

The stimulation of gastric secretion is usually divided into three phases (Fig. 30.5).

1. *Cephalic (neural) phase.* The sight, smell, taste and even the thought of food activates the

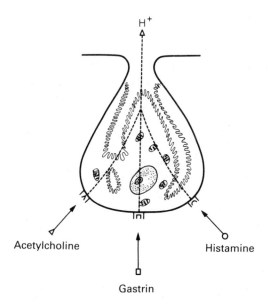

Fig. 30.4 Diagrammatic representation of the parietal cell showing receptor sites for the three major stimulants of acid secretion

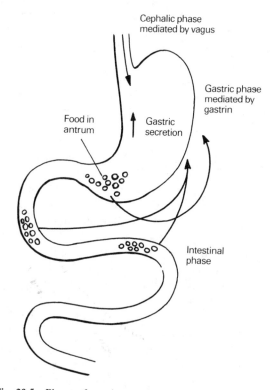

Fig. 30.5 Phases of gastric secretion

vagal centre. Impulses then pass down both vagal nerves to stimulate the parietal and peptic cells directly by releasing acetylcholine, and indirectly by releasing gastrin from the antrum. The indirect mechanism is less important than the direct one.

2. *Gastric phase*. Food in the stomach initiates acid and pepsin secretion by releasing gastrin from G-cells in the antrum. Antrectomy without vagotomy reduces the maximal acid response to histamine by 50–80%. Protein constituents are particularly effective releasers of gastrin. Luminal pH regulates the gastric phase in that gastrin secretion is reduced by antral acidification: the gastrin response to a protein meal when luminal pH is 2.5 is 80% less than that at pH 5.5. This inhibitory feedback mechanism is important in preventing inappropriate acid and pepsin secretion.

Gastric distension also stimulates gastric acid and pepsin secretion. Local intramural reflexes involving acetylcholine release are probably responsible.

3. *Intestinal phase*. This phase commences as food enters the duodenum and persists for some hours after a meal. The mechanism responsible is uncertain but may involve release of gastrin from cells in the duodenum, release of other hormones from the small intestine, or neural reflexes. Increased acid secretion follows extensive resection of the small intestine, suggesting that important inhibitory mechanisms are also triggered by food in the intestine.

PEPTIC ULCERATION

Peptic ulceration results from an imbalance between gastric secretion and the ability of the mucosa of the upper gastrointestinal tract to withstand peptic digestion. The proteolytic enzyme pepsin is responsible for mucosal digestion and ulceration; acid secretion is important only in that it provides an environment conducive to peptic activity. Pepsin enjoys optimal activity at around pH 2, is inactive when pH exceeds 4.8, and is irreversibly inactivated above pH 7.

Excessive or inappropriate acid and pepsin secretion is implicated in duodenal ulceration in that the mean maximal secretory capacity of duodenal ulcer patients exceeds that of normal subjects. However, there is considerable overlap between the groups and many individuals with duodenal ulceration have secretory capacities within or below the normal range. Hypersecretion is not of primary importance in the development of gastric ulceration. Defective mucosal defence is believed to be a major factor leading to ulceration in individuals with normal or reduced secretory capacity. However, ulceration does *not* occur in the absence of acid and pepsin secretion. At least some secretion is essential to exploit defective or damaged mucosal defences and cause ulcer formation. The role of the organism *Campylobacter pylori* in the aetiology of peptic ulceration is likely to prove important.

Peptic ulceration produces a wide spectrum of clinical disorders. For example, the ulcer may be acute or chronic, may heal spontaneously or exhibit alternating periods of remission and exacerbation. It may also give rise to complications such as bleeding, perforation or stenosis. Stress ulceration is an acute form of gastric or duodenal ulceration encountered during severe illness or injury, and will be considered separately. The incidence of peptic ulcer in this and other western countries is declining for reasons which are not understood.

Sites of peptic ulcer

Peptic ulceration may occur in the duodenum, stomach, oesophagus and jejunum, and rarely in relation to a Meckel's diverticulum as a result of ectopic acid-secreting mucosa (Fig. 30.6).

Duodenum

Ulceration of the first part of the duodenum is the commonest form of peptic ulcer. Ulceration of other parts of the duodenum is exceptional but may occur in the rare Zollinger-Ellison syndrome (see p. 465).

Stomach

Gastric ulceration is the second commonest form of peptic ulcer. Three types of gastric ulcer are described (Fig. 30.7).

Type I or primary gastric ulcers account for the

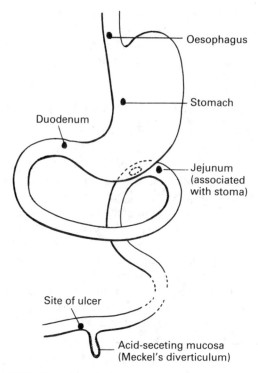

Fig. 30.6 Sites of peptic ulceration

association with duodenal ulcers and arise because of gastric stasis due to duodenal deformity.

Type III ulcers are found in the pyloric channel or immediate prepyloric area and are believed to have more in common with duodenal than gastric ulceration. Thus they are associated with normal or increased levels of gastric secretion.

Oesophagus

Oesophageal ulceration is relatively rare and is due to reflux of acid and pepsin from the stomach (see Ch. 26). These ulcers are small and superficial unless they occur on columnar mucosa, when they may be large and penetrating.

Jejunum

Jejunal ulceration is uncommon. It occurs as a form of recurrent ulceration when gastric contents have been diverted into the jejunum by gastrojejunal anastomosis, and may be a manifestation of the Zollinger-Ellison syndrome (see later).

majority and arise because of damaged mucosal defences. The ulcer is often on the lesser curve, is usually associated with gastritis, and develops at the junction between acid-secreting and non-acid secreting mucosa.

Type II or secondary gastric ulcers are found in

Symptoms of peptic ulceration

Pain

The clinical features of peptic ulceration are dominated by epigastric pain. As the stomach and duodenum, in terms of their visceral embryonic

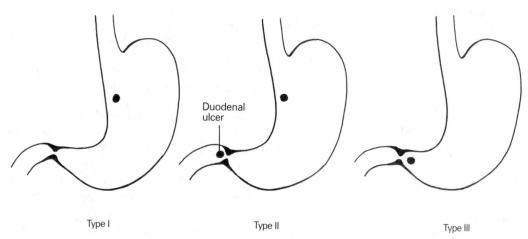

Fig. 30.7 Types of gastric ulcer

innervation, are midline structures, the pain is felt in the midline of the epigastrium and is of vague, boring and deep-seated type. The main characteristics of peptic ulcer pain are periodicity and its relationship to food.

1. *Periodicity*. 'Good spells and bad spells' are typical. Usually symptoms occur every 3–6 months and last for 7–10 days, but the time, both of the attacks and period of remission, is variable. No clear explanation has yet been given for this typical pattern.

2. *Relationship to food*. During an attack, the pain of peptic ulceration is related to food. Typically, the pain occurs when the stomach is empty and is relieved within minutes of taking food. It is truly a 'hunger pain'. If symptoms are severe, the pain wakens the patient during the night, usually around 02.00–03.00 o'clock when, as at other times, a drink of milk will rapidly abate the symptoms. Alkali has a similar effect.

Accompanying symptoms

Pain apart, peptic ulcer causes symptoms of hyperacidity with heartburn (burning pain in the midline of the lower chest), waterbrash (sudden flow of saliva) and a general feeling of upper abdominal unease. Vomiting of small quantities of fluffy secretions tinged with foodstuffs (which often relieves the pain) is typical. A feeling of fullness accompanied by inability to eat large quantities of food is a common symptom which can cause embarrassment.

'*Retention vomiting*' due to pyloric obstruction may occur after a long period of peptic ulcer symptoms, but is less common than that occurring during an acute attack as described above.

The role of surgery in peptic ulceration

Peptic ulcer patients may come under the care of the surgeon:

1. for the management of ulcer disease suspected or diagnosed by general practitioners and other hospital physicians;

2. for treatment of acute complications of peptic ulcer, namely bleeding, perforation or stenosis;

3. for treatment of long-term complications of previous ulcer surgery; and

4. for treatment of stress ulceration, which may occur as a consequence of injury, operation or severe illness.

ELECTIVE SURGICAL MANAGEMENT OF PEPTIC ULCERATION

Patients may be referred directly to the surgeon by their general practitioner or referred for surgery by a physician. Patients coming to hospital for the first time may have had little or no investigation of their symptoms, whereas those referred by a physician have usually undergone thorough investigation and a trial of medical management. Regardless of the mode of referral, the surgeon must address the following issues:

1. Is the diagnosis of peptic ulcer correct and have all necessary investigations been completed?

2. Are there sufficient indications for surgical rather than continued medical management?

Barium meal examination may have been carried out previously, but it should be borne in mind that the ulcer may not be seen in some 25% of patients.

Endoscopy is indicated in patients with 'X-ray negative dyspepsia' and is mandatory in all cases of gastric ulcer so that the ulcer can be inspected and biopsied to exclude malignancy. Endoscopy is still not carried out as a routine by some clinicians in patients with a radiologically proven duodenal ulcer. However, full endoscopy is recommended in patients being considered for surgery, not only to confirm the diagnosis, but also to detect unsuspected oesophageal lesions or secondary gastric ulceration.

Acid secretory studies are no longer performed as a routine. Most surgeons have abandoned selective surgery policies in which the type of operation performed was determined by the patient's maximal acid secretory capacity. Determination of basal acid output and maximal response to pentagastrin was once used to diagnose the Zollinger-Ellison syndrome and to exclude achlorhydria in patients thought to have benign gastric ulceration. However, gastrin radioimmunoassay has replaced secretory studies in the diagnosis of the Zollinger-Ellison syndrome, while endoscopy is now used to inspect and biopsy all gastric ulcers to exclude malignancy.

Serum gastrin levels are measured under fasting conditions and in response to secretin injection whenever the Zollinger-Ellison syndrome is suspected (see later).

Oral cholecystography or ultrasonic scanning is always advisable because of the frequency with which peptic ulcer and cholelithiasis coexist.

Indications for surgery in duodenal ulceration

Failure of medical management

Reduction of gastric secretion and ulcer healing can now be achieved in the majority of patients by the histamine H_2-receptor antagonists cimetidine or ranitidine. However, while these drugs speed ulcer healing and can sustain remission, they do not remove the underlying ulcer diathesis. Although cimetidine and ranitidine appear to be relatively safe drugs, the consequences of long-term therapy are as yet unknown, and many physicians are reluctant to prescribe more than two 6-week courses of the drug or to persist with maintenance therapy for more than 12 months. For these reasons surgery is usually recommended when these drugs fail to control ulcer symptoms (uncommon), when a patient is unwilling or unable to comply with the prescribed medical regimen (uncommon), or when symptoms recur after two full courses of the drug or after a sustained period of maintenance therapy. Even more effective histamine H_2-receptor blockers have been introduced recently, and are under clinical assessment. Omeprazole, possibly the most potent gastric secretory inhibitor, acts by ATPase inhibition, thus impairing the action of the gastric proton pump, and is also currently under clinical trial.

The severity of symptoms varies considerably from patient to patient and the duration of history alone should not necessarily influence the decision to advise surgery. Patients should no longer have to 'earn their operation' by years of discomfort and misery. Factors which favour early recourse to operation include:

onset in adolescence
a strong family history of duodenal ulceration

high levels of acid secretion
a previous complication (see below)
occupational factors
intercurrent disease

Loss of time from work is usually regarded by patient and surgeon as a factor favouring operation. In the Armed Forces, peptic ulceration leads to automatic medical downgrading with adverse effects on promotion prospects. Patients likely to spend long periods without easy access to medical care should be advised to have surgery.

Patients who require long-term anticoagulant or steroid therapy and who have an ulcer should have this treated surgically before starting therapy if this is feasible.

Development of complications

A previous history of perforation or ulcer bleeding is a strong indication for elective operation in patients with recurrent symptoms. Pyloric stenosis is an absolute indication for surgery. Patients with combined duodenal and gastric ulcers are advised to have operation because the response to medical management is usually poor.

Psychological factors

Patients with marked psychological disturbance or personality disorder pose a difficult problem in management, and some surgeons are reluctant to recommend operation. However, the prospects for ulcer healing after operation are just as good as in other patients, and this group should not be denied surgery. It is essential to make certain that the patient's symptoms are due to duodenal ulcer, and this requires endoscopic visualization of an active ulcer crater during a symptomatic period. All concerned must be made aware of the fact that surgery is unlikely to influence the underlying psychological problem, and continued collaboration with a psychiatrist may be necessary.

Indications for surgery in gastric ulceration

Patients with gastric ulceration are more likely to require operation than those with duodenal ulcer. The indications for surgery are summarized below.

Suspicion of malignancy

Approximately 10% of ulcers diagnosed as benign on barium meal examination prove to be malignant. Malignant transformation of a benign peptic ulcer is now considered unlikely, and many cases of 'malignant transformation' merely reflect failure to detect the underlying malignant nature of the ulcer. Endoscopic inspection and multiple biopsies to exclude malignancy are essential prerequisites of the medical treatment of gastric ulceration, and any course of treatment must be followed by full reassessment to reduce diagnostic error. Ulcers at sites other than the lesser curvature are regarded with particular suspicion, but vigilance cannot be relaxed when the ulcer is located on the lesser curve.

Failure of medical management

Failure of ulcer healing after a 6-week course of therapy suggests that there may be underlying malignancy and is a strong indication for surgery. *Recurrence of ulceration* is an absolute indication for operation.

Development of complications

A history of previous perforation or bleeding, or the development of fibrous contraction and an 'hour-glass stomach' are indications for operation.

Indications for surgery in endocrine adenopathies

Peptic ulceration occurs in some 15% of patients with hyperparathyroidism and may be due to hypergastrinaemia and gastric hypersecretion consequent on hypercalcaemia. In the majority of cases the peptic ulcer heals following surgical treatment of hyperparathyroidism, and direct ulcer surgery is only indicated if ulceration persists. The surgical management of the Zollinger-Ellison syndrome is discussed later in this Chapter.

Preparation for elective operation

The patient is prepared as for any elective major abdominal operation. A nasogastric tube is passed on the morning of operation to ensure that the stomach remains empty, to aid the surgeon in mobilization of the oesophagus for vagotomy, and to prevent postoperative gastric distension.

The patient is warned to expect a hospital stay of about 7–10 days and should remain off work for about 6 weeks.

Principles of surgery

The aim of surgery is to reduce acid and pepsin secretion to levels no longer associated with peptic ulceration. The ideal operation should achieve this consistently and safely with an acceptably low incidence of postoperative side effects. A number of operations are available for the surgical cure of gastric and duodenal ulcer but no one operation is ideal and different surgeons may vary in their choice of procedure.

Choice of operations for duodenal ulcer

Truncal vagotomy and drainage

Division of the anterior and posterior vagal trunks just beneath the oesophageal hiatus reduces acid and pepsin secretion at the expense of impaired receptive relaxation and diminished antral motility. These undesired effects led to significant stasis in approximately half of the patients subjected to truncal vagotomy alone, and for this reason truncal vagotomy is now combined routinely with a procedure to facilitate gastric drainage and prevent stasis. The drainage procedure may consist of pyloroplasty or gastroenterostomy (Fig. 30.8). Gastroenterostomy is preferred if there is marked duodenal inflammation or scarring, but otherwise there is little to choose between the two procedures.

Truncal vagotomy and drainage is safe in that the operative mortality is below 1%, but approximately 10% of patients develop recurrent ulceration (see below). Failure to define and divide all vagal trunks is usually responsible. The integrity of the vagus can be tested by the induction of insulin hypoglycaemia, which with intact vagi stimulates a brisk secretory response. Postoperative insulin tests show that vagotomy is incomplete in 30–40% of patients. The insulin test

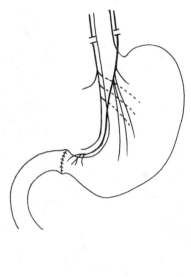

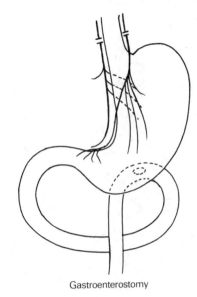

Pyloroplasty

Gastroenterostomy

Fig. 30.8 Truncal vagotomy and drainage

is often unpleasant for the patient, is potentially dangerous, and is no longer performed routinely.

In addition to gastric denervation, truncal vagotomy denervates the other abdominal organs supplied by the vagus. Diarrhoea may follow vagotomy and drainage, although it poses a serious problem in only about 3% of patients. At one time, diarrhoea was considered to be a consequence of the vagotomy but it may well be due to the drainage procedure and uncontrolled gastric emptying. The *dumping syndrome* may also be a consequence of uncontrolled gastric emptying. Bilious vomiting is a common side effect of truncal vagotomy and drainage and results from regurgitation of bile through the pyloroplasty or gastroenterostomy.

Despite these shortcomings, its relative safety and ease of performance have made truncal vagotomy and drainage the most commonly performed duodenal ulcer operation in this country.

Selective vagotomy and drainage

This operation was introduced to avoid vagal denervation of abdominal organs other than the stomach in the hope that the incidence of side effects would be lower than that after truncal vagotomy. Only the gastric branches of the vagus were divided (Fig. 30.9) and it was hoped that the more detailed dissection would ensure complete gastric vagotomy and a reduced incidence of recurrent ulceration. These hopes have not been realized and this operation is now seldom performed.

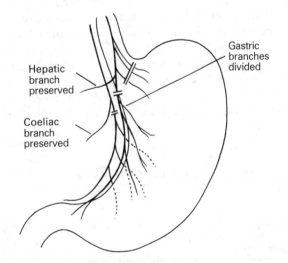

Hepatic branch preserved

Coeliac branch preserved

Gastric branches divided

Fig. 30.9 Selective vagotomy

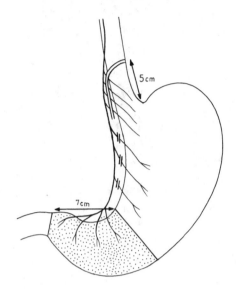

Fig. 30.10   Highly selective vagotomy

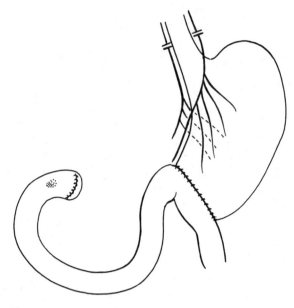

Fig. 30.11   Truncal vagotomy and antrectomy (Billroth II)

Highly selective vagotomy (proximal gastric vagotomy)

This operation has been used over the past two decades and has increased in popularity. Only those vagal fibres innervating the body of stomach are divided, while those supplying the antrum and other abdominal organs are spared (Fig. 30.10). Acid and pepsin secretion are reduced to about the same extent as after truncal vagotomy, but the antrum and pylorus remain innervated so that there is no need to carry out a drainage procedure. The operation is safe, the incidence of side effects such as diarrhoea, bilious vomiting and dumping is minimal, and the rate of recurrent ulceration is little greater than that after truncal vagotomy and drainage (Table 30.1). The operation is now considered by many surgeons to be the procedure of choice.

Truncal vagotomy and antrectomy

As vagal denervation is combined with removal of the major gastrin-producing area, this operation has a recurrent ulcer rate of only 1%. It is associated with a greater operative mortality than truncal vagotomy and drainage, or highly selective vagotomy. The incidence of other side effects is similar to that of truncal vagotomy and drainage (see Table 30.1).

Intestinal continuity after antrectomy is restored by gastroduodenal (Billroth I) or gastrojejunal (Billroth II) anastomosis (Fig. 30.11).

Partial gastrectomy

Partial gastrectomy was once the standard operation for duodenal ulcer but has been largely

Table 30.1   Results of surgery for duodenal ulcer

	Highly selective vagotomy	Truncal vagotomy + drainage	Truncal vagotomy + antrectomy	Partial gastrectomy
Operative mortality	0.3%	0.6–0.8%	1.0–1.5%	2%
Satisfactory long-term results*	86%	75%	85%	75%
Recurrent ulceration	10%	10%	1%	3%

*Visick grades I and II. The Visick grading system has four categories: I and II are often combined as 'satisfactory', while III and IV are 'unsatisfactory'.

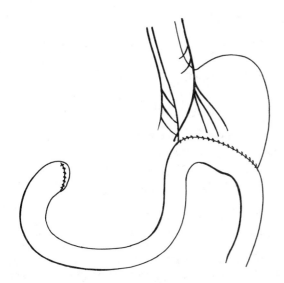

Fig. 30.12 Partial gastrectomy for duodenal ulcer (Polya or Billroth II)

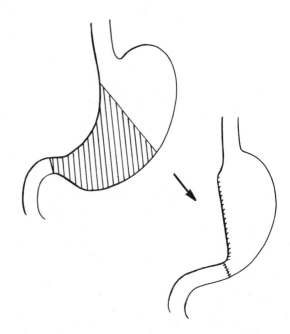

Fig. 30.13 Partial gastrectomy for gastric ulcer (Billroth I)

superseded by the various operations involving vagotomy. The operation consists of removing the antrum plus a proportion of the body of the stomach, leaving only one-quarter to one-third of the stomach intact. Intestinal continuity is restored by gastrojejunal anastomosis, the so-called Billroth II procedure; the commonest variation of this procedure is that described by Polya (Fig. 30.12). The more extensive the resection, the lower the risk of recurrent ulceration. The surgeon has to balance the desire to avoid recurrence against the undesirable consequences of a small gastric remnant (see below). Partial gastrectomy carries an overall operative mortality of approximately 2%. Leakage from the duodenal stump after Billroth II procedures is the commonest cause of death. The results of the different operations for duodenal ulcer are summarized in Table 30.1.

Choice of operations for gastric ulcer

Type I gastric ulcer (see Fig. 30.7)

The choice rests between Billroth I partial gastrectomy (Fig. 30.13) and truncal vagotomy with drainage. Partial gastrectomy reduces acid and pepsin secretion by removing about 60% of the stomach, including the ulcer. The results of the operation are usually excellent. Operative mor-

tality is about 2% and recurrent ulceration is rare (Table 30.2). As the ulcer is removed for complete histological examination, there is no risk of leaving a malignant ulcer in situ.

Truncal vagotomy and drainage is a less certain method of reducing acid and pepsin secretion, and recurrent ulceration is a problem in some 10% of patients (see Table 30.2). The operation carries a lower operative mortality than partial gastrectomy but there is a real risk that a malignant ulcer may be missed and left in situ. If truncal vagotomy and drainage is used, the stomach must be opened and the ulcer subjected to multiple biopsy or excision.

Most surgeons now favour partial gastrectomy for gastric ulceration because of the possibility of

Table 30.2 Results of surgery for gastric ulcer

	Truncal vagotomy + drainage	Partial gastrectomy
Operative mortality	1.5%	2%
Satisfactory long-term results*	70%	75%
Recurrent ulceration	10%	3%
Risk of retained cancer	Not known	None

*Visick grades I and II.

malignancy. Truncal vagotomy and drainage is usually reserved for poor-risk patients or those in whom the ulcer is situated so high on the lesser curvature that gastric resection would be extensive or difficult and incur serious risk of complications.

Highly selective vagotomy is not recommended for gastric ulceration.

Type II gastric ulcer

This type of gastric ulcer is secondary to duodenal ulceration and the surgeon carries out the operation he favours for duodenal ulcer. If the gastric ulcer is to be left in situ, adequate biopsy is advised. However, it is exceptional for gastric cancer to coexist with duodenal ulceration.

Type III gastric ulcer

From the point of view of surgical management, pyloric channel and prepyloric ulcers are regarded as variants of duodenal ulcer and are treated accordingly.

Postoperative care

Patients are liable to the complications of any abdominal operation but the postoperative course is usually smooth. The nasogastric tube is normally removed by the second postoperative day and drinking allowed. By the time of discharge (about 1 week after operation) the patient should be eating the normal hospital diet. He is advised initially to eat small meals at frequent intervals, rather than attempt two or three large meals in the course of a day.

'Ulcer diets' are not necessary after operation. No restrictions are placed on food content. However, the patient should be warned to avoid fruits such as oranges with a strong pith. The pith may pass undigested through a wide or incontinent gastric outlet and occlude the small intestine, causing a 'bolus' obstruction.

Complications of surgery

The following complications may arise in the immediate postoperative period.

Chest infection

This is common because the upper abdominal incision restricts lung expansion and coughing, and many ulcer patients are cigarette smokers.

Suture line haemorrhage

This occurs during the first 24 hours and is recognized by bright red blood in the nasogastric aspirate. It usually ceases spontaneously, but transfusion may be needed. Reoperation is rarely required.

Stomal hold-up

Stomal hold-up with obstruction of the gastric outlet is suspected if the patient continues to have large volumes of nasogastric aspirate. An X-ray examination with Gastrografin will confirm stomal obstruction. Oedema is the usual cause, and hypoproteinaemia and electrolyte upsets may contribute. Mechanical factors such as malposition of the stoma, kinks or adhesions are occasionally responsible.

Hypoproteinaemia and electrolyte imbalance are corrected, nasogastric aspiration is maintained, and parenteral nutrition is instituted. The majority of patients settle with these conservative measures, but hold-up persisting beyond 10–14 days usually requires reoperation and refashioning of the stoma.

Anastomotic leakage

This is most likely to occur at the suture line of the duodenal stump following Billroth II partial gastrectomy (Fig. 30.14). Oedema or kinking at the gastrojejunal anastomosis causes an increase in pressure in the afferent loop which compromises duodenal blood supply and impairs healing of the duodenal suture line. Duodenal stump 'blow-out' becomes evident on the 4th or 5th day after operation. The patient looks and feels unwell, experiences pain in the right hypochondrium, has a fever and discharges bile-stained fluid through the wound or drain track. Local adhesions usually prevent generalized peritonitis, but subphrenic or subhepatic abscess formation is common and a persistent fistula forms. Duodenal fistula can

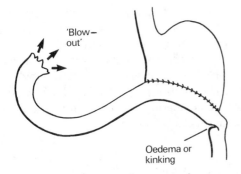

'Blow—out'

Oedema or kinking

Fig. 30.14 Duodenal leakage following Billroth II partial gastrectomy

rapidly lead to fluid and electrolyte imbalance, wasting, and excoriation of the skin around the fistula. Urgent treatment is therefore required.

1. *Ensure that external drainage is adequate* and that duodenal content is not accumulating within the abdomen. Reoperation may be needed to place a large drain down to or into the leaking duodenum. Repair of the fistula is usually not feasible at this stage.

2. *Maintain fluid and electrolyte balance* by recording daily fluid and electrolyte intake and loss, and replacing any deficit via an intravenous infusion line. The volume of loss from the fistula varies greatly but may exceed 3 litres a day.

3. *Prevent excoriation of the skin* around the fistula site by the proteolytic enzymes in pancreatic juice. The skin is protected by applying a leak-proof adhesive (Stomahesive) pad and attaching a colostomy bag to collect the fistula fluid. Alternatively, a sump suction drain may be placed in the fistula track or the patient can be nursed in the prone position.

4. *Maintain nutritional intake.* Oral intake may be continued when the output from the fistula is small, and this may be supplemented by an elemental diet. If the volume of output increases, food residue appears in the discharging fluid or the patient is progressively losing weight and deteriorating, parenteral nutrition is necessary.

5. *Ensure that there is no distal hold-up* preventing healing of the duodenum.

In the majority of patients, the fistula will heal on conservative management within 2 weeks.

Failure to heal suggests persisting afferent loop obstruction, and contrast radiology followed by reoperation may be required.

TREATMENT OF COMPLICATIONS OF PEPTIC ULCERATION

Haemorrhage

Bleeding occurs in about 20% of ulcer patients, and peptic ulcer is the commonest cause of acute upper gastrointestinal blood loss. Its investigation and management are discussed in more detail later in this Chapter.

Perforation

Clinical features

Perforation of a duodenal ulcer is ten times more common than perforation of a gastric ulcer. No age group is immune but the peak incidence is in the fourth and fifth decades of life.

Perforation can occur without significant preceding dyspepsia and may be stress-related. On the other hand, the patient may have had a long dyspeptic history with previous episodes of bleeding or perforation.

Treatment is influenced by whether the ulcer is 'acute' or 'chronic'. For practical purposes, a duodenal ulcer is regarded as chronic when the history exceeds 3 months. A gastric ulcer which perforates is regarded as chronic.

Clinically, perforation of a peptic ulcer usually presents as an acute abdominal catastrophe with sudden severe epigastric pain which rapidly becomes generalized throughout the abdomen. The precise time of onset is clearly recalled. Retching may have occurred at the onset of pain but vomiting is rare.

The patient lies still, being afraid to move for fear of exacerbating the pain. Abdominal tenderness, guarding and board-like abdominal rigidity are characteristic and denote peritonitis. In some patients the full clinical picture does not develop because the perforation is sealed rapidly by omentum, so that the signs remain localized. In others, fluid leaking from the perforation down the right

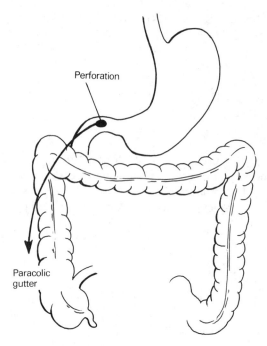

Fig. 30.15 Perforated duodenal ulcer showing leakage down the paracolic gutter

paracolic gutter (Fig. 30.15) produces clinical findings resembling those of acute appendicitis.

Leaking gastric and duodenal fluid is irritant and causes a chemical peritonitis with marked exudation of fluid. This dilutes the leaking fluid so that abdominal pain and other signs often become less after some hours. The peritoneal fluid is initially sterile but secondary bacterial invasion occurs within 6 hours. Bacterial peritonitis follows.

The overall mortality of perforated peptic ulcer is about 10%. This increases with delay in diagnosis and management. Mortality is greatest in the elderly and those ill from intercurrent disease.

Diagnosis

The clinical diagnosis is confirmed in approximately two-thirds of patients by the presence of air beneath the diaphragm on a chest X-ray or erect abdominal films. Lateral decubitus films may also reveal free peritoneal gas and are of particular value in shocked or debilitated patients. Absence of peritoneal gas does not rule out a perforation. If the diagnosis is in doubt, e.g. when the perfor-

ation is into the lesser sac or rapidly seals and air is not seen on a plain X-ray, an emergency Gastrografin meal should be ordered.

Acute pancreatitis should always be considered in the differential diagnosis of a perforated ulcer. The serum amylase concentration should be determined, remembering that moderate elevation may occur in a perforation.

Initial management

A nasogastric tube is passed as soon as the diagnosis is suspected. Emptying the stomach prevents further peritoneal contamination and may relieve pain. Adequate analgesia should be provided, haematology, urea and electrolyte concentrations checked, the patient's blood group determined, and an intravenous infusion of crystalloid solution commenced. If the patient is seriously shocked on presentation, this must be corrected before operation.

Contraindications to surgical management

Perforated peptic ulcer is managed by operation unless:

1. the patient is extremely ill on admission, there having been a long delay between perforation and diagnosis, with the development of bacterial peritonitis;

2. the perforation has sealed, as indicated by an absence of generalized abdominal signs and confirmed by Gastrografin examination; or

3. facilities for surgical treatment are not available.

The patient should then be managed conservatively by regular nasogastric aspiration, intravenous fluid therapy, antisecretory drugs, and broad spectrum antibiotic cover if there are signs of peritonitis. Conservative management was once a popular alternative to operation and gave comparable results in terms of mortality. However, there was a higher incidence of subphrenic or local abscess after conservative management, and occasionally a more serious cause of peritonitis, e.g. strangulated bowel, was wrongly treated. Operation is now preferred.

Operative management of perforated duodenal ulcer

Simple closure. The abdomen is opened through a short right paramedian or midline incision. All foreign material is aspirated from the peritoneal cavity, the peritoneum is lavaged with saline, and the perforation is closed by three absorbable sutures incorporating a tag of omentum (Fig. 30.16). The abdomen is then closed without drainage.

Following simple closure of an *acute ulcer*, one-third of patients have no further dyspepsia, one-third experience mild symptoms easily controlled medically, and one-third eventually require definitive ulcer operation.

Vagotomy and pyloroplasty. Simple closure of a *chronic* ulcer is most likely to be followed by recurrent dyspepsia requiring later definitive surgery. It is therefore better to carry out definitive surgery at the emergency laparotomy. Truncal vagotomy and pyloroplasty is then the procedure of choice. The perforation is excised or incorporated into the pyloroplasty. If gross scarring or duodenal friability makes pyloroplasty difficult, a gastrojejunostomy is performed after closure of the perforation.

Emergency definitive surgery is not advised (1) in poor-risk patients with severe intercurrent disease; (2) when the perforation is more than 12 hours old and bacterial contamination is likely to be heavy; and (3) when an experienced surgeon or anaesthetist is not available. Age by itself is not a contraindication. Given correct patient selection and appropriate surgical expertise, the mortality of an emergency vagotomy and pyloroplasty should be no greater than that of simple closure.

Operative treatment of perforated gastric ulcer

Perforated peptic gastric ulcers are usually chronic and definitive surgery is preferred to simple closure. Approximately 15% of perforated gastric ulcers are malignant and, provided an experienced team is available, Billroth I gastrectomy is the procedure of choice. Excision of the ulcer with truncal vagotomy and pyloroplasty is a satisfactory alternative in those cases where the position of the ulcer makes gastrectomy difficult.

Simple closure after adequate biopsy of the ulcer is justifiable in poor-risk patients, but careful follow-up for ulcer recurrence is mandatory.

Pyloric stenosis

The stenosis is usually located in the first part of the duodenum rather than at the pylorus, but the term pyloric stenosis is time-honoured. Obstruction results from oedema during an acute exacerbation of ulceration, from fibrous scarring during repair, or from a combination of the two. Muscle spasm may play a role in some patients, notably those in whom the ulcer is located within the pyloric channel. Pyloric stenosis is less common than ulcer bleeding or perforation.

A rare form of pyloric stenosis due to hypertrophy of the pyloric musculature which is unassociated with peptic ulceration also occurs in adults. This is similar to the congenital pyloric stenosis in infants, and may be a mild and chronic form of that disease.

Clinical features

The symptoms of pyloric stenosis are insidious and consist of upper abdominal distension following meals, eructations and bad breath. Intermittent bouts of diarrhoea may occur. The character of the peptic ulcer pain may change, initially becoming continuous and intractable and later less intense or even disappearing. Vomiting occurs late, and classically is of retention type. Every few days the

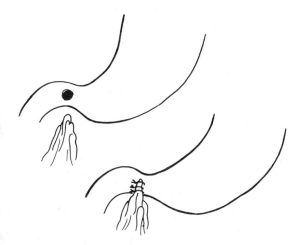

Fig. 30.16 Closure of duodenal perforation

patient vomits copious quantities of gastric juice containing partially digested food which he recognizes having eaten some hours or days before. The site of the obstruction is reflected by the fact that the vomitus never contains bile.

On examination the classical clinical feature is that of gastric distension. The stomach may be visibly enlarged, and gentle side-to-side shaking of the patient elicits a succussion splash. In long-standing stenosis from duodenal ulceration visible peristalsis is not a feature. A plain abdominal X-ray may show a large fluid-filled stomach. This is confirmed by a barium meal, which will show a grossly distended stomach, hypertrophied mucosa and mixing of barium and retained foodstuffs giving a frothy or thumb-print appearance.

Pyloric obstruction may also be caused by conditions other than chronic duodenal ulcer, e.g. a distal carcinoma. The cause of the obstruction is not always obvious on barium studies or on endoscopy and definition of the cause may have to await laparotomy.

Biochemical changes

The initial biochemical changes in long-standing pyloric stenosis are due to starvation. Sodium is retained by the kidney, and water and salt balance is preserved. However, the obligatory excretion of potassium leads to hypokalaemia. Intracellular potassium is lost and replaced by sodium and hydrogen ions so that there is an intracellular acidosis and extracellular alkalosis.

With vomiting there is loss of acid gastric juice, this leading to intensification of the alkalosis and hypokalaemia and loss of salt and water. The patient becomes severely dehydrated. Chloride ions are also lost and replaced by bicarbonate. The urine is alkaline.

As stores of potassium become progressively exhausted the kidney excretes hydrogen rather than potassium ions and paradoxical aciduria may occur. This is a sign of severe biochemical upset.

It should be noted that if the obstruction is due to a carcinoma, there is likely to be hypochlorhydria of the gastric juice so that the disturbance of acid-base balance is less severe.

Reduced intake of protein leads to hypoproteinaemia. As this is a hazard to healing after surgery the plasma proteins must always be estimated preoperatively.

Treatment

The treatment of pyloric stenosis is surgical relief of the obstruction. This is not an emergency procedure and several days of preparation for the operation are usual. Dehydration, electrolyte and acid-base balance are corrected by intravenous infusion of saline and potassium chloride monitored by urine volume, serum levels of electrolytes and blood gas estimations. Anaemia occurs in about one-quarter of patients with pyloric stenosis and should be rectified.

A large-bore (32Fr) nasogastric tube is passed to empty the stomach of food residue and allow lavage. Once the aspirate is clear, the tube can be replaced by one of smaller diameter which is kept in place until operation. Regular aspiration avoids gastric retention and allows the gastric muscle to regain tone.

Operation is usually undertaken after some 4–5 days of intravenous therapy and aspiration. Truncal vagotomy and gastrojejunostomy is the procedure of choice. In the rare case of a pyloric carcinoma this should be resected.

Nasogastric intubation is continued for some days after the operation to avoid gastric retention and encourage the gastric muscle to regain tone. However, in cases with long-standing and chronic retention, gastric dilatation may persist.

Recently, an alternative to operation has been introduced. The patient is endoscoped and if possible a balloon catheter is passed through the stenotic area. The balloon is then inflated to dilate the area of stenosis. The technique is similar to that of balloon angioplasty (see Ch. 21) but its long-term effectiveness is not yet known.

LONG-TERM COMPLICATIONS OF PEPTIC ULCER SURGERY

Recurrent ulceration

Gastric ulcer. Recurrence of gastric ulcer after gastrectomy is uncommon (see Table 30.2) and may require further resection. Recurrence of a gastric ulcer after truncal vagotomy and drainage is treated by partial gastrectomy.

Duodenal ulcer. The incidence and site of recurrent ulceration after surgery for duodenal ulcer is influenced by the type of operation used (see Table 30.1). After a pyloroplasty or gastroduodenal anastomosis, recurrent duodenal ulceration may occur, whereas following a gastrojejunal anastomosis the ulcer is on the jejunal side of the anastomosis. The ulcer recurs because the initial operation failed to reduce acid and pepsin secretion sufficiently. Recurrent ulcer is associated with renewal of ulcer symptoms but the periodicity of the pain may be atypical. The diagnosis is confirmed by endoscopy. Barium studies may be difficult to interpret because of the previous surgery.

Reoperation is advisable, the aim being to ensure that acid and pepsin secretion are reduced further. Patients with recurrence after vagotomy and drainage or highly selective vagotomy are treated by attempting to complete the vagotomy in association with antrectomy. Recurrence after partial gastrectomy is best dealt with by the addition of a truncal vagotomy. Recurrence after truncal vagotomy and antrectomy is rare and is treated by searching for and dividing any remaining intact vagal fibres and more extensive gastric resection. Although rare, the Zollinger-Ellison syndrome may present as recurrent ulceration. A fasting gastrin level should be measured routinely to exclude this possibility.

Long-term therapy with histamine H_2 antagonists may be used in patients unfit for, or unwilling to undergo, further surgery.

Ulcers on the anastomotic site may be associated with the use of non-absorbable sutures at the initial operation. The levels of acid and pepsin secretion are not high. On endoscopy a suture is seen in the base of the ulcer, removal of which results in healing. Some now recommend that only absorbable sutures are used in gastric anastomoses.

In addition to causing renewed pain and dyspepsia, recurrent ulcers may be complicated by bleeding, perforation or the development of a gastro-jejuno-colic fistula (Fig. 30.17). Bleeding and perforation occur more frequently than with primary ulcers, but fistula formation is relatively rare. This usually arises after gastrojejunal anastomosis, particularly when the anastomosis has been retrocolic. The communication between

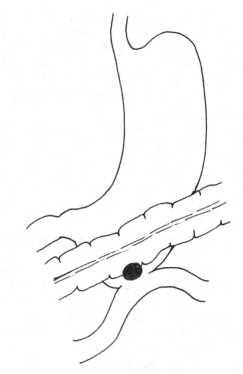

Fig. 30.17 Gastro-jejuno-colic fistula

stomach and large bowel allows colonization of the stomach and small bowel by faecal organisms which produces severe diarrhoea and malabsorption and leads to rapid weight loss. Only small amounts of food pass directly from stomach to colon so that the diagnosis is confirmed most readily by barium enema.

Should a fistula form, early operation after bowel preparation is indicated. The fistula is disconnected, the colon repaired, and an appropriate recurrent ulcer operation is carried out. These aims are usually achieved at one operation, but preliminary transverse colostomy may be required to divert the faecal stream, relieve symptoms and allow nutritional status to improve in poor-risk patients.

Bilious vomiting

Occasional bilious vomiting occurs in about 30% of patients after gastric surgery. In a small proportion the vomiting is frequent and persistent due to bile reflux into the stomach causing severe gastritis. Bile lying in an empty stomach overnight gives rise to a complaint of morning nausea. Vomiting is often precipitated by eating a cooked breakfast. Many patients with bilious vomiting are heavy smokers and/or drinkers. If so, abstinence or moderation is the single most effective measure in its management.

In a few patients, bilious vomiting is the result of afferent loop obstruction after a gastrojejunal anastomosis. Pressure building up in the loop causes colicky upper abdominal pain; when the obstruction is overcome, bile and pancreatic juice are discharged rapidly into the stomach and vomited.

Persistent troublesome bilious vomiting may respond to antacid or cimetidine therapy, which reduces the amount of acid available to exploit the damaged gastric mucosal defences. Metoclopramide improves gastric emptying. If such medical management fails to relieve symptoms, an operation to divert bile from the stomach using a Roux-en-Y anastomosis (Fig. 30.18) is indicated. The Roux loop should be at least 45 cm long to prevent bile refluxing into the stomach.

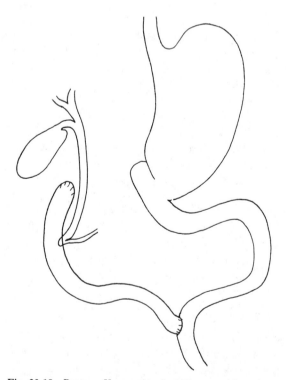

Fig. 30.18 Roux-en-Y operation for bilious vomiting

Following gastrectomy for ulcer, there may be a small increase in the incidence of gastric carcinoma in which chronic biliary gastritis has been implicated. Highly selective vagotomy is not associated with increased biliary reflux and may not increase the risk of carcinoma in this group.

Food vomiting

Vomiting of food may be due to fibrosis and narrowing of the stoma or to faulty siting of a gastroenterostomy. A diagnosis of stomal malfunction can be confirmed radiologically or endoscopically. Revisional surgery is required.

Occasional patients develop gastric hypotonia despite an adequate anastomosis. Food vomiting may be relieved by metoclopramide, an antiemetic which coordinates and improves gastric emptying.

Dumping

The dumping syndrome consists of uncomfortable epigastric fullness after food associated with flushing and sweating, marked lassitude, increased peristalsis with borborygmi, and sometimes diarrhoea. These symptoms commence within 10–15 minutes of eating and usually settle within 30–60 minutes. The patient frequently has to lie down until symptoms pass.

Epigastric fullness after eating an average-sized meal occurs in about 40% of patients after gastric surgery. Impaired receptive relaxation is believed to be responsible. This symptom alone does not constitute dumping. It usually improves spontaneously in a few months and can be avoided by taking small meals without fluids.

The dumping syndrome proper is due to rapid emptying of hyperosmolar solutions, particularly of carbohydrates, into the small bowel (Fig. 30.19). It can be induced by jejunal instillation of hypertonic glucose and is believed to be due to the osmotic attraction of large amounts of fluid into the lumen of the small bowel. There is transcellular flux of potassium and other ions and extracellular fluid volume is reduced. Distension of the jejunum creates a sensation of fullness and stimulates peristalsis. Release of 5-hydroxytryptamine and bradykinin may also be implicated.

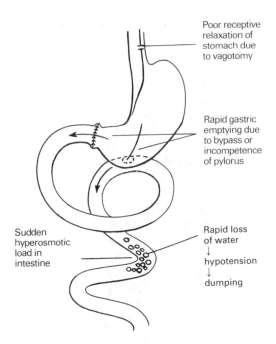

Poor receptive relaxation of stomach due to vagotomy

Rapid gastric emptying due to bypass or incompetence of pylorus

Sudden hyperosmotic load in intestine

Rapid loss of water
↓
hypotension
↓
dumping

Fig. 30.19 Dumping syndrome

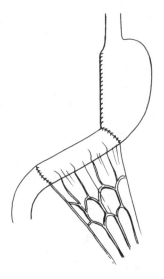

Fig. 30.20 Jejunal interposition to relieve symptoms of dumping

The symptoms of dumping may be ameliorated by reducing the size of meals (which are taken more frequently), reducing carbohydrate consumption, and avoiding liquids during meals. Otherwise the medical treatment of dumping has proved unsatisfactory. If troublesome symptoms persist after dietary modification, operation may be required. If the previous operation has been a truncal vagotomy with drainage, reconstruction of the pylorus (in pyloroplasty patients) or taking down of a gastrojejunostomy should be undertaken. If the previous operation has been a gastrectomy, conversion of a gastrojejunal to a gastroduodenal anastomosis may help; if the gastric remnant is small, interposition of a segment of jejunum between stomach and duodenum should be considered (Fig. 30.20). It is advisable to wait for at least one year after the primary operation, as (1) symptoms often improve spontaneously and (2) the long-term results of surgery for dumping are disappointing.

Reactive hypoglycaemia

Reactive hypoglycaemia was once erroneously known as 'late dumping', but this term is no longer used. Rapid absorption of glucose from the upper small bowel produces hyperglycaemia and causes excessive insulin secretion with subsequent reactive hypoglycaemia. Tremor, tachycardia, palpitation and sweating develop about 90–120 minutes after a meal and are potentiated by exercise. Approximately 5–10% of patients experience this symptom at some time after surgery, but in the great majority such hypoglycaemia is mild, transient and easily avoided.

Patients are advised to reduce carbohydrate consumption and to carry glucose sweets to take if symptoms arise. Revisional surgery is rarely required.

Diarrhoea

Diarrhoea may occur after any type of gastric operation but is now most common after truncal vagotomy and drainage. Mild transient diarrhoea occurs in over 20% of patients and severe diarrhoea in 3–4%. When severe, the diarrhoea is episodic and unpredictable. It is associated with great urgency and may result in incontinence, disrupting the patient's professional and social life. Steatorrhoea and malabsorption are rare.

The cause is not certain but loss of gastric continence is now considered to be a major factor. In some patients specific foods are incriminated, and their avoidance 'cures' the problem.

Patients with dumping are given appropriate advice (see above). Symptomatic treatment of diarrhoea with kaolin, codeine phosphate or diphenoxylate with atropine (Lomotil) often helps. If diarrhoea is severe and does not respond to treatment, operation may be advised, the aim being to restore gastric continence either by refashioning the pylorus or taking down a gastrojejunostomy or, if necessary, performing a jejunal transposition to enlarge a small gastric remnant. In some patients, conversion of a gastrojejunal to a gastroduodenal anastomosis improves the symptoms.

Malabsorption

Failure to gain weight is a constant complication of extensive gastric resection. The degree of weight loss is proportional to the extent of resection and in the majority is due to inadequate intake. Fear of precipitating dumping may be responsible. Dietary advice may be all that is required.

True malabsorption with steatorrhoea and weight loss is relatively rare. It may be caused by lactose intolerance, the blind loop syndrome or a gastro-jejuno-colic fistula.

The blind loop syndrome is encountered occasionally after Billroth II gastrectomy or gastrojejunostomy with vagotomy. The diagnosis is confirmed by the demonstration of high jejunal bacterial counts and a good response to antibiotics. Conversion of the gastrojejunal to a gastroduodenal anastomosis, or replacement of a gastrojejunostomy with a pyloroplasty can give permanent relief.

Anaemia

Iron deficiency anaemia is common after all forms of peptic ulcer surgery. It is particularly prevalent after gastrectomy. Premenopausal women, because of menstrual blood loss, are particularly susceptible to this complication. The common causes are:

1. patients leaving hospital with a degree of anaemia due to operative or preoperative blood loss;

2. reduced acid secretory capacity with less efficient absorption of dietary iron; and

3. chronic blood loss from gastritis.

Any patient who is anaemic at the time of hospital discharge should have a 3-month course of oral iron. Haemoglobin levels should be monitored thereafter. All premenopausal women requiring gastric surgery are advised to take prophylactic iron during one month in three.

Anaemia due to vitamin B_{12} deficiency is relatively uncommon after gastric surgery in those without steatorrhoea. It is seen most frequently after gastric resection but can occasionally follow truncal vagotomy and drainage and may complicate gastritis. Parenteral vitamin B_{12} administration is required for life.

Calcium malabsorption

This may develop in association with steatorrhoea, but can also occur 10–15 years after operation in some patients without steatorrhoea. Partial gastrectomy enhances calcium malabsorption and postmenopausal women who frequently lack calcium are particularly prone to develop osteomalacia. For this reason, partial gastrectomy is avoided if possible in female patients.

Tuberculosis

Patients with a history of tuberculosis are prone to relapse following gastric resection and must be carefully followed up.

STRESS ULCERATION

Acute superficial ulcers may develop in the stomach or duodenum after operation, injury or severe illness. The ulcers are frequently multiple, are usually small, and are sometimes described as erosions. The cause of stress ulceration is not clear but reduced mucosal resistance is probably important. Resistance is impaired during periods of ischaemia with reduced gastric mucosal blood flow, by bile reflux, by exposure to drugs such as aspirin or other non-steroidal anti-inflammatory drugs, and by increased output or administration of glucocorticoids.

Ulceration of the duodenum in patients with severe burns (Curling's ulcer) or of the stomach and duodenum after neurosurgical illness or operation (Cushing's ulcer) are specific forms of stress ulceration. Cushing's ulcers are unusual in that gastric secretion is increased, possibly because of increased vagal activity associated with increased intracranial pressure.

All forms of stress ulceration can cause bleeding which may be life-threatening. Except in Cushing's and Curling's ulcers, perforation is uncommon because of the superficial nature of the lesions. Suppression of gastric secretion by cimetidine or continuous administration of alkali in high dosage is of value in prevention and treatment of stress lesions, and surgery should be avoided if at all possible.

If bleeding fails to respond to medical management, operation usually consists of vagotomy and drainage with direct suture of larger erosions. Vagotomy reduces gastric secretion and favours the opening of arteriovenous shunts which divert blood from the engorged mucosa. The management of bleeding is discussed in detail later in this chapter.

ZOLLINGER-ELLISON SYNDROME (GASTRINOMA)

The Zollinger-Ellison syndrome is a rare entity in which autonomous secretion of gastrin leads to gastric hypersecretion and a fulminant form of peptic ulceration (Fig. 30.21). The tumour (gastrinoma) usually arises from gastrin-secreting cells (G cells) in the islets of the pancreas but may also arise in the stomach or duodenum. About two-thirds of gastrinomas are malignant and more than three-quarters of patients have multiple tumours.

Men are more commonly affected than women (in a ratio of 3:2) with a peak incidence between 20 and 50 years of age.

G-cell hyperplasia is a very rare condition in which hypergastrinaemia is due to hyperplasia of G cells in the antrum, and not to tumour formation.

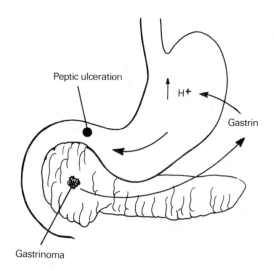

Fig. 30.21 Zollinger-Ellison syndrome

Clinical features

The classical presentation is one of severe fulminating ulcer dyspepsia refractory to routine forms of therapy. Many patients first have only mild dyspepsia which is slowly progressive. Bleeding (33%), perforation (25%) and pyloric obstruction (10%) are common. Ulceration often occurs at more than one site in the stomach, duodenum or proximal jejunum.

One-third of patients have diarrhoea. This is usually due to underlying steatorrhoea caused by destruction of lipase by the high luminal acid content of the small bowel, and should be distinguished from the watery diarrhoea of the WDHA syndrome (watery diarrhoea, hypokalaemia and achlorhydria; see Ch. 37). Diarrhoea may be the first symptom of a gastrinoma.

One-quarter of gastrinoma patients have other endocrine abnormalities. Parathyroid adenomas commonly coexist and in some patients there is multiple endocrine neoplasia (see Ch. 23).

Diagnosis

A high index of suspicion is essential if the diagnosis is to be established or even entertained before or at the time of primary operation. This should be prompted by:

1. chronic duodenal ulceration associated with gastric hypersecretion and a ratio of basal to maximal acid output which exceeds 0.6:1;

2. duodenal ulceration occurring in childhood or youth;

3. stomal ulceration developing rapidly after surgery for duodenal ulcer, particularly when a gastrectomy or truncal vagotomy and antrectomy has been performed;

4. peptic ulceration involving unusual sites such as the distal duodenum or jejunum;

5. peptic ulceration associated with unexplained diarrhoea; and

6. associated endocrine abnormalities such as hyperparathyroidism.

Gastric secretory studies are no longer the mainstay of diagnosis. Emphasis now is placed on radioimmunoassay of gastrin in the circulating blood. The normal range for fasting serum gastrin levels in most laboratories is below 150 ng/l. All gastrin values above this level are viewed with suspicion. The higher the fasting gastrin, the more likely the diagnosis of gastrinoma, and levels in excess of 500 ng/l are strongly suggestive. Provocation tests may be employed for confirmation. A rapid intravenous bolus injection of secretin causes a marked rise of serum gastrin in gastrinoma patients.

Selective angiography may help to localize the tumour and detect hepatic metastases. Selective venous sampling using a catheter passed through the liver into the splenic vein is also useful for detecting high local venous gastrin levels and so localizing tumour deposits.

Before accepting the diagnosis of a gastrinoma, other causes of hypergastrinaemia must be excluded. These are: pernicious anaemia, achlorhydria or hypochlorhydria due to gastritis, gastric outlet obstruction, short bowel syndrome, and renal insufficiency.

Management

The availability of the histamine H_2-receptor antagonist cimetidine (and more recently other antisecretory drugs) has offered a feasible alternative to surgery in many patients. Although doses of the order of 2400 mg/day may be required, gastric hypersecretion can usually be controlled.

Ideally an attempt should then be made to resect the tumour and so remove the cause of the hypergastrinaemia. However, this is frequently thwarted by the fact that the majority of tumours are multiple and/or malignant.

If the acid hypersecretion cannot be controlled by drugs, total gastrectomy is likely to prove necessary. Following this operation 60% of patients survive 5 years and 40% for 10 years, the pancreatic tumour remaining stable or rarely even regressing. Cytotoxic therapy may be of some value for the treatment of recurrent malignant disease.

GASTRIC NEOPLASMS

BENIGN GASTRIC NEOPLASMS

Benign tumours of the stomach may arise from epithelial or mesenchymal tissue. Adenomatous polyps are the commonest neoplasm to arise from epithelium and may be single or multiple. The risk of malignant transformation increases with polyp size and when there are multiple polyps.

Leiomyoma is the commonest benign mesenchymal tumour. Neurogenic tumours, fibromas and lipomas are rare.

Benign tumours are frequently discovered as an incidental finding on barium meal examination, but may give rise to bleeding or intermittent pyloric obstruction with vomiting. Intussusception through the pylorus is exceptionally rare.

The benign nature of the polyp is confirmed by endoscopy with biopsy. Some pedunculated polyps can be removed endoscopically using a diathermy snare, but operative removal is indicated for large polyps in view of the risk of malignant transformation. Multiple polyps are treated by gastric resection, and total gastrectomy is required on rare occasions for diffuse gastric involvement.

MALIGNANT GASTRIC NEOPLASMS

Cancer of the stomach

The stomach is the second commonest site for cancer of the gastrointestinal tract. In the UK, each year 50–60 persons per 100 000 are affected by the disease, which accounts for 10% of cancer deaths. Present-day methods of treatment have done little to alter its appalling mortality, with less than 10% of all patients surviving for 5 years.

Cancer of the stomach is curable by surgery only if it is confined to the stomach wall. Such favourable cases are relatively uncommon and generally detected only through the screening of normal persons. By the time most patients experience symptoms related to the disease it has already spread through and beyond their stomach, and cure by local treatment is no longer possible, although considerable palliation of symptoms may be achieved.

In an attempt to reduce the high mortality of gastric cancer, air contrast barium studies and endoscopy are being used to screen asymptomatic persons. This allows detection of lesions which are confined to the mucosa and which, following gastrectomy, have a high likelihood of cure. Recent survival figures from Japan, where screening is widely practised, suggest that 95% of such patients live for 5 years or more.

In Britain, routine screening for gastric cancer is limited to individuals at high risk, e.g. those with atrophic gastritis or pernicious anaemia, in whom annual contrast barium studies or endoscopy should be arranged.

Aetiological factors

There are marked geographical differences in the incidence of gastric cancer. In Japan, Iceland, South America and Eastern Europe it is much more common than in the UK or North America. There may also be differences in incidence within a country. In England and Wales the line between the Severn and the Wash divides the country into northern high incidence and southern low incidence areas.

It is believed that these differences are due to environmental factors, a view supported by the striking reduction in incidence in the United States during the past 40 years. A similar trend has occurred in Britain, in which the peak incidence for the disease occurred in the decade 1930–1940.

Cancer of the stomach is twice as common in males as in females and most common in unskilled social groups. Its incidence increases with age (mean age 56 years), although 1 in 15 cases still occur in patients under 40 years of age.

Certain occupations increase the risk of gastric cancer. For example, miners, and rubber and asbestos workers are prone to develop the disease.

Family history is relevant. Blood relatives of patients with the disease are at increased risk. Those of blood group A are more prone to develop gastric cancer than other blood-group types.

The incidence of gastric cancer is increased by three to four times in patients with pernicious anaemia or other atrophic states affecting the gastric mucosa. Hypochlorhydria, by altering the distribution of bacteria in the gastrointestinal tract, is believed to be one factor. Intestinal metaplasia of the gastric mucosa is another. Adenomatous gastric polyps, particularly when multiple, are prone to become malignant; recent evidence suggests that the incidence may be as high as 20%.

A benign gastric ulcer occasionally undergoes malignant change, but in general the relationship between benign and malignant ulceration is not strong. Gastrectomy for peptic ulcer may increase the risk of gastric cancer, believed again to be associated with reduction in acid secretion. The incidence of gastric cancer in patients treated by antisecretory drugs is under review.

The main factors which lead to the development of gastric cancer are believed to be dietary in origin. For example, an association between human cancer of the stomach and a high intake of nitrate salts has been described. On reduction to nitrites by bacterial action, N-nitrosation of amino compounds occurs in the stomach to form N-nitroso compounds (nitrosamines) which are known to be carcinogenic. Bacteria also catalyse the N-nitrosation of secondary amine groups, a factor of particular importance in the achlorhydric stomach.

Pathology

Cancers of the stomach are adenocarcinomas derived from mucus-secreting cells of gastric glands. They can occur in any part of the stomach but are most common in the pyloric antrum and on the lesser curvature. They are classified as (1) ulcerating; (2) proliferating (encephaloid or polypoidal); and (3) infiltrating, depending on the degree of penetration of the gastric wall and growth into the lumen. Combinations of these types occur. Diffuse infiltration of the whole of the stomach accompanied by a fibrous reaction causes the so-called leather-bottle stomach (linitis plastica).

The common modes of spread are:

1. direct extension to neighbouring organs (e.g. liver, pancreas, colon);

2. transcoelomic spread within the peritoneal cavity to form seedling deposits on peritoneal and omental surfaces, on the ovaries (Krukenberg tumour) and in the rectovesical pouch (forming a so-called rectal 'shelf');

3. lymphatic spread to regional lymph nodes in the perigastric tissues, along the splenic and hepatic vessels, and in the porta hepatis (occasionally the disease spreads along the course of the thoracic duct to involve the left supraclavicular nodes and form a hard mass in the neck); and

4. blood-borne spread via the portal vein to the liver and occasionally to the lungs and other sites.

As with cancers elsewhere, lymph node involvement is a bad prognostic sign. When a tumour is confined to the gastric wall, 5-year survival after resection approximates 45%. Involvement of local lymph nodes reduces this figure to under 20%.

An international system of clinical and pathological staging using TNM (tumour, nodes, metastases) categories is described but is not commonly used in this country. A system of classification has also evolved for those early gastric cancers discovered in asymptomatic patients by double contrast (air and barium) studies or endoscopic examination.

Clinical features

The classical symptoms of gastric cancer (anorexia, vomiting, anaemia, eructations, ill-health and loss of weight) are those of late disease.

Early symptoms are referable to the gastrointestinal tract and are similar to those caused by a variety of minor digestive ailments. Epigastric pain, vague indigestion or fullness are typical. A history of recurrent dyspepsia or relief by alkali does not rule out the diagnosis of cancer.

Frank haemorrhage from a gastric cancer is rare. Slow oozing of blood from its surface is common and causes anaemia with lassitude, pallor and breathlessness. Anaemia should never be treated without investigation for chronic blood loss.

Rarely, the initial symptoms of a gastric cancer can be acute with pyloric stenosis, perforation or severe haemorrhage. In some cases, the first symptom may be caused by metastatic deposits, e.g. in the liver, supraclavicular nodes or peritoneal cavity.

Diagnosis

Those with symptoms of early disease do not usually have clinical signs. In such patients the faeces must be tested for occult blood.

By the time most patients are referred to hospital, loss of weight is obvious. An epigastric mass may be found on abdominal examination. The liver, supraclavicular nodes and pelvic floor must be carefully examined for metastatic disease. A full blood examination is requested and a barium meal arranged. Double contrast studies are now routine in patients in whom gastric cancer is suspected.

In an established tumour, ulceration, a filling defect and rigidity of the stomach wall are typical features of the disease. In linitis plastica, the stomach is contracted to a narrow rigid tube which empties rapidly into the duodenum.

Early lesions form a mucosal 'plaque', a small superficial ulcer or disrupted mucosal folds. These appearances are detected only by double contrast techniques or endoscopy.

Differentiation of a malignant from a benign gastric ulcer on radiological grounds can prove difficult. Irregularity of the base, interruption and rigidity of the mucosal folds, and a crater which does not penetrate beyond the confines of the stomach are signs suggesting cancer. Ulcers on sites not usually affected by peptic ulceration, e.g. greater curve, are also suspicious.

All patients with X-ray findings suggesting the possibility of cancer of the stomach should be gastroscoped and the lesion biopsied. It is also advisable to gastroscope all patients over middle age with recent dyspepsia and a negative barium examination. Smears of surface cells for cytological examination may be made by brushing the gastric mucosa through the endoscope. Gastric secretion studies and blind cytology (e.g. by gastric lavage) are no longer used for diagnosis.

Differential diagnosis. A carcinoma of the stomach must be differentiated from other infiltrating lesions. Of particular importance is non-Hodgkins lymphoma which may cause a large apparently inoperable tumour which, nevertheless, is amenable to therapy. Giant hypertrophy of the gastric mucosa may be associated with clinical and radiological features similar to those of cancer. In all cases gastroscopy should be performed.

The differentiation between a benign and malignant gastric ulcer is now made primarily on histological grounds.

Treatment

The primary treatment of gastric cancer is surgical. Unless there is gross clinical evidence of metastatic disease or general illness severe enough to contraindicate surgery, the abdomen should be explored.

The first duty of the surgeon is to confirm the diagnosis. This is usually obvious but a small lesion may be difficult to palpate through the gastric wall. Opening the stomach (gastrotomy) and palpation within the lumen is advocated but is no substitute for precise preoperative definition of the lesion by endoscopic biopsy.

Next, the surgeon should determine the extent of the disease. Peritoneal seedlings of tumour, ascites and gross liver metastases indicate that this is incurable and that operative procedures will not help. Small liver metastases and extensive lymph node invasion are also signs of incurable disease, but if the patient has obstructive symptoms, surgical removal of the tumour may be worthwhile. In this situation, some surgeons perform a simple bypass procedure (gastroenterostomy), but the palliation achieved is poor. Histological examination (if not previously done) is mandatory even in apparently inoperable cases since, if the diagnosis proves to be that of lymphoma, radiotherapy and/or chemotherapy can give excellent remission of disease.

In the absence of obvious spread to other sites, a gastric resection should be performed unless the cancer is so fixed to surrounding structures that it is irremovable.

The operation. The standard operation for cancer of the distal stomach is a partial gastrectomy removing the distal three-quarters of the stomach and the first 2–3 cm of the duodenum. As regional lymph nodes should be included with the specimen, blood vessels are ligated and divided at their origins and the omentum is removed with the stomach. A gastrojejunal (Polya) reconstruction is usual.

For cancers of the body of stomach, or the cardia, a total gastrectomy will be required including removal of the lower 2–3 cm of the oesophagus. In some cases this is combined with resection of the spleen and the distal end of the pancreas. Reconstruction is by the anastomosis of a loop of proximal jejunum to the oesophagus usually by the Roux-en-Y technique. The length of ascending limb should exceed 45 cm to prevent alkaline oesophagitis. Total gastrectomy is best performed through a thoracoabdominal approach, extending the abdominal incision over the costal margin, opening the chest and dividing the diaphragm down to the oesophageal hiatus.

Adjuvant therapy. Radiotherapy has little place in the management of adenocarcinoma of the stomach. Combination chemotherapy may achieve remissions in some patients with advanced disease, and adjuvant chemotherapy at the time of primary surgery is under study. In advanced cases simple palliative measures usually suffice.

Gastric lymphoma

Lymphomas account for 2% of all malignant gastric tumours. The presenting symptoms and signs resemble those of gastric carcinoma but are often mild relative to the size of the neoplasm. The tumour may be misdiagnosed radiologically as gastric cancer, and endoscopy with biopsy is essential.

Radical subtotal gastrectomy followed by radiotherapy results in a 5-year survival rate approaching 50% if lymphoma is localized, and tumour size should not be taken as a contraindication to surgery. If local extension prohibits resection, radiotherapy often gives worthwhile palliation, while diffuse disease may respond to chemotherapy.

Gastric leiomyosarcoma

These tumours account for less than 1% of malignant gastric neoplasms. The lesion may protrude into the gastric lumen, remain within the gastric wall, or even bulge into the peritoneal cavity. The luminal surface frequently ulcerates due to central necrosis, and bleeding is common.

The tumour grows slowly and metastasizes late. The 5-year survival rate is around 50% after partial gastrectomy. The tumours are not radio-sensitive so that prognosis is poor if the lesion cannot be resected.

UPPER GASTROINTESTINAL HAEMORRHAGE

Bleeding from the upper gastrointestinal tract is common. If mild and chronic, it may go unnoticed for many months until the development of anaemia raises the suspicion of chronic blood loss. If severe, it can cause acute hypovolaemia and shock requiring urgent treatment in hospital. The blood may be vomited (haematemesis), when it may be bright red and fluid, have a coffee-ground appearance, or contain clots. If it passes down the gastrointestinal tract and is excreted in altered form in the faeces (melaena), it is black and treacly.

Causes

Peptic ulceration of the stomach or duodenum, or gastritis with erosions are responsible for the majority of massive upper gastrointestinal bleeds. Oesophageal varices complicating portal hyper-tension, and Mallory-Weiss tears at the gastro-oesophageal junction account for most of the remainder. A rare cause of acute bleeding is a chronic gastric ulcer complicating a para-oesophageal hernia. Sliding hiatus hernia with erosive oesophagitis may cause chronic bleeding but not acute haemorrhage.

Clinical assessment

History

A history of peptic ulceration, of liver disease or of previous operations may prove helpful in sug-gesting a likely source of bleeding. A recent story of severe vomiting may indicate the likelihood of mucosal tears in the region of the cardia (Mallory-Weiss syndrome). Previous upper gastrointestinal

barium studies may have shown a chronic peptic ulcer or duodenal scarring and should be enquired after.

Ingestion of non-steroidal anti-inflammatory compounds (e.g. aspirin or indomethacin), steroids or anticoagulants predisposes to gastrointestinal haemorrhage, and specific enquiry regarding such drugs must be made. Recent or chronic alcohol abuse is also important. However, the history is not always helpful and may even be misleading. No less than 40% of patients with known upper gastrointestinal disease will prove to have bled from another cause or from a different site.

Clinical examination

A thorough clinical examination is mandatory. Particular attention is paid to detecting any signs of chronic liver disease (liver palms, spider naevi, jaundice) and/or portal hypertension (palpable spleen, ascites, distended collaterals). It is also im-portant to seek evidence of such rare conditions as hereditary telangiectasia.

An important part of the initial clinical assess-ment is to determine the likely amount of blood loss. This is frequently underestimated so that blood replacement is often too little, too late and too slow.

Pallor, tachycardia, hypotension or anaemia in-dicate a loss of at least 1 litre and the need for transfusion.

Principles of management

There are three vital steps in the care of a patient with massive gastrointestinal haemorrhage.

1. Early replacement of blood loss so that ex-sanguination is prevented and hypovolaemia promptly corrected.

2. Detection of the nature and site of the bleed-ing lesion.

3. Control of the bleeding point.

It is important to appreciate that all patients with an acute upper gastrointestinal bleed, even if apparently minor, should be referred urgently to hospital for investigation and treatment. Any minor bleed may become major within a few hours, causing severe hypovolaemia and shock.

Ideally, all patients should be admitted to the care of a haematemesis team which includes a surgeon. Otherwise, delay in reaching a diagnosis or failure to appreciate a serious risk of exsanguinating haemorrhage and the need for surgery may compromise survival. Unlike bleeding from an external site, severe bleeding into the gastrointestinal tract is not directly visible. The sense of urgency is much less.

Initial manoeuvres

The aim of immediate treatment is to restore the circulation and provide a reserve against continued or recurrent bleeding. An intravenous line is immediately established and 1 litre of crystalloid solution (saline or Ringer lactate) is infused while the patient's blood is grouped and cross-matched. Urea, electrolyte and haemoglobin concentrations and packed cell volume (haematocrit) are measured. A platelet count and prothrombin ratio should be requested on the first blood sample. Arterial Po_2, Pco_2 and hydrogen ion concentrations are determined if the patient is severely shocked.

Pulse and blood pressure are monitored and, if the patient is consistently hypotensive, a central venous line and urinary catheter are inserted. A large nasogastric tube is introduced and intermittent suction is instituted. This helps to prevent aspiration of gastric contents and may detect fresh bleeding. As the stomach may contain blood clot, it is important to maintain patency of the tube by repeated irrigation with saline.

Replacement of blood volume

As soon as it is available, whole blood is infused through a free-flowing line. Pulse rate, central venous pressure and arterial blood pressure must be adequate, as judged by monitoring of volume and rate. If the patient is elderly, has cardiac failure or chronic respiratory disease, monitoring of pulmonary wedge pressure by a Swan-Ganz catheter may prevent pulmonary overload. If massive blood replacement is required, the blood must be warmed adequately and citrate acidaemia avoided by monitoring blood gases and pH and administering bicarbonate if necessary.

Impaired haemostasis is to be expected in patients needing massive transfusion and in those with deranged liver function. The administration of stored blood quickly results in deficiencies of labile factors V and VIII, but these defects can be restored by fresh frozen plasma (FFP), using one pack for every 3 litres of blood transfused. Clotting screens to determine thrombin time, prothrombin time, kaolin-cephalin coagulation time and platelet count are of value in patients with massive bleeding. Vitamin K_1 (5–50 mg intravenously) is given routinely to all patients who are jaundiced or when the prothrombin time is prolonged. FFP is needed in patients with liver disease unresponsive to vitamin K.

Urine output is monitored and maintained at more than 50 ml/hour by restoration of circulating blood volume.

It should again be stressed that all patients admitted to hospital with major upper gastrointestinal bleeding should be seen by a surgeon shortly after admission. This enables a balanced decision to be taken regarding further management and allows optimal timing of surgery if operation is required to control haemorrhage.

Detection of nature and site of the bleeding lesion

As soon as the blood volume has been restored, an attempt should be made to detect the site of bleeding, even if the patient appears to have settled completely. Patients rarely die from their initial bleed but the death rate from recurrent haemorrhage is significant and the opportunity to determine the source of bleeding must not be lost. As indicated above, a history of chronic peptic ulceration or radiological demonstration of a long-standing lesion, e.g. duodenal scarring, is not always helpful in defining the cause of bleeding. At one time a barium meal was used as the standard investigation for acute haemorrhage, but most clinicians now believe that the place of barium studies lies in detecting chronic gastrointestinal disease and not a site of acute bleeding. As barium in the gastrointestinal tract compromises both endoscopy and arteriography, it is now no longer used as the initial investigation in acute gastrointestinal haemorrhage.

Endoscopy is now preferred as the first investigation. With an end-viewing instrument the bleeding site is detected in 80–90% of cases. Even if the actual site of bleeding is not identified, oesophageal varices, gastric ulcer and gastric erosions are readily ruled out.

Arteriography detects bleeding into the gastrointestinal tract when this exceeds 1–2 ml/min. It is not used as a primary investigation but is indicated when the site of bleeding has not been identified on endoscopy and recurrent or continued bleeding demands surgical intervention. Should the arteriogram demonstrate the bleeding vessel, embolization may be successful and avoid operation.

Control of bleeding

The majority of patients admitted with massive upper gastrointestinal haemorrhage stop bleeding spontaneously. In this case, the patient gradually and steadily improves, and within 24–48 hours is able to take a light diet. Although H_2 antagonists have not proved helpful in the control of acute haemorrhage from an ulcer, patients with peptic ulceration should be prescribed full therapeutic doses so that their ulcers heal.

If the continued need for blood replacement (more than 5 units) indicates continuous bleeding, or if there is overt recurrent bleeding, surgery may be required to control haemorrhage. Patients with chronic peptic ulceration are more likely to continue to bleed than those with erosive gastritis, and patients past middle age are also more prone to further haemorrhage. The elderly are at particular risk in that they are least able to contend with the physical demands of repeated or recurrent major haemorrhage. Certain endoscopic appearances also denote an increased risk of further bleeding from peptic ulcer. These include a visible artery in the ulcer base and adherent fresh clot or black slough.

Management of specific lesions

Erosive gastritis

If endoscopy reveals that bleeding is due to gastritis or erosions, intensive antacid and/or antisecretory therapy is instituted. If bleeding persists, the erosion can be coagulated endoscopically using a laser or diathermy. On rare occasions bleeding persists and surgery is required. There is some debate about what constitutes the best surgical procedure but truncal vagotomy is an essential part because of its effect on the gastric blood flow. It may be combined with partial gastrectomy or a drainage procedure.

Peptic ulceration

If conservative measures fail to arrest haemorrhage, surgery is required. On opening the abdomen, the presence of a chronic ulcer is first sought by inspection and palpation of the entire stomach and proximal duodenum. If no lesion is detected, a gastrotomy is performed, incising the front wall of the stomach longitudinally midway between the greater and lesser curvature. Clot is evacuated and the gastric mucosa palpated and inspected. If no lesion is found, the incision is closed and a longitudinal incision made through the pylorus so that the proximal duodenum can be inspected (pylorotomy).

A bleeding duodenal ulcer is treated by underrunning the bleeding vessel with non-absorbable sutures. The pylorotomy is sutured transversely as a pyloroplasty and the operation is completed by truncal vagotomy.

A chronic gastric ulcer is best treated by gastric resection with a gastroduodenal (Billroth I) anastomosis. If the gastric ulcer is located high on the lesser curvature, it may be preferable to underrun it with non-absorbable sutures and then perform a vagotomy and pyloroplasty. In this event an adequate biopsy (with frozen section examination if possible) must be taken. Excision of the ulcer is the best form of biopsy but this is not always possible.

In all cases in which a peptic ulcer remains in situ, the patient must be carefully observed during the postoperative period for possible recurrence of haemorrhage. In this event further surgery may be required, usually with partial gastrectomy.

Trials with endoscopic coagulation (by laser, heat or sclerotherapy) of bleeding peptic ulcer suggest that this mode of therapy may prove to be a useful alternative to emergency surgery.

Oesophageal varices

These are discussed in detail in the context of portal hypertension (see Ch. 36).

Carcinoma of the stomach

This is a rare cause of acute gastrointestinal haemorrhage. If severe and exsanguinating, an emergency operation may be required. Gastrectomy is the only feasible method of controlling the haemorrhage.

Anastomotic ulcer

Massive haemorrhage from an anastomotic ulcer may require surgery. Primary control of the haemorrhage may be achieved by direct suture but it may be necessary also to modify the stoma, depending on the extent of local deformity and the nature of the previous operation. If definitive surgery is required, vagotomy (if not previously performed) combined with antrectomy is ideal.

Haemorrhage from an anastomotic ulcer following gastrectomy demands vagotomy with consideration of further resection.

In all cases of anastomotic ulcer the possibility of the Zollinger-Ellison syndrome should be remembered. The pancreas should be palpated at operation, and any suspicious lymph nodes biopsied. Serum gastrin levels should be determined in the postoperative periods.

MISCELLANEOUS DISORDERS OF THE STOMACH

Gastric diverticula

These are rare but may be mistaken radiologically for ulceration or neoplasia. Endoscopy resolves the diagnosis.

Bezoars

A bezoar is a concretion formed in the stomach or intestine (Fig. 30.22). Trichobezoars consist of hair and are seen in young girls or demented patients who chew and swallow their hair. Phytobezoars are less common and consist of ag-

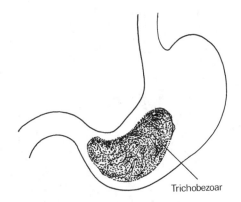

Fig. 30.22 Bezoar

gregations of vegetable material such as orange pith, fruit skin and seeds. Patients after gastric surgery are particularly at risk due to reduced levels of gastric secretion and gastric motor activity. Rare forms of bezoar include semi-solid bezoars of *Candida albicans* and shellac bezoars in painters or furniture makers.

All bezoars may attain large size before causing symptoms due to obstruction, gastritis and bleeding. The diagnosis is made by barium meal examination and surgical removal is advisable.

Swallowed foreign bodies

Accidental or deliberate ingestion of foreign bodies is common. The majority are radio-opaque and their progress can be followed radiologically. Most foreign bodies will pass through the alimentary tract without incident but operation is indicated if the object is deemed too large to leave the stomach, if signs of peritonitis develop, or if obstruction occurs.

Gastric volvulus

Volvulus is usually a sequel to development of a para-oesophageal hiatus hernia (see Ch. 26) or eventration of the diaphragm, the stomach rotating upwards around its longitudinal axis (Fig. 30.23). The patient develops localized epigastric pain, severe nausea but inability to vomit, and epigastric distension. It proves impossible to pass a nasogastric tube into the stomach, and the diag-

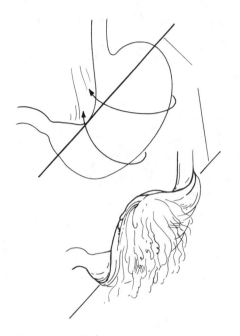

Fig. 30.23   Gastric volvulus

nosis is confirmed by plain films of chest and abdomen followed by a Gastrografin meal.

Immediate laparotomy is advisable to avoid gastric necrosis with perforation and haemorrhage. The volvulus is reduced and the oesophageal hiatus in the diaphragm is repaired. Resection is indicated if the stomach has undergone necrosis.

MISCELLANEOUS DISORDERS OF THE DUODENUM

Duodenal obstruction

Pyloric stenosis (see p. 459) is the commonest cause of duodenal obstruction. Neoplastic obstruction due to carcinoma of the pancreas (see Ch. 37) or mesenteric lymph nodes is relatively uncommon. Rare causes of duodenal obstruction include duodenal diverticula, duodenal atresia, annular pancreas and chronic duodenal ileus (Fig. 30.24).

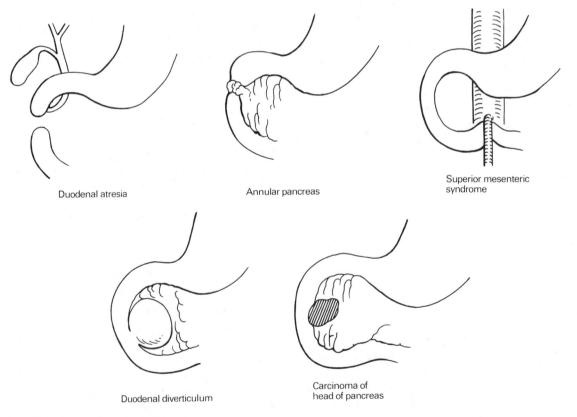

Duodenal atresia

Annular pancreas

Superior mesenteric syndrome

Duodenal diverticulum

Carcinoma of head of pancreas

Fig. 30.24   Causes of duodenal obstruction

Symptomatic diverticula are excised, while obstruction due to atresia or annular pancreas is usually bypassed by duodenojejunal or gastrojejunal anastomosis. Chronic duodenal ileus denotes recurrent duodenal obstruction in the absence of an anatomical or pathological cause, and often affects visceroptotic females in the fourth and fifth decade or rapidly growing thin children around puberty. Epigastric and right hypochondrial pain are accompanied by vomiting, and adoption of the knee-elbow position sometimes brings relief. The explanation for the condition is not known but some believe that the superior mesenteric vessels may cause obstruction as they cross the third part of the duodenum (see Fig. 30.24). Bypass using duodenojejunal anastomosis is indicated if ileus persists. In children the condition is usually self-limiting.

Duodenal diverticula

The duodenum is the second commonest site for diverticula formation in the gastrointestinal tract. They are rare before the age of 40 years, usually affect the second part of the duodenum, and are often adjacent to the entry of the common bile duct. They are usually discovered as an incidental finding on barium meal examination, but can cause obstruction and bleeding or become inflamed (diverticulitis). Symptomatic diverticula are excised.

Duodenal trauma

Duodenal injury usually follows severe crushing trauma, which also tends to affect the pancreas. Rupture of the duodenum is often retroperitoneal and its detection and treatment are discussed in more detail in Chapter 14.

31. The small intestine

Functional anatomy

The small bowel extends from the pylorus to the ileocaecal valve. Disorders of the duodenum are discussed elsewhere (see Ch. 30). The remainder of this chapter is devoted to the 500 cm of small intestine distal to the ligament of Treitz. The upper two-fifths of this section of the intestine constitute the jejunum, the lower three-fifths the ileum; there is no clear demarcation between them.

The jejunum and ileum are completely invested by peritoneum, with the exception of the narrow strip between the layers of the mesentery. The intestinal wall consists of an outer layer of longitudinal muscle, an inner layer of circular muscle, a strong fibroelastic submucosa, and the mucosa.

The mucosa consists of a single layer of columnar cells interspersed with mucous cells, Paneth cells and APUD cells. The columnar cells are renewed constantly by proliferation of cells in the crypts of Lieberkühn which take some 4–7 days to migrate to the tips of the villi.

The root of the small bowel mesentery extends from the left side of the body of L2 to the right sacroiliac joint.

The mesentery contains fat, blood vessels, lymphatics, lymph nodes and nerves. The superior mesenteric artery supplies the jejunum and ileum by a series of straight arteries which originate from arterial arcades in the mesentery. These vessels enter the mesenteric border of the gut. The antimesenteric border has a less profuse arterial supply and is more susceptible to ischaemia. Venous blood from the jejunum and ileum drains to the superior mesenteric vein and from there to the portal vein.

Lymphoid aggregates in the submucosa (Peyer's patches) are more numerous in the ileum than the jejunum. Lymph from the small intestine drains to regional nodes in the root of the mesentery before passing to the cisterna chyli. The mesentery contains both parasympathetic and sympathetic nerve fibres, but intestinal pain is mediated only by sensory afferents which follow the course of the sympathetic nerves.

Function of the small intestine

While the principal function of the small intestine is absorption, it also has important secretory and digestive functions which supplement those of the stomach, duodenum, liver and pancreas. The total area for absorption is 200–500 m^2. To achieve this absorptive area, the mucosa is thrown into circular mucosal folds (plicae semilunares) and surface villi (Fig. 31.1). In addition, microvilli form finger-like projections on the surface of the epithelial cells.

Ingested fluid and the secretions of the salivary glands, stomach, pancreas, liver and intestine present the jejunum with some 5–8 litres of fluid each day. In normal circumstances only 1–2 litres pass on into the colon (Fig. 31.2).

DIVERTICULA OF THE SMALL INTESTINE

Meckel's diverticulum

Meckel's diverticulum is the commonest congenital abnormality of the gastrointestinal tract and results from persistence of the intestinal end of the vitello-intestinal duct (Fig. 31.3). The diverticulum arises from the antimesenteric border of

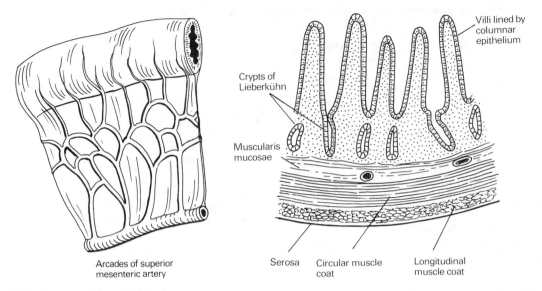

Villi lined by
columnar
epithelium

Crypts of
Lieberkühn

Muscularis
mucosae

Serosa   Circular muscle   Longitudinal
coat   muscle coat

Arcades of superior
mesenteric artery

Fig. 31.1   Anatomy of the small intestine

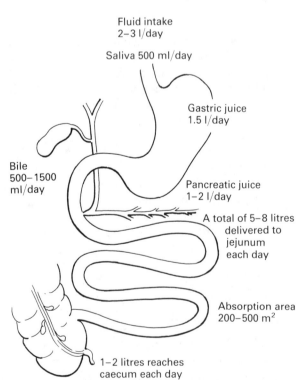

Fluid intake
2–3 l/day

Saliva 500 ml/day

Gastric juice
1.5 l/day

Bile
500–1500
ml/day

Pancreatic juice
1–2 l/day

A total of 5–8 litres
delivered to
jejunum
each day

Absorption area
200–500 m²

1–2 litres reaches
caecum each day

Fig. 31.2   Fluid shift in the small intestine

the ileum some 60–70 cm from the ileocaecal valve, is 5 cm long (range 1–12 cm), and is present in about 2% of all people. As it contains all layers of the bowel wall, it is a true diverticulum. The tip of the diverticulum is usually free, but in 10% of cases it is connected to the umbilicus by a fibrous cord representing the remaining portion of the vitello-intestinal duct. Heterotopic tissue is found in 50% of symptomatic diverticula. Most often this is gastric mucosa containing parietal (acid-secreting) cells. Other heterotopic tissues include pancreatic, colonic and duodenal mucosa.

Clinical features

Only 5% of Meckel's diverticula cause symptoms. The patients are usually infants, children or young adults. *Bleeding* from a Meckel's diverticulum is the commonest cause of severe gastrointestinal bleeding in childhood. This is due to acid secretions from heterotopic gastric mucosa causing 'peptic ulceration' in the nearby ileum.

Intestinal obstruction may be caused by intussusception of the diverticulum, volvulus around a band extending to the umbilicus, or a loop of bowel becoming trapped beneath such a band to form a 'closed loop'. Strangulation usually follows before operation can be performed.

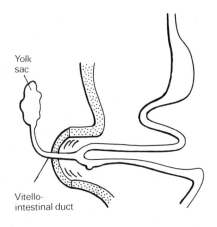
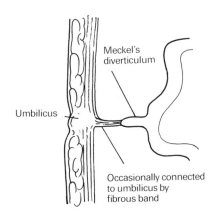

Fig. 31.3 Persistence of the vitello-intestinal duct giving rise to Meckel's diverticulum

Acute diverticulitis may give rise to abdominal pain and tenderness, pyrexia and leucocytosis. This cannot usually be distinguished clinically from acute appendicitis. Perforation is a common complication.

Management

Symptomatic Meckel's diverticula should be excised (Fig. 31.4). Asymptomatic diverticula discovered as an incidental finding at laparotomy for unrelated disease need not be excised unless they have a narrow neck and are therefore liable to obstruction or if nodularity indicates that abnormal mucosa is present. In patients with gastrointestinal haemorrhage from a Meckel's diverticulum it is unusual to demonstrate the diverticulum by barium studies. However, heterotopic gastric mucosa within a diverticulum may be detected by scintiscanning following injection of ^{99m}Tc-labelled sodium pertechnetate, which is concentrated in parietal cells.

Acquired diverticula

False diverticula of the jejunum and (less often) ileum may develop with advancing age. The diverticula are usually multiple wide-mouthed sacs caused by herniation of mucosa between the layers of the mesentery at the sites of vessel penetration of the gut wall (Fig. 31.5), and this position may make them difficult to recognize at laparotomy.

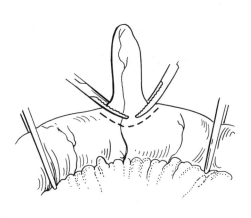

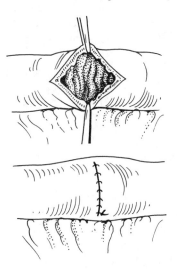

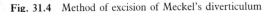

Fig. 31.4 Method of excision of Meckel's diverticulum

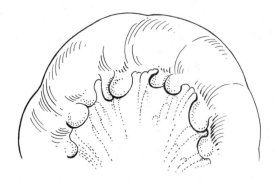

Fig. 31.5 Jejunal diverticulosis

The diverticula may cause bleeding, diverticulitis or, if extensive, malabsorption due to accumulation of intestinal organisms within them. Occasionally they perforate. They can be demonstrated by barium studies. If symptoms develop, the affected segment of bowel should be excised.

CROHN'S DISEASE

Crohn's disease was first described in 1932 by Crohn and his colleagues at the Mount Sinai Hospital, New York, as a disease which affected the terminal ileum, hence the alternative name of 'regional ileitis'. With the recognition that the jejunum could also be affected, the disease became known as 'regional enteritis'. When it was realized that it could also affect the colon as a distinct entity (as opposed to ulcerative colitis), it became clear that any part of the gastrointestinal tract could be involved. The name of the disease then reverted to Crohn's disease.

Crohn's disease is rare (less than one new case per 100 000 per year), but appears to be increasing in incidence in the UK. Its cause is unknown.

Pathological features

The diagnosis of Crohn's disease rests on recognition of its characteristic features on gross and microscopic examination. These include a 'cobblestone' appearance of the mucosa due to intercommunicating crevices or fissures surrounding islands of mucous membrane, which become raised through underlying inflammation and oedema. Serpiginous ulceration may also occur. Fibrosis leads to the formation of strictures which may be single or multiple, short or long.

Multiple lesions within the intestinal tract are common and are classically discontinuous, with intervening segments of normal bowel ('skip' lesions). Because of the penetrating nature of the disease process, the serosa may be inflamed or studded with small tubercle-like lesions. Sinus or fistula formation is common.

In approximately one-quarter of patients with small bowel disease and three-quarters of those with disease of the large bowel, anal lesions occur at some time. These include chronic fissure, ulceration, oedematous anal tags and anal fistulas. These skin lesions may spread onto the perineum and occasionally occur at other sites.

Microscopically, the most valuable diagnostic feature is the presence of non-caseating granulomas similar to those found in sarcoidosis; these are distinguishable in 50% of all cases. Other microscopic features include fissures or clefts passing deeply into the bowel wall, transmural inflammation with oedema and infiltration of inflammatory cells, and foci of lymphocytes.

Clinical features

The clinical presentation of Crohn's disease is varied. Continuous or episodic diarrhoea associated with recurrent abdominal pain, lassitude and fever is common. Declining general health, malabsorption, weight loss and, in children, retardation of growth are other non-specific signs. Specific features may give rise to the following complications.

Intestinal obstruction. Excessive fibrosis results from chronic granulomatous inflammation and lymphoedema. All layers of the bowel wall become thickened, leading to stenosis and partial intestinal obstruction. The tendency to obstruction is increased by adhesions between the inflamed bowel and neighbouring structures. The clinical presentation is often one of intermittent bouts of incomplete intestinal obstruction, on which complete obstruction may supervene.

Fistula formation. Adhesions between inflamed loops of bowel predispose to fistula formation. Internal fistulas may form between loops of small or large intestine, and between bowel and non-alimentary viscera such as bladder. External fistulas are often a consequence of surgical intervention and most often involve the anterior abdominal wall or perineum.

Abscess formation. Free perforation is uncommon but subclinical bowel perforation often leads to abscess formation. The usual clinical and laboratory evidence of an abscess may be masked by steroid therapy, and considerable clinical judgment is needed to detect these complications, which require prompt treatment.

Anal complications. Anal fissures and fistulas are a common complication of Crohn's disease. The fistulas are frequently multiple and indolent. They commonly open in the perianal region but may involve any part of the perineum, including the vagina or scrotum.

Radiological features

Radiology plays an essential role in the diagnosis of Crohn's disease. Proliferative changes with thickening of the bowel wall, narrowing of the lumen and separation of bowel loops coincide with evidence of tissue destruction with ulceration, spike-like fissures and a cobblestone appearance of the mucosa. With developing fibrosis, short and long strictures occur which give rise to the typical 'string sign' in the terminal ileum.

Management

Uncomplicated Crohn's disease should be managed conservatively. Rest, a high-protein low-residue diet, medium-chain triglycerides and vitamins improve nutritional state. Hydrophilic colloid preparations and codeine phosphate may help diarrhoea. Cholestyramine has been used to bind bile salts and this may also reduce diarrhoea.

Steroids are used in the acute phase and may reduce inflammatory manifestations. Long-term steroid therapy is not recommended. Sulfasalazine is of more value in the treatment of large bowel Crohn's disease (see p. 501). Azathioprine has been used with limited success.

About 90% of patients with Crohn's disease will require surgery at some stage. Since surgery is not curative, it is usually reserved for complications, but operation may be indicated for patients with intractable disease causing severe systemic problems.

The best surgical procedure is resection of the responsible segment(s) of intestine with restoration of continuity if feasible. Extended radical operations are no longer advised. The recurrence rate after resection is determined more by the natural history of the individual's disease than by the extent of surgery. Bypass of an affected segment is no longer recommended, as the majority of patients continue to experience major recurrent problems which ultimately require resection.

The overall recurrence rate after resection for Crohn's disease involving ileum is around 33% (compared to less than 20% when the disease is confined to the colon). Fistulas are uncommon when all involved bowel is resected, but are a frequent complication of laparotomy alone or bypass. In view of the high recurrence rate multiple operations may be necessary.

Mortality of surgery

The immediate postoperative mortality is about 5% in Crohn's disease. Late deaths related to operation bring the overall mortality to around 10%.

EXTERNAL FISTULAS OF THE SMALL INTESTINE

A fistula is an abnormal communication between two surfaces lined by epithelium (Fig. 31.6). Fistulas involving the small intestine are among the most difficult to manage. However, the principles of management of all fistulas arising from the digestive tract are the same.

Clinical features

External small bowel fistulas are usually a complication of surgery (in over 90% of cases) but can arise spontaneously, notably in patients with Crohn's disease. Development of a fistula following gastrointestinal surgery is usually heralded by unexplained pyrexia and tachycardia in the early postoperative period. Abdominal pain and tenderness follow, and are associated with signs

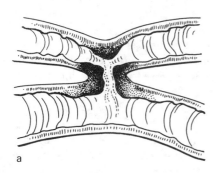
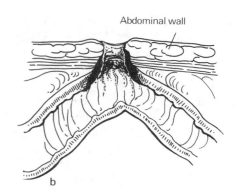

Abdominal wall

a

b

Fig. 31.6 Intestinal fistula. (a) Internal; (b) external

suggesting a simple wound infection or abscess. On rupture, frank discharge of intestinal content occurs through the wound or drain track. The escaping intestinal fluid can cause severe excoriation of the surrounding skin, particularly when the fistula originates from the upper small bowel and the fluid contains activated pancreatic secretions. Fistulas are classified as 'high-output' and 'low-output' according to the amount of fluid lost. 'High-output' fistulas develop from the upper small intestine, and 'low-output' fistulas from the lower small intestine and colon.

Management

The principles of management of external small bowel fistulas are: (1) replacement of fluid and electrolyte losses; (2) adequate external drainage to control sepsis; (3) nutritional support; (4) radiology to exclude distal obstruction; and (5) skin care.

Replacement of fluid and electrolyte losses. An accurate fluid balance chart is established with daily measurement of serum urea and electrolyte concentrations. Intravenous fluids are essential. High intestinal fistulas may be associated with losses of 3–4 litres of fluid each day leading to rapid dehydration and serious electrolyte deficits ('high-output fistula').

Adequate external drainage. Material escaping from the intestine must have free egress from the abdomen; otherwise intra-abdominal abscess formation or disseminated peritonitis with septicaemia will occur. Surgery may be required to establish drainage but at this stage does not include an attempt to close the internal site of leakage. When there is doubt about the formation of an abscess, a small amount of water-soluble contrast should be injected into the external opening during radiological screening.

Nutritional support. Parenteral nutrition has made a major impact on the mortality following fistula formation. In patients with low-output fistulas it may be possible to maintain nutrition by oral elemental diets, but in patients with high-output fistulas it is advisable to stop all oral intake until closure has been achieved. Patients with complicated inflammatory bowel disease may be suitable for long-term home parenteral nutrition.

Radiology. The majority of alimentary fistulas close on conservative management provided there is no distal intestinal obstruction. Contrast radiology is used to investigate the distal intestine but is usually deferred until the patient's condition is stable in terms of fluid and electrolyte balance, sepsis and nutritional support.

Fistulas associated with Crohn's disease or neoplasia are exceptions in that they are unlikely to close until the affected segment of bowel has been resected.

Skin care. Effective suction drainage minimizes skin excoriation in high-output intestinal fistulas. Stomahesive and Karaya gum are particularly useful in preventing damage to the skin around the external opening, and an ileostomy appliance is often useful.

Role of surgery. Definitive surgery (other than that to establish adequate external drainage) is required when there is distal obstruction preventing spontaneous closure, persisting underlying intestinal disease (e.g. Crohn's disease), or when healing fails to take place despite adequate conservative therapy for a number of weeks.

SHORT BOWEL SYNDROME

Effects of massive intestinal resection

The considerable functional reserve of the small bowel may be overcome by massive resection for trauma or for conditions such as mesenteric vascular disease, Crohn's disease, radiation enteritis or neoplasia. The consequences of resection are determined in part by the length and position of the segment removed, the nature of the underlying cause, the state of the ileocaecal valve (whether intact or removed), and the ability of the remaining bowel to increase its absorptive capacity by the compensatory process known as adaptation. The problem of loss of absorptive surface area is compounded by rapid intestinal transit, disturbances in the normal neurohormonal regulation of pancreatic and biliary secretion, continued loss of bile salts from the body's bile salt pool, and reflux of bacteria from the colon with overgrowth in the remaining small bowel. Nutritional consequences are usually severe when more than 75% of the small bowel is lost. Loss of the jejunum impairs absorption of fat, carbohydrate and protein, although the ileum can compensate to some extent. Loss of the terminal ileum results in permanently impaired absorption of bile salts and vitamin B12.

Some patients develop massive gastric hypersecretion, due possibly to loss of intestinal hormones capable of inhibiting gastric secretion. The problem improves with time, but can compound malabsorption in that pH is lowered in the intestinal lumen, with resultant inactivation of lipase and trypsin.

The characteristic clinical course after massive small bowel resection is one of rapid and profound fluid and electrolyte loss from severe diarrhoea. The severity usually diminishes after a few weeks, during which time adaptation of the remaining bowel takes place. The mucosa becomes hyperplastic, the villi increase in length, the crypts of Lieberkühn deepen, and the entire wall of the bowel becomes thickened.

Patients who undergo massive ileal resection but retain the colon are at risk of developing calcium oxalate calculi in the urinary tract because of excessive oxalate absorption from the colon. Resection of the terminal ilium also increases the risk of gallstone formation due to depletion of the bile salt pool.

Management

Immediate postoperative management is directed at intravenous replacement of fluid and electrolyte loss, and provision of parenteral nutrition. Diarrhoea can be combated with codeine phosphate. Oral feeding should not be attempted while severe diarrhoea persists. Antisecretory drugs are useful if gastric hypersecretion is present.

As diarrhoea abates, oral isotonic fluids are commenced cautiously. Elemental diets are used in dilute form and are best given at controlled rates by an infusion pump connected to a fine-bore nasogastric or nasoenteric tube. Such tubes are usually well tolerated and their use avoids problems caused by the lack of palatability of elemental diets. The rate and concentration of the alimentary intake is gradually increased, bearing in mind that adaptation may continue for 12–24 months.

Parenteral nutrition is discontinued once an adequate oral intake can be tolerated, but long-term parenteral nutrition may be unavoidable in some patients. Vitamins A, D and K are prescribed routinely in patients with persisting malabsorption. Vitamin B12 is prescribed for life after extensive ileal resection.

As indicated above, the development of nutritional support units and programmes of home-nutrition has greatly improved the care of such patients. An indwelling venous catheter is inserted through which the patient 'feeds himself' during sleep from a 3-litre bag containing all essential nutrients (see Ch. 5).

PARTIAL ILEAL BYPASS FOR HYPERLIPIDAEMIA

Hyperlipidaemia (hypercholesterolaemia and hypertriglyceridaemia) increases the risk of atherosclerosis and its complications. Hyperlipidaemia may be reduced by dietary modifications, drugs (e.g. clofibrate, cholestyramine) and/or partial ileal bypass. Bypass reduces cholesterol absorption and by depleting the bile acid pool further reduces hyperlipidaemia as cholesterol is increasingly converted to bile acids to maintain pool size. Serum cholesterol is reduced by about half following bypass and even further if the diet is modified to reduce cholesterol intake. Xanthelasma and xanthoma generally decrease in size or disappear and angina pectoris often becomes less troublesome. Diarrhoea is an almost inevitable complication of surgery but tends to improve with time. Vitamin B12 supplements are advisable but malabsorption of other essential nutrients is seldom a problem and body weight is usually unaffected.

INTESTINAL ISCHAEMIA

Acute intestinal ischaemia

Superior mesenteric artery occlusion

Thrombotic or embolic occlusion of the superior mesenteric artery is an acute abdominal emergency with a high mortality. In most patients, thrombosis is the final event in atheromatous narrowing of the vessel. Emboli account for occlusion in one-third of cases and usually originate from intracardiac thrombus in patients with atrial fibrillation or recent myocardial infarction.

Occlusion occurs most commonly in elderly patients affected by cardiac failure. Delay in diagnosis remains a problem, and most patients do not come to surgery until necrosis of the bowel is advanced and peritonitis is established.

It is important to appreciate that abdominal pain and vomiting *in the absence of abdominal signs* may precede peritonitis and collapse for several hours or even some days. Bowel ischaemia proceeds from mucosa to serosa, and peritonitis does not develop until all layers are involved. The majority of infarctions affect the ileum.

Management. Successful management requires early diagnosis and operation to restore blood flow before irreversible changes occur in the bowel wall. Plain abdominal films usually show no intestinal abnormality in the critical early period. Lateral aortography under local anaesthesia or selective superior mesenteric arteriography can be used to confirm the diagnosis of occlusion but must be carried out promptly.

For superior mesenteric artery thrombosis, an aortomesenteric bypass graft using autogenous vein is preferred. All gangrenous bowel must be resected, as well as any segments of doubtful viability. A 'second look' operation 24–48 hours later to confirm viability of remaining bowel is now routine practice in many clinics. Antibiotics, oxygen, peritoneal lavage and adequate fluid replacement are essential parts of management.

Should the occlusion be due to an embolus, embolectomy and closure of the arteriotomy with a vein patch graft may restore the mesenteric circulation and avoid the need for or minimize the extent of gut resection.

Mesenteric venous occlusion

Mesenteric venous occlusion is much less common than arterial occlusion but equally devastating. Any disease predisposing to intravascular coagulation can cause venous occlusion and sporadic cases have been reported in pregnancy, in the puerperium and in young women taking oral contraceptives. The arterial supply to the midgut is normal but there is thrombosis of the mesenteric veins followed by venous gangrene of the bowel. Treatment consists of anticoagulation and bowel resection as required. Only occasionally is venous thrombectomy helpful. The mortality from this condition is high.

Non-occlusive infarction

Intestinal infarction may occur without demonstrable occlusion of major vessels, as for example in low flow states in severe shock. Conservative treatment is recommended and resection is only undertaken when there is obviously necrotic bowel.

Chronic intestinal (mesenteric) ischaemia

Chronic midgut ischaemia is a rare condition which gives rise to pain in the midabdomen after eating, diarrhoea due to malabsorption, and weight loss. A bruit in the para-umbilical region is an occasional sign and supports the diagnosis. Occult blood is present in the faeces. Arterial narrowing revealed at angiography may be relieved by surgical reconstruction.

NEOPLASMS OF THE SMALL INTESTINE

Small bowel neoplasms are rare, comprising less than 5% of all gastrointestinal neoplasms. Benign lesions are 10 times as common as malignant lesions.

Benign tumours

Solitary small bowel tumours include adenomatous or villous polyps, hamartomas, lipomas, haemangiomas and leiomyomas. Multiple hamartomatas occur in the familial Peutz-Jeghers syndrome in association with mucocutaneous pigmentation and diffuse gastrointestinal polyposis. Operation is indicated if any benign small bowel neoplasm causes symptoms such as bleeding or intussusception.

Malignant tumours

Adenocarcinoma

Small bowel adenocarcinomas are extremely rare when one considers the length of the small intestine. Yet they are still the commonest malignant tumour of the small bowel. Symptoms are usually due to obstruction, but by the time they occur the disease is usually advanced. Treatment consists of laparotomy and resection of the affected segment and its mesentery. If the lesion is irresectable, useful palliation may be achieved by bypass surgery.

Lymphoma

Lymphoma may originate in the small intestine. Resection of a single involved segment is indicated if obstruction or bleeding develops, but the disease should be regarded in the same light as lymphoma arising elsewhere, and appropriately staged before planning further treatment. Small deposits of lymphoma can cause perforation of the bowel wall, the patient then being admitted to hospital with peritonitis. At operation a small punched-out hole is discovered in the small gut. In such cases biopsy by excision of the perforation must precede closure.

Carcinoid tumours

Carcinoid tumours most frequently arise in the appendix. The small intestine is the second-commonest site of carcinoid formation and one-third of tumours have metastasized by the time of presentation. Symptoms may be produced by obstruction or bleeding, and some 10% of patients present with the carcinoid syndrome. Biologically active tumour products are normally inactivated by the liver, but once hepatic metastases develop these substances are secreted directly into the systemic circulation. The syndrome comprises periodic flushing attacks, diarrhoea, bronchoconstriction, and right-sided heart disease, notably pulmonary stenosis. Urinary levels of 5-hydroxyindoleacetic acid (5-HIAA) are elevated in the majority of patients with the syndrome. Treatment of carcinoid tumours consists of excising all accessible tumours in the small bowel and its mesentery. Hepatic metastases have been treated by hepatic lobectomy in some patients but the role of such radical surgery and the chemotherapy is as yet uncertain. The recently available analogue of somatostatin (SMS 201–995) may give valuable symptomatic relief but has to be given parenterally.

32. The large intestine

Surgical anatomy

The large intestine extends from the ileocaecal valve to the anorectal junction. Embryologically it is derived from the distal part of the midgut, the entire hind gut and portions of the cloaca. It is supplied by branches of the superior and inferior mesenteric artery (Fig. 32.1). The rectum receives an additional suply from branches of the median sacral artery, and middle and inferior rectal branches of the internal iliac artery. The *ileocaecal* valve is on the medial wall of the caecum. It has two pouting lips and functions as a one-way valve, preventing reflux of caecal content into the terminal ileum.

The *caecum* is a blind pouch in the right iliac fossa which overlies the iliacus and psoas muscles and the femoral nerve. It is covered by peritoneum on both sides and on the anterior surface. However, a peritoneal reflection may also cover the posterior surface, creating a retrocaecal space. The *appendix* opens at the base of the caecum in the

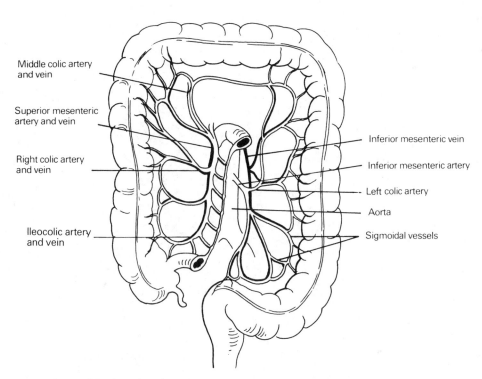

Fig. 32.1 The blood supply of the large intestine

embryo, but as a result of differential rates of growth of the caecal wall, it comes to open on the posteriomedial wall in the adult.

The *ascending colon* extends upwards from the ileocaecal valve for approximately 15 cm to the *hepatic flexure*. It is covered by peritoneum on its anterior and lateral surfaces and lies lateral to the right ureter. The hepatic flexure usually overlies the lower pole of the right kidney. The *transverse colon* is suspended by mesentery and is approximately 45 cm long. The antimesenteric surface is attached to the greater omentum. The *descending colon* passes from the *splenic flexure* to the pelvic brim, is covered by peritoneum on its anterior and lateral surfaces, and lies lateral to the left ureter. The superior mesenteric artery supplies the colon almost as far as the splenic flexure, while the distal colon is supplied from the inferior mesenteric artery.

The *sigmoid colon* varies greatly in length, but is usually less than 50 cm long. Like the transverse colon, it is invested by peritoneum on all sides and has a mesentery. This sigmoid mesocolon forms an inverted 'V' attached to the pelvic brim overlying the left ureter as it crosses the bifurcation of the left common iliac artery.

The *rectum* commences as the colon loses its mesentery. It is approximately 15 cm long and passes downwards in the hollow of the sacrum to end at the anorectal junction. The upper third of the rectum is covered on the front and on both sides by peritoneum, the middle third is peritonealized only in front, and the lower third lies beneath the peritoneal floor of the pelvis. The posterior aspect of the rectum is bound loosely to the sacrum by a condensation of connective tissue (the fascia of Waldeyer), behind which lies the pelvic plexus of autonomic nerves. Laterally the rectum is attached to the side walls of the pelvis by lateral ligaments which contain the middle rectal arteries.

The wall of the large bowel consists of an outer longitudinal layer and inner circular layer of smooth muscle. In the colon, the longitudinal muscle is condensed into three bands (taeniae) which lie anterior, posteromedial and posterolateral and which meet at the base of the appendix. Over the rectum these bands coalesce to form a continuous investment of longitudinal muscle. The

inner circular layer is continous throughout, but is thickened in the anorectal canal to form the internal sphincter.

The *appendices epiploicae* are small pedunculated fat pads attached to the bowel wall between the taeniae.

The *mucosa* consists of columnar epithelium with crypts passing down to the muscularis mucosae, and numerous goblet cells which secrete mucus. Beneath the muscularis mucosae is a submucosa of fibrous connective tissue. The arteries supplying the large bowel anastomose in the mesentery close to the bowel to form a continuous *marginal artery* from which vessels pass to encircle the bowel. These circumferential arteries give off numerous small branches which pierce the muscle coat. The mucosal protrusions of diverticular disease lie immediately adjacent to the points of vessel penetration (Fig. 32.2). The venous drainage of the large bowel accompanies the arterial supply.

Lymph drains from the colon to epicolic nodes on the bowel wall, and then to paracolic nodes between the marginal artery and the bowel (Fig. 32.3). Lymph then drains to intermediate

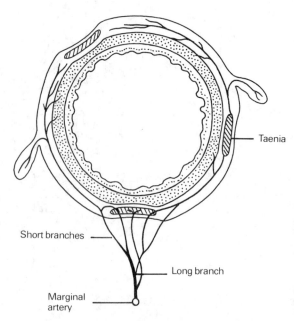

Fig. 32.2 The circumferential arteries of the large bowel

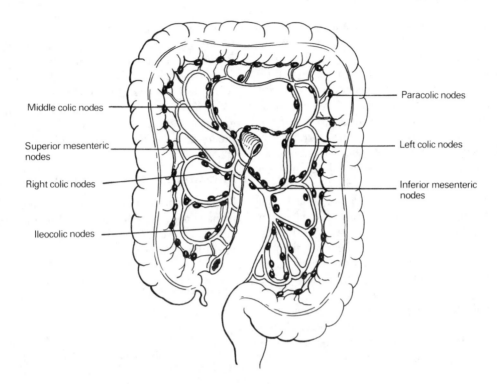

Middle colic nodes

Superior mesenteric nodes

Right colic nodes

Ileocolic nodes

Paracolic nodes

Left colic nodes

Inferior mesenteric nodes

Fig. 32.3 Lymphatic drainage of the colon

nodes on the main vessels, and to principal nodes alongside the origin of the superior and inferior mesenteric vessels. Lymph from the rectum drains upwards to superior rectal and inferior mesenteric nodes, or laterally along the middle rectal vessels to the internal iliac nodes. Downward spread to inguinal lymph nodes is exceptional from the rectum. However, drainage of the anal canal and perianal skin is to the inguinal nodes.

Function of the large bowel

The large bowel mucosa actively absorbs sodium and water from the faeces and actively secretes potassium, though usually not in any significant quantity. The right side of the large bowel is the main site of water absorption, while the left side acts as a reservoir for solid faeces until defaecation is appropriate. Mucus secreted by the large bowel mucosa acts as a lubricant. Irritation increases mucus secretion to the extent that in inflammatory disease it becomes visible as a covering layer on solid faeces or as a mucous discharge.

Investigation of large bowel disease

History and physical examination

Diseases of the large bowel may present with abdominal pain, alteration in bowel habit (which may consist of constipation, diarrhoea or alternating bouts of each) and the passage of blood or mucus per rectum. Abdominal pain may be accompanied by nausea. In patients with obstruction it is often associated with abdominal distension and, later, vomiting. Weight loss, malaise and anaemia are important non-specific features. A detailed case history must be obtained and combined with a thorough physical examination, including inspection of the oral mucous membrane, hands and finger nails. Examination of the abdomen may reveal distension, an obvious mass or visible peristalsis. The caecum is often palpable in thin subjects, and the descending colon and sigmoid colon may be palpable when loaded with faeces. The lower two-thirds of the rectum is palpable on rectal examination. Other parts of the large bowel are not normally palpable.

Differentiation between faeces and solid tumour may be difficult. Faeces can sometimes be indented by the examining fingers, whereas a solid tumour can not. Impacted faeces often constitute a large part of the palpable mass in patients with obstructing large bowel cancer. Abdominal auscultation will determine the presence and quality of bowel sounds, and may reveal arterial bruits.

Hepatomegaly may be due to hepatic metastases in patients with cancer. Digital rectal examination is mandatory. Three-quarters of rectal carcinomas and up to one-third of all colonic carcinomas can be felt rectally. The finding of an empty rectum in a patient with palpable faecal masses in the pelvic colon raises the suspicion of rectosigmoid obstruction. A tumour in this region may more readily be palpated through the rectal wall if the patient turns onto his *right* side.

The withdrawn finger is always inspected to determine the colour of faeces and to detect blood or mucus. A specimen of faeces is tested for occult blood if blood staining is not obvious.

Further investigation

Proctoscopy and *sigmoidoscopy* are undertaken routinely when large bowel pathology is suspected or when there is a history of bleeding per rectum. The sigmoidoscope can usually be passed painlessly up to the level of the rectosigmoid junction without special preparation and allows visualization of the whole of the rectum at the patient's first attendance. A small-diameter short instrument (20 cm) is preferred by some. To examine the sigmoid colon a flexible sigmoidoscope can now be used but meticulous bowel preparation is required. A rectal biopsy taken by punch forceps is painless and furnishes material for histological diagnosis.

Barium enema is the routine method for detecting gross abnormalities in the bowel lumen. Air-contrast studies allow better mucosal definition and are used to detect polyps and ulcers. A barium enema should not be carried out within 5 days of rectal biopsy to avoid perforation of the bowel at the weakened biopsy site. As the rectum is not easily visualized by a barium enema, sigmoidoscopy should also be carried out.

Fibreoptic colonoscopy is used to observe and biopsy specific areas of any part of the large bowel. Polyps can be removed with a diathermy snare.

Examination of the stool by direct microscopy will reveal any parasites and their ova, and culture is used to isolate bacteria. The toxin of *Clostridium difficile*, one of the causal agents of pseudomembranous colitis, may also be detected.

PRINCIPLES OF LARGE BOWEL SURGERY

Certain principles of preoperative preparation and management are common to all operations on the large intestine. These may have to be modified if operation is required urgently.

Preoperative preparation

Patient counselling

The type of operation to be undertaken must be discussed as fully as possible with the patient. Particular efforts must be made to explain the need for a temporary or permanent artificial stoma. If a stoma is planned, the site is chosen before the operation by trial-fitting of an appliance. A stoma-care nurse is invaluable in preoperative preparation and subsequent care, and a visit from a member of a local ileostomy or colostomy association can provide valuable reassurance.

Improving nutritional status

Patients with inflammatory or malignant disease of the large bowel are often malnourished and anaemic. Anaemia is readily corrected by transfusion, but malnourishment may take weeks to correct by a high-calorie, high-protein diet. The dangers of delaying operation have to be balanced against the potential benefits of improved nutritional status. In such patients the timing of surgery requires experience and sound clinical judgement.

Bowel preparation

The risk of anastomotic leakage and wound sepsis is reduced if the large bowel is empty at the time of resection. Antimicrobial prophylaxis is of secondary value.

Mechanical bowel preparation. The large bowel can be emptied by a combination of purgatives and enemas during the 2–3 days before operation. Mannitol 100 g in 1000 ml is used as an osmotic aperient. Picolax is an alternative stimulant laxative.

Alternatively, the bowel can be emptied by whole-gut irrigation on the day before operation. A nasogastric tube is inserted and, with the patient sitting upright, 2–4 litres of balanced crystalloid fluid are instilled each hour until the effluent from the anus is clear. A padded commode or flush-toilet is an advantage. Metoclopramide 10 mg and frusemide 20 mg are given intramuscularly at the start of the procedure to accelerate gastric emptying and reduce the risk of pulmonary oedema. This technique is used less frequently than formerly, and is contraindicated in patients with known cardiac or renal disease and in those with obstructing lesions.

Low-residue diet. Patients may be admitted 5 days before elective large bowel surgery and placed on an elemental low-residue diet such as Vivonex or Flexical. A large-bowel enema is given on the day before operation. Elemental diets are absorbed entirely in the small bowel and reduce bacterial density in the large bowel. Their unpleasant taste may be hidden by flavouring, or they can be given through a nasogastric tube. In most units a two-day 'no-residue, fluids only' regimen is preferred.

Antibiotic prophylaxis. Mechanical cleansing of the large bowel is usually combined with an attempt to reduce the density of bacteria. A 5-day oral course of non-absorbable sulphonamide in combination with a final 48-hour course of neomycin or kanamycin was the standard method to reduce the bacterial flora in the past. However, this did not reduce the number of anaerobic organisms (notably Bacteroides) and it is now customary to include metronidazole (Flagyl) in preoperative antibiotic prophylaxis.

The use of oral antibiotics in prophylaxis is associated with an increased incidence of post-operative enterocolitis due to overgrowth of resistant organisms. Many surgeons now prefer to use antibiotics parenterally, starting at the time of induction of anaesthesia. A cephalosporin plus metronidazole 500 mg is administered intra-venously every 8 hours for three doses. Although expensive, such regimens reduce the incidence of postoperative infection without the risk of enterocolitis. Metronidazole may be given, less expensively, by suppository.

Urinary tract preparation

Ureteric damage is one of the hazards of large bowel surgery, and large bowel cancer may invade and obstruct the ureter. An excretion urogram should be obtained before elective operation to detect any ureteric obstruction and confirm the presence of two functioning kidneys. Any decision at operation to sacrifice an involved ureter and kidney can then be made on rational grounds.

A urinary catheter is inserted prior to operation to ensure that the bladder does not impede access to the pelvis. Postoperatively the catheter is left in place to prevent urinary retention. Measurement of hourly urine output provides a valuable guide to the need for fluid replacement.

Preparation for emergency surgery

In patients presenting with obstruction, perforation, toxic dilatation or massive bleeding from the large bowel, emergency surgery may be required. Adequate resuscitation is essential before anaesthesia. In intestinal obstruction large volumes of extracellular fluid may be lost by accumulation in the gastrointestinal lumen and by vomiting. Perforation allows fluid to escape into the peritoneal cavity, and associated ileus results in further fluid loss into the lumen of the small bowel. Fluid replacement is essential (using 0.9% saline with added potassium to replace crystalloid loss). Loss from massive bleeding is best replaced by blood, although colloids or plasma can be used until blood becomes available (see Ch. 4).

Severe bleeding from the large bowel is difficult to localize. If time permits, mesenteric arteriography may define the source. Otherwise, the surgeon may have to rely on peroperative colonoscopy (using the 30 cm sigmoidoscope inserted through a colotomy) to inspect the bowel lumen. This, however, is associated with significant morbidity and may not define the source of bleeding.

Operative technique

The extent of resection in both elective and emergency surgery is governed by the arterial blood supply and the disease process. In malignant disease, it is essential to remove as much of the draining lymphatic system as possible (Fig. 32.4), and division of peritoneal attachments allows adequate mobilization of the bowel on its mesentery. Preliminary high ligation of the main vessels supplying the involved segment is desirable to prevent embolization of tumour cells during handling of the bowel. Similarly, it is wise to place occluding tapes on either side of the growth to avoid luminal dissemination of tumour cells.

Anastomoses must be made without tension. Stapling is used increasingly as an alternative to hand suture.

Many surgeons place a soft tube drain down to colonic anastomoses so that any bowel content that may leak from the anastomosis can escape directly to the surface without contaminating the peritoneal cavity or abdominal wound. Leakage is usually manifest by the 5th postoperative day. Drains should be left in situ until at least that time.

Intestinal stoma

A permanent intestinal stoma is best sited on a line between the umbilicus and the anterior superior iliac spine, sufficiently far from both to allow easy fixation of an appliance. Temporary colostomies may have to be positioned at other sites to allow subsequent resection.

Ileostomy

The commonest reason for an ileostomy is proctocolectomy carried out for ulcerative colitis or Crohn's disease. The stoma is fashioned so that a nipple of small bowel protrudes from the skin, facilitating direct delivery of the irritant small bowel content into an appliance. Excoriation of surrounding skin is prevented by a well-fitting appliance and the use of a protective skin barrier such as Karaya gum.

Conventional ileostomies are incontinent, but a continent ileostomy can be made by constructing a reservoir (Kock pouch) from a loop of small bowel and valve by artificial intussusception of a length of small bowel (Fig. 32.5). The pouch is emptied by passing a soft plastic tube through the valve to syphon off the pouch contents. A continent ileostomy can be fashioned at the time of primary surgery or an incontinent ileostomy can be converted to a continent one at subsequent surgery. Such reservoir ileostomies are contraindicated in Crohn's disease because of the risk of development of Crohn's disease in the bowel forming the reservoir. The recent development of methods to restore continuity by constructing an ileal pouch and anastomosing it to the anal canal has greatly reduced the need for continent ileostomies in ulcerative colitis.

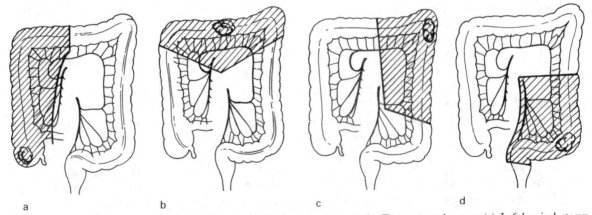

| a | b | c | d |

Fig. 32.4 Types of resection for cancer of the colon. (a) Right hemicolectomy. (b) Transverse colectomy. (c) Left hemicolectomy. (d) Sigmoid colectomy

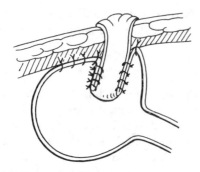

Fig. 32.5 Continent ileostomy with Kock pouch (intussusception or 'nipple' valve reservoir)

Colostomy

A colostomy may be permanent, e.g. after removal of the distal large bowel and rectum, or temporary following partial colonic resection, when later restoration of continuity is envisaged. If an anastomosis is performed at the time of resection, a temporary proximal colostomy may be used to deflate and defunction the distal bowel until healing of the anastomosis has been confirmed by radiological examination. This is particularly useful in resections of the rectosigmoid region, when the anastomosis may be low down in the pelvis.

Two types of colostomy are commonly used. A *loop colostomy* (Fig. 32.6), which is usually temporary, is constructed by bringing a loop of colon to the surface. An *end colostomy* may be permanent or temporary and is constructed by bringing the divided end of the bowel to the surface (Fig. 32.7).

A caecostomy is used occasionally for temporary decompression of the large bowel. The caecum may be brought up to the anterior abdominal wall and anastomosed to skin, but more commonly a tube is passed through the anterior abdominal wall into the lumen of the caecum. Caecostomy produces only limited decompression of the large bowel and does not completely divert the fluid faecal stream to the surface. Regular flushing of the tube caecostomy with water is needed to promote continued drainage of faeces.

Care of the colostomy. Two methods are used to cope with a colostomy, which forms an 'incontinent anus' on the abdominal wall. Most commonly patients accept that spontaneous colon movements will occur, and are willing to collect the motions in a suitable colostomy bag. A variety of disposable adherent appliances are available which can be kept in position for several days at a time and emptied when required. These are either manufactured in one piece, with an adherent fenestrated patch incorporated into the back of a plastic bag; or in two pieces, i.e. a separate adherent moulded flange with a groove into which a bag can be fixed. An air vent is incorporated. Neither is perfect, and the skin surrounding the stoma is prone to irritation.

The alternative is to wash out the colon through the colostomy every 24 hours. As this empties the colon, the colostomy does not act spontaneously during the day. A simple dressing is then all that is required. The wash-out regimen involves the patient in a fairly troublesome routine requiring the availability of a douche can, tubing and catheters. In the UK this method is generally advised only if a colostomy appliance has proved unsatisfactory.

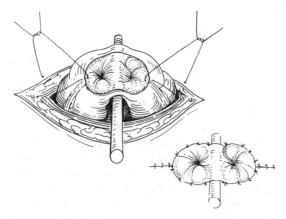

Fig. 32.6 Loop colostomy (the rod is kept in place for approximately 7 days)

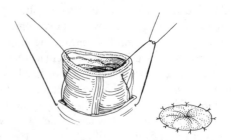

Fig. 32.7 End colostomy

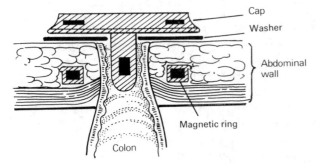

Fig. 32.8 Continent colostomy using a magnetic ring and plug

With both types of colostomy care, the patient needs to adjust his diet to avoid foods which are known to cause upset. Fruit, vegetables, beers and wines are particularly liable to cause looseness and should be avoided altogether or taken only in small quantities. Foods which cause excess flatus (e.g. onions, spices, curries) are also best avoided.

Attempts to create continent colostomies include implantation of a magnetic ring around the emerging bowel in order to hold in place a close-fitting plastic-covered metal plug (Fig. 32.8). A carbon filter allows escape of gas. This method has had varying success and is not in common use.

COMPLICATIONS OF LARGE BOWEL SURGERY

Shock

Unrecognized or undertreated preoperative hypovolaemia favours the development of hypovolaemic shock during operation. Most anaesthetic agents encourage peripheral pooling of blood and compound the problem. The splanchnic vascular bed is a 'low-priority area' in shock and, by impairing local blood flow, hypovolaemia may have a critical effect on anastomotic healing. Adequate preoperative volume replacement is essential. *Septicaemic shock* is a potential consequence of spillage of bowel contents during operation. Spillage is more likely to occur in poorly prepared or obstructed patients. Lavage of the peritoneal cavity with saline or tetracycline solution (1 g/l) is indicated. Treatment consists of crystalloid and colloid replacement, oxygen administration and systemic antibiotic therapy.

Anastomotic leakage

Minor degrees of anastomotic leakage can be demonstrated radiologically in up to 50% of distal colonic anastomoses. In only 5% of patients are these leaks of clinical significance. Leakage may result in intra-abdominal collection of faecal material, septicaemia and shock. Treatment consists of surgical drainage after appropriate resuscitation, with formation of a defunctioning colostomy or exteriorization of both ends of the leaking anastomosis. Anastomotic leaks can also give rise to a faecal fistula with escape of faeces along the drain track or through abdominal and perineal wounds. If there is no distal obstruction and the patient is otherwise well, the fistula may be treated conservatively in the expectation that it will close spontaneously. Closure is hastened by creation of a proximal diverting colostomy or institution of an elemental or parenteral diet to reduce fistula output and maintain adequate nutrition.

Wound infection

Despite antibiotic prophylaxis, wound infection rates of 15% are common. Endogenous gut bacteria are almost always responsible. Infection delays healing, may cause secondary bleeding, and favours wound dehiscence and incisional hernia.

Genitourinary damage

The commonest postoperative urinary problem is retention of urine. This may be due to pre-existing prostatic disease in males or development of partial prolapse in females.

Damage to the parasympathetic nerves (nervi erigentes) as they pass through the pelvis results in loss of bladder motor activity, postoperative retention, and overflow incontinence. Following resection of the lower sigmoid colon or rectum, a catheter should be left in the bladder for 4–5 days. If retention is evident on removal, it should be replaced. If the prostate is not the seat of the trouble, cystometric studies should be arranged.

Prostatic enlargement may require transurethral resection, whereas neurogenic bladder dysfunction can usually be managed by parasympathomimetic drugs and teaching the patient to empty the bladder by straining. Bladder neck resection may be required in some patients.

The ureters may be damaged during mobilization of the colon, while the prostatic and membranous urethra may be damaged during excision of the anorectum.

After rectal excision for cancer, one-third of males become impotent due to division of the nervi erigentes. A further third are unable to ejaculate due to division of sympathetic nerves in the pelvis plexus. It is important to warn male patients of this complication before obtaining their consent to this operation.

DISEASES OF THE LARGE INTESTINE

DIVERTICULAR DISEASE

With the exception of solitary diverticula of the caecum (see below), diverticula of the large bowel are rare before the age of 35 years. By the age of 65 years at least 30% of the general population are affected. There is a slight male preponderance.

The diverticula, which are of the pulsion type, emerge between the mesenteric and antimesenteric taeniae, and are most common in the sigmoid colon (Fig. 32.9). They result from herniation of the large bowel mucosa through the circular muscle at the sites of penetration of small blood vessels. Their wall consists only of mucosa and serosa.

Diverticular disease is associated with increased intraluminal pressure in the large bowel and hypertrophy of both circular and longitudinal muscle layers. Muscle hypertrophy precedes the development of diverticula and this 'prediverticular state' may be detected radiologically. In general, the disease is uncommon in societies whose usual diet is high in roughage.

Clinical features and treatment of uncomplicated diverticular disease

Diverticular disease may be asymptomatic, or it may produce central or left iliac fossa pain, alteration in bowel habit and occasional bleeding from the rectum. The diagnosis is confirmed by a barium enema which shows evidence of muscle thickening and multiple diverticula.

Medical treatment

Most patients improve on a high-fibre diet (with added bran or hydrophilic colloids) and antispasmodics (e.g. propantheline bromide 15 mg four times a day) if spasm is thought to be a major feature. Codeine phosphate may be necessary to control diarrhoea.

Elective surgery

Elective surgery is indicated only if the patient continues to have repeated attacks of acute diverticular disease despite taking a high-residue diet and bulk laxatives. Sigmoid colectomy is usually performed, with immediate end-to-end anastomosis to restore intestinal continuity. A temporary loop colostomy can be used to protect the anastomosis if bowel preparation has been inadequate.

Sigmoid myotomy was once proposed as an alternative to sigmoid colectomy in the elective treatment of diverticular disease. This involved division of the circular muscle of the affected segment in order to reduce intraluminal pressure. The myotomy was made longitudinally through one of the antimesenteric taeniae until mucosa bulged through the incision. Good results were reported

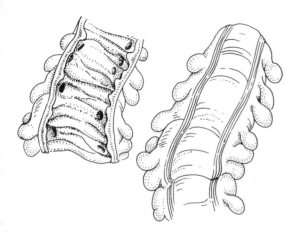

Fig. 32.9 Macroscopic appearance of diverticular disease

initially, but the operation may be complicated by leakage and has fallen into disuse.

Complications of diverticular disease

Inflammation

Patients with diverticular disease may develop peridiverticulitis due to inflammation of a diverticulum and spread of infection through its wall. This results in severe localized abdominal pain, nausea, vomiting, pyrexia and leucocytosis. There is evidence of local peritonitis with tenderness and guarding in the left iliac fossa. The patient should be confined to bed and given intravenous fluids and antibiotics. The condition usually settles after a few days of this treatment. If not, one should suspect the development of a pericolic abscess, which may become palpable and require drainage. About 40% of patients have no further attacks following resolution of inflammation and less than 10% eventually require some form of surgery.

Perforation

Diffuse peritonitis from rupture of a pericolic abscess may complicate peridiverticulitis. The peritoneal contents are then purulent. Alternatively, faecal peritonitis may occur from free perforation of the colon at the site of a diverticulum, a complication associated with a 50% mortality rate.

This is an emergency requiring urgent resection of the affected segment of bowel. Immediate anastomosis of the large intestine is usually contraindicated and both ends of the cut bowel are exteriorized (one as an end colostomy, the other as a mucus fistula) to await restoration of intestinal continuity as an elective procedure (Fig. 32.10). Alternatively, only the proximal end is exteriorized as a colostomy and the distal end is closed and allowed to drop back into the abdomen (Hartmann's procedure). Continuity is restored at a later date. The peritoneal cavity should be irrigated before closure and many surgeons use a solution of tetracycline in saline for this purpose.

Obstruction

An acute attack of diverticular disease may present as intestinal obstruction. This may be due to oedema or fibrosis of the large bowel, or to small bowel loops adhering to the inflamed colon. At operation it may be difficult to differentiate the lesion from carcinoma of the colon, and the true diagnosis may not be known until after the resection, when the results of histological examination become available.

A staged procedure is necessary to relieve the obstruction and restore intestinal continuity.

1. In the classical three-stage operation the obstruction was overcome by fashioning a temporary proximal loop colostomy. Resection of the

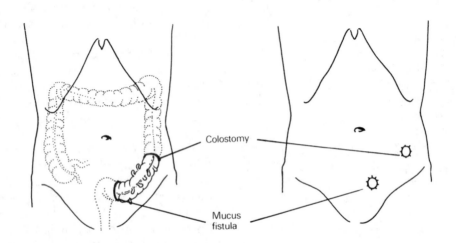

Colostomy

Mucus fistula

Fig. 32.10   Principles of emergency resection for perforated diverticular disease. Intestinal continuity is restored at a later date

affected segment of bowel with end-to-end anastomosis was then carried out at a second elective operation, and closure of the colostomy deferred for a further 4–6 weeks to allow anastomotic healing.

2. Experienced surgeons may be able to use a two-stage procedure instead, resecting the affected segment of colon at emergency operation and restoring intestinal continuity at a subsequent elective operation.

3. If the patient is fit and the surgeon experienced, immediate anastomosis may be considered. As this requires an empty proximal colon, 'on-table' bowel lavage with warmed saline solution must first be carried out. This is instilled through a catheter inserted into the colon through the appendix stump or terminal ileum. Irrigation is continued until the effluent from the cut end of colon runs clear. Primary anastomosis is then undertaken.

Stricture formation

Recurrent attacks of diverticular disease may result in stenosis which is demonstrable by barium enema. The most important consideration is to exclude cancer. In stricture from diverticular disease the involved segment is longer than in cancer, there is gradual (not abrupt) transition from normal bowel, and the mucosa remains intact (Fig. 32.11). The presence of diverticula on a barium enema does not necessarily indicate that stenosis is due to diverticular disease. Cancer and diverticular disease frequently coexist, as both conditions are common in older patients.

Fistula

Diverticular disease may give rise to fistulas between the sigmoid colon and the bladder, small bowel (Fig. 32.12) or vagina. It is the commonest cause of a colovesical fistula, a complication commoner in males than in females, in whom the uterus is interposed between the sigmoid colon and bladder. The patient usually gives a history of intractable cystitis with pneumaturia or the passage of faeces per urethram. The diagnosis is confirmed by barium enema or cystography. The fistula is treated surgically. After removal of the affected

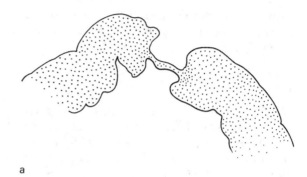

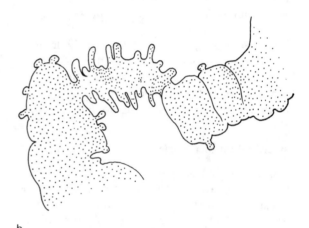

Fig. 32.11 Radiological appearance on barium enema of stricture due to (a) carcinoma and (b) diverticular disease of the sigmoid colon

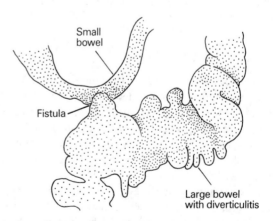

Fig. 32.12 Radiological appearance on barium enema of internal fistula

bowel the bladder defect usually closes satisfactorily if adequate urinary drainage is provided temporarily with a urinary catheter.

Bleeding

Until recently it was believed that massive rectal bleeding was most likely to be due to diverticular disease. Angiographic investigations have now shown that in two-thirds of such cases the bleeding is due to other causes. Even if diverticula are present in the sigmoid colon, bleeding is equally likely to arise from another lesion. Angiomatous malformations, polyps and diverticula of the right colon are likely causes.

Preoperative angiography is now advisable in all patients with massive rectal bleeding so that the lesion can be localized and then resected. If no lesion is seen and bleeding continues, 'blind' total colectomy with ileorectal anastomosis is advised.

Diverticulum of the caecum

A solitary diverticulum of the caecum is a congenital lesion. It arises from the medial wall of the caecum close to the ileocaecal junction and may extend upwards retroperitoneally. If obstructed by a faecolith, it may become acutely inflamed, producing a clinical syndrome similar to that of acute appendicitis. Repeated attacks of inflammation may lead to fibrosis of the diverticulum, leaving a residual (solitary) ulcer of the caecal mucosa. The condition is often difficult to distinguish from carcinoma at operation but right hemicolectomy is usually required in any event.

ULCERATIVE COLITIS

This disease, the aetiology of which is unknown, has an incidence of 5 new cases per 100 000 population per year. It most commonly affects young adults, particularly women, in a male-to-female ratio of 1 : 1.5. Although more common in first degree relatives, 90% of patients have no family history.

It is primarily a disease of the large bowel. Systemic manifestations (iritis, arthritis, hepatitis, pyoderma gangrenosum) are described but these often disappear completely when all of the affected bowel has been removed. In 95% of cases ulcerative colitis is a diffuse disease, starting in the rectum and extending proximally for a variable length. The whole of the colon may become involved, and so-called 'backwash' through the ileocaecal valve can cause ileitis. In 5% of patients the disease is segmental and the rectum is spared. Because of the frequency of rectal involvement, sigmoidoscopy is the key to diagnosis.

The characteristic histological feature is the formation of crypt abscesses in the depths of the glandular tubules with a surrounding inflammatory infiltrate. The abscesses coalesce to form ulcers which undermine the mucosa and penetrate as far as the muscularis mucosae. The intervening mucosa becomes oedematous and swollen, and in severe cases forms inflammatory pseudopolyps. The bowel wall loses its haustrations and becomes thickened and rigid as a result of muscle hypertrophy. The thickening is less severe than in Crohn's disease and stricture formation is uncommon. During an acute attack the bowel may become paper-thin and grossly dilated, resulting in the so-called *toxic megacolon* or *toxic dilatation*. This complication is believed to be due to destruction of the myenteric nerve plexus.

Other complications include perforation, massive bleeding, anorectal suppuration, and carcinoma of the colon. These are considered in more detail below.

Clinical features

Ulcerative colitis usually presents with attacks of diarrhoea and passage of blood and mucus per rectum. With extensive disease these symptoms are severe, the patient passing up to 10–15 motions daily. Urgency to defaecate can be incapacitating. Severe attacks may be associated with abdominal pain, tenderness and pyrexia.

Most attacks are mild, and patients with rectal bleeding may initially come to the surgeon with a request to assess and treat haemorrhoids. The importance of sigmoidoscopy in the assessment of such patients cannot be overemphasized. Rectal examination should include careful inspection for anal complications of fissure and fistula. The rectal mucosa may feel thickened and boggy. On sigmoidoscopy the mucosa is red, matt and granular, and there may be punctate haemorrhages or spontaneous bleeding. Contact bleeding, produced by gently rubbing the mucosa with a gauze pledget, is a typical feature.

Plain films of the abdomen are of value in the acute attack. Pseudopolyps in the gas-filled colon strongly support the diagnosis and avert the need for barium enema at this stage. If there is any suspicion that toxic dilatation may be developing, daily plain films should be taken to monitor progress; they allow much more accurate assessment than measurements of abdominal girth.

A barium enema is of value in assessing the extent of the disease but is contraindicated in the acute phase because of the danger of perforation. Typical changes include loss of haustrations and reduction in the calibre of the bowel, irregular fluffy outline of the mucosa, pseudopolyps and, rarely, strictures (Fig. 32.13). Widening of the retrorectal space is a constant feature of chronic disease. The disease must be differentiated from amoebic colitis, Crohn's disease and, in the elderly, ischaemic colitis.

The course of ulcerative colitis is almost invariably one of relapse and remission but a chronic continuous form is also described. In some patients the initial attack is fulminating, and toxic dilatation of the colon with exacerbation of systemic and abdominal symptoms may occur at any time.

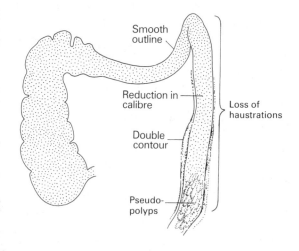

Fig. 32.13 Radiological changes of ulcerative colitis seen on barium enema

Smooth outline

Reduction in calibre

Double contour

Pseudo-polyps

Loss of haustrations

Treatment

Medical treatment

Initial treatment of an attack of ulcerative colitis relies on medical measures. With fluid replacement, correction of anaemia, adequate nutrition and steroid therapy, 97% of patients survive their initial attack, but 70% are destined to have further attacks. Long-term treatment with sulfasalazine (0.5–1 g orally every 6 hours) has been shown to reduce the incidence of relapse. Topical steroids (administered as suppositories or prednisone retention enemas) will usually control mild attacks, but systemic steroids (prednisone 10–15 mg orally every 6 hours) are needed during an acute relapse.

Some 15% of patients eventually require surgery, which may be elective or emergency. It has been calculated that 1 in 50 patients with mild proctitis, 1 in 20 with moderate colitis and 1 in 3 with extensive disease will come to surgery.

Indications for elective surgery

Failure to thrive. Failure to thrive despite adequate medical management is reflected in retardation of growth and sexual development in children, and by malnourishment and anaemia in adults.

Anorectal complications. These occur in almost 20% of cases and include recurrent abscesses and fistulas. They usually remit following removal of the affected colon.

Benign strictures. Less than 10% of patients develop benign strictures and half of these are found in the rectum. Stricture is due to submucosal fibrosis and causes acute or subacute obstruction. Strictures are more common in Crohn's disease and that diagnosis must be considered. Carcinoma must also be excluded. Colonoscopy may be useful in clarifying the diagnosis when the stricture is outwith the reach of the sigmoidoscope.

Polyp formation. Severe polyp formation with the typical 'sea-wrack' appearance indicates that the bowel is likely to be permanently and severely involved.

Carcinoma. The risk of developing carcinoma of the large bowel is greatly increased by ulcerative colitis. At least 10% of patients who have had colitis for 10 years and 20% of those who have had it for 20 years develop cancer. Malignant change is more likely in patients with extensive disease and those with early-onset colitis. The average age of development of cancer in patients with colitis is 43 years, compared to 63 years in the general population.

The detection of malignant change is difficult as the symptoms remain those of colitis. Patients with longstanding disease should be screened annually by colonoscopy and biopsy of any suspicious lesion, or by sigmoidoscopy and regular barium enema studies to detect early signs of stenosis. Carcinoma in ulcerative colitis is usually poorly differentiated and has a poor prognosis.

Systemic complications. A variety of systemic complications occur in ulcerative colitis. These include erythema nodosum, pyoderma granulosum, eye lesions, hepatitis and cirrhosis of the liver, sclerosing cholangitis, and ankylosing spondylitis. Provided permanent changes have not occurred, removal of the colon leads to resolution of some of these associated systemic disorders.

The procedure. The patient is prepared as outlined earlier in this chapter, except that mechanical bowel cleansing with enemas is usually avoided. The classical approach is to remove the large bowel including the rectum (panproctocolectomy) and create an ileostomy. Great care is taken to protect the parasympathetic and sympathetic nerves in the sacral plexus by dissecting as close as possible to the rectum. In the rare cases shown to have only segmental disease on barium enema and a histologically normal rectum, the rectum may be left in situ and an ileorectal anastomosis performed. However, even in such cases it is safer to perform an ileostomy and bring the proximal end of the rectal stump to the surface as a mucus fistula. If subsequent sigmoidoscopy shows no evidence of continuing rectal disease, an ileorectal anastomosis can be used to restore continuity and continence. Sigmoidoscopy is still carried out regularly to check that the rectal stump is not becoming involved.

In recent years there has been a trend to preserve the anal sphincters and form a 'pouch' of the terminal ileum by anastomosing loops in a 'J' or 'W' fashion, which is then anastomosed to the anal canal. The colon and proximal rectum are removed in the normal way. The mucosa of the distal rectum is dissected off the remainder of the rectal wall using a transanal approach, and the prepared pouch is brought down through the rectal tube for anastomosis to the anal canal. A temporary ileostomy is fashioned to protect the anastomosis until healing has been demonstrated by Gastrografin enema.

Such procedures are associated with significant early postoperative morbidity and are best performed in specialized centres. By one year after operation most patients will be fully continent, but will pass on average five to six motions per day. This procedure should therefore be reserved for younger fit patients who wish to avoid an ileostomy. It is contraindicated in patients with Crohn's colitis.

If surgery is undertaken in patients with malignant change, the resection is more extensive in that regional lymph nodes are also removed.

Indications for urgent and emergency surgery

Acute fulminating ulcerative colitis. This refers to a florid initial attack during which there is marked deterioration in the patient's symptoms associated with pyrexia and toxaemia. Medical treatment should always be tried first, but if aggressive therapy fails to control the disease or there is no significant improvement within five days, urgent surgery is indicated.

Toxic megacolon. Acute dilatation of the colon affects 5% of patients with ulcerative colitis. It may occur during any attack and is associated with abdominal distension, local or diffuse tenderness, feeble or absent bowel sounds and cramping abdominal pain. A plain X-ray shows dilatation of the colon, which is usually most evident in the transverse colon. Although one may try to persist with conservative treatment, most advise urgent operation. Metronidazole has recently been used in its treatment in addition to standard medical measures.

Perforation. This complication also occurs in 5% of patients. It is most commonly associated with toxic dilatation of the colon, complicating one-third of such cases. Perforation is notoriously difficult to diagnose but should be suspected when there is rapid deterioration despite vigorous medical treatment. Abdominal pain and guarding may be absent. Free gas on a plain abdominal X-ray is diagnostic. Surgery is indicated as soon as perforation is suspected.

Massive bleeding. This is a rare indication for emergency surgery.

The technique. Emergency colectomy and total proctocolectomy carry a high operative mortality (20%). It is usual to leave the rectal stump as a mucous fistula and remove it subsequently if active disease persists. In severely ill patients with toxic megacolon, ileostomy with decompression of the sigmoid and transverse colon by establishing colostomies is reported to carry a lower mortality than subtotal colectomy with ileostomy; most surgeons still favour colectomy.

CROHN'S DISEASE

Although it was originally believed that Crohn's disease affected predominantly the terminal ileum, it is now recognized that it can occur in any part of the gastrointestinal tract. Both small and large bowel are affected in one-half of all cases and in a further quarter the large bowel alone is affected. The large bowel is usually affected segmentally, with thickening of the bowel wall and fissuring of the mucosa to produce a cobblestone appearance.

Histologically the most reliable feature is the occurrence of granulomas, although these are not invariable. In 50% of cases the rectum is involved by the disease and 70% of these patients have anal lesions. Fistula-in-ano, abscesses and fissures are much commoner in Crohn's disease than in ulcerative colitis. Anal ulceration appears to be specific to Crohn's disease with rectal involvement. There is some evidence that carcinoma is more frequent in a colon affected by Crohn's disease.

Clinical features

The clinical features of Crohn's disease are similar to those of ulcerative colitis. However, diarrhoea is usually less severe, abdominal pain is more common, and tenderness, an abdominal mass and internal or external fistulas are more frequent signs. If the rectum is involved, sigmoidoscopy may reveal the typical cobblestone appearance or patchy ulceration. On barium enema the lesions may be separated by normal bowel ('skip lesions') and show irregularity of the mucosa, rigidity of the bowel and fine radiating spikes due to fissuring. Internal fistulas are common in Crohn's disease but do not occur in ulcerative colitis.

As in about half of all cases the small bowel is also affected, a small bowel enema or barium meal and follow-through examination should also be carried out. Rectal biopsy alone may not add useful information. Biopsy during colonoscopy is more helpful and may be used to assess the extent of the disease.

Although less common than in ulcerative colitis, toxic dilatation is a recognized complication of Crohn's disease. Carcinoma of the colon is a rare complication of longstanding disease.

Treatment

Medical treatment

Every attempt is made to correct anaemia and malnourishment. There are no specific therapeutic agents available for the treatment of Crohn's disease. Recent controlled trials have confirmed that the response of active symptomatic disease to prednisone (20–60 mg daily by mouth) or sulfasalazine (3–4 g daily by mouth) is significantly better than that to placebo. In general, patients with large bowel Crohn's disease are more likely to respond to sulfasalazine (the compound is metabolized by colonic bacteria to its active principals sulfapyridine and 5-aminosalicylate), whereas those with small bowel disease are more likely to respond to steroids. Combination of the two drugs does not appear to confer benefit, and neither agent is capable of preventing relapse or recurrence once the disease has become quiescent or has been treated surgically.

Indications for surgery

Failure to thrive. In some cases chronic ill-health with intractable symptoms demands operation. In others a severe exacerbation of the disease may fail to respond to medical treatment and surgery then offers the only hope of inducing a remission. The incidence of cancer in the colon affected by Crohn's disease is not sufficiently high to merit surgery as a prophylactic measure.

Obstruction. This is due to cicatricial stenosis. It usually develops insidiously, presenting as subacute or intermittent obstruction.

Perforation. Perforation occurs in about 20% of patients with large bowel Crohn's disease, but preceding fibrosis and adhesions tend to limit spread and result in a walled-off abscess. The patient presents with a swinging temperature, toxaemia, local tenderness, and sometimes a palpable mass. Free perforation of the colon resulting in faecal peritonitis is rare, but an abscess may secondarily rupture into the peritoneal cavity to produce purulent peritonitis.

An abscess can also perforate into a neighbouring viscus to form an internal fistula. The presence of a fistula between loops of intestine is almost diagnostic of Crohn's disease and sudden development of diarrhoea strongly suggests such fistula formation.

While an abscess may resolve with antibiotic therapy, surgical drainage may be required. This results in an enterocutaneous fistula unless the affected segment of bowel is also resected.

Fistula. Formation of a fistula, either enterocutaneous or entero-enteral, occurs in 20% of patients with small and large bowel Crohn's disease and in 10% of those with large bowel disease alone.

Most fistulas eventually require surgery. Immunosuppressive therapy with azathioprine is now rarely used. Preoperative preparation with parenteral nutrition is a valuable means of restoring nutritional status before surgery.

Patients with colonic fistula can be fed an elemental diet that is completely absorbed in the upper gastrointestinal tract. The management of colovesical fistula has been discussed on p. 497. Early surgery is indicated to avoid chronic urinary tract infection and impairment of renal function.

Principles of surgery for Crohn's disease

The main aim of surgical treatment for Crohn's disease is conservation and differs from that of ulcerative colitis in that the ileum is more commonly resected and the rectum spared. Ileorectal anastomosis is associated with a high incidence of

breakdown and leakage, and it may be advisable to perform a temporary ileostomy. In patients with obstruction, ileostomy is usually advised.

If only a small segment of colon is involved, it may be possible to resect this locally, together with a margin of approximately 10 cm of normal bowel. A primary anastomosis may be performed, but if there is any doubt about involvement of the ends by the disease, they are better exteriorized. Bowel which has perforated or fistulated must be excised. The extent of the resection depends on the site and extent of involvement.

PSEUDOMEMBRANOUS COLITIS

This condition was once believed to be due to superinfection of the bowel with staphylococci, but it is now known that *Clostridium difficile* is more commonly the organism responsible.

Pseudomembranous colitis is associated with the use of oral antibiotics, particularly clindamycin and lincomycin. There is necrosis of the mucous membrane of the colon associated with profuse watery diarrhoea, toxaemia, shock and collapse. The stools are watery green, foul-smelling and often blood-stained and contain fragments of pseudomembrane (mucosal sloughs). The pseudomembrane is usually evident on sigmoidoscopy and the diagnosis is confirmed by histological examination. The diagnosis is confirmed by demonstration of the toxin of *Cl. difficile* in the stool or in pseudomembrane obtained by rectal biopsy. Treatment consists of intravenous fluid replacement and vancomycin. Both staphylococci and clostridia are sensitive to vancomycin and it is not absorbed in the small bowel.

OTHER INFLAMMATORY CONDITIONS OF THE LARGE BOWEL

Hypertrophic tuberculous colitis

This condition is rare except in the tropics and Asia. The wall of the colon becomes thickened due to granulomatous infiltration, fibrosis and caseation. Stricture may occur and the mucosa may appear cobblestoned and ulcerated.

The patient usually presents with abdominal

pain, alteration in bowel habit and occasional passage of blood and mucus. A mass may be palpable in the right iliac fossa. The disease must be differentiated from Crohn's disease and from carcinoma. The treatment of choice is antituberculous chemotherapy, but resection is often the only way of excluding carcinoma. Antituberculous chemotherapy is commenced if tuberculosis is confirmed histologically.

Infections of the large bowel with *Schistosoma mansoni* (bilharzia), *Entamoeba histolytica* or *Chlamydia* (lymphogranuloma venereum) all result in inflammation which may progress to stricture formation and require surgical resection.

Irradiation proctitis

External and internal radiation for the treatment of cancer of the cervix or bladder can result in proctocolitis. An acute granular proctitis occurs as an early reaction and can lead to delayed ulceration, stricture formation and a rectovaginal fistula. Loose stools, tenesmus, urgency, pain and bleeding are typical clinical features.

On sigmoidoscopy the changes are most prominent on the anterior wall of the rectum and may be confined to this area. In early cases topical steroids may give symptomatic relief, but resection of the rectum or defunctioning colostomy is usually indicated if stricture or fistula formation have occurred.

VOLVULUS

Volvulus denotes rotation of a loop of bowel and its mesentery around a fixed point. It results in closed loop obstruction of the rotated loop and also obstruction of the proximal bowel. The circulation to the involved loop is impaired, and strangulation with gangrene may follow. The sigmoid colon is the commonest part of the intestinal tract to be affected, but unusual mobility of the right colon may also allow volvulus of the caecum and terminal ileum.

Sigmoid volvulus is common because of the proximity of the limbs of the sigmoid loop at their point of fixation to the pelvic brim, and because of the solid and relatively heavy contents of this part of the gut. The condition is particularly common in countries where diets rich in roughage are consumed, e.g. Africa, Eastern Europe, Russia. The bowel usually rotates in an anticlockwise direction (Fig. 32.14).

The patient presents with symptoms of large bowel obstruction, i.e. colicky pain, constipation and distension. Distension is asymmetrical and the outline of the distended colon may be visible. A plain X-ray shows a grossly distended sigmoid

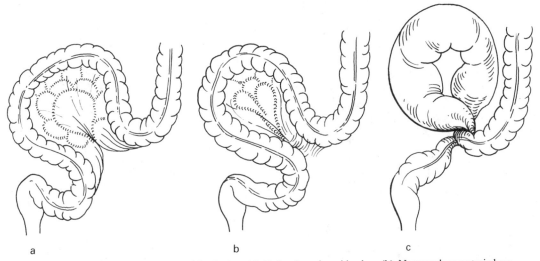

a   b   c

Fig. 32.14 Stages in the development of sigmoid volvulus. (a) Redundant sigmoid colon. (b) Narrowed mesenteric base. (c) Volvulus

loop rising out of the pelvis to occupy the whole of the abdominal cavity. Multiple fluid levels may also be present in the distended proximal large and small bowel.

Deflation of the twisted sigmoid colon is attempted by sigmoidoscopy and passage of a soft well-lubricated rectal tube. Successful passage of the tube through the twist results in rapid decompression. The tube is left in situ for 48 hours and is gently irrigated to prevent its blockage.

If the tube cannot be passed or if there are signs suggesting strangulation, laparotomy is performed. If the loop is necrotic, it is resected and the ends of the colon are exteriorized for later restoration of continuity. If the bowel is not strangulated, the decision to resect depends on the general condition of the patient. Guiding the rectal tube into the distended loop may be all that is required in patients unfit for more major surgery. As volvulus of the sigmoid colon has a 40% recurrence rate, definitive treatment by *elective* sigmoid colectomy should be performed wherever possible.

MEGACOLON

Hirschsprung's disease

This congenital condition affects 1 in 5000 babies. It is due to an absence of ganglion cells in Auerbach's and Meissner's plexus of the large bowel so that there is loss of peristalsis in the affected segment. Usually, the distal large bowel is affected over a short segment of 5–20 cm, but occasionally longer segments and even the whole large bowel may be involved. Bowel proximal to the affected segment becomes grossly distended.

Hirschsprung's disease may present as neonatal large bowel obstruction, which must be differentiated from meconium ileus. Digital examination of the rectum may result in initial apparent 'cure', but the condition recurs either immediately or later in childhood and causes constipation with gross gaseous distension. Ischaemic colitis may complicate the disease and must be differentiated from ulcerative colitis.

In children, Hirschsprung's disease must be distinguished from acquired megacolon due to chronic constipation (Fig. 32.15). Barium enema (which is performed without preparation) shows a dilated segment above the narrowed aganglionic distal segment. Histological confirmation and assessment of the limit of the abnormal area can be made by a full thickness rectal biopsy. It should be noted that ganglia are normally absent for about 1.5 cm above the anal verge.

In neonates, treatment consists of irrigation of the bowel with saline solution followed by an operation designed to bring ganglionated bowel down to the anal verge. This is carried out at the

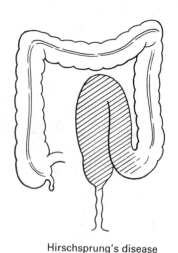

Hirschsprung's disease

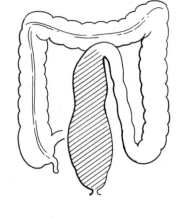

Acquired megacolon

Fig. 32.15 Radiological appearance on barium enema of Hirschsprung's disease and acquired megacolon

age of about 6 weeks. In older children presenting with obstruction, a preliminary colostomy is followed by definitive operation some 3 months later.

Acquired megacolon

Chronic constipation in childhood may result in *acquired megacolon* and *megarectum*. The initial complaint may be of faecal soiling. On abdominal examination, the large bowel is full of palpable faeces, and rectal examination reveals faeces in a dilated rectum. Although it may be associated with enuresis, and psychological or psychiatric upset, chronic constipation is more commonly the result of bad toilet training or the presence of an anal fissure.

The aim of treatment is to keep the large bowel and rectum empty so that normal muscular tone can be regained. This requires faecal disimpaction under general anaesthesia and regular colonic washouts.

Megacolon due to neurotoxicity may complicate vincristine therapy.

ISCHAEMIC COLITIS

The chief causes of ischaemic colitis are summarized in Figure 32.16. The vascular supply to the large intestine may be impaired by:

1. operative division of its main feeding vessels, e.g. of the inferior mesenteric artery during resection of an abdominal aortic aneurysm, or the middle colic artery during resection of the stomach or pancreas;

2. spontaneous occlusion of a main artery by atherosclerosis or embolic disease;

3. occlusion of the small mesenteric vessels due to distal arterial disease or to an episode of hypotension-associated diminished perfusion; or

4. mesenteric venous thrombosis, often affecting small veins.

Provided the arterial system is healthy, occlusion of one main vessel is unlikely to have any untoward effects. However, if the circulation is already compromised by atherosclerosis, ischaemic changes may occur. These may be unremitting or transient.

If unremitting, the large bowel becomes gangrenous, leading to perforation and peritonitis. This is an emergency necessitating urgent operation.

Transient ischaemia results in abdominal pain, diarrhoea and bleeding. Sigmoidoscopy may show friable, oedematous and granular mucosa, starting above the level reached by the rectal blood supply, i.e. 12–15 cm from the anal verge.

Barium enema will demonstrate a narrowed segment with an irregular contour, sacculation and

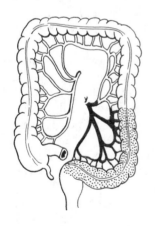

Operative division
of main vessel

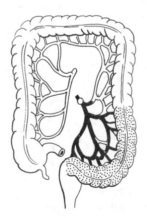

Spontaneous occlusion
by embolus or thrombus
of main vessel

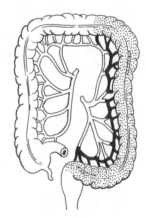

Occlusion of small
mesenteric vessels

Fig. 32.16   Causes of ischaemic colitis

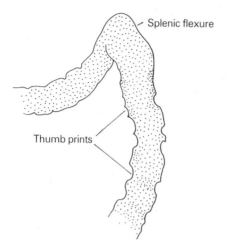

Fig. 32.17 Radiological appearance on barium enema of ischaemic colitis

'thumb-printing' due to oedematous change in the mucosa. This is most commonly seen at the junction between superior and inferior mesenteric blood supplies close to the splenic flexure (Fig. 32.17).

These changes may either resolve or proceed to the formation of a fibrous stricture, which may cause a delayed obstruction.

POLYPS

Polyps of the large intestine are common and take several forms. They may be inflammatory (as in ulcerative colitis), hamartomatous (as in Peutz-Jeghers syndrome) or neoplastic (adenomas or papillomas). While single polyps do occur, most are multiple.

Juvenile polyps

These hamartomas are found in children (usually under the age of 10 years) and are mostly single. They are commonest in the rectum and sigmoid colon. The polyps are pedunculated, and consist of a vascular core with an inflammatory cell infiltrate which is covered by normal mucosa. Symptoms arise because of bleeding due to torsion of the pedicle or as a result of surface trauma, and because of prolapse of the polyp through the anus. The polyps should be removed by snaring and

dividing the pedicle at colonoscopy. The polyps recur in about 10% but there is no risk of malignancy.

Peutz-Jeghers syndrome

This is a congenital abnormality characterized by brown or blue pigmented spots on the lips, buccal mucosa, fingers and toes, and multiple hamartomatous polyps throughout the whole of the gastrointestinal tract. The polyps may be sessile or pedunculated, and the abnormal muscularis mucosae forms a tree-like structure covered by normal epithelium. As the polyps are not true neoplasms, there is no potential for malignant change. They may cause symptoms through bleeding or intussusception, and local resection may then be required.

Adenomatous polyps

These are true neoplasms, accounting for 90% of neoplastic polyps of the colon. They vary from small sessile seed-like excrescences to large pedunculated masses several centimetres in diameter. They are most commonly pedunculated. Histologically they are formed by a mass of glandular tubules fed by a central fibrovascular core and covered by a mucous membrane of varying degrees of differentiation. In approximately one-third of cases the polyps are multiple. Their distribution is similar to that of carcinoma: about 80% are found in the sigmoid colon or rectum.

It is estimated that at least 5% of the normal population have adenomatous polyps in the colon. Most of these are symptomless, but rectal bleeding, intussusception and prolapse through the anus can occur. Over one-third of polyps can be seen at sigmoidoscopy. Air-contrast barium enema will reveal others, provided they are over 0.5 cm in size. Colonoscopy is used both for diagnosis and to remove the polyp by diathermy snare.

The risk of malignant change increases with polyp size. While only 1% of polyps under 1 cm in diameter undergo malignant change, the comparable figure for polyps over 1 cm is 5%. Thus all polyps over 1 cm in size should be removed. Histological examination includes a search for malignant change and for invasion of the stalk.

Polyp formation signals that the mucosa is liable to develop further polyps or carcinoma, and these patients must be followed up by regular air-contrast barium enema studies or colonoscopy for the rest of their lives.

In view of the distribution of adenomatous polyps and their propensity for malignant change, it has been suggested that most cases of carcinoma of the colon develop from pre-existing polyps. Satellite polyps are present in one-third of patients with carcinoma of the large bowel. It is for this reason that some surgeons recommend colonoscopy with prophylactic removal of polyps even when they are asymptomatic.

Villous adenoma

This tumour accounts for 10% of neoplastic polyps of the large bowel. It is most commonly found in the rectum and sigmoid colon and only rarely in the caecum and ascending colon. It forms a soft shaggy sessile growth which spreads to involve a considerable area of mucosa (Fig. 32.18). The central connective tissue core bears numerous frond-like branches covered with colonic mucosa. It is generally accepted that this is a premalignant lesion; invasive cancer is found in at least 30% of cases.

Rectal bleeding is a late symptom and suggests malignant change. Typically there is excessive

mucus secretion and a troublesome mucous discharge. Some patients present with dehydration, hypokalaemia, weakness, oliguria and alkalosis due to excess loss of mucus. If in the rectum, the villous adenoma will be palpable and is seen through the sigmoidoscope as a coarsely granular or shaggy plum-coloured area of mucosa. Areas of induration should raise the suspicion of malignant change. Villous adenomas of the colon are diagnosed by barium enema and colonoscopy. Biopsy is undertaken to confirm the diagnosis, but a report of benign tumour does not exclude cancer, as malignant change is usually focal. For this reason all villous adenomas should be excised.

Rectal adenomas can be removed through the anus with diathermy provided they are not too large. For large tumours, a formal posterior approach to the rectum is required. The rectal wall is split and the tumour is excised with surrounding mucosa (Fig. 32.19). The finding of invasive cancer is an indication for formal resection of the affected portion of bowel.

Familial polyposis

This rare hereditary disease is transmitted by an autosomal dominant gene. Thus males and females are at equal risk, and the chances are that half the children of a given family will be affected. The genetic abnormality is always expressed, so that the disease is transmitted only by those who suffer from it. Sessile and pedunculated adenomas develop during childhood in the large bowel. There may be a few scattered lesions or many hundreds of adenomas. The rectum is almost always involved. Symptoms usually develop between the ages of 10 and 15 years, and consist principally of rectal bleeding, diarrhoea and mucus discharge. Malignant change is inevitable in individuals who develop polyposis but is virtually unknown before the age of 20 years.

Familial polyposis is treated by total colectomy. At one time most surgeons also removed the rectum and established an ileostomy, but the current trend is to preserve the rectum and perform an ileorectal anastomosis. The rectum is freed from polyps by diathermy and kept under permanent surveillance by sigmoidoscopy because the risk of

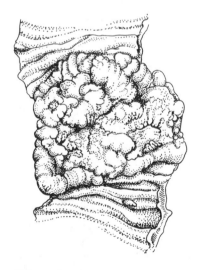

Fig. 32.18 Villous adenoma

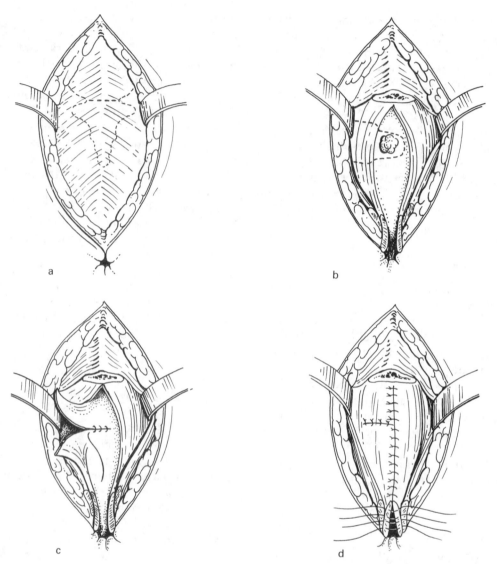

Fig. 32.19   Removal of a large rectal adenoma via a posterior (transphincteric) approach. (a) Exposure. (b) Anal sphincter divided (the interrupted line indicates the extent of tumour excision). (c) Closure of defect in rectal wall. (d) Individual layers of sphincter carefully rejoined

malignancy remains. It is essential to examine all other members of the family so that those with polyposis can be treated before cancer supervenes. The ideal time for operation is around school-leaving age.

Gardner's syndrome is a related condition in which sebaceous cysts, dermoid cysts, bony exostosis and connective tissue tumours are found in association with multiple adenomas. The incidence is one-tenth that of familial polyposis.

CARCINOMA OF THE COLON AND RECTUM

Carcinoma of the colon and rectum is second only to lung cancer as a cause of death from cancer in Western society. Scotland has the highest incidence of colorectal cancer in the world. Within its population of 5 million there are 39 new cases per 100 000 population each year and 1800 deaths each year.

It is predominantly a disease of older people and is uncommon before the age of 40, although the young are not immune. Overall, males and females have an equal chance of developing the disease. However, there is a sex difference in its distribution. Cancer of the rectum is more common in males while cancer of the caecum is more common in females. This suggests that the aetiology of these two conditions is different.

Two-thirds of large bowel cancers originate in the rectum and sigmoid colon, 10% occur in the caecum, and the remainder are distributed through the rest of the large bowel (Fig. 32.20). It is a multifocal disease; 3% of cases have synchronous tumours elsewhere, while 1% of patients will develop a further tumour of the colon with each 10 years of follow-up.

Aetiology

Cancer of the large bowel is rare in Africa, the Orient and South America. Its incidence parallels that of coronary artery disease and breast cancer. Environmental factors are considered to be im-

portant. It is suggested that diets low in fibre and bulk are associated with a higher incidence of the disease. A high dietary fibre content increases the speed of intestinal transit so that any carcinogen in the diet and faeces will be in contact with the mucosa for a shorter time. The high incidence of cancer of the sigmoid colon and rectum supports the theory that a contact carcinogen is involved. Bile salts are also thought to be implicated, and clostridia and coliform organisms with dehydrogenating activity can convert bile salts to carcinogenic sterols.

Other factors associated with large bowel cancer include ulcerative colitis, adenomatous polyps, familial polyposis and villous adenoma (see above).

Pathology

Three gross types of tumour are described: polypoidal, ulcerating and stenosing (Fig. 32.21). Infiltrating tumours spread circumferentially to cause an annular 'napkin ring' or 'string' stricture. The lesions are adenocarcinomas derived from the columnar epithelium of the bowel and show a wide spectrum of differentiation. A small proportion have a colloid or gelatinous structure; these lesions tend to occur in younger patients and are associated with a poor prognosis.

The cancer may spread by the following routes.

1. *Direct spread* occurs circumferentially and radially in the bowel wall. The muscle coats are penetrated and perforation may occur.

2. *Transperitoneal spread* occurs when tumour cells liberated into the peritoneal cavity form seedling deposits in the peritoneum.

3. *Lymphatic spread* leads to nodal involvement in 40% of all cases coming to operation. The affected nodes lie in the mesocolon and para-aortic region.

4. *Spread via the blood stream* gives rise to overt liver metastases in 10–20% of patients coming to operation.

Classification of tumour. Carcinoma of the large bowel can be divided into four stages using a modification of Duke's classification (Table 32.1). More detailed classifications have been devised, e.g. the TNM system, but these are not commonly used.

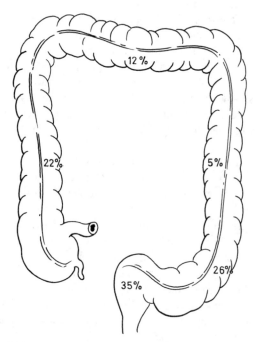

Fig. 32.20 Cancer of the colon: tumour distribution within the colon

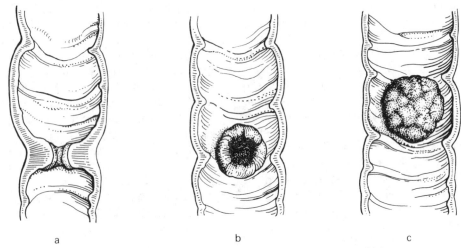

a   b   c

Fig. 32.21 Pathological types of large bowel cancer. (a) Stenosing. (b) Ulcerating. (c) Polypoidal

Table 32.1 Stages of cancer of the large bowel (modified Dukes' classification)

Stage	Definition
A	Growth confined to bowel wall
B	Spread through bowel wall
C	Involvement of regional lymph nodes
C_1	Few nodes involved near primary growth but some glands in chain free from metastases below the ligature on main regional vessels
C_2	Continuous string of nodes containing metastases right up to ligature on main regional vessels
D	Distant metastases

As might be expected, tumours of category A have the best prognosis. However, neither this classification nor the histological features of the tumour allow an accurate prognosis in individual patients. Tumour resectability is also an important prognostic indicator and is determined by the degree of local extension and fixation.

Clinical features

The key clinical features of carcinoma of the colon are alteration of bowel habit and bleeding from the rectum. The nature and degree of these complaints depends on the site of the tumour.

Right colon. As the contents of the caecum and ascending colon are fluid, altered bowel function or obstructive symptoms are associated only with large tumours. In most patients there is at most mild diarrhoea. Chronic blood loss, although usually unrecognized by the patient, causes anaemia and there is deterioration in general health and loss of weight. Vague right iliac fossa pain may be present and a mass may be palpable.

Left colon. As the left colon is narrower and has more solid contents, obstruction is relatively common. Increasing constipation (requiring progressively larger doses of aperients) and alternating bouts of diarrhoea are characteristic. Distension, audible borborygmi and colicky pain are common, and blood and mucus are often passed per rectum. The patient may feel unwell and lose weight.

Rectum. Bleeding is a prominent feature of rectal carcinoma. The patient often believes that he has piles and it is only on complete examination that the cause of the bleeding is found to lie higher in the rectum. The presence of a tumour in the rectum causes persistent bowel symptoms. A classical feature is early morning diarrhoea. This is spurious diarrhoea in that the patient experiences the desire to defaecate but passes only a little slime and blood. This may be repeated several times before a motion is passed and some relief obtained. Urgency, tenesmus and a feeling of incomplete evacuation of the bowel are also common symptoms. The general health may remain good.

Complications

Cancer of the colon may present with intestinal obstruction (20% of cases), perforation (10%), formation of enterocolic or vesicocolic fistula, or massive bleeding (rare). Although chronic bleeding from a carcinoma is the rule, serious and life-threatening haemorrhage rarely occurs.

Investigation

Almost half the patients will have a palpable mass at the time of presentation, either on abdominal or rectal examination. One-third of colorectal cancers lie within reach of a finger on rectal examination. As half of all colorectal tumours lie in the rectum, sigmoidoscopy is an essential investigation in all patients with altered bowel habit or rectal bleeding, and mandatory in patients who complain of piles.

Barium enema examination complements sigmoidoscopy. The tumour appears as a short irregular filling defect with shouldering where it meets normal bowel. Even if a rectal cancer is discovered on direct examination, it is important to examine the bowel radiologically after a barium enema to exclude a second tumour situated more proximally.

Liver function tests, liver scans and chest X-rays are necessary to exclude overt metastases. If the tumour is likely to be close to the ureter, an intravenous urogram should be obtained.

All tumours within reach of the sigmoidoscope are biopsied. For others, a colonoscopic biopsy is performed if the diagnosis is in doubt.

Treatment

Intra-abdominal spread and resectability can only be assessed adequately at laparotomy. This is required in all cases except those who are unfit for general anaesthesia and in whom there is no obstruction. The operation performed depends on the condition of the patient and the site and extent of the tumour. For tumours in the caecum, ascending or transverse colon, a right hemicolectomy or extended right hemicolectomy with ileocolic anastomosis is carried out (Fig. 32.22). More distal colonic lesions are resected by left hemicolectomy

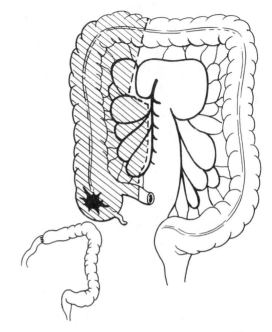

Fig. 32.22 Right hemicolectomy for carcinoma of the caecum

or sigmoid colectomy, removing as much of the regional lymphatic supply as practicable.

Cancers of the upper third of the rectum are treated by resection of the sigmoid colon and upper rectum, with anastomosis of the colon to the rectal stump. Carcinoma of the middle third of the rectum can usually be sufficiently mobilized to allow anterior resection with primary anastomosis between the proximal sigmoid colon and lower rectum (Fig. 32.23). If bowel preparation is inadequate or the integrity of the anastomosis in doubt, a temporary proximal colostomy may be performed to prevent leakage.

Carcinomas of the lower third of the rectum are usually treated by a combined abdominal and perineal approach (abdominoperineal resection) in which the rectum including the anal canal is completely removed. The pelvic colon is then brought to the surface as a permanent colostomy. In females the posterior vaginal wall may be removed with the rectum. In males, care must be taken not to damage the urethra or prostate. Damage to autonomic nerves in the presacral or pelvic plexus is unavoidable in many cases.

At one time carcinomas lower than 12 cm from

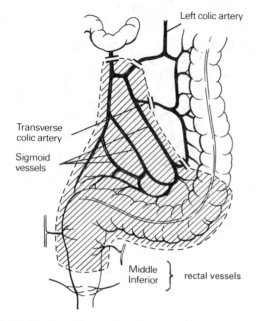

Fig. 32.23 Anterior resection of rectum for carcinoma of the middle third of the rectum

the anal verge were treated routinely by abdomino-perineal resection. However, modern stapling guns allow much lower anastomosis so that even tumours lying as low as 7 cm from the anus can now be removed by anterior resection. There may also be a place for local diathermy in the treatment of some well-differentiated rectal cancers, avoiding the need for either extensive operation or permanent colostomy.

Prognosis

The overall operative mortality in patients with large bowel cancer used to be around 10% but better results are now achieved in specialist centres. Elective procedures carry an operative mortality below 5%, whereas the operative mortality of emergency surgery is 20%.

The overall 5-year survival of patients with large bowel cancer barely reaches 25%. Approximately 50% of patients have resectable lesions and half of these patients will be alive 5 years after operation. Survival is related to the Dukes stage of the tumour, and varies from 80% at 5 years in those without lymph node involve-

ment (Dukes A and B) to 30% in those with metastases in lymph nodes. If distant metastases are present, survival rarely exceeds 1–2 years.

Pre- and postoperative radiotherapy have been employed in attempts to improve the results of surgery for rectal cancer, but the value of this approach is still controversial.

Radiotherapy can also be used in the palliation of large bowel cancer. Chemotherapy with 5-fluorouracil and nitrosoureas has proved disappointing, both in the treatment of advanced metastatic disease and as adjuvant systemic therapy in patients undergoing resection.

Presymptomatic diagnosis of large bowel cancer

There has been an improvement in survival rates following the increased public awareness of the potential significance of altered bowel habit and rectal bleeding. Measures to detect the disease in asymptomatic patients are also under study.

1. A haemoccult test may be used to detect occult blood in the faeces. The patient is given three cards impregnated with guaiac on which to place a smear of faeces on successive mornings. The cards are posted to the laboratory, where an oxidizing agent is added. This produces a blue colour if blood is present. Patients with positive tests are investigated further, initially to determine whether they are truly positive and thereafter by full sigmoidoscopic and barium enema examination of the colon. More specific and sensitive tests are under investigation.

2. In some American screening centres routine sigmoidoscopy, barium enema and colonoscopy are used to examine asymptomatic patients. Such investigations are costly and not generally available.

3. Carcinoembryonic antigen (CEA) is found in most adenomas and large bowel carcinomas, and serum concentrations are raised in a proportion of patients presenting with large bowel cancer. However, CEA has proved disappointing as a tumour marker for diagnostic purposes, being associated with a high false positive rate. Serial estimates may be more useful to detect recurrence following apparently curative bowel resection.

33. The appendix

Surgical anatomy

The appendix normally develops as a conical true diverticulum from the dependent pole of the caecum. Agenesis is rare. As a result of differential caecal growth during infancy the origin of the appendix is pushed medially until it eventually originates from the medial wall of the caecum some 2 cm below the ileocaecal junction (Fig. 33.1). The taeniae coli converge on the root of the appendix and so aid in its localization at laparotomy.

Despite its constant point of origin from the caecum, the position of the appendix varies greatly. In most individuals it lies behind the caecum or hangs down over the pelvic brim (Fig. 33.2). In 1–5% of subjects, the appendix lies in front of or behind the terminal ileum. Malrotation of the colon and complete situs inversus are uncommon developmental abnormalities in which the appendix is found in the upper abdomen or left iliac fossa. The position of the appendix has an important influence on the clinical picture of appendicitis.

The appendix is lined by colonic epithelium and has no known function in man. The development of lymphoid tissue in its wall during childhood suggests that it may then have an immunological function. The lymphoid tissue regresses in adolescence. The appendix lumen is frequently obliterated by fibrosis in older patients.

ACUTE APPENDICITIS

Incidence

Acute appendicitis is predominantly a disease of Western civilization and is uncommon in Africa and Asia. The condition may be becoming more common in developing countries because of their adoption of low-residue Western-style diets. Its incidence in Britain has fallen dramatically over the past 30 years.

Acute appendicitis remains the commonest abdominal surgical emergency in childhood, adolescence and early adult life. Less than 2% of cases occur in infants under 2 years; the incidence is highest during the second and third decades of

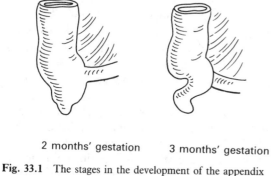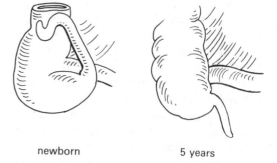

| 2 months' gestation | 3 months' gestation | newborn | 5 years |

Fig. 33.1 The stages in the development of the appendix

513

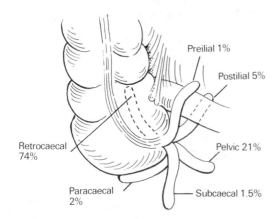

Preilial 1%

Postilial 5%

Retrocaecal
74%

Pelvic 21%

Paracaecal
2%

Subcaecal 1.5%

Fig. 33.2   Variations in the position of the appendix

life. Thereafter it declines and less than 5% of cases occur in patients over 60 years.

Aetiology

A combination of stasis and infection is required to produce experimental appendicitis. The typical onset with abdominal colic suggests that obstruction is a major factor in man. Obstruction causes accumulation of secretion and distension, leading to pressure necrosis of the mucosa and invasion of the wall by bacteria. The age of peak incidence of appendicitis parallels that of maximal development of lymphoid tissue. Lymphoid hyperplasia within the wall predisposes to obstruction in younger patients and may also account for the frequency of mesenteric adenitis at that age. In older patients inspissated faeces forming faecoliths are a major cause of obstruction. Less common causes of obstruction include kinks, adhesions and neoplasia. Appendicitis is not caused by specific bacteria. The majority of organisms concerned are normal gut inhabitants. Threadworms can produce signs and symptoms resembling mild appendicitis but are incriminated in only a few cases.

The inflammatory process may resolve spontaneously. More commonly, however, progressive infection and obstruction lead to impairment of blood supply. The antimesenteric border is most vulnerable, and patchy gangrene appears first in its midportion. Morbidity rises sharply once the blood supply has been compromised, and even before frank perforation occurs bacteria migrate

through the damaged wall into the peritoneal cavity. The increased morbidity of appendicitis in the elderly is partly explained by the more rapid development of gangrene and perforation.

Once perforation has occurred, the outcome depends on the ability of the omentum to contain the infection. If it can be contained, an appendix mass or abscess results; if not, generalized peritonitis ensues. The omentum is not fully developed in infants, and localization of infection is less effective than in older children and adults. However, in all age groups, *delay* in diagnosis and treatment remains the most important factor which worsens prognosis.

Clinical features

Many of the so-called 'typical' signs and symptoms of acute appendicitis are not always present or may appear only in the late stages of the disease. These vary according to the position of the appendix.

Symptoms

Pain is usually the first and most impressive symptom. In the 'typical' case, it begins as periumbilical colic which may be severe or amount to no more than an aching discomfort. The colic is a true *visceral* pain due to appendiceal obstruction. In children there may appear to be little wrong between the bouts of pain.

Classically, the pain remains periumbilical for several hours before shifting to the right iliac fossa. This shift denotes the development of *somatic* pain due to parietal peritonitis. This somatic pain is sharply localized, and causes discomfort on moving or coughing. In one-third to one-half of cases, the pain commences and remains in the right iliac fossa without preceding visceral pain. When the appendix is retrocaecal, somatic pain is perceived in the flank and loin rather than in the right iliac fossa. A pelvic appendix may not be associated with any somatic pain.

Anorexia is almost invariable. Hunger usually indicates that the patient does not have appendicitis. Nausea occurs in most patients and precedes vomiting which is seldom a prominent feature. Alteration of bowel habit may be noted.

Some patients complain of a sense of fullness and may have taken aperients in an attempt to gain relief; others have constipation which precedes the attack. Diarrhoea may occur in younger children and is a feature of pelvic appendicitis which irritates the neighbouring rectum.

Signs

Fever and tachycardia are *not* early signs of appendicitis. Pulse and temperature may not rise significantly until perforation has occurred. Foetor often accompanies appendicitis, but is not invariable and occurs in many other acute abdominal conditions.

The abdominal signs vary according to the position of the appendix. Tenderness and muscle guarding localized to the right iliac fossa are the most consistent findings. Tenderness is often maximal over McBurney's point (Fig. 33.3), which lies one-third of the way along a line drawn between the right anterior superior iliac spine and the umbilicus, and is associated with rebound tenderness and hyperaesthesia. Other signs include Rovsing's sign (pressure on the left iliac fossa producing right-sided pain) and the psoas sign (pain during passive extension of the right hip) but these are of doubtful value (see Ch. 29).

Retrocaecal appendicitis is notoriously difficult to diagnose in its early stages. Nausea, vomiting and diarrhoea may be the only symptoms. Perforation, abscess formation or the development of a mass may occur before diagnosis. Tenderness, if present, is maximal in the right flank or loin.

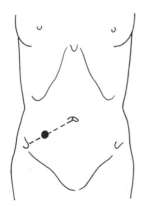

Fig. 33.3 McBurney's point

Pelvic appendicitis often produces little tenderness or guarding on abdominal examination, but tenderness is usually present on digital rectal examination.

Perforation of the appendix with diffuse peritonitis leads to generalized tenderness, guarding and rigidity. Even at this stage, tenderness is often still maximal in the right iliac fossa.

Bowel sounds are normal or only slightly reduced in frequency in the early stages of appendicitis.

In some cases a mass is palpable in the abdomen or on rectal examination. This inflammatory mass consists of omentum and neighbouring viscera which have adhered to the inflamed appendix.

Digital rectal examination reveals tenderness in approximately one-third of patients with appendicitis. It is a valuable means of detecting gynaecological causes of abdominal pain. If the faecal occult blood test is positive, an alternative diagnosis (neoplasia or Crohn's disease) should be considered.

Diagnosis

The diagnosis of acute appendicitis is essentially clinical and rests heavily on the finding of pain, tenderness and guarding in the right iliac fossa. Most patients have a polymorphonuclear leucocytosis of $10-15 \times 10^9/l$ on admission, but as this is a feature of many other causes of the acute abdomen it is not diagnostic. Urinalysis is usually normal in appendicitis, although a few pus cells and red cells may be present if the inflamed appendix lies adjacent to the ureter. Gross pyuria indicates primary urinary tract infection rather than appendicitis; while significant haematuria is more likely to be associated with a ureteric calculus. The range of differential diagnoses is wider in women than in men (see below). Females are more likely to have a normal appendix removed, especially between the ages of 15 and 20 years.

Plain abdominal X-rays are of value in diagnosis primarily as a means of excluding other causes of abdominal pain such as perforated peptic ulcer, ureteric calculi and intestinal obstruction. There are no pathognomic features of acute appendicitis but some patients have fluid levels in the right iliac fossa, a radio-opaque appendiceal faecolith (10%

of cases), increased soft tissue density in the right iliac fossa with obliteration of the psoas border, or gas bubbles in the region of the appendix (indicating perforation).

Acute appendicitis is seldom absent from the differential diagnosis of acute abdominal pain. Fortunately the majority of conditions which are confused with appendicitis also require laparotomy. However, 'medical' causes of abdominal pain such as basal pneumonia and diabetic ketosis, for which laparotomy is positively contraindicated, must be excluded. The diagnosis of acute appendicitis is notoriously difficult in the young and elderly, and this undoubtedly contributes to the high incidence of gangrene and perforation in these age groups.

Differential diagnosis

The following should be noted.

1. Central abdominal colic in the early stages of appendicitis may suggest gastroenteritis or mechanical intestinal obstruction. The key to the diagnosis of gastroenteritis is that nausea, vomiting and diarrhoea usually precede or accompany pain. Tenderness is seldom localized to the right iliac fossa and the patient may have symptoms of a viral illness, such as headache, myalgia and photophobia.

2. The clinical features of intestinal obstruction depend on the level of the obstructing lesion. High intestinal obstruction is characterized by profuse vomiting and relatively little abdominal distension, whereas low obstruction causes marked distension and late onset of vomiting. Regardless of the level of the lesion, tenderness is seldom localized to the right iliac fossa.

3. While right iliac fossa pain and tenderness are the most consistent clinical features, they can be produced by a large number of conditions, including mittleschmerz, acute mesenteric adenitis, acute terminal ileitis and inflammation of a Meckel's diverticulum. Although the presence of these conditions may be suspected clinically, all can mimic appendicitis closely, and laparotomy is usually indicated if pain and tenderness persist.

4. Acute salpingitis can produce right iliac fossa tenderness, but the condition is often bilateral and causes suprapubic or diffuse lower abdominal tenderness. Fever is usually higher in salpingitis than in appendicitis and the systemic upset is less marked than from a comparable fever in the late stages of appendicitis. Vaginal examination reveals a hot, tender cervix and a vaginal discharge is present in most cases of salpingitis.

5. Ureteric colic can be associated with pain and tenderness on deep palpation over the ureter, but the severity and radiation of the pain in the presence of haematuria usually indicate the true diagnosis. Abdominal X-rays and an intravenous urogram are likely to show the calculus.

6. Pelvic appendicitis may be simulated by salpingitis, diverticular disease or perforation of a colonic carcinoma. Differentiation between these colonic diseases and appendicitis may be difficult, especially when the sigmoid colon is redundant and lies in the right iliac fossa. As a general rule, tenderness is more diffuse and the involved colon may give rise to a palpable mass.

7. Retrocaecal appendicitis causes pain and tenderness which is higher and situated more posteriorly than usual, and may mimic perinephric abscess, acute pyelonephritis, perforated colon cancer or acute cholecystitis. High fever and chills are more typical of perinephric abscess and acute pyelonephritis than of appendicitis, and pyuria and costovertebral angle tenderness are usually present. Cholecystitis is associated with gallbladder tenderness and a positive Murphy's sign in most cases. Mild icterus and a palpable mass in the region of the gallbladder also suggest cholecystitis.

8. The presence of a mass in the right iliac fossa raises the question of intussusception in young children, acute terminal ileitis and Crohn's disease in older children and adults, ovarian cysts in women, and neoplasia of the bowel in older patients.

9. In patients who develop diffuse peritonitis as a result of appendicitis, the original site of infection may be difficult to define. However, tenderness may still be maximal in the right iliac fossa.

10. Perforated peptic ulcer can simulate appendicitis, particularly when escaping gastric and duodenal contents run down the right paracolic gutter and give rise to pain and tenderness in the right iliac fossa. Free perforation of the appendix

rarely produces radiological evidence of gas under the liver or diaphragm, in contrast to perforation of a peptic ulcer or perforated diverticular disease.

11. Acute pancreatitis can mimic appendicitis at all stages, but upper abdominal or diffuse pain in pancreatitis is associated with copious vomiting and retching, back pain, and hyperamylasaemia.

12. Ruptured ectopic pregnancy can also simulate all stages of appendicitis, beginning with cramping pain in the iliac fossa and proceeding to spreading pain and tenderness as blood disseminates throughout the peritoneal cavity. The true diagnosis may be suggested by a history of menstrual irregularity, vaginal bleeding and shoulder-tip pain which may be induced by elevation of the foot of the bed.

Problem areas in diagnosis

Appendicitis in infancy

Appendicitis in infancy is uncommon, diagnosis is difficult, and the average delay between onset and definitive diagnosis is around 4 days. This delay is reflected in the high incidence of positive radiological signs, abscess formation or generalized peritonitis at the time of surgery. These occur in virtually all infants under 1 year of age. Appendicitis is more common in children with Hirschsprung's disease.

In infants and young children, early appendicitis causes irritability and anorexia. Vomiting, pain, fever and loose bowel movements may develop as the disease progresses.

Clinical examination is difficult and tenderness cannot be localized readily. The development of fever in an infant, if associated with any abdominal tenderness, should always raise the suspicion of acute appendicitis.

Appendicitis during pregnancy

Acute appendicitis is as common in pregnant as in non-pregnant women (it complicates 1 in 2000 pregnancies) and should always be borne in mind when acute abdominal pain develops during pregnancy.

Early diagnosis is vital but difficult, especially in the third trimester, as the appendix is then dis-placed upwards by the gravid uterus so that pain and tenderness are higher than expected. Rectal or vaginal signs are absent. The white cell count is normally elevated in pregnancy and abdominal X-rays are usually contraindicated.

Delay is so harmful to mother and unborn child that, provided urinary tract infection has been excluded, operation should be carried out as early as possible. Maternal and fetal deaths do not result from appendicectomy but from peritonitis. The fetal mortality in uncomplicated appendicitis is 3%, that following perforation 30%. The incidence of appendicitis is uniform throughout pregnancy, although the risk of maternal mortality increases as pregnancy progresses.

Difficulty in diagnosis, reluctance to operate on pregnant women and avoidable delay account for the high risks of appendicitis in pregnancy.

Appendicitis in the elderly

Appendicitis has a more rapid course in the elderly. Gangrene and perforation are five times as common in patients over 60 years of age, primarily due to delay in diagnosis. The 'classical' features of appendicitis are often lacking, pain being a less prominent feature. Appendicitis may not even be considered as a cause of the patient's symptoms. Awareness of the rising incidence of appendicitis in the elderly, its atypical presentation and a willingness to undertake laparotomy promptly are the keys to successful management.

Appendicitis developing in hospital

Hospitalized patients are not immune to appendicitis and may develop the condition while undergoing investigation and treatment for unrelated medical conditions, or while recovering from other forms of surgery. Lack of awareness may cause avoidable delay in treatment.

Treatment of uncomplicated acute appendicitis

The aim of treatment is to remove the appendix before gangrene and perforation occur. Preoperative resuscitation is not generally required unless there is generalized peritonitis.

Appendicectomy is carried out under general

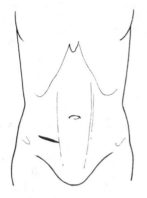 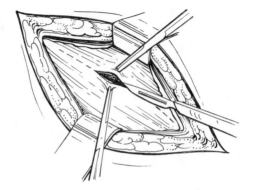

Fig. 33.4 'Gridiron' incision for appendicectomy

anaesthesia. The abdomen is entered through a small transverse incision centred over McBurney's point in the right iliac fossa (Fig. 33.4). A right paramedian incision does not give as good access for appendicectomy, but is used if the diagnosis is in doubt.

The muscles of the anterior abdominal wall are split in the line of their fibres as each layer is encountered ('gridiron' incision). The peritoneal cavity is entered and the caecum is identified and delivered through the wound. The appendix often emerges with the caecum but may require mobilization if adherent to neighbouring structures. If the organ cannot be identified readily, the taeniae coli should be traced to its base.

The mesoappendix is divided and its contained appendicular artery ligated. The appendix is ligated at its base and removed. The appendix stump is invaginated into the caecum using a purse-string suture.

The appendix is sent for histological examination to confirm the diagnosis and to exclude the presence of a carcinoid tumour. A swab for bacteriological culture is taken from the peritoneal cavity in all cases.

The wound is closed in layers. Local antiseptic agents such as povidone-iodine reduce the incidence of subsequent wound infection. Many surgeons now prefer to use metronidazole (500 mg intravenously or 1 g as a suppository with premedication) as a means of reducing the incidence of wound infection. Drainage of the peritoneal cavity or wound is indicated only if

there is gangrene and perforation or a localized abscess.

Problems during appendicectomy

The normal appendix

Depending on the policy of the surgeon, an apparently normal appendix will be removed in up to 20% of emergency appendicectomies. Attempts to improve diagnostic accuracy by delaying operation may be hazardous and lead to an unacceptable increase in morbidity and mortality from gangrene and perforation.

If the appendix is seen not to be acutely inflamed, other pathology must always be excluded. If peritoneal fluid is present, it may give a clue to the correct diagnosis. Mesenteric adenitis may be associated with clear yellow free peritoneal fluid, perforation of a peptic ulcer with bile-stained fluid, colonic perforation with faecal content, and infarction of bowel with blood-stained fluid. Free blood suggests rupture of a vessel or an ectopic pregnancy. If there is any uncertainty, the wound is extended or an additional incision made.

If no pathology is immediately apparent, the distal ileum is withdrawn and examined to exclude a Meckel's diverticulum, terminal ileitis, Crohn's disease or mesenteric adenitis. Both ovaries and tubes are inspected and an attempt is made to visualize the sigmoid colon. Even if other pathology is present, a normal appendix should be removed when operating through a gridiron incision, otherwise confusion may occur later because the patient bears an appendicectomy scar.

Lumps in the appendix

At operation there may be a mass palpable within the appendix. Faecoliths are the commonest cause. In obstructive appendicitis they may lose their mobility and be mistaken for neoplasms until the removed organ is incised and inspected. Neoplasms are rare (see later).

Mucocele of the appendix

This rare condition results from chronic obstruction of the appendix with accumulation of mucin resulting in cystic dilatation (Fig. 33.5). The obstruction is usually due to fibrous tissue but sometimes to a malignant mucous papillary adenocarcinoma. Simple mucoceles are cured by appendicectomy.

Pseudomyxoma peritonei is a rare complication of mucocele of the appendix (or ovarian neoplasm). Mucin-producing cells are disseminated throughout the peritoneal cavity. Extreme care should be taken to avoid rupture during removal.

Acute terminal ileitis and appendicectomy

Acute terminal ileitis used to be regarded as a manifestation of Crohn's disease. It is now realized that it is due to a self-limiting infection with

Yersinia enterocolitica or *Y. pseudotuberculosis*. Acute ileitis mimics appendicitis clinically, but at laparotomy the terminal ileum is red and thickened, mesenteric adenitis is obvious, and the caecum and appendix appear normal. Histological examination of the enlarged nodes and the appendix reveals non-specific changes. The diagnosis can be confirmed by serology or node culture.

At one time appendicectomy was thought to be contraindicated because of the risk of a fistula from the inflamed bowel, but it is now recommended to leave the ileum alone and to remove the appendix. Even in true Crohn's disease of the ileum, the appendix can safely be removed, provided it is not itself involved.

Further treatment is not required after appendicectomy for acute terminal ileitis, except in the rare event of yersinia septicaemia, when tetracycline is prescribed. An outpatient barium meal and follow-through should be performed to exclude true Crohn's disease elsewhere.

Meckel's diverticulum

Inflammation in a Meckel's diverticulum cannot be distinguished clinically from acute appendicitis. Laparotomy is required for both conditions and an acutely inflamed Meckel's diverticulum should be resected.

A diverticulum is sought routinely if the appendix is not inflamed, but this is best avoided in the presence of an inflamed appendix. Meckel's diverticula discovered incidentally need not be removed as a routine (see Ch. 31).

Postoperative complications

Complications are uncommon following early removal of an inflamed appendix. The incidence and severity of complications rises with gangrene and perforation.

Bleeding in the immediate postoperative period is rare. It is usually due to technical error, and results from slipping of ligatures on the meso-appendix or within the layers of the wound. Reoperation may be required.

Urinary retention may be a problem and require catheterization.

Wound infection used to occur in approximately

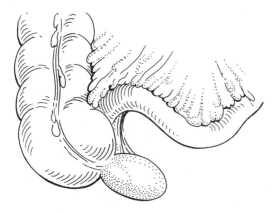

Fig. 33.5 Mucocele of the appendix

one-third of appendicectomy wounds. The incidence was higher following removal of a gangrenous or perforated appendix. The use of topical antiseptics and metronidazole has reduced this risk (see above).

Contamination of the wound with purulent material during surgery is an indication for delayed primary suture. Only the deeper layers of the wound are closed. The skin and subcutaneous tissues are left open for some 4–5 days. Once it is clear that the wound is healthy and uninfected, it is closed.

The development of pyrexia with erythema, pain and tenderness around a closed appendicectomy wound is an indication to remove skin sutures to allow free drainage.

Intraperitoneal abscesses can occur at any site in the peritoneal cavity following perforation of the appendix. An abscess is especially common in the pelvis. This may take some days to develop, and there is usually swinging pyrexia with tachycardia, deep seated pelvic pain and diarrhoea. A tender boggy mass is palpable rectally and may discharge pus spontaneously. Surgical drainage may be required if the patient becomes increasingly toxic or the mass becomes palpable suprapubically. The abscess can usually be drained through the rectum.

Leakage from the appendix stump is a rare complication of uncomplicated appendicectomy. It may cause spreading peritonitis, when reoperation is urgently indicated or discharge through the wound to form a chronic faecal fistula. This is likely to close spontaneously. Persistence of the fistula should raise the suspicion of disease of the caecum, e.g. chronic inflammation (tuberculosis or actinomycosis), Crohn's disease or cancer.

Intestinal obstruction may follow laparotomy for acute appendicitis. If it occurs early in the postoperative period, conservative management with nasogastric suction and intravenous fluids is justifiable, at least initially. Obstruction later in the postoperative course usually requires operation.

Prognosis in acute appendicitis

Uncomplicated appendicitis has an overall mortality of less than 0.1%. Gangrene and perforation increase both morbidity and mortality to the region of 5%. The very young and the very old are at particular risk, but in these, as in all age groups, the risk can largely be avoided by earlier diagnosis and treatment.

Complications of acute appendicitis

The complications of appendicitis are avoided by prompt diagnosis and early appendicectomy.

Perforation

It is unusual for the appendix to perforate within 12 hours of onset of inflammation. Gangrene and perforation occur more rapidly in the elderly, and are hastened in all age groups by ill-advised use of aperients or enemas in the early stages of the disease. Pain sometimes eases temporarily after perforation, but diffuse pain and tenderness with increasing pyrexia, tachycardia and clinical deterioration follow.

Management. Prompt appendicectomy is essential to prevent further spread of infection and deterioration in the patient's general condition. Preoperative resuscitation may be needed in some cases and must be vigorous so that further delay is avoided. A nasogastric tube is inserted, intravenous fluids are commenced, and systemic antibiotics (metronidazole and gentamicin) are administered. The technique of appendicectomy remains identical to that described for uncomplicated appendicitis. It is particularly important to take a swab for bacteriological culture, to avoid leaving portions of necrotic appendix behind, and to use lavage to aspirate all infected free fluid and pus from the peritoneal cavity. Many surgeons drain the peritoneal cavity after removing a perforated appendix, and all take precautions to reduce the incidence of wound infection (see above).

Appendix abscess formation

The development of an abscess is usually associated with increasing pyrexia, pain and the presence of a mass. The patient's general condition remains good. The mass is tender and, when situated in the right iliac fossa, palpable on abdominal examination. A pelvic abscess produces few abdominal signs but is detectable as a tender swelling on digital rectal examination. An abscess behind the caecum or terminal ileum is difficult to detect.

Management. Drainage of the abscess with appendicectomy is the treatment of choice. Great care is taken not to disseminate infection by unnecessary mobilization. Drainage with delayed interval appendicectomy is now standard practice when the appendix cannot be readily removed.

Conservative management used to be popular in patients with a well-defined abdominal mass. This approach is now only used in the occasional patient with a history extending over several days who presents with a well-defined mass, an otherwise soft, non-tender abdomen and no evidence of toxaemia. The patient is confined to bed, given parenteral fluids and nothing by mouth. Progress is monitored by regular recording of vital signs and twice daily measurement of the mass.

The aim is to allow inflammation to settle and to permit easy interval appendicectomy. Conservative treatment is abandoned if the mass increases in size, the general condition deteriorates, or there is evidence of dissemination of infection. In these circumstances adequate drainage is the main object of surgery, but the appendix is removed whenever possible. Conservative treatment is inadvisable in young children, the elderly and pregnant women.

Portal pyaemia

This is now rare. Suppurative thrombophlebitis of the portal vein produces recurring chills, drenching sweats, high swinging pyrexia and icterus, and there are multiple hepatic abscesses. Gas within the portal system is produced by anaerobic organisms and may be detected radiologically.

Management. Vigorous antibiotic treatment offers the only hope of survival.

CHRONIC APPENDICITIS

It is conceivable that some cases of intermittent 'grumbling' pain in the right iliac fossa are due to recurring bouts of low-grade appendicitis. The condition remains something of a diagnostic scapegoat, but such patients may be cured of their symptoms by elective appendicectomy. This should be advised only when other investigations prove negative.

TUMOURS OF THE APPENDIX

Carcinoid tumours

The appendix is the commonest site for carcinoid tumours of the gastrointestinal tract, which arise from the argentaffin cells of neuroectodermal origin (APUD cells). Carcinoid tumours account for 85% of appendix neoplasms and are found in 0.5% of appendices removed for other reasons. They are submucosal tumours of distinct yellow colour usually near the tip of the appendix. Most are benign and first noted as an incidental finding at appendicectomy. A malignant carcinoid tumour may infiltrate the muscle wall, spread to the mesoappendix and metastasize to regional lymph nodes. Liver metastases are very rare, and the carcinoid syndrome virtually unknown.

Small tumours are treated by appendicectomy. If the tumour is larger (more than 2 cm) or involves the caecal wall, or if there is associated lymph node involvement, a right hemicolectomy should be considered.

Adenocarcinoma

An adenocarcinoma of the appendix is a highly malignant form of colonic neoplasm, doubtless because of its rapid spread to regional lymph nodes. It usually presents as acute appendicitis or an appendix abscess. Right hemicolectomy is indicated in all cases.

34. Intestinal obstruction

Intestinal obstruction can be classified (1) according to the level of obstruction of the gastrointestinal tract (high or low small-bowel, colonic); (2) according to the rate of progression of the obstruction (acute, subacute, chronic or acute-on-chronic); or (3) on the basis of the pathological process responsible (intraluminal, mural, extramural).

It is important to differentiate causes which may impair the blood supply and cause strangulation from those which only cause simple occlusion of the lumen. Should strangulation of a segment of bowel occur, urgent surgical intervention is mandatory and the prognosis is more serious. For example, prompt operation on an inguinal hernia causing simple mechanical occlusion of the intestine carries little hazard to life. If operation is delayed and strangulation supervenes, significant mortality results.

It is also important to recognize that obstruction may be associated with perforation of the bowel wall in the absence of devascularization from strangulation. This can be due to the causative lesion penetrating the bowel wall, or simply to overdistension of bowel proximal to the obstruction. Thus, obstruction of the colon from carcinoma may be complicated by perforation at the site of the tumour. Rupture of a grossly distended caecum can occur and is believed to have an ischaemic basis.

While most obstructions occur at only one point, a loop of bowel may be occluded at both ends. In this event the contents of the loop cannot get out in either direction so that there is rapid distension of the loop with a much higher chance of strangulation than in a simple obstruction. Examples of such 'closed-loop' obstruction are

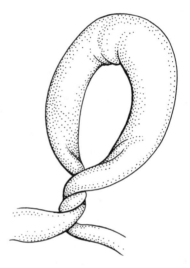

Fig. 34.1 Volvulus — an example of closed-loop obstruction

obstructed external or internal hernia, volvulus of the small or large intestine (Fig. 34.1), and colonic obstruction in the presence of a competent ileo-caecal valve. In this event small bowel material may continue to enter the loop but cannot leave it.

The frequency of the various causes of intestinal obstruction changes with age. Atresia of the bowel and other congenital defects are found mainly in infancy; hernias and adhesions occur at any age; and carcinoma of the colon is a disease of the elderly. Geographic and racial factors are other determinants. In the UK, approximately one-third of intestinal obstructions are due to hernias, one-third to large bowel cancer, and the remaining third to bands and adhesions. Volvulus is a rare cause, whereas in some parts of Africa and Russia sigmoid volvulus is common and second only to hernia as a cause of acute intestinal obstruction.

Obstruction due to tuberculous disease is common only in developing countries and that due to amoebiasis in the tropics.

Pathophysiology

Simple mechanical obstruction

The bowel above the obstructing lesion becomes distended with fluid and gas, and this stimulates excessive peristalsis, producing colic. The gas which accumulates is mainly swallowed air with a small and variable contribution from putrefaction within the bowel lumen. As distension increases, the blood vessels in the bowel wall become stretched and their diameter narrowed, so that blood flow is impaired. The mucosa is the first part of the bowel wall to show the effects of ischaemia. There is diminished absorption by the gut and net excretion of water and electrolytes into the lumen, resulting in depletion of extracellular fluid (ECF) and hypovolaemia. Some of the ECF passing into the gut lumen is lost by vomiting. Substantial 'hidden' losses are also inevitable as fluid accumulates in the bowel. As a rough guide, a loss of 2 litres of ECF can be assumed prior to vomiting. With established vomiting and dehydration, this increases to approximately 4 litres. If there is circulatory collapse with hypovolaemic shock, the deficit is of the order of 6 litres.

The fluid lost is isotonic with ECF but has a relatively high potassium concentration. If the obstruction is at or near the pylorus, there is also loss of acid, and metabolic alkalosis develops. If the obstruction is lower in the intestine, the lost fluid is slightly alkaline and there is no significant acid-base imbalance unless there is gross hypokalaemia (metabolic alkalosis) or shock (metabolic acidosis).

In simple mechanical obstruction, shock occurs late and is due to progressive depletion of ECF. The patient becomes increasingly dehydrated and there is tachycardia, falling central venous pressure and hypotension. Hypoxia may occur and is exacerbated by intestinal distension elevating the diaphragm and embarrassing ventilation.

Bacteraemia is not an important factor in the causation of shock associated with simple intestinal obstruction. Although there is an increase in luminal bacterial content, the peritoneal fluid remains sterile unless the bowel wall becomes ischaemic.

Strangulation obstruction

The initial stage of strangulation is venous occlusion with the development of oedema in the bowel wall. Arterial blood continues to enter the bowel until prevented from doing so by increasing back pressure. The bowel then becomes infarcted. Losses of plasma and blood are substantial and usually overshadow the loss of ECF due to preceding mechanical obstruction. Blood and plasma losses are particularly marked in strangulated sigmoid volvulus, when up to 70% of the total blood volume can be sequestered in the infarcted segment. The development of shock is accelerated by bacteraemia. Bacteria and their toxins pass through the ischaemic bowel wall into the peritoneum and are absorbed into the blood stream.

Clinical features of intestinal obstruction

Symptoms and signs

Abdominal colic is the cardinal symptom of obstruction. Its distribution reflects the region of the bowel which has been obstructed. With small bowel obstruction, the bouts of colic are felt in the midline of the abdomen around the umbilicus and become more frequent and more severe with time. In contrast to patients with acute peritonitis, who are afraid to move for fear of exacerbating the pain, those with abdominal colic are restless and move around during an attack. The development of constant and more localized pain associated with tenderness heralds the onset of *strangulation* and is an indication for urgent operation.

Strangulation is notoriously difficult to detect clinically in its early stages. It can never be excluded confidently without laparotomy and, except in a few specific instances (see below), urgent surgical intervention is advised in all patients with mechanical intestinal obstruction. The development of severe constant localized pain with tenderness and guarding suggests local peritonitis due to strangulation. This suspicion is increased if the patient appears more ill than might be expected from the length of history, particularly when there is associated pallor or circulatory collapse.

In large bowel obstruction the patient complains of vague lower abdominal pain with periodic exacerbations.

Vomiting occurs early in a high intestinal obstruction but may be absent in low small bowel or colon obstruction. Initially, the vomitus contains foodstuffs but later it becomes fluid and bilious before turning brown. This is due to the reflux of small bowel contents and not, as at one time believed, to the vomiting of faecal matter. As the obstructed small gut may be contaminated with faecal organisms, the smell of the vomitus can be offensive.

Absolute constipation is the rule with complete obstruction but this symptom may be late, particularly in high obstructions. Even in colonic obstruction, bowel movements or the passing of flatus may continue until the distal bowel is empty of faeces and gas. In low small bowel or colon obstructions the patient may complain of increasing girth due to intestinal distension.

Physical examination

Examination of the abdomen. Abdominal distension is described as a cardinal feature of intestinal obstruction. However it may be absent in a high obstruction. In low small bowel or colon obstructions visible loops of small intestine may form a 'ladder' pattern across the abdomen. Occasionally, peristalsis may be visible.

Ascites and gross obesity can confuse the picture but gaseous distension of the bowel gives a resonant note on percussion of the abdomen.

Auscultation during an attack of colic reveals a run of exaggerated bowel sounds. When the bowel becomes distended with fluid and gas, bowel sounds become high-pitched and tinkling.

Examination of the abdomen may reveal the cause of obstruction. An abdominal scar raises the possibility of adhesion obstruction or may indicate previous surgery for a disease which can cause recurrent obstruction (e.g. Crohn's disease). The hernial orifices must always be carefully examined.

The danger of overlooking a small groin hernia, particularly a femoral hernia, cannot be over-emphasized. There may be little local pain or tenderness. Central abdominal colic tends to focus attention away from the causal lesion and an obese, patient may not even be aware of its presence.

Digital rectal examination. Digital rectal examination is essential. Faecal impaction is a frequent cause of obstruction in the elderly, and an obstructing cancer of the rectum may be palpable. A mass in the rectovesical pouch suggests widespread abdominal neoplasia.

Proctoscopy and sigmoidoscopy. Proctoscopy and sigmoidoscopy should always be performed when large bowel obstruction is suspected. In some cases of sigmoid volvulus, sigmoidoscopy may result in relief of obstruction.

Radiological investigation

Plain films of the abdomen will reveal gaseous distension of the bowel with fluid levels on the erect or lateral decubitus views. Exceptions are high intestinal obstructions, when little or no gas is seen (except in the stomach) and a gastric fluid level may be detected.

The site of obstruction may be deduced from the plain abdominal film. Obstructed small bowel occupies the centre of the abdomen, has markings which extend across the whole diameter of the bowel (valvulae conniventes) and does not become as grossly distended as the colon. Obstructed large bowel occupies a peripheral position, has haustral indentations and may become grossly distended, particularly when the obstruction is of the closed loop type. In some cases, the level at which obstruction has occurred can be seen by a 'cut-off' in the pattern of gaseous distension.

Contrast radiology

Contrast radiology is seldom indicated in acute intestinal obstruction unless the diagnosis is in doubt. As undiluted barium can compound obstruction, only Gastrografin or dilute (half-strength) barium should be used. Barium must never be used when perforation is suspected.

MANAGEMENT

Prompt diagnosis and operation are essential to reduce the risk of strangulation. Specific indications for conservative treatment of intestinal obstruction are outlined below.

Resuscitation

It is essential to restore the circulatory state and correct fluid and electrolyte deficits before operation. In the presence of strangulation, there may not be enough time for adequate resuscitation and the benefits of delaying operation to allow resuscitation must then be balanced against the risk of progressive impairment of the blood supply to the obstructed bowel. The decision when best to operate may thus be difficult.

Principles of surgery

Small bowel obstruction

Extrinsic lesions (e.g. hernias, bands, adhesions) are the commonest cause of small bowel obstruction. Hernias are reduced and repaired, while adhesions and constricting bands are divided. Lesions within the bowel wall are less common and require resection of the involved segment. Obstruction due to an intraluminal mass, e.g. a bolus of food, is rare. It is initially managed by 'milking' the affected segment in order to move the obstructing material on into the large bowel. If this is not possible, enterotomy is needed to remove the cause of the obstruction. A bypass operation or resection is sometimes required to deal with an irremoveable obstruction (Fig. 34.2). Strangulated bowel is blue-black in colour, lacking in sheen, papery in consistency and does not show peristalsis when flicked or squeezed. If there is any doubt about its viability, the involved loop must be resected, usually with an end-to-end anastomosis of the remaining bowel.

Large bowel obstruction

Obstructing lesions of the right side of the colon can usually be managed by right hemicolectomy with immediate ileocolic anastomosis. Bypass without resection with an ileocolic anastomosis

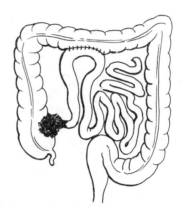

Fig. 34.2 Ileo-transverse anastomosis to bypass an irresectable lesion at the ileocaecal valve

may be considered as a palliative measure if the patient has non-resectable carcinoma. It may also be performed as a preliminary to later resection if the patient's general condition is poor.

The management of obstructing lesions of the left side of the large bowel is more difficult. Emergency resection with immediate anastomosis carries a high risk of anastomotic leakage and is generally not advised. The classical three-stage approach (Fig. 34.3) is now less frequently employed than in the past. This consists of (1) an emergency transverse colostomy to relieve obstruction. (2) Following adequate preparation, an elective resection of the affected segment of bowel is usually carried out some weeks later. The transverse colostomy is retained to divert the faecal stream until anastomotic healing has been confirmed radiologically after instillation of barium through the distal loop. (3) The transverse colostomy is closed, usually about 4–6 weeks after the second stage.

Several alternatives to this procedure have been introduced to allow completion of the operative treatment in two stages.

1. The initial decompressing colostomy can be placed close to the tumour so that at a second (and final) stage a radical resection can be performed which includes removal of the tumour and the colostomy with restoration of continuity by end-to-end anastomosis (Fig. 34.4).

2. Alternatively, the segment of bowel containing the tumour can be resected at the initial

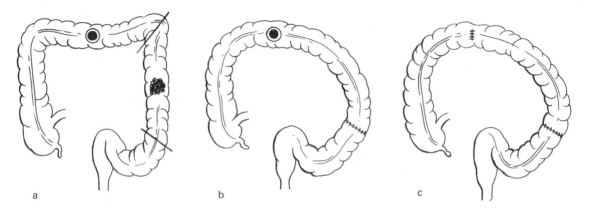

Fig. 34.3 Three-stage resection of large bowel. (a) Emergency transverse colostomy (the site of subsequent resection is also shown). (b) Elective resection of large bowel segment, retaining the colostomy to protect the anastomosis. (c) Closure of colostomy

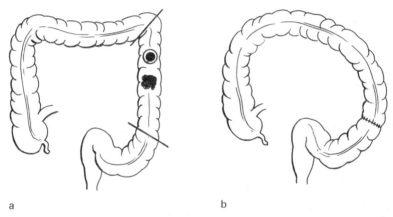

Fig. 34.4 Two-stage resection of large bowel. (a) Initial defunctioning colostomy adjacent to obstructing lesion. (b) Subsequent resection with end-to-end anastomosis

operation, with exteriorization of the proximal and distal cut ends of the bowel (Fig. 34.5). Continuity is restored at a later, second operation. The Hartmann procedure is a variation used when the tumour is in the lower pelvic colon or rectum. Following primary resection, only the proximal cut end is brought to the surface as a colostomy, the distal limb of the bowel being oversewn and allowed to drop back into the abdomen (Fig. 34.6). Continuity may be restored later.

Recently, a one-stage procedure has been advocated in which resection of the affected bowel is followed by immediate anastomosis. An essential aspect of this operation is 'on-table' colonic lavage to prepare the bowel for the anastomosis. This operation requires great surgical skill and is only recommended in fit patients or those unwilling or unable to cope with even a temporary stoma.

After resection of an appropriate length of bowel containing the obstructing lesion, a Foley catheter (24 Fr) is inserted into the caecum via the base of the removed, appendix and secured by a purse-string suture. It is then connected to an irrigation system containing isotonic saline solution (Fig. 34.7a & b). A wide-bore collecting tube is tied into the proximal cut end of the colon and led to a collecting vessel of suitable size before irrigation is commenced (Fig. 34.7c). The saline washes faeces from the colon into the collecting system, although harder scybala may require assistance by

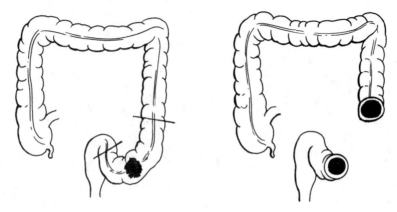

Fig. 34.5   Resection of a segment of large bowel with exteriorization of both ends. Continuity is restored at a later stage

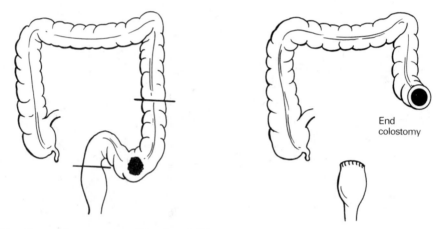

End
colostomy

Fig. 34.6   Hartmann's procedure: resection of large bowel with proximal end colostomy and oversewing of the rectal stump. Continuity may be restored later

manual massage. Irrigation is continued until the effluent is clear. As much as 10–12 litres of saline may be required. The anastomosis can then be constructed safely. The Foley catheter is brought out in the right iliac fossa to act as a temporary caecostomy for a few days and the abdominal incision is closed (Fig. 34.7d).

Resection is always necessary if strangulation is present. Right hemicolectomy with an ileocolic anastomosis remains the procedure of choice for right-sided lesions. Immediate anastomosis is not normally recommended following resection of strangulated segments of the left colon or rectum, and either both ends of the cut bowel should be exteriorized or a Hartmann's procedure performed (see above).

Rarely, a patient with large bowel obstruction is unfit for laparotomy. A blind caecostomy may then be performed under local anaesthesia. A large-bore tube is inserted into the caecum with the object of decompressing the proximal large bowel. The tube has to be irrigated at intervals to prevent blockage.

Conservative treatment

Non-operative treatment of mechanical intestinal obstruction is indicated, at least initially, in the following circumstances.

Adhesion obstruction. If a patient has already undergone multiple operations for episodes of obstruction due to peritoneal adhesions, further

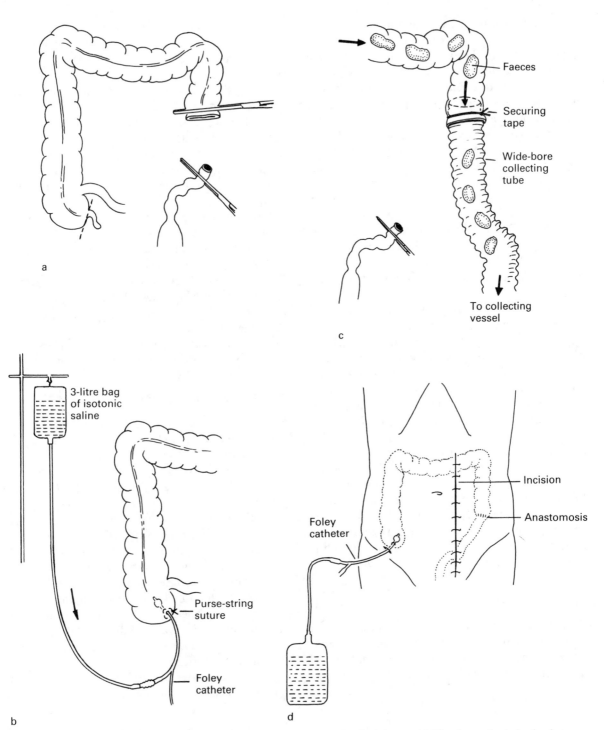

Fig. 34.7 Principles of one-stage resection and anastomosis using 'on-table' colonic lavage. (a) The obstructing lesion has been resected. (If present, the appendix is also removed.) (b) A Foley catheter is inserted through the appendix stump, secured by a purse-string suture and connected to the irrigating system. (c) Faecal content is washed from the colon into the collecting system. (d) The anastomosis has been made, the Foley catheter led out from the caecum to form a temporary caecostomy, and the abdomen closed

surgery carries little prospect of long-term success and may be hazardous because of the risk of inadvertent entry into the bowel lumen. Conservative treatment with fluid replacement and nasogastric suction is preferred but must be abandoned if there are signs suggesting strangulation or if obstruction persists.

Widespread intra-abdominal malignancy. In a patient with known carcinomatosis, intestinal obstruction is treated by operation only if the surgeon, in consultation with the patient and relatives, believes that this is in the patient's best interest. Usually it is not.

Crohn's disease. Crohn's disease affecting the small intestine is often complicated by bouts of subacute obstruction. These usually resolve on conservative management, but, if not, operation is required.

Postoperative obstruction. While abdominal distension, vomiting, failure to pass flatus and other changes during the postoperative phase are generally attributed to paralytic ileus, mechanical obstruction can follow any intra-abdominal operation. It is most commonly due to adhesions or to the bowel becoming trapped in peritoneal or mesenteric defects. If signs of mechanical intestinal obstruction persist for more than 2–3 days after the operation, laparotomy is undertaken.

Sigmoid volvulus. Non-operative decompression by sigmoidoscopy and insertion of a soft lubricated rubber tube through the twisted loop is usually attempted first. Only if this fails or if strangulation is suspected, should laparotomy be performed (see Ch. 32). Caecal volvulus, which is rare, is best treated by right hemicolectomy.

PARALYTIC ILEUS

Paralytic ileus may complicate mechanical obstruction or it may arise as a result of peritonitis, retroperitoneal bleeding or acute pancreatitis. It is due to interference with splanchnic nerve function and commonly occurs in response to a direct toxic effect on the bowel wall (e.g. in peritonitis). Gross electrolyte depletion (notably of potassium and magnesium), hypoxia and shock can also cause ileus.

In contrast to a mechanical obstruction, intestinal colic is not a feature. The abdomen is distended, there is little tenderness and no guarding on palpation. Bowel sounds are absent. Vomiting or nasogastric aspirations are often copious. Plain films show gaseous distension with multiple fluid levels throughout the whole length of the gut.

Treatment. Paralytic ileus is treated conservatively by nasogastric aspiration and intravenous replacement of fluid and electrolytes. Parasympathomimetic drugs have been used but are not generally advised. Surgery is contraindicated, but the patient must be reviewed twice daily so that a positive decision can be made to persist with conservative therapy. Any suggestion of mechanical intestinal obstruction, strangulation or persisting general or local infection demands operation.

PSEUDO-OBSTRUCTION

Pseudo-obstruction is a syndrome in which gross gaseous distension of the abdomen, obstructive bowel sounds and fluid levels on X-ray all suggest mechanical obstruction of the large intestine without a mechanical obstructing factor being present. The condition is occasionally seen in patients with respiratory or renal disease, and may occur after major trauma or major operation, not necessarily on the gastrointestinal tract.

In some cases, gas may be seen extending into the rectum on plain abdominal X-ray but, if not, an enema with dilute barium confirms the absence of an obstructing lesion. Treatment is conservative and laparotomy is advised only if the diagnosis is in doubt or if the distension is so gross as to raise fear of caecal perforation.

Colonoscopic decompression of the distended bowel has been used successfully in a few patients.

35. Anorectal conditions

Surgical anatomy

Musculature

The anal canal is 3–4 cm long and consists of two muscular tubes: the inner tube, which is a continuation of the smooth muscle of the gut, and the outer tube, which consists of a sheath of striated muscle (Fig. 35.1).

Inner tube. The internal sphincter is the final condensation of the circular layer of gut muscle, and as such is controlled by the autonomic nervous system. The longitudinal muscle of the gut becomes fibrous as it passes between the internal and external sphincters, ending as a series of bands which radiate to the perianal skin (see Fig. 35.1).

Outer tube. The puborectalis fibres of the levator ani originate from the back of the pubic symphysis and form a U-shaped sling which blends with the outer layer of the bowel as it passes through the pelvic floor. This sling helps to maintain the 80° angle between the axes of the rec-

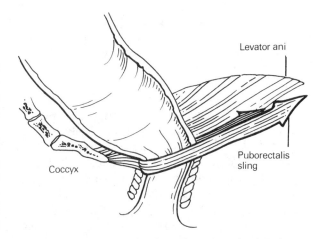

Fig. 35.2 Puborectalis sling establishing the perineal angle

tum and anal canal (Fig. 35.2) and also compresses the anal canal into an anteroposterior slit.

The lower border of puborectalis is in continuity with the external sphincter (see Fig. 35.1), both muscles being striated and under voluntary control. The *anorectal ring* is the condensed ring of muscle formed by the puborectalis and the upper edges of the internal and external sphincters. The ring can be felt rectally and is vital to continence.

The lining of the anal canal

The anal valves are crescentic mucosal folds which form a serrated or 'pectinate' line around the lumen some 2 cm from the anal verge (Fig. 35.3). The pectinate line corresponds to the line of fusion between endoderm of the embryonic hindgut and ectoderm of the anal pit. The canal above this line has a mucosal lining innervated by the autonomic nervous system, whereas beneath the pectinate line

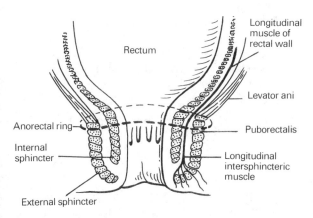

Fig. 35.1 Musculature of the anorectal region

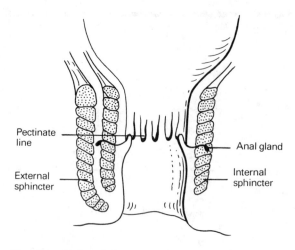

Fig. 35.3   Lining of the anal canal

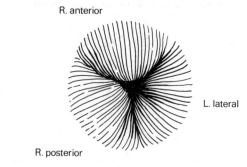

Fig. 35.4   The anal cushions

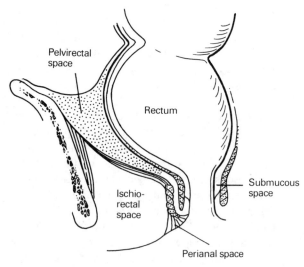

Fig. 35.5   Tissue spaces in relation to the anorectal region

it is lined by modified skin innervated by the peripheral nervous system. Histologically there is a gradual transition from mucus-secreting columnar mucosa to stratified squamous epithelium. Keratinization and epidermal appendages appear only beyond the anal verge.

The mucosa above the pectinate line is thrown into vertical folds, or anal columns, the distal ends of which fuse to form the anal valves. Each valve encloses an anal crypt, and an anal gland opens into the floor of some of the crypts. These glands ramify in the submucosa to reach the internal sphincter, some of them penetrating to the intersphincteric plane (see Fig. 35.3). The glands are important in the spread of anorectal infection.

The submucosa of the anal canal forms three pads of vascular connective tissue, the so-called 'anal cushions'. These lie in the left lateral, right posterior and right anterior positions and impart a Y-shaped configuration to the lumen (Fig. 35.4).

Tissue spaces in relation to the anorectal region

1. *The ischiorectal fossa* is the pyramidal space bounded laterally by the side wall of the pelvis, medially by the external anal sphincter and superiorly by the levator ani (Fig. 35.5). The fossa contains fatty connective tissue and is crossed by the inferior rectal vessels. The two fossae communicate behind the anal canal.

2. *The perianal space* lies below the inferior mar-

gins of the anal sphincters and is loculated by fibrous septae.

3. *The submucous space* lies between the internal sphincter and the mucocutaneous lining of the upper two-thirds of the anal canal, and contains the internal haemorrhoidal venous plexus.

4. *The pelvirectal space* is a potential space between the upper surface of the levator ani and the pelvic peritoneum, and contains the lateral ligaments of the rectum.

Blood supply

The superior rectal artery is the continuation of the inferior mesenteric artery and according to classical descriptions forms three branches (two right, one left) which descend the rectum to the anal canal. However, the arterial anatomy is very variable. The anal canal is also supplied by branches of the internal iliac artery. The middle rectal artery enters the rectum above the levator ani, while the inferior rectal artery traverses the ischiorectal fossa. There are profuse anastomoses between the three rectal arteries (Fig. 35.6).

The superior rectal vein drains upwards into the portal system, while the middle and inferior rectal veins drain laterally into the systemic venous system. Venous anastomoses in the submucosa form the internal haemorrhoidal plexus above the pectinate line, and the external haemorrhoidal plexus below.

Lymphatic drainage

Carcinoma of the rectum spreads upwards along the superior rectal lymphatic vessels, although lesions in the lower extraperitoneal rectum occasionally spread laterally to the internal iliac glands. Metastasis to inguinal glands occurs only when carcinoma involves the skin of the lower anal canal or perianal region (Fig. 35.7).

Surgical physiology

Anal continence

The internal sphincter provides resting anal tone but relaxes following distension of the rectum by flatus or faeces. The external sphincter is contracted voluntarily if defaecation has to be postponed, and, although contraction can only be maintained for a minute or so, the rise in rectal pressure usually abates if the call to stool is resisted.

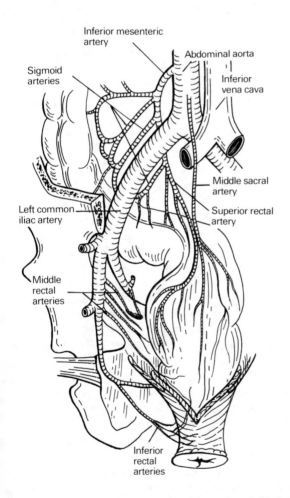

Fig. 35.6 Blood supply of the rectum (shown from behind)

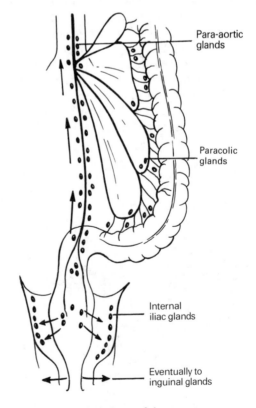

Fig. 35.7 Lymphatic drainage of the rectum

Continence depends on (1) intact rectal and pelvic floor innervation to appreciate rectal distension; (2) intact anal sensation to determine the nature of the rectal contents; and (3) intact innervation of anal sphincters and levator ani. Division of the lower portion of one or both anal sphincters produces only minor defects in continence, but division of the anorectal ring causes disastrous loss of control.

The following mechanical factors may contribute to continence.

1. The 80° angle between the rectum and anal canal (see Fig. 35.2) means that increases in intra-abdominal pressure tend to press the anterior rectal wall down onto the anal canal. This prevents inadvertent escape of flatus or faeces when intra-abdominal pressure rises during coughing and exercise.

2. The anal canal has been likened to a flutter valve as it passes through the pelvic diaphragm. The canal walls are kept in apposition by the internal sphincter and the puborectalis sling so that continence can be maintained without conscious effort during rises in intra-abdominal pressure. When pressure rises *within the rectum*, the valve opens and contraction of the external sphincter is needed to preserve continence (Fig. 35.8).

3. The striated muscle of the external sphincter and puborectalis is maintained in a state of tonic contraction. This is important for maintaining the two mechanisms described above.

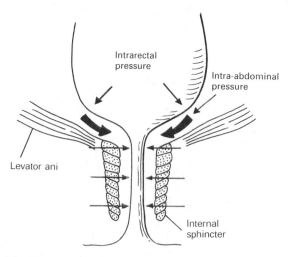

Fig. 35.8 Mechanism of continence

4. The bulk of the anal cushions may contribute to closure. Minor defects in continence occur in about one-quarter of patients following haemorrhoidectomy.

Control of defaecation

An increase in intrarectal pressure is followed, over a few minutes, by relaxation or 'accommodation' of the rectum. During this period there is a feeling of fullness if the rectum is sufficiently distended. At the same time, the internal anal sphincter partly relaxes, thus allowing rectal contents to reach the upper part of the somatic sensory epithelium. Gas can be detected by a voluntary slight increase in intra-abdominal pressure which allows a small amount of gas to escape. However, if stool is present, the external sphincter is rapidly contracted until accommodation in the rectum has been completed. During defaecation there is a release of cortical inhibition and a voluntary increase in intra-abdominal pressure. The angle between rectum and anal canal is straightened and the sphincters and pelvic floor relax. There is reflex contraction of pelvic colon and rectum.

ANAL INCONTINENCE

Anal incontinence may result from any of the following causes.

Congenital abnormalities. Incontinence is a feature of some congenital abnormalities such as anorectal agenesis with rectocloacal fistula.

Trauma. Division of the sphincters and anorectal ring may follow accidental injury, obstetric tears or operative trauma.

Neurological and psychological disease. Various diseases affecting the nervous system (e.g. spina bifida, spinal trauma, spinal tumours, multiple sclerosis, tabes dorsalis) can give rise to anal incontinence. Incontinence of faeces is a common manifestation of behavioural problems in children, senile dementia and all other forms of psychotic illness.

Anorectal disease. Rectal prolapse, third degree piles, chronic inflammatory bowel disease and anorectal cancer may cause incontinence by stretching, infiltrating or destroying the sphincter mechanism.

Faecal impaction. Impaction of faeces leads first to constipation and then to overflow incontinence of faeces with a feeling of incomplete evacuation of the bowel. Faecal impaction in elderly and bed-bound patients is the commonest cause of incontinence in surgical practice.

Treatment

There is no satisfactory treatment for many causes of incontinence. The management of congenital abnormalities is outwith the scope of this book. Traumatic division of the sphincter mechanism can be repaired surgically under cover of a temporary defunctioning colostomy. If there is gross contamination at the time of injury, it is advisable to limit initial treatment to wound toilet and colostomy, and defer definitive repair until the acute inflammation has subsided. Obstetric tears can often be dealt with by primary suture, but may require subsequent repair of the perineum.

Laxity of the anal sphincters may be reduced by suture if the sphincter muscle has been partially or completely divided. A preliminary defunctioning colostomy is advisable. Sphincteroplasty operations are also available to tighten the sphincters and puborectalis muscle. Insertion of an encircling Thiersch wire may be considered in elderly unfit patients. These various surgical manoeuvres often fail. A permanent colostomy is then required.

Faecal impaction demands manual or instrumental disimpaction followed by enemas and aperients to restore normal bowel action.

HAEMORRHOIDS

Aetiology

Haemorrhoids (piles) remain one of the commonest ailments of Western society, although their aetiology remains uncertain. Piles commonly develop or increase in size during pregnancy and are associated with constipation and straining at stool. There are no valves in the portal venous system, and it may be that increases in intra-abdominal pressure dilate unsupported anal canal veins. Refined low-residue Western diets with a consequent need to strain at stool may be a contributory factor.

However, there are a number of facts which do not support the varicose vein theory of origin. The development of piles in pregnancy could equally be due to increased laxity and vascularity of the pelvic tissues. Piles are not more common in patients with portal hypertension. Rectal cancer is said to predispose to pile formation by obstructing venous drainage, but it is just as likely that these two common conditions coexist fortuitously.

Alternative explanations for haemorrhoidal formation include hyperplasia of a submucosal vascular network, straining at stool with attenuation of the supporting framework of the anal cushions, and development of constricting fibrous bands within the anal canal.

Classification

Internal piles

These originate as bulges in the upper anal canal and lower rectum. The piles contain the internal haemorrhoidal plexus, but thickened mucosa and connective tissue often contribute to the pile mass. Progressive enlargement involves the skin-lined lower anal canal with its underlying external haemorrhoidal plexus. At this stage the piles become visible externally.

The piles lie in the left lateral, right anterior and right posterior positions relative to the anal canal (see Fig. 35.4). Smaller accessory piles are often present between the three main masses. Piles which bulge into the lumen without prolapsing through the anus are called first-degree, those which prolapse on defaecation but return spontaneously second-degree, and those which remain prolapsed, third-degree piles. Some long standing piles cannot be returned to the anal canal and are sometimes called fourth-degree piles.

Thrombosed internal haemorrhoids. This acute painful condition is often described by patients as 'an attack of piles'. It occurs when the anal sphincters contract around prolapsed piles and so prevent their return to the anal canal and obstruct venous return. Congestion and thrombosis follow and the piles become hard and tender, in contrast to uncomplicated third-degree piles.

Necrosis may follow. The skin-covered part of the piles and the perianal skin become oedematous and overhanging, hiding the swollen mucosal component. Proctoscopy is usually impossible because of discomfort, and is not needed to establish the diagnosis. The term 'strangulated piles' is commonly used to describe this sequence of events.

External piles

These originate outside the anal canal and are quite distinct from the internal haemorrhoids described above. The term is used to describe anal haematomas and skin tags, but is confusing and best avoided.

Clinical features

1. *Bleeding* is traditionally the first symptom. While this remains true for first degree piles, many patients with prolapsing piles consider prolapse to occur first. Bleeding is usually first noted as a bright red streak on the toilet paper or stool surface after a bout of constipation, but often increases in frequency and severity until a steady drip or squirting of blood accompanies defaecation. Severe secondary anaemia is uncommon.

2. *Prolapse* produces symptoms in the majority of patients. It is at first a transient feature on defaecation, but then occurs with increasing frequency until third degree piles result.

3. *Mucous discharge* occurs when the columnar mucosa of the upper anal canal is exposed. Associated *skin tags* are common and may cause excoriation and pruritus.

4. *Pain* is rare in uncomplicated piles. Many patients experience discomfort and some consider this to be their main complaint.

5. *Thrombosed piles* can cause severe pain in relation to the pile-bearing areas.

Assessment and diagnosis

A careful history and abdominal examination must precede anorectal examination. Anal bleeding cannot be attributed to piles until other anorectal pathology, particularly a neoplasm, has been excluded.

Inspection of the perianal area is carried out with the patient in the left lateral position. First-degree piles produce no outward abnormality. Separation of the buttocks often reveals the skin-covered component of second-degree piles, and the piles may prolapse when the patient is asked to strain. In prolapsed third-degree piles, the red columnar anal mucosa is usually visible, separated by a furrow from the skin-lined component.

Digital rectal examination may reveal no abnormality, unless the piles are of long standing and thickened. Proctoscopy is the key diagnostic investigation, the piles bulging into the lumen as the instrument is withdrawn. The patient is asked to strain during withdrawal so that vascular engorgement is produced and the degree of prolapse can be determined. Sigmoidoscopy is essential to exclude coexisting rectal pathology which might mimic bleeding from piles. Barium enema is indicated when symptoms cannot be explained by proctoscopic and sigmoidoscopic findings. With thrombosed piles the skin around the anus is swollen and oedematous in relation to the pile-bearing areas. Gentle separation of these allows a glimpse of the thrombosed pile masses, which may be red, blue or, if necrotic, black.

Treatment of internal piles

Conservative treatment

Small asymptomatic first-degree piles which are discovered as an incidental finding should be left alone. Symptomatic piles merit treatment but there is little place for 'medical' treatment by local ointments or suppositories. A high-residue diet or bulk laxative should be prescribed to combat habitual constipation, and this may be all that is needed to cure the condition.

Specific treatments

Injection therapy. First-degree piles are easily treated by injection. A trial of injection is also worthwhile in second-degree piles but not in those of third degree, which cannot be cured by this means. However, when operation is contra-indicated in patients with such prolapsing piles, injections may give some relief.

The object of injection therapy is to produce

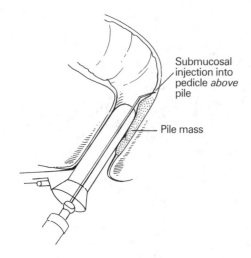

Submucosal injection into pedicle *above* pile

Pile mass

Fig. 35.9 Injection sclerotherapy for haemorrhoids

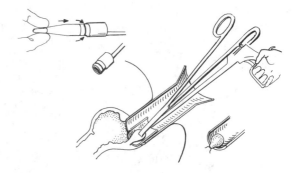

Fig. 35.10 Rubber-band ligation of haemorrhoids. A conical applicator is used to slide a rubber band over the end of the banding instrument. The pile is drawn downwards into the instrument and the rubber band is slipped around its pedicle

submucosal fibrosis in the upper anal canal and lower rectum, constricting vascular spaces within the pile and decreasing mucosal mobility. A Gabriel syringe is filled with sclerosant (e.g. 5% phenol in almond oil) and, using a proctoscope, 3–5 ml is injected into each pile pedicle at or just above the anorectal ring (Fig. 35.9). Transient deep-seated aching sometimes follows injection of sclerosant but the technique is usually painless when performed correctly.

Complications such as ulceration and necrosis at the injection site, submucosal abscess, haematuria, prostatic abscess, and transient inflammatory narrowing of the anal canal are all rare.

Bleeding should cease within 24–48 hours of successful injection. Injection may be repeated if symptoms recur but operation is then usually advised.

Rubber-band ligation. This technique provides an increasingly popular alternative to injection. The pile mass is pulled down through a proctoscope and a rubber band is applied around the mucosa-covered part of pedicle (Fig. 35.10). One pile is ligated at each visit, further banding being carried out at 3-week intervals. Approximately one-third of patients require medication for discomfort. Banding is not suitable for the skin-covered component of piles or associated skin tags.

Cryodestruction. Cryosurgery has been used to treat second- and third-degree piles without anaesthesia. A profuse offensive discharge persists for about 10 days but the patient can usually return to work on the day after treatment.

Infrared photocoagulation. A fibreoptic probe connected to a source of infrared radiation is applied to the haemorrhoid and one or two short pulses of irradiation are delivered. This causes coagulation within the haemorrhoid, with consequent reduction in size. The technique can be carried out as an outpatient procedure, is simple and effective and, as the equipment is inexpensive, is steadily gaining in popularity.

Manual anal dilatation under general anaesthesia (Lord's technique). Manual dilatation of the anal canal and lower rectum to four fingers' width can be used to treat piles of any degree. A moist sponge is inserted for 1 hour after the procedure to prevent haematoma formation and the patient is allowed home after recovery from anaesthesia. He is provided with a bulk laxative and an anal dilator to prevent recurrent anal constriction. Mild incontinence of flatus may occur after dilatation, but faecal incontinence is rare. The technique enjoyed some popularity in the past but is now infrequently practised as an alternative to formal haemorrhoidectomy.

Haemorrhoidectomy. Several operations are described to treat internal piles. Most commonly practised is ligation and excision of each pile mass following its dissection from the anal canal (Fig. 35.11).

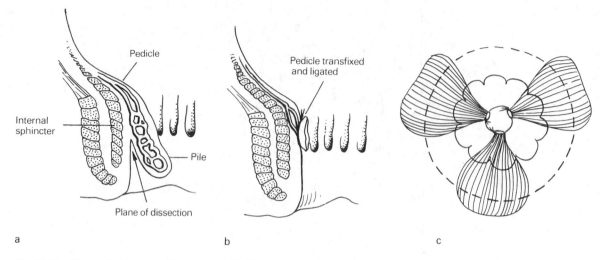

Fig. 35.11 Haemorrhoidectomy. (a) Anatomy. (b) Haemorrhoid excised. (c) Anus at end of operation showing raw areas

The plane of dissection passes just within the internal sphincter, which is carefully preserved. Each vascular pedicle is transfixed and ligated, and the piles are excised to leave three raw areas separated by bridges of skin and mucosa. Epithelialization of the raw areas takes place in 3–4 weeks and prevents excessive fibrosis or anal narrowing. Modification of this technique, including submucosal dissection, makes little difference to the overall results.

Complications. Postoperative pain is the commonest problem, and considerable discomfort accompanies the first bowel motion. It is advised that stools should be kept soft (e.g. by methyl cellulose) for 3–4 weeks while epithelialization takes place. Male patients occasionally have difficulty in micturition but catheterization is rarely needed. Reactionary haemorrhage occurs in less than 2% of patients, and secondary haemorrhage 7–10 days after operation in just over 1%. Anal stenosis, fissure, abscess and fistula are rare complications. The late results show that while only 5% of patients have recurrent symptoms, two-thirds will have first-degree piles on proctoscopy. On careful questioning some patients admit to intermittent flatus incontinence or soiling of underwear, but significant faecal incontinence is rare.

Treatment of thrombosed internal haemorrhoids

In the early stages it may be possible to return prolapsed piles to the anal canal and allow the congestion to settle. This is seldom feasible by the time the majority of patients present, although anal dilatation performed under general anaesthesia may promote reduction. Conservative treatment includes bed rest, local application of dressings soaked in hypertonic saline, analgesics and mild aperients.

Resolution takes about 10 days. Although haemorrhoidectomy is usually required at some future date, in some cases the attack of thrombosis will have cured the piles. Immediate haemorrhoidectomy is now seldom advised.

Conclusions regarding the treatment of haemorrhoids

Banding is probably now the mainstay of treatment for symptomatic first-degree and early second-degree piles. Haemorrhoidectomy is still practised widely for third-degree piles and those second-degree piles which are unsuitable for injection or fail to respond. Photocoagulation avoids inpatient treatment, is painless and has gained in popularity. Haemorrhoidectomy is probably best reserved for those cases in which photocoagulation fails. Thrombosed piles are best treated conservatively at first.

Perianal haematoma

This common condition (also referred to as thrombosed external pile) is due to rupture of a vein at the anal verge with haematoma formation. A small painful lump develops rapidly, often appearing after an episode of straining at stool. The lump is tense, blue, well circumscribed and exquisitely tender. The haematoma is readily distinguished from thrombosed internal haemorrhoids by its restricted size, and from perianal abscess by its colour.

Spontaneous resolution takes some days and often leaves a skin tag at the site. Occasionally the haematoma ruptures or becomes secondarily infected.

Operation is generally advised to relieve pain and tenderness and to speed recovery. The haematoma is evacuated under local anaesthesia and the wound is left to granulate.

RECTAL PROLAPSE

Three types of rectal prolapse are described.

Type I is an *incomplete, partial* or *mucosal* prolapse in which the mucous membrane lining the anal canal is lax and protrudes through the anus.

Type II is a *complete prolapse* in which intussusception of the rectum results in the whole thickness of the bowel protruding through the anus.

Type III is also a *complete prolapse* involving the whole thickness of the rectal wall, but in this case due to a sliding hernia of the pouch of Douglas. If there is associated vaginal prolapse, the term *procidentia* is applied.

Any type of prolapse can occur at any time of life. However, incomplete (type I) prolapse is common in young children, whereas complete (type II and III) prolapse is commoner in adults. Approximately 85% of affected adults are women, and older females are particularly at risk.

Aetiology

Partial prolapse. Prolapse in childhood is favoured if the sacral curve of the rectum is lacking so that the rectum and anus form a vertical tube. Excessive straining at stool is a major factor, and malnourishment contributes by reducing the amount of fat in the supporting ischiorectal and pararectal tissues.

Partial prolapse in adults may complicate haemorrhoid formation or may follow damage to the anal sphincters during labour or anal surgery.

Complete prolapse. Most patients with complete prolapse have deficient muscle tone in the pelvic floor and anal canal, which can now be confirmed by neurophysiological testing. Many female patients have had previous hysterectomy or other gynaecological procedures. Additional factors may include lack of fixation of the rectum to its sacral bed, intussusception of the rectum and an abnormally deep rectovaginal or rectovesical pouch.

Clinical features

Prolapse is first noted during defaecation. For a time it will reduce spontaneously once straining ceases. Discomfort during defaecation is common, and there may be bleeding and mucus discharge from the engorged mucosa. The prolapse recurs with increasing ease and may even be caused by mild exertion such as coughing and walking. The bowel habit becomes irregular, and laxity of the musculature coupled with impaired rectal sensation leads to incontinence of both flatus and faeces. Such incontinence is the main reason for patients seeking help. Associated uterine prolapse compounds the problem by causing incontinence of urine.

The prolapse may not be apparent until the patient is asked to bear down and strain. The anus is usually patulous and can be opened widely simply by drawing the buttocks apart. Digital rectal examination reveals poor sphincter tone, and two or more fingers can be inserted without apparent discomfort. The prolapse appears progressively on straining but seldom protrudes for more than 10 cm. The mucosa is thickened, engorged and corrugated but mucosal folds may be ironed out as the prolapse emerges. The thickness of the prolapse is judged between finger and thumb to decide whether it is partial or complete. Partial prolapse seldom protrudes for more than 5 cm. The mucosa is smooth.

The complications of rectal prolapse include irreducibility with ulceration, bleeding and gangrene, and rarely rupture of · the prolapsed bowel.

The diagnosis of rectal prolapse is usually straightforward. The appearance can be confused with large third-degree piles, and occasionally with prolapse of a rectal neoplasm.

Treatment

In children operation is rarely required. Prolapse responds to conservative measures in most cases and rarely persists beyond the age of 5 years. Constipation and straining at stool should be avoided, and the buttocks may be strapped together to discourage prolapse during defaecation. If these measures fail, submucosal injection of phenol may be used to fix lax mucosa to underlying tissues.

In adults, the choice of treatment depends on the type of rectal prolapse.

Partial prolapse

Provided sphincter tone is satisfactory, partial prolapse in adults can be treated by excising prolapsing mucosa using a technique similar to that used for the dissection and ligature of haemorrhoids. Patients with poor sphincter tone are unlikely to benefit from this procedure as their main complaint is incontinence rather than the prolapse. Various methods of improving sphincter tone have been described although none is entirely satisfactory. These methods include voluntary exercise of sphincter muscle, electrical stimulation, and perineorrhaphy to tighten the puborectalis muscle. Education of bowel habit is an important part of treatment, and insertion of a Thiersch wire (see below) may be considered in frail elderly patients.

Complete prolapse

Various methods are available for the treatment of complete prolapse; none is ideal.

Narrowing of the anus. The simplest form of surgery consists of inserting a Thiersch wire of stainless steel or synthetic monofilament material around the anal canal (Fig. 35.12), but this procedure is rarely successful in complete prolapse. The incidence of faecal impaction is high so that regular stool softeners need to be taken indefinitely. Although some surgeons advise this procedure for all elderly patients, most can tolerate abdominal repair surprisingly well.

Repair of pelvic structures and fixation of rectum. A variety of repairs can be carried out through the abdomen. These are successful in an anatomical sense in that they prevent further prolapse, but some degree of incontinence persists in about 30% of patients. Most methods include thorough mobilization of the rectum, fixation of the rectum to the sacrum, suture of the levator ani muscles in front of the rectum, and obliteration of the deep pouch of Douglas. Mobilization of the rectum favours extensive adhesion formation and prevents further prolapse by fixing the rectum to the sacrum. Additional fixation can be achieved by attaching a sheet of Ivalon sponge to the front of the sacrum and wrapping this sheet around the mobilized rectum, or by placing non-absorbable sutures between the rectum and periosteum of the

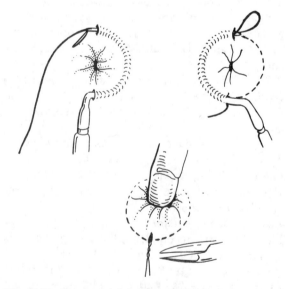

Fig. 35.12 Treatment of rectal prolapse by insertion of a Thiersch wire using an aneurysm needle (the wire is tightened around one finger)

sacrum. Repair without bowel resection is advised whenever possible, but anterior restorative resection may be required. If incontinence persists after a satisfactory anatomical repair, sphincter function may be improved by a *post-anal repair* in which, through an incision posterior to the anus, the posterior part of the sphincters is strengthened by sutures and the margins of the puborectalis are sutured together behind the rectum to increase the angle between the rectum and the anal canal. Abdominoperineal resection of the rectum is a last resort in patients with gross incontinence who fail to respond to less radical measures. In very frail patients a colostomy alone may suffice.

PRURITUS ANI

Aetiology

This is a common condition which occurs more frequently in men, especially between the ages of 30 and 60 years. Causal factors can be identified in only 50% of patients. It is assumed that psychogenic problems, chemical irritation by some constituent of faeces, or food allergy are responsible in the remainder. Defined causes of pruritus ani include the following.

Skin disease. Skin lesions may be localized to the perianal area or, as in the case of psoriasis and lichen planus, there may be lesions elsewhere. Contact eczema can be caused by local application of steroid, antibiotic, local anaesthetic or lanolin ointment or creams. Premalignant keratosis is a rare cause of perianal itching.

Infective conditions. Candidiasis must be considered in diabetics and those who have received prolonged courses of corticosteroid or broad spectrum antibiotics. Fungal infections occur occasionally. Threadworms are common in children but not in adults. Anal warts are commonly complicated by pruritus.

Gastrointestinal conditions. Pruritus can be a feature of anorectal disorders which cause a rectal discharge. Such disorders include piles, fissure, fistula, proctitis, polyps and rectal cancer. Frequent bowel movements in the irritable bowel syndrome, ulcerative colitis or malabsorptive disorders also predispose to pruritus.

Miscellaneous conditions. Some drugs such as quinidine and colchicine cause pruritus when taken for prolonged periods. Obesity increases the risk of pruritus.

Clinical features

The itching varies from a minor nuisance to a source of overwhelming misery. The urge to scratch is often irresistible so that the skin is damaged, causing local discomfort or pain. Symptoms are worst after defaecation and at night, regardless of the cause of pruritus.

The perianal skin may show no abnormality on examination, but more often appears raw and excoriated with linear cracks, ulcers and lichenification. Psoriasis and fungal infection often have a well-defined border.

Investigation is aimed at establishing the underlying cause. The entire skin surface is inspected, and proctoscopy and sigmoidoscopy are performed. The urine is examined for glucose. Candidiasis and fungal infection can be confirmed on skin scrapings.

Treatment

Underlying causes such as psoriasis, diabetes and infections are treated in the usual manner. Abnormalities of the anal region such as skin tags, fissures and fistulas should be surgically corrected.

In the large number of patients in whom no cause can be defined, a number of useful symptomatic measures can be introduced. First, all local applications are discontinued. Attention to anal hygiene is essential, as there may be primary or secondary sensitivity to faeces or rectal mucus. The region should be washed with lukewarm water in the morning and evening, and immediately after defaecation. Medicated soaps are avoided as their contained antiseptic may cause irritation. Excessive use of any form of soap is discouraged. After washing, the area is patted dry with a soft towel. It must not be rubbed vigorously. Application of talcum powder may be useful in warm weather to combat excessive sweating, and shaving of the perianal skin may be worthwhile. Woollen and nylon underwear favour sweating and should be replaced by cotton mesh garments.

It may be possible to identify certain items of diet which exacerbate pruritus, e.g. beer, red wine, coffee, curries, fruit and milk. Ingestion of mineral oil may favour pruritus by causing anal leakage, and advice on laxatives is essential. Bulk laxatives are preferred as a means of achieving a regular soft motion.

Considerable will power is needed to stop scratching during waking hours. Involuntary scratching during sleep can be reduced by sedation with phenothiazines. Postmenopausal women may benefit from oestrogen therapy, particularly if there is associated genital pruritus.

Continuing support is essential. Regular review ensures that the prescribed measures are being carried out.

Surgical treatment by denervation of the perianal skin through two curved incisions, one on either side of the perianal verge, has been described. The results are variable.

ANORECTAL ABSCESS

Aetiology

Anorectal abscesses are a common cause of admission to hospital. They are two to three times more common in males, the highest incidence occurring in the third and fourth decades.

There is no apparent cause for abscess formation in the majority of patients. It has been suggested that infection arises in an anal gland, passes to the intersphincteric space, and can then track (1) downwards to present as a perianal abscess, (2) outwards to form an ischiorectal abscess, or (3) upwards to produce a high intermuscular abscess (Fig. 35.13). Intersphincteric abscesses undoubtedly occur, but are less common than this concept suggests.

Associated underlying diseases such as Crohn's disease, ulcerative colitis, rectal cancer, HIV infection and active tuberculosis are sometimes present and should always be considered in patients with recurrent anorectal infection.

Anorectal abscess may lead to the development of a fistula-in-ano or, conversely, may complicate the presence of a fistula. In all recurrent abscesses this underlying cause should be kept in mind.

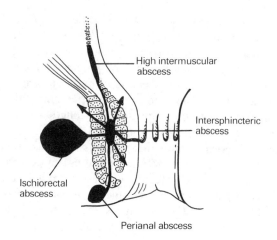

Fig. 35.13 Sites of anorectal abscess

Clinical features

Perianal abscess is common and presents as an acute painful tender swelling at the anal verge. Systemic upset is minimal.

Ischiorectal abscess is also common and produces a brawny diffuse induration lateral to the anus. The swelling is painful and tender but fluctuation occurs late. Systemic upset is pronounced. The swelling may be palpable on digital rectal examination and infection may extend behind the anal canal as a 'horseshoe abscess' involving both ischiorectal fossae.

Intersphincteric abscess is uncommon. Continuous throbbing anal pain is exacerbated by defaecation. There are few external signs unless the abscess is complicated by perianal or ischiorectal suppuration. Discharge into the anal canal leads to the passage of pus and blood. On digital rectal examination there is a boggy tender swelling under the mucosa.

High intermuscular abscess is rare and resembles an intersphincteric abscess in its presentation.

Pelvirectal abscess originates from pelvic sepsis.

Treatment

Perianal and ischiorectal abscesses are incised and drained under general anaesthesia. A specimen of pus is taken for bacteriological examination. The cavity walls are probed gently to detect any communication with the anal lumen. Fistulous connections can be demonstrated in up to one-third of patients but many such 'fistulas' are caused by injudicious probing. Assuming that no communication is detected, the abscess is deroofed by making a cruciate incision and excising the four triangles of skin (Fig. 35.14). The excised skin and a biopsy of the abscess wall are sent routinely for histological examination. A minority of surgeons suture the wound under antibiotic cover.

Problems in the treatment of anorectal abscess

1. *Fistula-in-ano.* If the internal opening of a fistula-in-ano is demonstrated on exploration and is below the pectinate line, the fistula should be laid open. This should only be performed by an experienced surgeon. If there is doubt about the level of the fistula, treatment should be deferred.

2. *Recurrence.* About one-quarter of patients presenting with an anorectal abscess develop recurrent abscess or a fistula, those with ischiorectal abscesses being most at risk. The rate of recurrence is not influenced by the primary treatment, i.e. whether primary suture is carried out or the wound is left to drain and heal by granulation.

3. *Inflammatory bowel disease.* Anorectal abscess may be the first manifestation of Crohn's disease,

ulcerative colitis or, much less commonly, tuberculosis. These abscesses are characteristically indolent and lined by pale grey granulation tissue. They should be incised and drained. Bacteriological and histological confirmation of the diagnosis is essential. Incision is frequently followed by fistula formation. Radical treatment should always be avoided in the first instance.

FISSURE-IN-ANO

An anal fissure is a tear in the sensitive skin-lined lower anal canal which produces pain on defaecation. The fissure commonly presents as an isolated primary problem but can be associated with other gastrointestinal diseases.

Classification

Primary fissure-in-ano

The aetiology of primary fissure-in-ano is uncertain but many patients first notice symptoms after passage of a hard constipated stool. The superficial fibres of the external sphincter are deficient posteriorly, and this may explain the frequency with which anal fissures occur in the posterior midline.

Secondary fissure-in-ano

Fissures are common in Crohn's disease and ulcerative colitis. Such secondary fissures are frequently multiple, occur at any point on the canal circumference, are broad-based and characteristically indolent. Fissures are a rare complication of anorectal operations such as haemorrhoidectomy.

Pathology of primary fissure

The typical primary fissure (Fig. 35.15) is a longitudinal tear extending from the anal verge to the pectinate line in the posterior midline. In 15% of female patients and in 1% of males the tear is in the midline anteriorly. The tear becomes a canoe-shaped ulcer, the floor of which contains the lower third of the internal sphincter. Inflammation

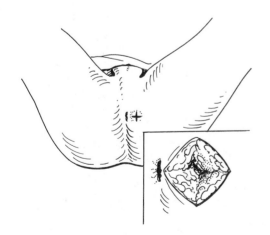

Fig. 35.14 Ischiorectal abscess showing treatment by cruciate incision. *Inset*: appearance of incision after excision of four skin triangles

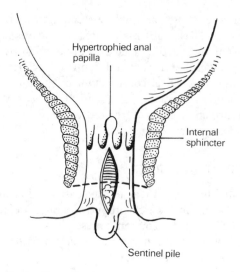

Fig. 35.15   Fissure-in-ano

causes swelling of the margins of the fissure, and an oedematous skin tag develops at the anal verge which is known as a *sentinel pile*. The swollen anal valve at the upper extent of the fissure is called a 'hypertrophied anal papilla'. Infection may produce a perianal abscess, incision of which results in a low anal fistula.

Anal fissures may heal spontaneously if untreated, or become chronic with fibrosis of the spastic internal sphincter.

Clinical features

The principal feature of a fissure is severe burning pain on defaecation which may persist for several hours. The pain may be so intense that defaecation is avoided. Bleeding sometimes occurs on defaecation, but is seldom profuse. The sentinel pile and associated serous discharge may cause excoriation and pruritus. Perianal abscesses and anal fistulas can complicate the fissure.

Recurrent or indolent fissures or fissures in an unusual site suggest the possibility of Crohn's disease or ulcerative colitis.

The diagnosis can usually be made on the history alone. Inspection reveals the sentinel pile, and traction on the anal skin may bring the lower part of the fissure into view. Digital rectal examination is painful and not often practicable. If the finger can be inserted, sphincter spasm is confirmed and

the indurated margins of the fissure are apparent. Maximal tenderness is elicited when the base of the fissure is palpable. Proctoscopy and sigmoidoscopy are essential to exclude other anorectal disease, but must be carried out under anaesthesia.

Treatment

Conservative treatment

Anal fissures can heal spontaneously. Conservative treatment with local anaesthetic ointments and suppositories has usually been tried without success by the time the patient is referred to hospital. Operative treatment allows a full anorectal examination, provides a rapid, more certain cure, and is generally advocated. Chronic fissures are unlikely to heal without operation.

Operative treatment

General anaesthesia is essential. The patient is placed in the lithotomy position, and the anal canal and rectum are examined thoroughly.

Anal dilatation. The majority of acute fissures respond to dilatation with dramatic relief of pain and spasm and subsequent healing. Transient impairment of anal control occurs in about a quarter of patients.

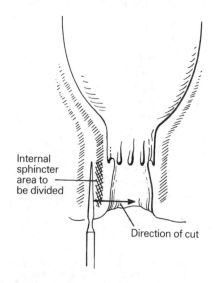

Fig. 35.16   Lateral subcutaneous internal sphincterotomy for fissure-in-ano

Lateral subcutaneous internal sphincterotomy. This operation gives a better guarantee of success as a first-line measure for both acute and chronic fissures. A tenotomy knife is introduced through the perianal skin on one side of the anal canal, and the internal sphincter is divided from the pectinate line downwards *without* entering the canal lumen (Fig. 35.16). The procedure gives immediate relief of pain. Open internal sphincterotomy and excision of the fissure is no longer practised.

FISTULA-IN-ANO

Aetiology

The aetiology of fistula-in-ano is uncertain. It may be that infection commences in an anal gland, spreads to produce an intersphincteric abscess and then tracks into the perianal or ischiorectal region. Surgical incision or spontaneous discharge completes the fistula, which is kept open by continuing infection from the anal lumen.

Anal fistulas have a well-recognized association with Crohn's disease, ulcerative colitis, tuberculosis, colloid carcinoma of the rectum, lymphogranuloma venereum and HIV infection.

Classification (Fig. 35.17)

Low anal fistula

This is the commonest anal fistula. The track does not extend higher than the anal crypts and usually enters the bowel at this level. The fistula may traverse both internal and external sphincters as it passes to the exterior, or descend in the intersphincteric plane.

High anal fistula

The track extends above the pectinate line but not above the anorectal ring. As with low fistulas, the track may traverse both sphincters or descend between them.

Anorectal fistula

These fistulas are rare. In the *ischiorectal* variety, the track extends above the anorectal ring but does

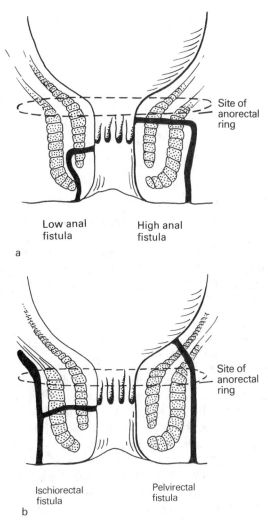

Fig. 35.17 Types of fistula-in-ano. (a) Anal fistulas. (b) Anorectal fistulas

not pass through the levator ani to enter the rectum.

Pelvirectal fistula

The rarer pelvirectal fistula does penetrate the levator, entering the rectum above the anorectal ring (see Fig. 35.17).

Goodsall's rule

Fistulas with an external opening in front of a transverse line through the anus generally open

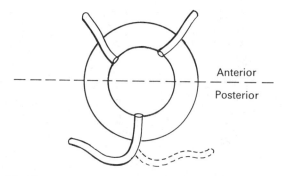

Fig. 35.18 Goodsall's rule

into the anal canal at the nearest point on its circumference. Fistulas with external openings behind this line tend to open internally in the posterior midline, and may extend behind the anal canal on both sides, forming a horseshoe fistula (Fig. 35.18).

Clinical features

Fistulas commonly present as abscesses, surgical incision of which completes the fistula. Alternatively, the patient notices a small discharging sinus with excoriation and pruritus. Once the fistula has formed, it is generally painless unless blockage leads to abscess formation. Carcinoma is a very rare complication of long-standing fisulas.

Examination reveals the external opening or openings. Digital rectal examination may reveal induration along the fistula track, while pressure on the indurated area expresses pus from the external opening. The internal opening may occasionally be seen on proctoscopy, and a malleable probe can be passed carefully along the fistula to define its course. Sigmoidoscopy is performed to exclude associated rectal disease.

Treatment

Fistulas associated with other anorectal disease are usually treated conservatively in the first instance. Those arising de novo rarely close spontaneously and operation is generally advised. The course of the fistula must be determined before embarking on surgery and the anorectal ring must be preserved. Disastrous permanent incontinence follows its inadvertent division.

Low anal fistulas are laid open along their entire length and allowed to heal by granulation and epithelialization. High anal fistulas and the ischiorectal type of anorectal fistula are treated in the same way provided the surgeon is certain that laying open the fistulas will not entail division of the anorectal ring. A two-stage procedure is sometimes used, passing a suture along the track and out through the anal canal. The suture is tied at the anal verge and this 'seton' allows fibrosis to occur before dividing the sphincteric muscle.

The rare pelvirectal fistula cannot be laid open without producing incontinence. The alternatives to a difficult formal repair are conservative treatment, long-term defunctioning colostomy, or excision of the rectum with permanent iliac colostomy.

BENIGN ANAL NEOPLASMS

The skin of the lower anal canal and perianal region may be affected by those benign neoplasms which affect the skin elsewhere.

Anal papillomas (anal warts, condylomata acuminata)

These deserve special mention. They arise from the anus or perianal skin, are often multiple, and often completely surround the anal region. Individual papillomas may be sessile or pedunculated, are often friable and bleed readily, and are usually associated with an offensive irritating discharge. The lesions are due to a viral infection and may present a serious problem in immunosuppressed patients.

Although they are particularly common in male homosexuals, these papillomas must not be confused with the flatter, smoother condylomata lata of secondary syphilis. Dark-ground illumination of the discharge fluid will reveal large numbers of spirochaetes and establish the diagnosis of syphilis if there is any uncertainty.

Treatment

Anal papillomas are treated by local application of podophyllin. Excision or diathermy may be needed if this fails to control the problem. In severe infections, interferon has been used with success.

MALIGNANT ANAL NEOPLASMS

Squamous cell carcinoma

This lesion accounts for at least 50% of malignant growths arising in the region of the anus and anal canal, but is rare compared to carcinoma of the rectum, which is about 50 times more common. Squamous carcinoma of the anus is more common in males. The aetiology of anal carcinoma is unknown but chronic irritation or infection may be a predisposing factor.

Clinical features

The patient usually presents with a localized ulcer or raised warty growth with an irregular ulcerated surface. A history of bleeding may give rise to an erroneous diagnosis of haemorrhoids. A profuse discharge results from ulceration and some patients develop incontinence due to involvement of the anal sphincter. Female patients may experience a vaginal discharge due to development of a fistulous communication with the vagina. The lesion is usually indurated, may spread around the anus, and is often fixed to underlying tissues by the time of presentation. Digital rectal examination may prove impossible because of stenosis or discomfort, but it is important to make certain that the lesion does arise from the anus or anal canal and is not a prolapsing or spreading adenocarcinoma of the lower rectum. The inguinal lymph nodes are examined carefully, as they receive lymph from the lower anal canal and perianal region and may be the seat of metastatic spread. Secondary sepsis produces nodes which are soft or firm, in contrast to the stony hard nodes of secondary neoplastic involvement.

The differential diagnosis of anal carcinoma includes anal papillomas, condylomata lata, primary syphilitic chancre, anal fissure, thrombosed piles, and Crohn's disease. The diagnosis must always be confirmed by biopsy.

Treatment

Anal carcinoma may be treated by radium implantation or X-ray therapy, but surgical excision is usually preferred if possible. Abdominoperineal excision of the anus, anal canal and rectum is the treatment of choice, particularly if the lesion extends above the pectinate line. In selected patients there may be a case for wide local excision if the lesion is confined to the anal margin or perianal area.

Treatment of the inguinal lymph nodes is controversial. Some 40% of patients will have nodal metastases at presentation and block dissection of obviously involved nodes is generally recommended once the patient has recovered fully from treatment of the primary anal lesion. If the nodes are not obviously involved, most surgeons would adopt a watching policy rather than carry out an unnecessary 'prophylactic' block dissection with its attendant hazards of sepsis, skin necrosis and lymphoedema. Radiotherapy offers an alternative method of treating involved inguinal nodes but many surgeons reserve this for patients with fixed inoperable nodes.

Results

The prognosis for patients with anal carcinoma is influenced by the extent of spread at the time of presentation, but in general the outlook is less good than that reported for carcinoma of the rectum. Five-year survival rates of around 50% can be achieved if excision is feasible, but few patients with obvious nodal metastases at presentation survive for more than five years.

Rare malignant tumours

Adenocarcinoma

Primary adenocarcinoma of the anal region is exceptionally rare but the neoplasm may arise in a long-standing fistula-in-ano, in the anal glands, or in the apocrine glands of the skin around the anal margin. Adenocarcinoma of the rectum may extend into the anal region and malignant cells from a colorectal cancer may implant in the raw wound following haemorrhoidectomy.

Primary anal adenocarcinoma is treated in the same way as squamous cell carcinoma, but in general the prognosis is poor.

Basal cell carcinoma

Basal cell carcinoma arising in the anal region is rare. The lesion has the same characteristics as basal cell carcinoma elsewhere and is treated by surgery or radiotherapy.

Malignant melanoma

Malignant melanoma of the anal region is rare.

PILONIDAL SINUS

A pilonidal sinus occurs predominately in the natal cleft of young adults. Pilonidal sinuses are also described in the hands of barbers and in the periumbilical area.

Typically a post-anal pilonidal sinus starts at an opening 2 cm posterior to the anus and extends subcutaneously in a headward direction for about 2–5 cm, expanding into a cavity. Secondary sinuses may arise from this and open onto the surface about 2 cm above the primary opening.

The opening of the sinus is lined by squamous epithelium but only for a few millimetres. Most of its wall is composed of granulation tissue. A typical feature of the sinus is its content of hairs. These are drawn into the sinus, tips first, and held in its depth by the direction of their scales.

Various theories have been proposed to explain the origin of a pilonidal sinus. These include congenital and traction dermoid cysts, remnants of vestigial glands, penetration by hairs due to the rolling action of the buttocks, and infection of hair follicles. They were common in US Army personnel during World War II — hence the term 'Jeep disease'.

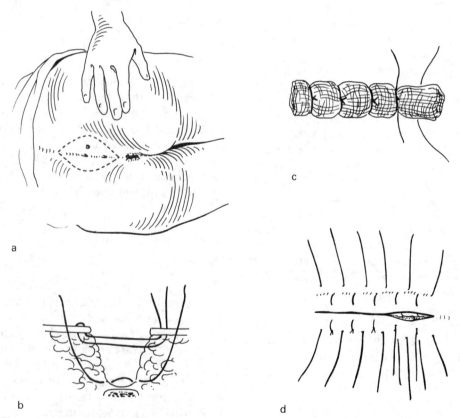

Fig. 35.19 Treatment of pilonidal sinus. (a) Elliptical incision to include all sinus openings. (b) Insertion of deep tension sutures down to the sacral fascia and placement of sutures in skin edges. (c) Skin sutures being tied. (d) Deep tension sutures tied over gauze roll to obliterate dead space

Clinical features

A pilonidal sinus does not usually become evident until infected. An acute or chronic abscess then develops, forming either a red tender hot swelling or a chronic discharge from the sinus. If seen in a quiescent phase the site of the external orifice is diagnostic.

Treatment

A pilonidal abscess is drained under general anaesthesia. The abscess cavity is deroofed and thoroughly cleaned out, removing all hair, granulation tissue and debris. It is left open to granulate and will heal over several weeks.

In a quiescent case, the sinus track is either excised or laid open. Excision of the sinus and its ramifications requires wide removal of tissue (Fig. 35.19). Primary suture is preferable but can be difficult without 'tenting' the skin over the underlying cavity. Rotation flaps can be used to facilitate primary healing.

When primary suture is not feasible or has failed, it is necessary to leave the wound open to granulate. Healing may then take many months. For this reason, marsupialization of the sinuses, i.e. laying them open and 'guttering' them by excising the skin edges, is preferred by many surgeons. The wound is left open, the skin edges being held apart by a pack or 'stent' of silicone foam so that they cannot reunite before healing occurs from the depths of the sinus.

Recently, destruction of granulations by injection of phenol into the sinus track has been reported to control symptoms.

Aftercare

Treated pilonidal sinuses are prone to recur. It is important that following any operative procedure for a pilonidal sinus the post-anal area is kept clean. In hirsute patients, regular shaving is advised.

36. The liver and biliary tract

THE LIVER

Anatomy

The liver is the largest abdominal organ, weighing approximately 1500 g. It extends from the fifth intercostal space to the right costal margin. It is triangular in shape, its apex reaching the left midclavicular line in the fifth space.

The liver is attached to the undersurface of the diaphragm by suspensory ligaments which enclose a 'bare area', the only part of its surface without a peritoneal covering. Its inferior or visceral surface lies on the right kidney, duodenum, colon and stomach.

Topographically the liver is divided by the attachment of the falciform ligament into right and left parts; fissures on its visceral surface demarcate two further lobes, the quadrate and caudate. These divisions are of little surgical import. From a practical standpoint it is the segmental anatomy of the liver, as defined by the distribution of its blood supply, which is important to the surgeon.

Vascular segmental anatomy

The portal vein and hepatic artery divide into right and left branches in the porta hepatis. Occluding either branch produces an easily visible line of demarcation which runs from the gallbladder bed to the inferior vena cava fossa and which separates the surgical lobes. Each surgical lobe is further divided into four segments corresponding to the main branches of the hepatic artery and portal vein. The left lobe can also be divided into a medial and lateral position by the attachment of the falciform ligament (Fig. 36.1).

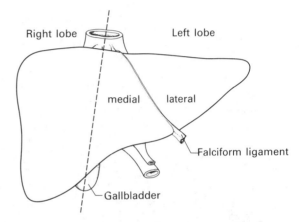

Fig. 36.1 Surgical anatomy of the liver

Blood supply

The liver normally receives 1500 ml of blood/min and has a dual blood supply: 65% comes from the portal vein and 35% from the hepatic artery. Because of its better oxygenation the hepatic artery supplies 50% of the oxygen requirements.

The venous drainage of the liver is by the right, middle and left hepatic veins, which leave the back of the liver to enter the vena cava (Fig. 36.2).

The functional unit of the liver is the hepatic lobule. Sheets of liver cells (hepatocytes) one cell thick are separated by interlacing sinusoids through which blood flows from the 'peripheral' portal tract to the 'central' branch of the hepatic venous system. The lobule forms a many-sided structure at each angle of which is a portal space containing a branch of the portal vein, hepatic artery and bile duct. Bile is secreted by the liver cells into small canaliculi which pass centrifugally

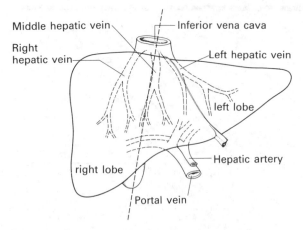

Fig. 36.2   Venous drainage of the liver

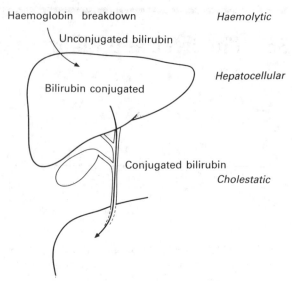

Fig. 36.4   Types of jaundice

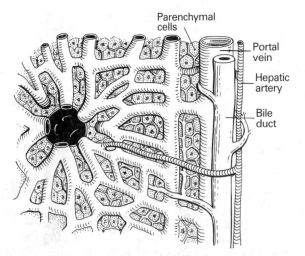

Fig. 36.3   The hepatic lobule: sinusoids drain into the central hepatic vein

through the lobule to drain into bile ductules leading to the right and left hepatic ducts (Fig. 36.3).

JAUNDICE

Jaundice is a yellowish discolouration of the tissues which is most obvious in those containing elastin, such as the skin and sclera. It is due to an increase in the level of circulating bilirubin and becomes obvious clinically when levels exceed 50 μmol/l. Jaundice may result from excessive destruction of red cells (haemolytic jaundice), from failure to remove bilirubin from the blood stream (hepatocellular jaundice), or from obstruction to

the flow of bile from the liver (cholestatic jaundice) (Fig. 36.4). Congenital non-haemolytic hyperbilirubinaemia is a relatively rare cause of jaundice due to defective bilirubin transport; the jaundice is usually mild and transient, the prognosis is excellent and the condition must not be confused with more serious causes of jaundice.

To the surgeon the most important type of haemolytic jaundice is that caused by hereditary spherocytosis, in which splenectomy may be necessary (see Ch. 38). Haemolytic jaundice may also occur after blood transfusion and after operative or accidental trauma where haematoma formation produces a pigment load which exceeds hepatic excretory capacity.

Hepatocellular jaundice is usually a medical as opposed to surgical problem although damage to liver cells can follow repeated general anaesthesia with halothane.

Cholestatic jaundice due to intrahepatic obstruction of bile canaliculi can be caused by drugs (e.g. chlorpromazine) and must be differentiated from extrahepatic obstruction, the cause of jaundice which has the greatest surgical relevance. Extrahepatic obstruction most commonly results from gallstones or cancer of the head of the pancreas. Other causes include cancer of the periampullary region or major bile ducts, iatrogenic biliary stricture, or extrinsic compression of the bile ducts by metastatic tumour.

Diagnosis

History and clinical examination

An accurate diagnosis of the cause of jaundice must be made as quickly as possible to allow prompt institution of appropriate treatment. The age, sex, occupation, social habits, drug and alcohol intake, history of injections or infusions, and general demeanour of the patient must all be considered. A history of intermittent pain, fluctuant jaundice and dyspepsia suggests calculous obstruction of the common bile duct, whereas a history of weight loss and relentless progressive jaundice favours a diagnosis of neoplasia. Obstructive jaundice is likely if there is a history of passage of dark urine and pale stools, and if the patient complains of pruritus (due to an inability to secrete bile salts into the obstructed biliary system). Hepatocellular jaundice is likely if there are stigmata of chronic liver disease such as liver palms, spider naevi, testicular atrophy and gynaecomastia. The abdomen must be examined for evidence of hepatomegaly or gallbladder distension, and for signs of portal hypertension such as splenomegaly, ascites and large collateral veins in the abdominal wall.

Biochemical investigations

Haemolytic jaundice is suggested if there are high circulating levels of unconjugated bilirubin but no bilirubin in the urine. Serum concentrations of liver enzymes are normal in these circumstances and the appropriate haematological investigations should be set in train.

In jaundice due to biliary obstruction, the circulating bilirubin is conjugated by the liver and rendered water-soluble; it can then be excreted in the urine and gives it a dark colour. As bile cannot pass into the gastrointestinal tract, the stool becomes pale and urobilinogen is absent from the urine. Obstruction increases the formation of alkaline phosphatase from the cells lining the biliary canaliculi and produces raised serum levels. In biliary obstruction the rise in serum alkaline phosphatase precedes that of bilirubin and its fall is more gradual once obstruction is relieved.

Serum transaminase and lactic dehydrogenase levels also often rise in obstruction. Conversely, swelling of the parenchyma in hepatocellular jaundice frequently produces an element of intrahepatic biliary obstruction and a modest rise in serum alkaline phosphatase concentration.

Serum hepatitis B surface antigen status should be determined in all jaundiced patients.

Radiological investigations

If the clinical picture and biochemical investigations suggest that jaundice is obstructive, radiological techniques can be used to define the site and nature of the obstruction.

Ultrasonography is the key investigation. It is safe, non-invasive and reliable in skilled hands. In the present context, it is used to define whether the patient has duct dilation due to obstruction and to confirm the need for more invasive investigation. Ultrasonography will also detect gallstones and space-occupying lesions in the liver and pancreas.

Endoscopic retrograde cholangiopancreatography (ERCP) involves outlining the biliary and pancreatic systems by injecting dye through a cannula inserted into the papilla of Vater by means of an endoscope passed into the duodenum. It gives more detailed information than ultrasonography and, as will be discussed later, also allows endoscopic treatment of gallstones, biopsy of periampullary tumours and relief of obstructive jaundice by insertion of stents.

Percutaneous transhepatic cholangiography (PTC) is used less often than formerly. It involves outlining the biliary system by dye injected through a slim flexible needle passed percutaneously into the liver. While diagnostic cholangiograms can be obtained in almost all patients with ductal obstruction, the technique may cause bleeding or bile leakage and can be complicated by bacteraemia and septicaemia. Coagulation status must be checked and the procedure covered by antibiotic administration (e.g. gentamicin). Facilities for emergency surgery should be available although they are seldom needed.

Computerized tomography can be used to identify hepatic, bile duct and pancreatic tumours in jaundiced patients.

Other radiological investigations are seldom needed. Isotopic liver scanning with ^{99m}Tc-labelled sulphur colloid may identify metastases but has been largely superseded by ultrasonography and CT scanning. Selective angiography is not used to diagnose the cause of jaundice but can be used to assess resectability if there is neoplastic obstruction. Barium meal examination and hypotonic duodenography are now obsolete investigations given the ready availability of ERCP. Nuclear magnetic resonance imaging may prove to be useful in the future.

Liver biopsy

Liver biopsy is a valuable diagnostic procedure in patients with unexplained jaundice in whom an obstructing lesion has been excluded by ultrasonography. It may be preceded by a CT scan to determine whether metastatic disease is present. If lesions have been identified, a 'target' liver biopsy can be conducted under ultrasonic or CT scanning control. Such techniques have diminished the need for target biopsy under laparoscopic control and general anaesthesia. Prothrombin time, platelet count and hepatitis B surface antigen status must always be determined and any clotting abnormalities corrected before biopsy is undertaken.

Laparotomy

Laparotomy is now seldom necessary to *establish* the cause of jaundice; its prime objective is to treat a causative lesion or relieve obstruction. Intraoperative ultrasonography and operative cholangiography may give useful additional information in patients with neoplasia and biliary obstruction. Appropriate preoperative preparation is particularly important in jaundiced patients (see Ch. 8).

CONGENITAL ABNORMALITIES

Polycystic disease is a rare cause of liver enlargement and may be associated with polycystic kidneys.

Cavernous haemangiomas are the most common benign tumours of the liver and may be con-genital and cause filling defects. Women are six times as commonly affected as men. Most of these haemangiomas are small solitary subcapsular growths found incidentally at laparotomy or autopsy.

Anatomical abnormalities of the extrahepatic bile ducts are common (see p. 565).

LIVER TRAUMA

After the spleen the liver is the solid organ most commonly damaged in abdominal trauma, particularly following road traffic accidents. Stab injuries and gunshot wounds of the liver are also increasing in incidence. These are considered in Chapter 14.

HEPATIC INFECTIONS AND INFESTATIONS

Hepatic abscess

Hepatic abscess may be classified as bacterial, parasitic or fungal. Bacterial abscess is the commonest problem in Western medicine but parasitic infestation is an important cause worldwide. Fungal abscesses are a rare cause of infection in patients with actinomycosis and those receiving long-term broad spectrum antibiotic treatment.

Pyogenic liver abscess

Bacterial infection may gain access (1) from the biliary system, (2) through the portal vein from abdominal sepsis, (3) by the hepatic artery from a septic focus anywhere in the body, (4) by direct spread from adjacent sepsis such as empyema of the gallbladder or a subhepatic abscess, or (5) following direct penetrating trauma. Calculous biliary obstruction is the commonest cause and portal spread from conditions such as appendicitis and diverticulitis is now rare. In some 50% of cases the abscess is 'cryptogenic' in that no cause can be found. The commonest infecting organisms are Gram-negative bacteria, notably *Escherichia coli*.

Pyogenic liver abscess is a relatively rare condition. The onset of symptoms is often insidious and the patient may present with a pyrexia of unknown origin. There is sometimes a history of sepsis elsewhere, particularly within the abdomen, and pain in the right hypochondrium. Other patients present with swinging pyrexia, rigors, marked toxicity and jaundice.

The liver may be enlarged and tender. Plain radiographs may show elevation of the diaphragm, pleural effusion and basal lobe collapse. Leucocytosis is usually present and there may be derangements in liver function tests. Ultrasonography or CT scanning is used to define the abscess, and ERCP may be useful if biliary obstruction is thought to be responsible.

Untreated abscesses often prove fatal because of spread within the liver to multiple sites, septicaemia and debility. Treatment consists of adequate drainage with appropriate antibiotic therapy. Some cases can be dealt with by percutaneous insertion of a catheter under ultrasonic guidance but formal surgical drainage under antibiotic cover is often needed. The drainage tube is left in place and the size of the cavity is monitored by serial X-rays following injection of contrast material.

Amoebic liver abscess

Entamoeba histolytica is a protozoal parasite which infests the large intestine and is endemic in many tropical regions. It is transmitted by cysts that are passed in the stools and which can survive for prolonged periods in moist surroundings. Overcrowding and insanitary living conditions favour ingestion of the cysts, which release trophozoites in the intestine. These probably penetrate the mucosa to gain access to the portal venous system and so spread to the liver. Hepatic cysts are usually solitary and situated in the right lobe. The abscess is large and thin-walled, and contains brown sterile pus resembling anchovy sauce.

Pain in the right upper quadrant is the most striking symptom. This is accompanied by anorexia, nausea, weight loss and night sweats. Over 90% of patients have tender enlargement of the liver. Other signs include basal pulmonary collapse, pleural effusion and leucocytosis. Ultrasonic and CT liver scans are used to demonstrate the site and size of the abscess.

The stool should be examined for amoebae or cysts. Direct and indirect serological tests to detect amoebic protein are available.

If untreated, an amoebic abscess may rupture into the peritoneal cavity or into a bronchus. Metastatic brain abscesses have been reported. Treatment consists of administration of an amoebicide (metronidazole and/or emetine) and usually results in rapid resolution. If there is no clinical response within 72 hours, the abscess should be aspirated by needle puncture although this is rarely necessary. Drainage by open operation is indicated only when there is secondary infection.

Hydatid disease

This is caused in man by one of two forms of tapeworm, *Echinococcus granulosus* and *Echinococcus multilocularis*. The adult tapeworm lives in the intestine of the dog, from which ova are passed in the stool; sheep or man serve as the intermediate host by ingesting ova (Fig. 36.5). The condition is common in sheep-rearing areas, e.g. Greece and Australia, where dogs, sheep and men live in close contact. Ova passed in the dog faeces may contaminate the food or fingers and so be ingested by man. They hatch in the duodenum and the embryos enter the portal venous system and pass to the liver, where they form a hydatid cyst. The cyst wall is surrounded by an adventitial layer of fibrous tissue and consists of a laminated membrane lined by germinal epithelium on which brood capsules containing scolices develop.

The disease may be symptomless, but chronic right upper quadrant pain with enlargement of the liver is the common presentation. The cyst may rupture into the biliary tree or peritoneal cavity, the latter sometimes causing an acute anaphylactic reaction from absorption of foreign hydatid protein. Other complications include secondary infection and biliary obstruction with jaundice.

Eosinophilia is common and serological tests such as the complement-fixation test are available to detect the foreign protein.

Hydatid cysts commonly calcify and may be seen on a plain film of the abdomen. Alternatively, they can be detected by ultrasonic or CT scanning of the liver. Treatment consists of isolating the cyst with packs, aspirating its contents and

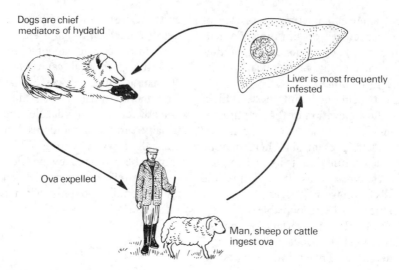

Fig. 36.5   Life cycle of *Echinococcus granulosus*

injecting a scolicidal agent (e.g. concentrated saline or 0.5% silver nitrate) to kill its contents. The cyst and its contained daughter cysts are then shelled out from the liver, taking care to remove the laminated membrane completely. Great care is taken not to spill the contents to avoid anaphylactic reactions and dissemination of viable scolices.

Mebendazole has been used as an alternative to surgical treatment but its value remains uncertain.

PORTAL HYPERTENSION

Portal hypertension is usually caused by increased resistance to portal venous blood flow, the obstruction being either prehepatic, hepatic or post-hepatic. Rarely it results primarily from an increase in portal blood flow. The normal pressure in the portal vein varies from 5 to 15 cm water. When the portal venous pressure is consistently raised above 25 cmH$_2$O, there may be serious clinical consequences. The causes of portal hypertension are shown in Table 36.1.

Portal vein thrombosis is a rare cause. It is most commonly due to neonatal umbilical sepsis, though the effects may not be manifest for many years.

By far the commonest cause of portal hypertension is cirrhosis of the liver. This results from chronic liver disease and is characterized by liver

Table 36.1   Causes of portal hypertension

Obstruction to portal flow

Prehepatic	Congenital atresia of the portal vein
	Portal vein thrombosis
	neonatal sepsis
	pyelophlebitis
	trauma
	tumour
	Extrinsic compression of the portal vein
	pancreatic disease
	lymphadenopathy
	biliary tract tumours
Intrahepatic	Cirrhosis
	Schistosomiasis
Posthepatic	Budd-Chiari syndrome
	Constrictive pericarditis

Increased blood flow (rare)

	Arteriovenous fistula
	Increased splenic blood flow
	in hypersplenism

cell damage, fibrosis and nodular regeneration. In micronodular cirrhosis there is an even distribution of nodules a few millimetres in diameter; in contrast, the nodules in macronodular cirrhosis are uneven in size and sometimes very large. Macronodules are usually found in end-stage cirrhosis, irrespective of its aetiology. The fibrosis obstructs portal venous return and portal hypertension develops. Arteriovenous shunts within the liver also contribute to the hypertension.

Alcohol is the commonest aetiological factor in Western countries and is increasing in prevalence. In North Africa, the Middle East and China schistosomiasis due to *Bilharzia mansonii* is a common cause. In alcoholic cirrhosis the abnormal resistance is predominantly postsinusoidal, as shown by an increase in wedged hepatic venous pressure. The hepatic veins become distorted by regenerative nodules, there is narrowing of the central veins by centrilobular collagen deposition, and swelling of the hepatocytes encroaches on the sinusoidal lumen. In schistosomiasis, granulomas from parasitic involvement are seen in the portal triads, and the hypertension is presinusoidal. Ultimately, as macronodules appear, the obstruction becomes postsinusoidal. Chronic active hepatitis, and primary and secondary biliary cirrhosis are relatively rare causes in this country. In a large number of patients the cause of cirrhosis remains obscure (cryptogenic cirrhosis).

Post-hepatic portal hypertension is rare. It is most frequently due to spontaneous thrombosis of the hepatic veins and this has been associated with neoplasia, oral contraceptive agents and polycythaemia. The resulting Budd-Chiari syndrome is characterized by portal hypertension, liver failure and gross ascites.

Effects of portal hypertension

As a result of gradual chronic occlusion of the portal venous system, collateral pathways develop between portal and systemic venous circulations. Eventually a large proportion of portal venous blood enters the systemic circulation directly and may give rise to portosystemic encephalopathy. Portosystemic shunting occurs (1) in veins at the junction of oesophagus and fundus of the stomach, (2) in retroperitoneal and periumbilical collaterals, and (3) in anastomotic veins in the anorectal region (Fig. 36.6).

The most important consequence of shunting is the development of *oesophageal varices*. The submucosal plexus of veins in the lower oesophagus and gastric fundus becomes variceal; oesophageal varices may then rupture to cause acute massive gastrointestinal tract bleeding. Such bleeding occurs in about 40% of patients with cirrhosis. The initial episode of variceal haemorrhage is fatal in

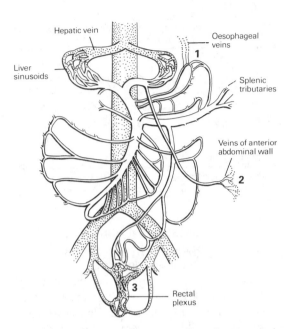

Fig. 36.6   The portal venous system. Sites of portosystemic shunting are marked **1–3**. Retroperitoneal communications also exist

about one-third of patients. At least two-thirds of those who survive their initial haemorrhage will bleed again.

Progressive enlargement of the spleen occurs from vascular engorgement and associated hypertrophy. Haematological consequences are anaemia, thrombocytopenia and leucopenia. (The resulting syndrome of *hypersplenism* is discussed in more detail in Ch. 38.) *Ascites* may develop and is due to an increased formation of hepatic and splanchnic lymph, hypoalbuminaemia, and salt and water retention. Increased aldosterone and antidiuretic hormone levels may contribute.

Portosystemic *encephalopathy* is due to an increased level of toxins such as ammonia in the systemic circulation. This is particularly likely to develop where there are large spontaneous or surgically created portosystemic shunts. Gastrointestinal haemorrhage increases the absorption of nitrogenous products and predisposes to encephalopathy.

Clinical presentation

Patients   with   cirrhosis   frequently   develop

Table 36.2 Assessment of patients with portal hypertension by modification of Child's criteria

Criterion	Points scored		
	1	2	3
Encephalopathy	None	Minimal	Marked
Ascites	None	Slight	Moderate
Bilirubin (μmol/l)	<35	35–50	>50
Albumin (g/l)	>35	28–35	<28
Prothrombin ratio	<1.4	1.4–2.0	>2.0

Grade A = 5–6 points; grade B = 7–9 points; grade C = 10–15 points. Shunts are contraindicated in group C.

anorexia, generalized malaise and weight loss. Clinical manifestations of liver disease may be present such as hepatosplenomegaly, ascites, jaundice and spider naevi. The serum bilirubin may be elevated and the serum albumin depressed. Anaemia may be present and the leucocyte count can be raised. The prothrombin time and other indices of clotting may be abnormal. Clinical and biochemical parameters are used as the basis of the Child's classification (Table 36.2). Patients allocated to Child's A have a good prognosis, whereas those in grade C have a poor prognosis and are not suitable for portosystemic shunting.

Patients with portal hypertension usually present to a surgeon (1) because of active bleeding from oesophageal varices; (2) to be considered for elective surgical treatment after recovery from an episode of acute haemorrhage; or (3) because of the discovery of varices which have not yet bled. Patients in this third group are usually kept under supervision although some surgeons now recommend prophylactic treatment of varices to avoid future bleeding.

Acute variceal bleeding

Patients presenting with acute upper gastrointestinal bleeding are carefully examined for evidence of chronic liver disease. The liver may be palpably enlarged and firm or nodular, the spleen may be enlarged, and ascites may be present. Jaundice, spider naevi, liver palms, opaque nails and finger clubbing are also sought. Distended collateral veins may be visible, particularly around the umbilicus, where they give rise to a 'caput Medusae'. Slurring of speech, a flapping tremor

or dysarthria may point to encephalopathy, and this may be precipitated or intensified by accumulation of blood in the gastrointestinal tract.

While a barium swallow and meal can detect oesophageal and gastric varices, the key investigation during an episode of active bleeding is endoscopy. This allows recognition of varices and defines whether they are or have been the actual site of bleeding. It is important to remember that peptic ulcer and gastritis are common complaints which occur in 20% of patients with varices. Even although a patient is known to have chronic liver disease and varices, bleeding cannot be assumed to be due to this cause.

Management

The priorities in the management of bleeding oesophageal varices are summarized in Table 36.3.

Active resucitation. Blood is withdrawn for grouping, cross-matching and a clotting screen; a free-flowing intravenous line is established, a urinary catheter is inserted to measure hourly urine output, pulse rate and blood pressure are monitored, and a central venous line is inserted to monitor central venous pressure. Large volumes of blood may be lost rapidly in these patients and the aim should be to replace blood loss quickly

Table 36.3 Priorities in the management of bleeding oesophageal varices

1. Active resuscitation
   Group and cross-match blood
   Establish i.v. infusion line(s)
   Monitor: pulse
             blood pressure
             hourly urine output
             central venous pressure
2. Assessment of coagulation status
   Thrombin time
   Kaolin cephalin clotting time
   Prothrombin time
   Platelet count
3. Urgent endoscopy
4. Control of bleeding
   Tamponade (Minnesota tube) or injection sclerotherapy
   Pharmacological measures (e.g. vasopressin)
5. Treatment of hepatocellular decompensation
6. Treatment/prevention of portosystemic encephalopathy
7. Prevention of further bleeding from varices
   Injection sclerotherapy
   Staple oesophagogastric junction
   Portosystemic shunting

with a view to urgent endoscopy. Many patients bleeding from varices will have coagulation defects from the outset and thrombocytopenia is common as a manifestation of hypersplenism. Fresh blood is preferred for transfusion purposes and the advice of the haematologist may be sought regarding the use of fresh frozen plasma or platelet transfusion.

Endoscopy. This is performed at the earliest opportunity, and in patients threatened by massive bleeding, active resuscitation is instituted and continued in the endoscopy suite. The tortuous varices are usually three in number and most prominent in the lower third of the oesophagus. If varices are the source of blood loss, this usually occurs from the lowest few centimetres of the oesophagus. Rarely, bleeding occurs from varices in the gastric fundus.

Control of bleeding. Medical agents used to lower portal venous pressure and arrest bleeding include vasopressin and somatostatin although their value is unproven. If variceal bleeding is apparent at the initial endoscopy, injection of ethanolamine is now used to arrest the bleeding. If haemorrhage is torrential and prevents direct injection, balloon tamponade is used to stop the bleeding.

The four-lumen Minnesota tube (Fig. 36.7) has largely replaced the three-lumen Sengstaken-Blakemore tube. The four lumina allow: (1) aspiration of gastric contents; (2) inflation of a gastric balloon with 150 ml of water to which a radio-opaque dye (Hypaque) has been added so that the balloon position can be checked radiologically (this balloon compresses the gastric fundus and oesophagogastric junction, so reducing the flow of blood into the oesophageal varices); (3) inflation of an oesophageal balloon with air to a pressure of 40 mmHg using a sphygmomanometer (this balloon applies direct pressure to the oesophageal varices); and (4) aspiration of the oesophagus and pharynx above the oesophageal balloon, so reducing the risk of aspiration pneumonitis and pneumonia.

Traction is applied to the Minnesota tube by pulling the gastric balloon up against the oesophagogastric junction and then taping a spatula to the tube as it emerges from the angle of the mouth. A trained nurse should be in constant

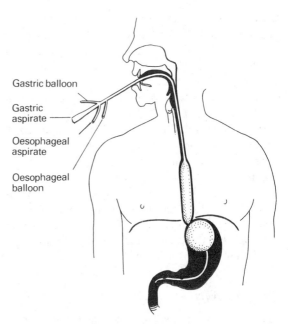

Gastric balloon

Gastric aspirate

Oesophageal aspirate

Oesophageal balloon

Fig. 36.7 Oesophageal tamponade using a Minnesota tube

attendance, and the pharynx and stomach are aspirated at 15–30 minute intervals. Balloon tamponade arrests bleeding from varices in over 90% of patients but the tube should not be left in place for more than 24–36 hours for fear of causing oesophageal necrosis. Tamponade should be regarded as a 'holding measure' which allows further resuscitation and treatment of hepatic decompensation. Unless more definitive measures are used to prevent further variceal bleeding (see below), two-thirds of individuals will rebleed while still in hospital and 90% will rebleed within a year.

Further resuscitation and treatment of hepatocellular decompensation. Control of variceal bleeding allows blood loss to be made good and permits full assessment of coagulopathy. Cimetidine (400 mg i.v. 6-hourly) is prescribed to reduce the risk of bleeding from gastritis or peptic ulceration, and may be combined with instillation of antacids down the gastric lumen of the Minnesota tube. A daily bowel washout is used to evacuate blood from the gut and reduce the risk of portosystemic encephalopathy. This endeavour can be assisted by prescribing aperients such as magnesium sulphate. Alternatively, magnesium trisilicate (30 ml 4-hourly) can be used for both its antacid and aperient properties. Lactulose (15–30 ml 8-hourly) is prescribed to reduce bacterial degradation of blood in the gut lumen and further reduce the risk of encephalopathy. Patients with oesophageal varices due to liver disease frequently have major defects in both the intrinsic and extrinsic clotting systems which may prove refractory to therapy. Vitamin K1 is prescribed to aid restoration of the extrinsic system, but fresh frozen plasma, factor concentrates and platelet transfusion may all be required to cover specific procedures such as sclerotherapy or surgery. It should be stressed that these transfusion measures have transient effects on blood coagulation and that the ultimate coagulation status depends upon restoration of hepatic function.

Prevention of further bleeding

A number of methods are now available to reduce the risk of further variceal bleeding. The method currently most frequently employed is repeated variceal sclerotherapy.

1. *Injection sclerotherapy* as described above is repeated at weekly or fortnightly intervals until the varices are completely sclerosed. Following complete ablation, fibreoptic examination is repeated periodically and any recurrent varices are injected. Multiple, excessive or too frequent injection, particularly into the wall of the oesophagus, may be complicated by ulceration and necrosis, sometimes with a fatal result. Controversy exists over whether the sclerosant should be injected directly into the varix or into the surrounding mucosa. The increased used of injection sclerotherapy has led to a substantial reduction in the number of patients submitted to shunt surgery. While sclerotherapy reduces the risk of further variceal bleeding, it is still uncertain whether it improves long-term survival prospects.

2. *Surgical disconnection* is usually reserved for patients who continue to bleed despite injection sclerotherapy. The left gastric vein and short gastric veins are ligated and the distal oesophagus is transected and re-anastomosed just above the cardia using a stapling gun (Fig. 36.8). Stapling is relatively easy to perform and the double row of staples inserted through the full thickness of the oesophageal wall occludes flow into the varices.

3. Emergency portosystemic shunting carries a high mortality and has been abandoned in most centres. On the other hand, *elective portosystemic shunting* is still used occasionally to decompress the portal system and reduce the risk of further

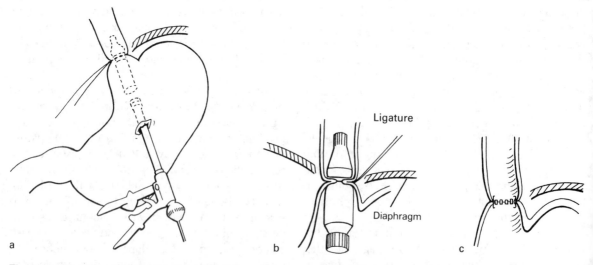

Fig. 36.8 Oesophageal stapling. (a) Gun inserted through an anterior gastrotomy. (b) Ligature tied just above the cardia, invaginating a flange of oesophageal wall between the two parts of the gun. (c) The gun has been fired, simultaneously resecting a full-thickness ring of oesophageal wall and anastomosing the cut ends with tantalum staples

variceal haemorrhage. Unfortunately, portosystemic encephalopathy can be a troublesome side effect and it is uncertain whether shunting prolongs life in patients with parenchymal liver disease. The indications for shunting are strict and in general the operation is only undertaken in patients whose condition is not complicated by jaundice, ascites or encephalopathy.

Portal venography is essential to define the anatomy of the portal venous system. It can be undertaken by percutaneous transplenic or transhepatic injection of contrast or by examining the venous phase after coeliac angiography. Ultrasonic and CT scans may also be used to examine the portal system.

Types of shunt procedure. There are several anatomical sites at which portosystemic shunts can be performed (Fig. 36.9). In a portacaval shunt the portal vein is anastomosed end-to-side or side-to-side to the inferior vena cava. Mesocaval shunts can be constructed between the superior mesenteric vein and inferior vena cava using autogenous saphenous vein or a synthetic graft. They are easier to perform but have a high incidence of thrombosis.

Splenorenal shunts, between the splenic and renal veins, are most appropriate when there is portal vein obstruction. The distal splenorenal (Warren) shunt selectively decompresses the lower oesophagus and upper stomach and maintains liver

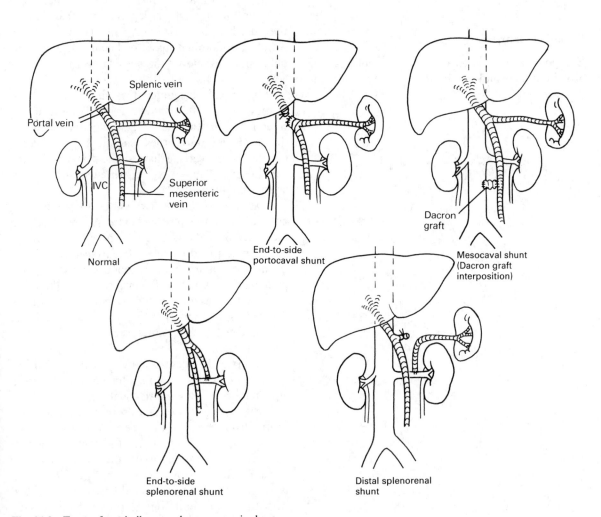

Fig. 36.9 Types of surgically created portosystemic shunts

blood flow, and is preferred by many surgeons. The incidence of encephalopathy is reported to be lower than after other shunt procedures.

The results of shunt surgery are very variable, depending chiefly on the liver function of the patient and the skill and experience of the surgeon.

Ascites

Ascites can be controlled by bed rest, salt and water restriction, and a diuretic such as the aldosterone inhibitor spironolactone. If refractory, ascites can be treated by inserting a peritoneojugular (LeVeen) shunt which allows one-way flow between the peritoneum and jugular vein (Fig. 36.10).

Encephalopathy

Encephalopathy is treated by witholding all protein intake and by bowel washouts and ad-

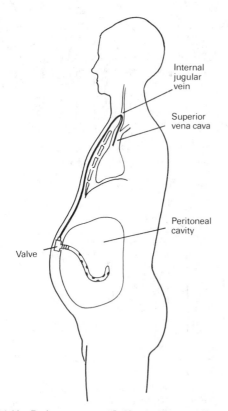

Internal jugular vein

Superior vena cava

Peritoneal cavity

Valve

Fig. 36.10   Peritoneo-venous (LeVeen) shunt to relieve ascites

ministration of oral lactulose to reduce bacterial decomposition of protein in the intestine. At least 1600 kcal of carbohydrate should be given daily, along with therapeutic amounts of vitamins.

TUMOURS OF THE LIVER

Hepatic tumours can be benign or malignant, primary or secondary. Primary tumours may arise from the parenchymal cells, the epithelium of the bile ducts or from the supporting tissues.

Benign hepatic tumours

Cavernous haemangioma is the most common benign liver tumour. Most are asymptomatic and are found incidentally at laparotomy. Occasionally they reach a large size and patients present with pain, an abdominal mass, or haemorrhage. Heart failure may develop if there is a large arteriovenous communication.

Symptomatic haemangiomas should be excised if they are small, or treated by radiotherapy if resection is hazardous. If discovered incidentally during laparotomy, they should be left alone; needle biopsy can be hazardous. Ligation of the hepatic artery may help in patients with a large arteriovenous fistula.

Liver cell adenomas, which occur almost exclusively in women, have increased markedly in incidence over the last decade, possibly as a result of the widespread use of oral contraceptives. Two-thirds are solitary. These tumours rarely become malignant and are well encapsulated. They are commonly asymptomatic, but occasionally produce right hypochondrial pain and may bleed spontaneously, sometimes in association with menstruation.

They may be identified by ultrasonography or CT scanning. Liver function tests and serum alphafetoprotein levels are usually normal.

Treatment usually consists of enucleation but formal liver resection may be necessary.

Focal nodular hyperplasia of the liver is a rare condition. The nodule is usually solitary and lies immediately beneath the liver capsule. The lesion is generally asymptomatic and has been associated with the use of oral contraceptives. Symptomatic lesions should be removed, but the condition is not premalignant and may regress once oral contraceptives are stopped.

Primary malignant tumours of the liver

Hepatocellular carcinoma (hepatoma)

Hepatocellular carcinoma (hepatoma) is relatively uncommon in the Western world but is common in Africa and the Far East. Environmental factors are probably important: in American negroes the incidence is the same as that in the white American population. The tumour is commoner in males. In the Western world about two-thirds of patients have pre-existing cirrhosis; many others have hepatitis B surface antigen in their blood. In Africa and the East, 'aflatoxin' (derived from the fungus *Aspergillus flavus*, which contaminates maize and nuts) is an important hepatocarcinogen. Viral hepatitis is also now regarded as an important aetiological factor.

Clinical features. The diagnosis is usually made late in the course of the disease. Common presenting features include abdominal pain, weight loss, abdominal distension, fever and intraperitoneal haemorrhage. In Westerners, sudden deterioration in a cirrhotic patient should lead to suspicion of tumour. Jaundice is uncommon unless the tumour is associated with advanced cirrhosis. On examination the liver is usually grossly enlarged.

Alphafetoprotein (an oncofetal antigen) is present in the serum of 80% of African patients with hepatocellular carcinoma, compared to only 30% of the white population with this disease. A filling defect is apparent on scintiscanning with ^{99m}Tc-labelled sulphur collid, while the same area shows an increased uptake when $[^{75}Se]$ selenomethionine is used. Plain X-ray may show calcification or detect pulmonary or other metastases. Ultrasonography, CT scanning and selective coeliac arteriography are valuable to determine the extent of the tumour and assess the feasibility of resection.

Treatment. The only prospect of cure lies in complete surgical resection of the tumour. This is only feasible when one lobe or segment of the liver is completely free of disease. As there is a tendency to multicentricity and for satellite lesions to surround a primary central tumour, cure is unusual. For advanced tumours, hepatic artery ligation or chemotherapy with doxorubicin (Adriamycin), methotrexate or 5-fluorouracil may have palliative value. The disease is usually advanced at the time of presentation and the 5-year survival rate is less than 10%. Liver transplantation has been used in the treatment of this tumour but with disappointing results.

Cholangiocarcinoma

This adenocarcinoma may arise anywhere in the biliary tree, including its intrahepatic radicles. It accounts for about 20% of malignant primary neoplasms of the liver in Western medicine. In the Orient it is most commonly associated with chronic parasitic infestation of the biliary tree.

Jaundice, pain and an enlarged liver are the common presenting features. Resection offers the only prospect of cure but is seldom feasible when cholangiocarcinoma arises in the liver substance. Cholangiocarcinoma arising from the extrahepatic bile ducts will be considered later.

Angiosarcoma

This is a rare tumour of the liver which arises after industrial exposure to vinyl chloride or exposure to the previously used radiological contrast medium Thorotrast.

The prognosis in patients with angiosarcoma is extremely poor and resection is seldom feasible.

Metastatic tumours

The liver is a common site for metastatic disease. Secondary liver tumours are 20 times more common than primary ones. In one-half of cases the original tumour is in the gastrointestinal tract; other common sites are the breast, ovaries, bronchus and kidney. Almost 90% of patients with hepatic metastases have tumour deposits in other organs.

Hepatomegaly and tenderness are distinctive features, and individual deposits may be palpable. The patient is often cachectic and ascites or jaundice may be present. Pyrexia occurs in 10–20% of patients with metastic tumours of the liver and may initially be regarded as pyrexia of unknown origin. Liver function tests are abnormal, particularly the alkaline phosphatase, lactate dehydrogenase and gamma-glutamyl transpeptidase, which are raised. Ultrasonic scans, scintiscans and CT scans may demonstrate multiple filling defects. The diagnosis is confirmed by aspiration cytology or needle biopsy. Target biopsy can be undertaken under ultrasonic control.

There is no effective treatment for most patients with hepatic metastases. Both lobes of the liver are usually involved, making surgical resection impossible. Hepatic artery ligation, radiotherapy and chemotherapy have all been used but the results have been disappointing.

Palpation of the liver for metastases should be carried out routinely during laparotomy. As benign cysts and adenomas may mimic small surface metastases, suspicious lesions should be biopsied if at all possible. In some tumours, notably those arising from the colon and rectum, apparently solitary metastases may be resected; reasonable survival periods have been reported after such resections.

LIVER RESECTION

The techniques of liver resection are complicated and operations such as hepatic lobectomy should be performed only by those with experience. Basically the vascular supply to the involved area of the liver is ligated and divided, following which the devascularized lobe or segment can be separated by 'finger fracture' of the parenchyma. Intervening biliary and vascular channels can be felt, defined and ligated. Adequate drainage of the area is essential following resection.

LIVER TRANSPLANTATION

This is considered in Chapter 15.

THE GALLBLADDER AND BILE DUCTS

Anatomy of the biliary system

The biliary 'tree' consists of fine intrahepatic biliary radicles, the right and left hepatic ducts, the common hepatic duct and the common bile duct. The right and left hepatic ducts converge to form the common hepatic duct. This is joined

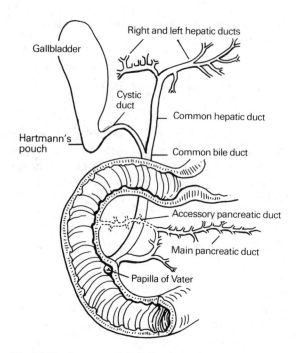

Fig. 36.11 Anatomy of the biliary tree

at a variable position by the cystic duct to form the common bile duct, which ends at the papilla of Vater, usually in the second part of the doudenum (Fig. 36.11).

The common bile duct is approximately 8 cm long and up to 10 mm in diameter. It lies in the free edge of the lesser omentum before passing behind the first part of the duodenum and through the head of the pancreas. The bile duct is usually joined by the pancreatic duct just before entering the duodenum.

The gallbladder lies in a bed on the undersurface of the liver between the right and left lobes. It is a muscular structure with a fundus, body and neck. Hartmann's pouch is a dilatation of the gallbladder outlet adjacent to the origin of the cystic duct in which gallstones frequently become impacted. The gallbladder is supplied by the cystic artery, a branch of the right hepatic artery.

Physiology

Bile acids and the enterohepatic circulation

Bile acids are sterols synthesized by the liver from cholesterol. The primary bile acids are chenodeoxycholic and cholic acid; these are conjugated with glycine or taurine to increase their solubility in water, and the conjugates (e.g. glycocholic and taurocholic acid) form sodium and potassium bile salts. In the intestine, bacterial action produces the secondary bile acids, deoxycholic and lithocholic acid.

Bile salts can combine with lipids to form water-soluble complexes called micelles (Fig. 36.12). Lecithin and cholesterol can be transported from the liver within such micelles. Bile salts are also detergents and reduction in surface tension allows fat to be emulsified in the intestine, thus facilitating its digestion and absorption. On reaching the distal ileum, 95% of the bile salts are reabsorbed, transported back to the liver and passed once again into the biliary system. This enterohepatic circulation (Fig. 36.13) allows a relatively small bile salt pool (2–4 g) to circulate some 6–12 times a day through the intestine. The daily faecal loss equals that of hepatic synthesis (0.2–0.6 g/24 h). When bile is excluded from the intestine, 25% of ingested fat may appear in the faeces and there is marked malabsorption of fat-soluble vitamins.

The gallbladder has a capacity of 50 ml and can concentrate bile by a factor of ten. It contracts in response to cholecystokinin (CCK), which is released from the duodenal mucosa by the presence of food, notably fatty acids. Gallbladder contraction is accompanied by reciprocal relaxation of the sphincter of Oddi. The secretion of

bile is promoted by the hormone secretin. The vagus nerve also stimulates bile secretion and gallbladder contraction.

CONGENITAL ABNORMALITIES

Congenital abnormalities of the gallbladder and bile ducts are common. The gallbladder may be absent (agenesis), double, intrahepatic, partitioned with a fold in the fundus (Phrygian cap) or multiseptate. The cystic duct may be absent or join the right hepatic duct rather than the common hepatic duct, and accessory ducts may be present. The cystic artery may be duplicated or may arise from the common hepatic or left hepatic artery. These anomalies are important in that great care must be taken to avoid inappropriate division of ducts and arteries in the course of cholecystectomy.

Biliary atresia

Failure of development of the duct system occurs once in every 20 000 to 30 000 births and is the commonest cause of prolonged jaundice in infancy. The condition may be acquired after birth rather than truly congenital in that it has not been described in autopsies of newborn infants. The site and extent of the atresia are variable and the duct system may be entirely replaced by solid fibrous strands. Fortunately, intrahepatic atresia is rare and the extrahepatic system is usually most affected.

Jaundice usually becomes apparent in the first 2–3 weeks of life, the urine is dark and the stools are pale. The liver and spleen usually enlarge. Liver function tests normally show an obstructive pattern although the serum transaminase levels are often elevated. Liver biopsy reveals cholestatic jaundice but differentiation from neonatal hepatitis is often surprisingly difficult.

In extrahepatic biliary atresia a Roux loop of jejunum is anastomosed to the intrahepatic duct system in the hilus of the liver (Kasai operation). Delayed treatment may allow progressive cirrhosis to develop, with consequent portal hypertension and ascites. The prognosis for infants with extra hepatic biliary atresia has improved although recurrent fibrosis and stricture may lead to

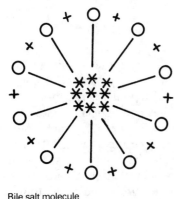

○   Bile salt molecule

✱   Cholesterol

✛   Phospholipid

Fig. 36.12 Cholesterol micelle

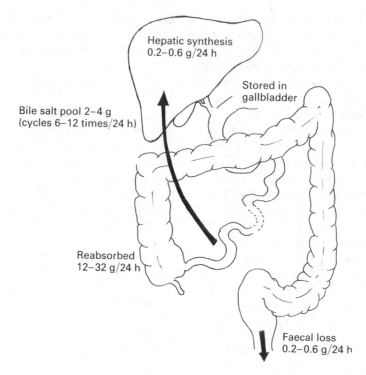

Fig. 36.13 The enterohepatic circulation

troublesome cholangitis and abscess formation. Intrahepatic atresia is rarely correctable. Liver transplantation should be considered in infants with progressive liver disease.

Choledochal cysts

Cystic transformation of the biliary tree (choledochal cyst) is rare. It is often associated with an anatomical abnormality in which the lower end of the common bile duct enters the pancreatic duct within the head of the pancreas. This may allow reflux into the biliary system and cause pain, inflammation and calculus formation. The abnormalities are probably congenital although diagnosis may be delayed until adult life.

The patient usually presents with intermittent pain and jaundice and may have attacks of pancreatitis. A mass may be palpable in the right hypochondrium. Ultrasonography and cholangiography (ERCP or PTC) establish the diagnosis. Excision of the cyst is advisable as there is a significant risk of malignant transformation.

Caroli's disease is a form of cystic biliary dilatation in which multiple cysts are found within the liver. Recurring infection may progress to cirrhosis and liver failure. Transplantation may be considered when medical treatment fails.

GALLSTONES

Pathogenesis

Gallstones are formed from the constituents of bile. The great majority of stones result from failure to keep cholesterol in micellar form in the gallbladder, and pigment stones (composed of calcium bilirubinate) are rare. Most cholesterol stones become mixed with bile pigments as they increase in size; such 'mixed' stones are much more common than pure cholesterol stones.

Gallstones are common in Europe and North America and less common in Asia and Africa. Their incidence increases with age. In 'developed' countries they occur in at least 20% of women over the age of 40; the incidence in males is about one-third of that in females. The disease has increased markedly in frequency and cholecystectomy is the commonest major elective abdominal operation in many Western countries.

Cholesterol stones

Cholesterol stones may occur in both sexes from the late teens onwards but are particularly common in middle aged, obese, multiparous females. Stone formation is encouraged if bile becomes supersaturated with cholesterol (i.e. lithogenic) either by excessive cholesterol excretion or by reduction in the amount of bile salt and lecithin available for micelle formation. Supersaturation is most likely to occur during the concentration of bile while it is within the gallbladder, and is favoured by stasis or decreased gallbladder contractility. The formation of cholesterol crystals is the key event, and this 'nuncleation' may be due to coalescence of cholesterol molecules or their precipitation around particles of mucus, bacteria, calcium bilirubinate or mucosal cells. Not all individuals with supersaturated bile develop gallstones so that other factors must be implicated. Pure cholesterol stones are yellowish-green with a regular shape but rough surface. They are usually solitary. In contrast, mixed stones are darker and are usually multiple.

Cholesterol stones are particularly common in some tribes of North American Indians, where more than 75% of women over 40 are affected. Such individuals have a small bile salt pool. Conversely, the high incidence of stones in Chilean women reflects high levels of cholesterol excretion.

Obesity and high-calorie or high-cholesterol diets favour cholesterol stone formation by producing highly supersaturated gallbladder bile. Drastic weight reduction and diets designed to lower serum cholesterol levels may also promote stone formation by mobilizing cholesterol and increasing its excretion.

Disease or resection of the terminal ileum and drugs such as cholestyramine may favour cholesterol nucleation by reducing the bile salt pool. Hormonal influences are reflected in an increased incidence of stone formation in women taking oral contraceptives or postmenopausal oestrogen replacement. Pregnancy may also have

an effect by increasing stasis within the gallbladder. Similarly, after vagotomy the gallbladder becomes flaccid and increases in volume. Hypercholesterolaemia as such is not associated with stone formation.

Pigment stones

Pigment stones consist of calcium bilirubinate and are usually multiple, small and amorphous. Stones found in Occidental patients are usually composed of black pigment, whereas brown pigment stones are common in Orientals. Pigment stones account for 25% of all gallstones in Western patients but for 60% of those in some Oriental countries such as Japan.

Chronic haemolysis favours pigment stone formation by increasing pigment excretion, and stone formation is common in congenital spherocytosis, haemoglobinopathy and malaria. Cirrhosis and biliary stasis are also important associations. Some patients with brown pigment stones have increased concentrations of unconjugated bilirubin in the bile. In Oriental patients this may be due to the action of beta-glucuronidase, which is produced by *E. coli* and which invades ductal systems infested with the parasites *Clonorchis sinensis* or *Ascaris lumbricoides*.

Pathological effects of gallstones (Fig. 36.14)

Inflammation

Inflammation of the gallbladder may be acute or chronic. Bacteria are cultivated from the bile of approximately one-half of patients with gallstones. The common organisms are *E. coli*, *Klebsiella aerogenes* and *Streptococcus faecalis*. Staphylococci, clostridia and salmonella are occasionally present.

Acute cholecystitis

This is usually produced by obstruction of the neck of the gallbladder or cystic duct by a stone. Prolonged obstruction in the presence of infected bile may produce an empyema. The thickened gallbladder becomes intensely inflamed, oedematous and occasionally gangrenous. The fundus of the distended, inflamed gallbladder may

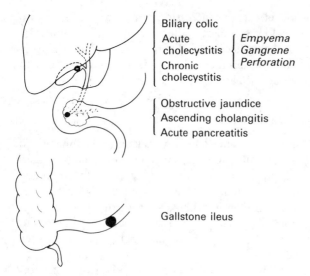

Biliary colic

Acute } cholecystitis { Empyema Gangrene Perforation

Chronic cholecystitis

Obstructive jaundice
Ascending cholangitis
Acute pancreatitis

Gallstone ileus

Fig. 36.14 Pathological effects of gallstones

perforate, giving rise to localized abscess formation and occasionally to biliary peritonitis.

Chronic cholecystitis

Infection may reach the gallbladder through the biliary tract or by lymphatic or haematogenous spread. Stasis predisposes to infection. Repeated bouts of biliary colic or acute cholecystitis culminate in fibrosis, contraction of the gallbladder and chronic inflammatory change with marked thickening of the wall. The gallbladder ceases to function. Chronic inflammatory change is commonly present in the gallbladders of typhoid carriers, which often harbour organisms for long periods of time.

Mucocele

A mucocele develops when the outlet of the gallbladder becomes obstructed in the absence of infection. The imprisoned bile is absorbed but clear mucus continues to be secreted into the distended gallbladder.

Choledocholithiasis

When gallstones enter the common bile duct they may pass spontaneously or give rise to obstructive jaundice, cholangitis or acute pancreatitis.

Gallstone pancreatitis most commonly occurs when a small stone becomes temporarily arrested at the ampulla of Vater. The exact mechanism whereby acute pancreatitis results is not clear. Reflux of infected bile into the pancreatic ducts may be responsible.

Gallstone ileus

This uncommon form of intestinal obstruction occurs when a large gallstone becomes impacted in the intestine. Stones large enough to block the gut are usually too large to pass through the sphincter of Oddi. They generally gain access by eroding through the wall of the gallbladder into the duodenum.

Carcinoma

The incidence of carcinoma of the gallbladder is increased in patients with long-standing gallstones.

Common clinical syndromes associated with gallstones

The majority of individuals with gallstones are asymptomatic or have only vague symptoms of distension and flatulence. Half of such patients will develop some symptoms or complications due to gallstones within 10 years. Gallstones may give rise to symptoms in several ways.

Biliary colic

Biliary colic is due to transient obstruction of the gallbladder from an impacted stone. There is severe gripping pain, often developing in the evening, and maximal in the epigastrium and right hypochondrium with radiation to the back. Though continuous, the pain may wax and wane in intensity over several hours. Vomiting and retching occur. Resolution follows when the stone falls back into the gallbladder lumen or passes onwards into the common bile duct. The patient recovers rapidly but repeated bouts of colic are common.

Acute cholecystitis

Acute cholecystitis results in a more prolonged and

severe illness. It usually begins with an attack of biliary colic, though its onset may be more gradual. There is severe right hypochondrial pain radiating to the right subscapular region, and occasionally to the right shoulder (from diaphragmatic irritation), together with tachycardia, pyrexia, nausea, vomiting and leucocytosis. Abdominal tenderness and rigidity may be generalized but are most marked over the gallbladder. Murphy's sign (a catching of the breath at the height of inspiration while the gallbladder is palpated) is usually present. A right hypochondrial mass may be felt. This is due to omentum 'wrapped' around the inflamed gallbladder.

In 85–90% of cases the attack settles within 4–5 days. In the remainder, tenderness may spread and pyrexia and tachycardia persist. Development of a tender mass associated with rigors and marked pyrexia signals empyema formation. The gallbladder may become gangrenous and perforate, giving rise to biliary peritonitis.

Jaundice can develop during the acute attack. Usually this is associated with stones in the common bile duct but compression of the bile ducts by the gallbladder may be responsible.

Acute cholecystitis must be differentiated from perforated peptic ulcer, high retrocaecal appendicitis, acute pancreatitis, myocardial infarction and basal pneumonia. Acute cholecystitis can develop in the absence of gallstones (acalculous cholecystitis). This is rare.

Chronic cholecystitis

Chronic cholecystitis is the common form of symptomatic gallbladder disease. It is almost invariably associated with gallstones. Recurrent flatulence, right upper quadrant pain and fatty food intolerance are common. The pain is worse after meals and is often associated with a feeling of distension and heartburn.

The differential diagnosis includes duodenal ulcer, hiatus hernia, myocardial ischaemia, chronic pancreatitis and gastrointestinal neoplasia.

Mucocele

A piriform swelling is palpable in the right hypochondrium. It is not tender and there is no pyrexia.

Choledocholithiasis

Stones are present in the common bile duct of 10–15% of patients with gallstones. There is little muscle in the wall of the bile duct and pain is not a symptom unless the stone impedes flow through the sphincter of Oddi. Then colic occurs. The vast majority of stones in the common bile duct originate in the gallbladder. 'Primary' duct stones are extremely rare.

Impaction of a stone at the sphincter causes obstruction to the flow of bile, with jaundice, the passage of pale stools, and dark urine. Obstruction commonly persists for several days but may clear spontaneously, either as a result of passage of the stone or its disimpaction. Small stones may pass through the common bile duct without causing symptoms.

In long-standing obstruction the bile ducts become markedly dilated. For the common bile duct a diameter of 10 mm is regarded as the upper limit of normal. A totally obstructed duct system becomes filled with clear 'white bile'; back pressure on the hepatocytes prevents clearance of bilirubin and mucus secretion is increased.

Infection of an obstructed biliary tract causes cholangitis with pain, pyrexia and jaundice (the so-called triad of Charcot). Long-standing obstruction of the biliary tract leads to secondary biliary cirrhosis.

Acute pancreatitis may be associated with a stone in the common bile duct. This is difficult to differentiate clinically from other forms of acute pancreatitis. A history of jaundice or cholangitis suggests that a stone was in the duct at the time of the attack.

Obstructive jaundice due to stones in the common bile duct has to be distinguished from other causes of obstructive jaundice, notably malignant obstruction and cholestatic jaundice. Acute viral or alcoholic hepatitis may occasionally be confused with obstructive jaundice.

Courvoisier's law. Fibrosed gallbladders which contain stones cannot distend when pressure increases in the obstructed biliary tree. Courvoisier's law states that if the gallbladder is palpable in the presence of jaundice, the jaundice is unlikely to be due to stone. This law is not inviolate.

Distended gallbladders are not always easy to

feel but can be detected readily by ultrasonic scans.

Acalculous conditions of the gallbladder

Cholesterosis

Cholesterosis or 'strawberry gallbladder' is a condition in which the mucous membrane of the gallbladder is infiltrated with lipid and cholesterol. It affects middle-aged and elderly patients of either sex.

Cholesterol stones are found in the gallbladders of half of these patients. Macroscopically the mucosa is brick-red and speckled with bright yellow nodules. Symptoms of acute and chronic cholecystitis may be produced, and cholecystectomy may be required.

Adenomyomatosis

This rare condition is characterized by mucosal diverticula (Rokitansky-Aschoff sinuses) which affect particularly the fundus and penetrate through the muscular layers to the serosa. Muscular hypertrophy and inflammatory cell infiltrates are present. The gallbladder often contains stones or biliary gravel. The condition is usually apparent on cholecystography and, if symptomatic, may require cholecystectomy.

Acute acalculous cholecystitis

About 5% of patients with acute cholecystitis have acalculous inflammation. The condition may be precipitated by major surgery, bacteraemia, trauma, pancreatitis or other serious illness. It may complicate the use of parenteral nutrition. The inflammatory reaction in the gallbladder wall may be intense and severe, leading to gangrene and perforation. Cholecystectomy is indicated and often has to be undertaken urgently.

Investigation of patients with suspected gallstones

Plain abdominal X-ray

As only 15% of gallstones contain enough calcium to be seen on a plain radiograph, this investigation is seldom used in diagnosis. Gas is occasionally seen outlining the biliary tree on plain X-ray; this usually denotes the presence of a fistula between the biliary tract and the gut. The fistula may have arisen spontaneously, as in gallstone ileus, or have been created surgically, as in choledochoduodenostomy.

Ultrasonography

Ultrasonography using a real-time scanner has become the mainstay of investigation. It permits inspection of the gallbladder, its wall and its contents, and demonstrates dilatation of the intrahepatic and extrahepatic duct systems. Stones reflect the ultrasonic wave and are thrown into prominence by the acoustic shadow they produce. The technique is extremely accurate in skilled hands. As it does not depend on hepatic excretion of contrast, it can be used both in jaundiced and non-jaundiced patients.

Oral cholecystography

An iodine-containing fat-soluble compound is taken orally, absorbed and excreted in the bile. After some hours the gallbladder becomes opacified and gallstones may be seen as filling defects within it. The technique will not outline the gallbladder when the serum bilirubin concentration is elevated, as sufficient contrast medium is not excreted. In non-jaundiced patients, failure to visualize the gallbladder may reflect obstruction of the cystic duct or the fact that the gallbladder is so grossly diseased that it has ceased to function. Occasionally non-opacification is due to vomiting, diarrhoea, pyloric stenosis or failure to take the tablets. Oral cholecystography is a reliable means of detecting gallstones in non-jaundiced patients but has been largely superseded by ultrasonography.

Intravenous cholangiography

This technique, which is now seldom used, involves intravenous injection of an iodine-containing compound which, within minutes, is excreted into the biliary system. Serial radiographs are taken, but visualization is often poor despite varying the depth of focus (tomography). Absence of gall-bladder opacification in the presence of normal liver function indicates that the cystic duct is blocked. The technique is of no value in jaundiced patients and the injection carries a small but definite risk of severe anaphylactoid reaction.

Endoscopic retrograde cholangiopancreatography (ERCP)

Using a side-viewing fibreoptic endoscope, the papilla of Vater may be seen and cannulated. Contrast is then injected to outline the biliary and pancreatic duct systems. If stones are detected in the common bile duct, they can be removed at the same time following endoscopic sphincterotomy.

Percutaneous transhepatic cholangiography (PTC)

In patients with obstructive jaundice the intra-hepatic biliary system can be entered per-cutaneously using a slim flexible needle through which radio-opaque dye is then injected. The site and nature of any obstruction can be defined. Ultrasonography is usually performed first to confirm that there is duct dilatation. PTC is virtually always successful when the ducts are distended and succeeds in two-thirds of patients who do not have a dilated duct system. Leakage of bile or bleeding from the puncture site are now rare complications but antibiotic cover (e.g. with gentamicin) is required during the procedure and the patient's coagulation status must be checked.

Isotope scanning

In acute cholecystitis, a gamma-camera can be used to scan the liver and biliary tree following intravenous injection of ^{99m}Tc-labelled HIDA (dimethyl-acetanilide-iminodiacetic acid). Failure to visualize the gallbladder within 2 hours suggests acute cholecystitis. The technique is no more ac-curate than ultrasonography and will not outline the biliary tree if the patient has significant jaundice.

Surgical treatment of gallstones

Patients with symptomatic gallstones are usually advised to undergo surgical treatment to relieve symptoms and avoid complications. Patients with asymptomatic gallstones diagnosed incidentally can be treated expectantly, particularly if they are elderly or suffering from other medical conditions likely to increase the risk of operation; in younger patients there may be a stronger case for surgery despite the absence of symptoms. The case is strengthened further if the stones are multiple and likely to cause complications such as acute pancreatitis.

Cholecystectomy

Surgical treatment of gallstones consists of remov-ing the gallbladder and its contained stones (cholecystectomy) and checking that there are no stones to be removed from the ductal system. Obese patients are advised to lose weight preoperatively.

The gallbladder is approached through a right subcostal, paramedian or midline incision. Follow-ing careful inspection and palpation of the abdominal contents, the cystic duct and cystic ar-tery are identified. Peroperative cholangiography is performed by cannulating the cystic duct (Fig. 36.15) and taking serial radiographs after

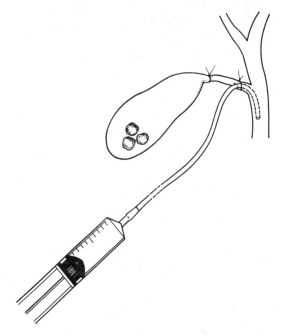

Fig. 36.15   Operative cholangiography

injection of contrast. The cholangiogram displays the anatomy of the duct system, identifies ductal stones and confirms that dye passes freely into the duodenum (Fig. 36.16). Once the films have been inspected, the gallbladder is removed after ligation and division of the cystic duct and cystic artery. A retrograde approach in which the gallbladder is mobilized 'fundus first' can be used when inflammation makes visualization of the biliary anatomy difficult. A few surgeons use peroperative cholangiography only if ductal stones are suspected by virtue of a history of jaundice, pancreatitis, dilatation of the common bile duct or multiple stones in the gallbladder, or if a stone is palpable in the duct system. Following removal of the gallbladder, haemostasis is secured and the wound is closed. Many surgeons leave a drain in the subhepatic space.

Recently laparoscopic cystectomy has been described; this takes much longer than 'surgical', but the hospital stay is short.

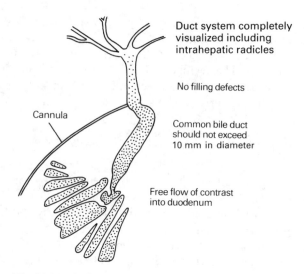

Fig. 36.16   Appearance of a normal cholangiogram

Exploration of the common bile duct

If stones are present in the duct system, the common bile duct is opened longitudinally between stay sutures (choledochotomy) and the stones are extracted with specially designed forceps (Desjardin forceps) or a Fogarty balloon catheter. Following exploration, further check cholangiogram films are obtained or the interior of the duct can be inspected with a rigid or fibreoptic choledochoscope. The best way of obtaining further films is to insert a small Foley catheter through the choledochotomy and use the inflated balloon to prevent escape of injected contrast medium (Fig. 36.17).

On completion of the procedure the opening in the common bile duct is closed around a T-tube, the long limb of which is brought out through a stab incision in the abdominal wall (Fig. 36.18). This serves as a 'safety valve' to allow safe escape

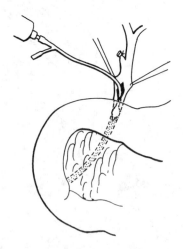

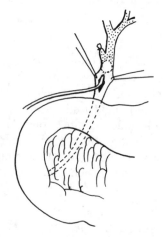

Fig. 36.17   Post-exploration cholangiography using the Foley catheter technique

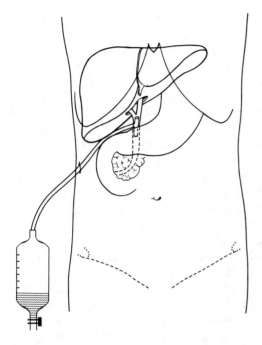

Fig. 36.18 T-tube drainage of the common bile duct

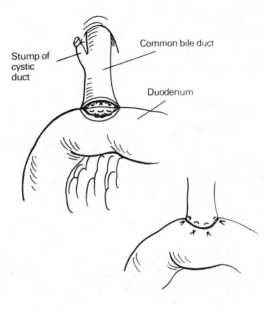

Fig. 36.19 Choledochoduodenostomy

of bile if there is a temporary obstruction to flow into the duodenum following duct exploration. It also allows instillation of iodine-containing dye to obtain a T-tube cholangiogram some 7–10 days after operation. If this shows free flow of dye into the duodenum and no residual duct stones, the T-tube can be removed.

If at operation there is gross ductal dilatation and the bile duct contains multiple stones and debris, some surgeons complete the duct exploration by anastomosing the common bile duct to a window cut in the adjacent duodenum (choledochoduodenostomy; Fig. 36.19).

If at operation a stone is firmly impacted at the lower end of the common bile duct, it may have to be removed through the duodenum. The sphincter of Oddi is incised (transduodenal

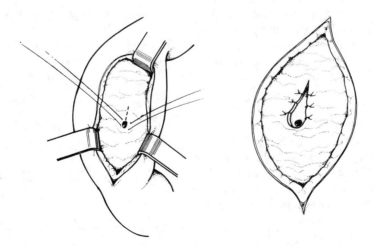

Fig. 36.20 Transduodenal sphincterotomy and sphincteroplasty. The opening of the pancreatic duct is visible within the open bile duct

sphincterotomy) to release the stone, and the operation is completed by suturing the duct mucosa to that of the duodenum (transduodenal sphincteroplasty; Fig. 36.20).

Complications of cholecystectomy

Operative mortality following elective cholecystectomy is low (0.2%) but is increased tenfold if there is obstructive jaundice or if the common bile duct has to be explored. The specific complications of cholecystectomy are as follows.

Haemorrhage

This may originate from the cystic artery or gallbladder bed. If the patient becomes shocked and bright red blood issues from the drain, re-exploration is mandatory.

Infective complications

Wound infection with organisms present in the bile (notably *E. coli*, *Klebsiella aerogenes* and *Strep. faecalis*) is a common potential danger. Its incidence after elective cholecystectomy can be reduced markedly by intravenous administration of an antibiotic such as a cephalosporin at the time of induction of anaesthesia. A longer course of antibiotics is usually prescribed when operating on patients with obstructive jaundice, cholangitis or complications such as acute cholecystitis or empyema. Collections of bile and/or blood readily become infected after cholecystectomy. Formal drainage may be needed if this progresses to the formation of a subhepatic or subphrenic abcess.

Bile leakage

This may be due to a ligature slipping off the cystic duct, accidental division of an unrecognized accessory duct, damage to the common bile duct, or retention of a duct stone after exploration. If substantial leakage continues, full radiological investigation and further surgery may be needed.

Retained stones

If the bile duct has been explored, the routine

postoperative T-tube cholangiogram (see above) may reveal that there is still a stone in the bile duct. Small stones can sometimes be flushed into the duodenum by irrigating the T-tube with saline; passage may be facilitated if agents such as caerulein are given to relax the sphincter of Oddi. Alternatively, cholesterol stones may be dissolved or made smaller by careful duct irrigation with agents such as methylterbutyl ether. If the duct cannot be cleared by irrigation, stones may be extracted under radiological control. The patient is discharged with the T-tube in place. This is removed 4–6 weeks later and a steerable catheter is passed along its track into the bile duct. A wire basket (Dormia basket) can be passed along the catheter to catch and withdraw the retained calculus (Fig. 36.21).

In some patients, unsuspected stones may be left in the bile duct at cholecystectomy. Such stones may remain asymptomatic but usually give rise to complications such as jaundice, cholangitis and pancreatitis in the months and years following cholecystectomy. ERCP can be used to confirm

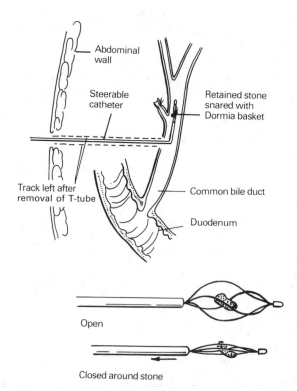

Fig. 36.21 Removal of a retained common bile duct stone

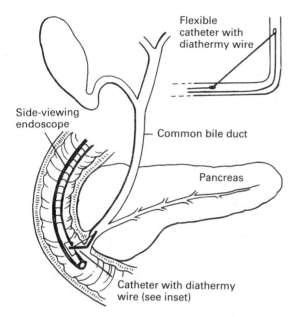

Fig. 36.22 Endoscopic papillotomy to remove retained stones

the presence of such retained stones and endoscopic papillotomy to recover them (Fig. 36.22). A diathermy wire attached to a cannula which is passed through the duodenoscope is used to divide the sphincter of Oddi. The stones can then be extracted with a Dormia basket or balloon catheter. The same method can be used to extract stones detected in the immediate postoperative period. If stones are too large to be withdrawn, a catheter can be left in the biliary system (nasobiliary catheter) and the stones can be dissolved (or at least reduced in size) by agents such as methylterbutyl ether (MTBE). It is now extremely uncommon to have to operate to retrieve retained bile duct stones.

Bile duct stricture

About 90% of benign duct strictures result from damage during cholecystectomy in which the duct is divided, ligated or devascularized. Common causes of injury include division of a ligated common bile duct which has been mistaken for the cystic duct, division of the right hepatic duct below the point of anomalous insertion of the cystic duct, and encirclement of the common bile duct by the ligature used to tie off the cystic duct. Strictures only occasionally result from abdominal trauma or erosion of the bile duct by a gallstone.

If the common bile duct is completely occluded, progressive obstructive jaundice develops in the postoperative period. If there is a partial stricture, attacks of pain, fever and obstructive jaundice signal the development of cholangitis. The serum alkaline phosphatase and transaminase concentrations are usually elevated, and blood cultures may be positive during attacks of fever. If left untreated, persistent cholangitis and obstruction progress to secondary biliary cirrhosis, hepatic abscess formation, portal hypertension and liver failure.

The site and extent of the stricture must be defined radiologically. After ultrasonography has been performed, PTC and/or ERCP are usually undertaken. Reconstructive surgery is undertaken in a specialist centre and usually necessitates bringing up a Roux loop of jejunum and anastomosing this to the distended biliary system above the stricture (Fig. 36.23).

Post-cholecystectomy syndrome

This term is used to embrace a group of complaints such as postprandial flatulence, fat intolerance, epigastric and right hypochondrial discomfort, and heartburn which may follow cholecystectomy. They tend to be more troublesome when cholecystectomy was performed in the absence of gallstones. Investigations are usually negative but some patients prove to have retained stones or other alimentary disorders such as peptic ulceration, gastritis and chronic pancreatitis. It is possible that some patients develop pain because of functional abnormalities of the sphincter of Oddi (see below).

Management of acute cholecystitis

Patients with acute cholecystitis are admitted to hospital. The pulse is measured hourly, blood pressure and temperature 4-hourly, and analgesics, intravenous fluid and a broad spectrum antibiotic such as a cephalosporin are prescribed. The patient is given nothing by mouth and a nasogastric tube may be passed, particularly if the

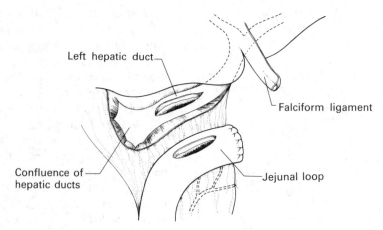

Fig. 36.23 Relief of bile duct stricture by anastomosis of a loop of jejunum to the distended biliary system above the stricture

patient is vomiting. The majority of patients settle on this regimen within a few days. Failure to settle suggests the presence of an empyema.

Some surgeons delay operation for about 6 weeks after the attack in the expectation that the acute inflammatory reaction will have resolved by then. Most now prefer to perform cholecystectomy within 72 hours of the onset of the attack. Provided the operation is carried out by an experienced surgeon and under antibiotic cover, such 'early' cholecystectomies are not associated with an increased incidence of complications. The duration of the illness and hospitalization are reduced and further attacks of acute cholecystitis during the waiting period for elective surgery are averted. It should be noted that this is a planned procedure carried out after appropriate investigation (usually ultrasonography) and with all facilities, on a routine elective list. 'Emergency' cholecystectomy at the time of admission is not advised except for empyema of the gallbladder or when there is evidence of spreading peritonitis.

If surrounding inflammation makes identification of the relevant anatomical structures difficult, cholecystostomy, i.e. drainage of the gallbladder with removal of gallstones, may be performed as an interim measure. Elective cholecystectomy is then usually performed approximately 2 months later.

Acalculous cholecystitis

Patients with an acute attack of acalculous cholecystitis require urgent cholecystectomy. Patients with long-standing symptoms and a radiological diagnosis of cholesterosis or adenomyomatosis are advised to undergo elective cholecystectomy. More difficulty arises with patients who have attacks of pain consistent with biliary colic but in whom investigations such as ultrasonography, oral cholecystography and ERCP reveal no abnormality. Some of these patients with 'acalculous biliary pain' may eventually prove to have non-biliary disease such as peptic ulceration, chronic pancreatitis or 'irritable' colon. In the majority, no explanation for the symptoms can be found, although recent evidence suggests that some may be suffering from a functional disorder of the sphincter of Oddi. Laparotomy may eventually have to be undertaken to exclude other pathology, confirm that there are no stones in the biliary tree, and remove the gallbladder as the potential source of symptoms. The results of cholecystectomy in these patients are extremely variable and many patients continue to have symptoms.

Non-surgical treatment of gallstones

In patients with smaller non-calcified cholesterol stones in a functioning gallbladder, surgery can be avoided by using chenodeoxycholic acid or the more recently introduced, ursodeoxycholic acid to expand the bile salt pool and so dissolve the stones(s). The exact mechanism of action of these drugs is not understood but both also appear to influence hepatic cholesterol metabolism. Treatment may have to be continued for a year to allow complete dissolution of stones, during which time the patient remains subject to any of the complications of gallstones. Diarrhoea and disordered liver function tests are dose-related side effects. On stopping treatment, bile returns to a supersaturated state in 1–3 weeks and gallstones may re-form. For these reasons, dissolution therapy has not become popular.

A new form of treatment currently under assessment is the percutaneous injection of methylterbutyl ether into the gallbladder to dissolve cholesterol stones. The efficacy and complications of this approach have yet to be evaluated. Similarly, destruction of stones by extracorporeal shock wave lithotripsy is currently being evaluated and is showing great promise.

OTHER BENIGN BILIARY DISORDERS

Asiatic cholangiohepatitis

This condition occurs in the Far East and is particularly common in coastal Chinese communities. Suppurative cholangitis develops and pigment stones form in the intrahepatic and extrahepatic biliary tree. Deconjugation of bilirubin glucuronide by bacteria may be implicated in stone formation, and *E. coli* and *Strep. faecalis* can often be isolated from the bile and portal blood.

The clinical features are those of obstructive jaundice, pain and fever, and liver abscesses may form. The condition is difficult to treat. Cholangitis is treated with antibiotics and stones within the duct are removed at operation. Ductal obstruction may be treated by choledochoduodenostomy or transduodenal sphincterotomy if this is appropriate. A T-tube left in the bile duct may be used for intermittent lavage to keep the ducts clear of debris. Hepatic lobectomy or segmental resection may be indicated if suppuration and obstruction have led to regional destruction of liver tissue.

Primary sclerosing cholangitis

Both intrahepatic and extrahepatic bile ducts may be affected by this condition and become in-

durated and irregularly thickened. There is a marked chronic inflammatory cell infiltrate and fibrous narrowing of the biliary tree. The aetiology of the condition is unknown but it may have an immunological basis. Over three-quarters of patients also suffer from ulcerative colitis. Other associated conditions include retroperitoneal fibrosis, immunodeficiency syndromes and pancreatitis. Rarely, bile duct carcinoma develops and obstruction can give rise to bacterial cholangitis and secondary biliary cirrhosis.

The condition frequently affects young adults and gives rise to intermittent attacks of obstructive jaundice, pruritis and pain. ERCP and liver biopsy are the mainstays of diagnosis. Treatment is generally unsatisfactory. Colectomy does not improve the cholangitis in patients with ulcerative colitis. Corticosteroids and D-penicillamine have been used but have no proven value. Duct strictures can sometimes be treated by surgical bypass or insertion of stents. The outlook is extremely variable; in some the disease appears to remit, yet progressive liver failure may ensue so that liver transplant is required.

TUMOURS OF THE BILIARY TRACT

Carcinoma of the gallbladder

Carcinoma of the gallbladder is rare and almost invariably related to the presence of gallstones. The condition is four times as common in females as in males. About 90% of lesions are adenocarcinomas, the remainder are squamous carcinomas.

Direct invasion commonly obstructs the bile duct or porta hepatis. Initial symptoms are indistinguishable from those of gallstones but jaundice is unremitting. A mass is frequently palpable.

Cholecystectomy is possible only in the early stages of tumour growth. Some surgeons recommend 'en bloc' wedge resection of an adjacent 3–5 cm of normal liver and dissection of regional lymph nodes. In most cases the condition is inoperable.

The 5-year survival rate is less than 5%.

Carcinoma of the bile ducts

Cholangiocarcinoma is a relatively uncommon lesion which affects the elderly and may be in-

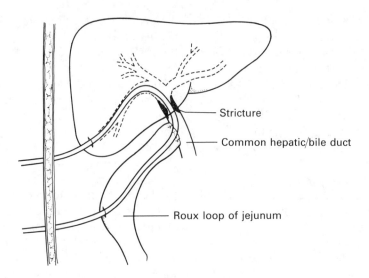

Stricture

Common hepatic/bile duct

Roux loop of jejunum

Fig. 36.24 U-tube biliary decompression

creasing in frequency. The cancer may arise from the intrahepatic or extrahepatic bile ducts and can be multifocal. The lesions are said to be slow-growing but this has been overemphasized.

Clinical features

Progressive obstructive jaundice and intermittent attacks of pain and cholangitis are the usual presenting features. The gallbladder may become obstructed because of cystic duct involvement and empyema can develop. Anorexia and weight loss are common but metastases are rare. Increasing biliary obstruction and cholangitis lead to liver failure, and portal hypertension may supervene. Pruritus is often a particularly distressing symptom.

Management

The diagnosis should be confirmed by per-cutaneous aspiration cytology or on material obtained at operation. Carcinoma of the common bile duct is treated by the Whipple operation (pancreaticoduodenectomy; see p. 590) if the tumour is localized and the patient is deemed fit for radical resection. Carcinoma of the upper biliary tract can only be resected in some 10% of patients; following resection the remaining biliary tree is anastomosed to a Roux loop of jejunum. In some patients palliation can be achieved by inserting a stent through the tumour by endoscopic or percutaneous transhepatic techniques. If this is not possible, a stenting tube can be inserted at operation (Fig. 36.24) or a Roux loop of jejunum can be anastomosed to a section of the left hepatic duct exposed by incising the left lobe of the liver. Following palliation, few patients with cholangio-carcinoma survive for more than a year.

37. The pancreas

Surgical anatomy

The pancreas develops from a ventral and a dorsal bud. These appear during the fourth week of fetal life, rotate and fuse thereafter. With rotation of the duodenum, the pancreas shifts to the left and takes up its definitive position. Most of the duct which drains the dorsal bud joins that from the ventral bud to form the main pancreatic duct (of Wirsung); the rest of the dorsal duct becomes the accessory pancreatic duct (of Santorini). This enters the duodenum 2.5 cm proximal to the main duct (Fig. 37.1)

The main pancreatic duct and the common bile duct converge as they enter the second part of the duodenum. The majority of individuals have a short common channel, and only 10% retain an ampulla of Vater into which these two ducts enter before joining the duodenum.

The pancreas lies behind the lesser sac and stomach and is relatively inaccessible for clinical and radiological examination (Fig. 37.2). The head of the gland lies within the C-shaped loop of the duodenum, with which it shares a common blood supply from the superior and inferior pancreaticoduodenal arteries. The superior mesenteric vein and splenic vein join behind the neck of the pancreas to form the portal vein, while the body and tail of pancreas lie in front of the splenic vein as far as the splenic hilum. The body and tail of the pancreas receive arterial blood from the splenic artery as it runs along the upper border of the gland. The pancreas is friable. This, and its intimate relationship to major blood vessels, explains why bleeding is the main cause of death after pancreatic trauma.

The common bile duct passes through the head of the pancreas, and obstructive jaundice is frequently due to neoplasia or inflammation involving this part of the gland.

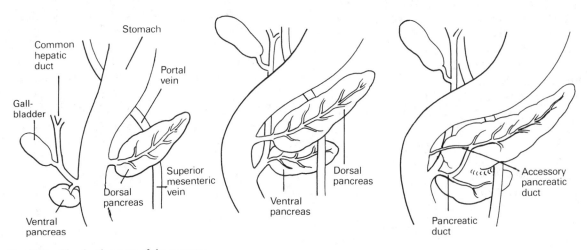

Fig. 37.1 The development of the pancreas

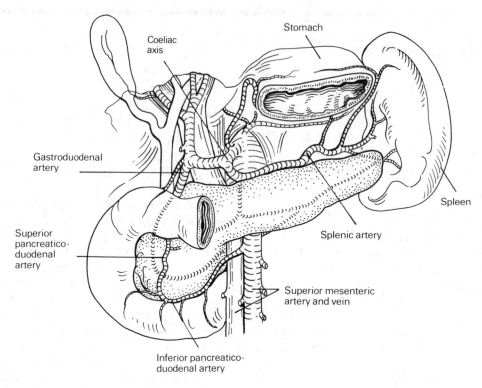

Fig. 37.2 Anatomical relationships of the pancreas

Surgical physiology

Exocrine function

The acinar cells of the pancreas secrete 1–2 litres of alkaline (pH 7.1–8.2) enzyme-rich juice each day. The enzymes are synthesized and stored in zymogen granules in the acinar cells. Lipase and amylase are secreted in an active form. Proteolytic enzymes are secreted as inactive precursors which are activated by duodenal enterokinase.

The exocrine secretion of the pancreas is stimulated by food in the duodenum and proximal jejunum, and by acid in the duodenum. Food-stimulated pancreatic secretion is mediated by cholecystokinin (CCK), while that induced by acid is mediated by secretin. Secretin stimulates watery alkaline secretion, whereas CCK stimulates secretion rich in enzymes. The vagus nerve also stimulates pancreatic secretion, and hormonal and neural factors interact to regulate pancreatic function.

Endocrine function

Endocrine functions of the pancreas are subserved by the cells which form the islets of Langerhans. A variety of cell types are now recognized: type A cells secrete glucagon, B cells secrete insulin, D cells secrete somatostatin, PP cells secrete pancreatic polypeptide, and D_1 cells may secrete vasoactive intestinal polypeptide (VIP). Only glucagon and insulin have established physiological roles and the significance of the other endocrine cells is uncertain. Gastrin-producing (G) cells are not found in the pancreas except in the rare Zollinger-Ellison syndrome (see Ch. 30).

CONGENITAL DISORDERS OF THE PANCREAS

Annular pancreas

This is a rare cause of duodenal obstruction (see p. 474).

Pancreas divisum

In approximately 5% of individuals the ducts draining the dorsal and ventral pancreas fail to fuse. This means that the majority of the secretion of the pancreas has to enter the duodenum through the smaller accessory duct. It is not certain whether this can give rise to acute and chronic pancreatitis.

Aberrant pancreatic tissue

Rests of heterotopic pancreas may be found at any point in the gastrointestinal tract, but are commonest in the duodenum, stomach and proximal jejunum. Many remain asymptomatic but they can cause ulceration, bleeding or obstruction. They may cause confusion in the interpretation of a barium meal.

Cystic fibrosis (mucoviscidosis)

Cystic fibrosis affects sweat glands, pancreas and bronchial mucous glands. Meconium ileus may follow and require relief of intestinal obstruction in neonates. Malabsorption becomes a feature as the disease progresses.

INFLAMMATORY DISORDERS OF THE PANCREAS

Pancreatitis may be acute or chronic. After an attack of acute pancreatitis the gland returns to anatomical and functional normality. Chronic pancreatitis is associated with permanent derangement of structure and function. Some patients suffer from recurrent (or relapsing) acute pancreatitis, enjoying relatively normal health between attacks, but their condition may progress to chronic pancreatitis.

Acute pancreatitis

In Britain there are 50–100 new cases of acute pancreatitis per million population each year. The incidence is increasing, possibly as a result of increasing alcohol consumption. All adult age groups may be affected. Acute pancreatitis is a serious condition with a mortality rate of around 10%.

Aetiology

The cause of acute pancreatitis is undefined. Premature activation of pancreatic enzymes with rupture of the duct system leads to autodigestion of the gland. Intraduct activation of enzymes such as trypsinogen, chymotrypsinogen, phospholipase, elastase and catalase unleashes a chain reaction of cell necrosis, further enzyme release and changes in the microcirculation. Reflux of duodenal juice and bile into the pancreatic duct or spasm at the sphincter of Oddi may be important causes of enzyme activation within the duct system.

Conditions associated with the development of acute pancreatitis are listed in Table 37.1. Biliary tract disease and alcohol are of overriding importance.

Biliary tract disease and acute pancreatitis. Gallstones are present in about 50% of patients who develop acute pancreatitis in Britain. The great majority of these patients have at least a short common channel involving the terminal portion of the common bile duct and pancreatic duct (Fig. 37.3). In the majority of patients stones ranging in diameter from 1 to 12 mm can be recovered from the faeces within a few days of the onset of pancreatitis. These stones have the same chemical composition as stones recovered from the gallbladder at subsequent surgery and it is believed that their transient impaction at the sphincter of Oddi

Table 37.1 Causes of acute pancreatitis

Non-traumatic causes (75%)	
Major factors	Biliary tract disease (50%)
	Alcohol (20%)
Minor factors	Pancreatic cancer
	Drugs (e.g. steroids)
	Renal transplantation
	Hyperlipidaemia
	Hyperparathyroidism
	Viral infection (mumps, Coxsackie)
	Scorpion bites (Trinidad)
	Hypothermia
	Periarteritis nodosa
	Pregnancy
	Previous Polya gastrectomy
Traumatic causes (5%)	
	Operative trauma
	Blunt or penetrating injury
	Investigation (ERCP or arteriography)
Idiopathic (20%)	

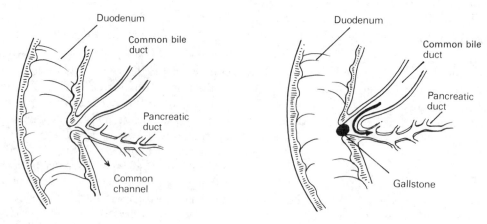

Fig. 37.3 A common channel shared by the bile duct and the pancreatic duct may allow gallstone pancreatitis

(see Fig. 37.3) is the cause of the attack of pancreatitis. Further support for a causal relationship between gallstones and acute pancreatitis is provided by the observation that further attacks of pancreatitis are exceptional once biliary tract disease has been eradicated.

Alcohol-associated pancreatitis. The proportion of cases of acute pancreatitis associated with alcohol varies greatly in different parts of the world. In Scotland the figure is around 30%, whereas in North America, South Africa and France it may be as high as 50–90%. The mechanism is uncertain. Suggested causes include a specific toxic effect, pancreatic protein hypersecretion with plug formation, spasm of the sphincter of Oddi and duodenitis.

Pathophysiology

Pancreatic inflammation ranges in severity from mild oedema to severe necrosis and haemorrhage. Proteolytic enzymes released from the gland are responsible for increased capillary permeability, protein exudation, retroperitoneal oedema and peritoneal exudation. Vasoactive kinins such as bradykinin and kallikrein are also released by proteolytic enzyme activity. Many of the circulatory changes in acute pancreatitis result from this fluid, electrolyte and protein loss. Possible other factors are:

1. development of acute renal failure, possibly due to local intravascular coagulation and release of a vasopressor substance affecting the renal vascular bed;

2. development of shock lung with atelectasis, left-sided pleural effusion, pulmonary oedema and right-to-left shunting of blood;

3. development of ECG changes suggesting ischaemia, possibly due to coronary vasoconstriction by a 'myocardial depressant factor'; and

4. consumptive coagulopathy.

Liver function may be disturbed in acute pancreatitis by obstruction of the common bile duct, cholangitis or direct hepatocellular depression. This may account for the unreliability of radiological investigation of the biliary tree in the 2–3 weeks following the attack.

Clinical features

Previous attacks of dyspepsia, biliary colic or transient jaundice may be described. Alcohol intake should be documented carefully, bearing in mind that an attack of pancreatitis is often delayed for some 24 hours after ingestion of alcohol or a large meal. The rarer causes of acute pancreatitis (see Table 37.1) are considered when there is no evidence of gallstones, alcohol intake or trauma. Agonizing pain in the epigastrium or right hypochondrium with radiation through to the back is common. Shoulder-tip pain is uncommon. Nausea and vomiting and retching are prominent. Severe pancreatitis is accompanied by shock (see Ch. 3).

Classically the clinical signs are less impressive than expected from the symptoms and this may prevent consideration of the correct diagnosis. There is little muscle guarding or rigidity, and tenderness is relatively slight. Bruising around the umbilicus (Cullen's sign) or in the loin (Grey Turner's sign) are rare late manifestations of pancreatitis.

Diagnosis

The key to the diagnosis of acute pancreatitis is a high index of suspicion and measurement of the serum amylase. With inflammation there is rupture of cells and parts of the ductal system, with release of amylase into the circulation. The normal range for serum amylase is 100–300 i.u./l and values above 1000 i.u./l strongly support the diagnosis of acute pancreatitis. False negative results occur in about 5% of patients with pancreatitis. A number of other conditions can give rise to 'false positive' results by causing hyperamylasaemia (Table 37.2).

In pancreatitis the rise in serum amylase is frequently transient, occurring within 6 hours of the attack and persisting for some 48 hours. Urinary amylase levels are also increased and persist after serum levels have returned to normal. Persistent hyperamylasaemia in the absence of abnormal urinary amylase levels suggests *macroamylasaemia*, a rare condition in which amylase is bound to globulin and forms a complex too large to be excreted by the kidney.

The amylase-creatinine clearance ratio (ACCR) is elevated (1–4% above normal) in most patients with acute pancreatitis. This may be a more reliable diagnostic test than measurement of serum amylase alone, but is seldom used in practice.

Table 37.2 Non-pancreatic disorders capable of causing hyperamylasaemia

Acute cholecystitis
Perforated duodenal ulcer
High intestinal obstruction
Mesenteric vascular occlusion
Bowel strangulation
Dissection of aortic aneurysm
Rupture of aortic aneurysm
Ruptured ectopic pregnancy

There are no pathognomic radiological signs of acute pancreatitis but plain films of the chest and abdomen may reveal:
1. left-sided pleural effusion (20% of cases);
2. blurring of the psoas margin by retroperitoneal inflammation (rare);
3. a bowel empty of gas apart from a 'sentinel loop' of jejunum resulting from local ileus in bowel overlying the inflamed gland (gas may be seen in the hepatic and splenic flexures but not in the transverse colon — the 'colon cut-off' sign); and
4. associated gallstones.

Gastrografin studies are not usually indicated but may be of value when ulcer perforation cannot be excluded clinically. The C-loop of the duodenum may be widened by inflammation in the head of the pancreas, the duodenal folds may be oedematous and coarse, and the papilla of Vater sometimes appears retracted (the 'reversed 3 sign') because of oedema of the medial wall of the duodenum.

Urea and electrolyte measurements reflect the state of hydration and are useful in the management of fluid and electrolyte balance. Liver function tests sometimes reveal hyperbilirubinaemia and elevation of liver enzymes. Hyperglycaemia and glycosuria may occur transiently.

Arterial blood gas measurement is essential in shocked patients and may reveal severe hypoxia. Moderate polymorphonuclear leucocytosis is common.

The serum calcium concentration should be estimated. Hypocalcaemia in acute pancreatitis is due partly to calcium soap formation as a consequence of fat necrosis, but mostly reflects a fall in serum albumin concentration and hence a reduction in protein-bound calcium levels. Marked reduction in the level of ionized calcium is unusual and frank tetany is exceptional.

Treatment

There is no specific treatment for acute pancreatitis. The majority of patients settle on conservative management, which should include the following.

Pain relief. Severe pain requires the administration of opiates. Morphine and pethidine both cause some spasm of the sphincter of Oddi and are contraindicated on theoretical grounds. In practice, pethidine is frequently prescribed and is effective.

Treatment of shock (see Ch. 3). Large volumes of crystalloid solution, plasma or dextran may be needed to maintain circulating fluid volume. Oxygen therapy is essential.

Suppression of pancreatic function. The patient is forbidden to drink or eat. Absence of food and acid from the duodenum prevents liberation of duodenal secretin and CCK and thus avoids stimulation of pancreatic secretion. A nasogastric tube may relieve vomiting but controlled trials have failed to show that outcome is affected by routine intubation. Anticholinergic drugs such as atropine inhibit vagal activity and relax the sphincter of Oddi, but there is no evidence of their value in acute pancreatitis.

Other medical measures. Some surgeons prescribe a broad spectrum antibiotic routinely for patients with pancreatitis. However, they are not of proven value and the majority of surgeons await evidence of infection. If there is associated cholangitis, an antibiotic should be given.

Although diabetes is rare, its development may require insulin therapy.

The kallikrein inhibitor aprotinin (Trasylol) has no proven therapeutic value and is no longer prescribed. Glucagon, once regarded as a useful means of suppressing pancreatic secretion, is also no longer used.

Peritoneal lavage with isotonic crystalloid solutions is a useful means of recovering peritoneal fluid when the diagnosis of pancreatitis is uncertain, and may have a therapeutic role. Lavage aims to remove fluid containing enzymes and vasoactive substances and so prevent their absorption into the blood stream. Preliminary results were encouraging, but recent controlled trials have not shown any reduction in morbidity or mortality in patients with severe acute pancreatitis.

Surgical treatment. There is general agreement that acute pancreatitis should be managed conservatively if possible. Laparotomy is indicated in the following circumstances.

1. *When the diagnosis is uncertain.* As shown in Table 37.2, a number of acute abdominal conditions may cause hyperamylasaemia and the majority of these may prove fatal if not treated surgically. Laparotomy is indicated if the diagnosis of acute pancreatitis is in doubt. If it reveals mild pancreatitis, the abdomen is closed without drainage. Drainage of the lesser sac with peritoneal lavage is considered if the pancreatitis is severe.

2. *When the patient fails to improve on conservative management.* If the general condition of the patient deteriorates despite intensive medical management, laparotomy should be performed. Necrotic pancreatic tissue is removed and the peritoneal cavity is irrigated with saline solution. Two large peritoneal drains are inserted and postoperative lavage is instituted. Resection of the pancreas in sick patients with multisystem failure is a formidable undertaking and carries a mortality of up to 50%. Contrast-enhanced CT scanning now provides a valuable guide to the development of pancreatic necrosis and may confirm the need for urgent surgery before multisystem failure becomes established.

3. *When the patient has gallstones.* In the past, patients thought to have gallstone pancreatitis were allowed to settle on conservative management before being investigated radiologically, and were then readmitted for elective biliary surgery some 6–8 weeks later. This approach has now been superseded by a policy of 'early' intervention during the first admission to hospital. Ultrasonography is used to confirm the presence of stones and surgery is undertaken once the attack of pancreatitis has settled. In patients with severe pancreatitis, endoscopic retrograde cholangiography may be more accurate than ultrasonography in diagnosing the presence of stones, and also allows removal of ductal stones following division of the sphincter of Oddi (endoscopic papillotomy), thus permitting resolution of the attack. It cannot be overemphasized that patients who have had an attack of gallstone pancreatitis should not be allowed to suffer another. When biliary surgery is undertaken it consists of cholecystectomy with operative cholangiography to determine whether stones are still present in the duct system and thus require removal.

Complications of acute pancreatitis

Pancreatic pseudocyst. A pancreatic pseudocyst is

a collection of pancreatic secretions and inflammatory exudate within a lining of inflammatory tissue rather than epithelium (true cyst). A pseudocyst is usually located in the lesser sac or retroperitoneal tissue around the pancreas. Pseudocysts develop in about 10% of patients and are most common following alcoholic or traumatic pancreatitis.

Small pseudocysts are often asymptomatic and usually resolve spontaneously. Larger collections displace and compress the stomach or duodenum, and may cause considerable discomfort.

Clinical features. Pseudocysts typically do not manifest themselves for some 2–3 weeks after the episode of pancreatitis. Persistent or intermittent hyperamylasaemia may signal their presence. Ultrasound is of great value in monitoring the progress of pancreatic inflammation and in detecting pseudocyst formation. Some cysts become so large that they are palpable.

Treatment. The presence of a pseudocyst is not in itself an indication for surgical treatment. Treatment is indicated only if the pseudocyst is enlarging, and aims to avoid infection of the contents, haemorrhage or rupture. It normally consists of drainage of the pseudocyst into the stomach (cystogastrostomy), the duodenum (cystoduodenostomy) or a Roux loop of jejunum (cystojejunostomy Roux-en-Y), whichever appears most appropriate (Fig. 37.4). Partial

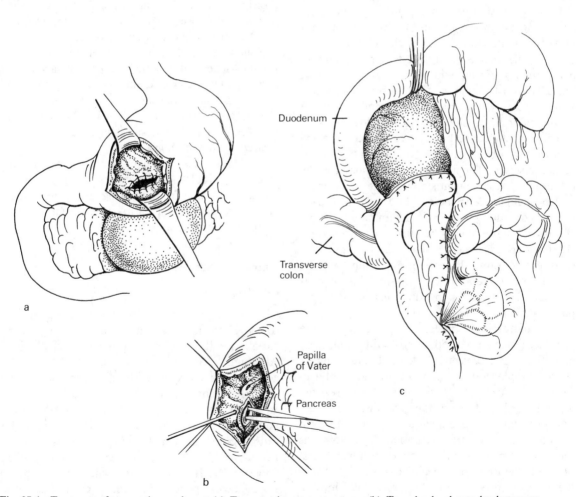

Fig. 37.4 Treatment of pancreatic pseudocyst. (a) Transgastric cystogastrostomy. (b) Transduodenal cystoduodenostomy. (c) Cystojejunostomy Roux-en-Y (note that the loop is usually brought retrocolic not antecolic as shown here)

resection of the pancreas is an alternative approach which is rarely indicated. As the tissues holding the sutures must be firm, it is wise to allow the pseudocyst time to 'mature' (i.e. 4–6 weeks) before operating, if this is feasible.

Ultrasonography allows puncture of the pseudocyst and insertion of a catheter for external drainage. However, this approach may allow infection to supervene and is waning in popularity.

Pancreatic abscess. The presentation may resemble that of pancreatic pseudocyst but the patient is usually ill, and has pyrexia and leucocytosis. The presence of an abscess is confirmed by ultrasound. Adequate drainage under antibiotic cover is mandatory and this usually necessitates laparotomy rather than percutaneous drainage.

Progressive jaundice. Persistent or progressively deepening jaundice may indicate that a gallstone is impacted at the lower end of the biliary tree or that the bile duct is compressed by pancreatic inflammation. Early operation is indicated. Calculous obstruction is treated by cholecystectomy, operative cholangiography, and extraction of the offending gallstone. If radiology fails to reveal a gallstone, the biliary tree is decompressed by insertion of a T-tube until pancreatic inflammation resolves. The finding of a pseudocyst in the head of pancreas demands appropriate treatment.

Persistent duodenal ileus. Protracted ileus usually reflects continuing pancreatic inflammation. In the absence of a pseudocyst requiring drainage, persistent duodenal ileus may be bypassed by gastroenterostomy. Parenteral nutrition or tube feeding (via a jejunostomy or nasoenteric tube) is often needed to maintain nutritional status while pancreatitis is resolving.

Gastrointestinal bleeding. Severe acute pancreatitis may be complicated by bleeding from gastritis, gastric erosions or acute duodenal ulceration. Prophylactic cimetidine is advisable in patients thought to have severe pancreatitis. Should bleeding develop, the guidelines for investigation and management are as outlined in Chapter 30. On rare occasions, laparotomy is required urgently for massive intraperitoneal bleeding due to erosion of blood vessels by the inflammatory process or for bleeding into a pseudocyst from microaneurysms.

Table 37.3 Factors used to predict severity of acute pancreatitis within 48 hours of admission

Age	>55 years
White cell count	>15 × 10^9/l
Blood glucose (no diabetic history)	>10 mmol/l
Serum urea (no response to i.v. fluids)	>16 mmol/l
Pao$_2$	<60 mmHg
Serum calcium	<2.0 mmol/l
Serum albumin	<32 g/l
Serum lactate dehydrogenase	>600 U/l
Serum aspartate aminotransferase/ alanine aminotransferase	>100 U/l

Prognosis

A number of clinical and laboratory criteria have been defined which have prognostic significance (Table 37.3). In the system shown, three or more positive criteria indicate severe disease. Such patients are more likely to develop complications, and the disease more often proves fatal.

Following resolution of the acute attack, the prognosis depends on the aetiological factor concerned. The biliary tree must be investigated in all cases. Gallstone-associated pancreatitis has an excellent long-term outlook once cholecystectomy has been carried out and gallstones have been cleared from the biliary tree.

The prognosis in alcohol-associated pancreatitis is less favourable. Many patients are unable or unwilling to abstain from drinking and suffer further attacks of acute pancreatitis with progression to chronic pancreatitis.

Chronic pancreatitis

Aetiology

Chronic pancreatitis is a relatively rare disease in the UK. Its incidence may be increasing in association with the growing problem of alcoholism. Although alcoholism is much the commonest aetiological factor, cholelithiasis is present in some 25% of patients and may have a contributory role. In India and Africa, where the disease affects younger patients, malnutrition is an important cause. Rarer causes include mucoviscidosis, hyperparathyroidism, haemochromatosis and familial pancreatitis. It is uncertain whether inadequate drainage of pancreatic secretions in pancreas divisum is a cause of chronic pancreatitis or whether pancreas divisum is merely an incidental finding.

Pathophysiology

Chronic inflammation leads to progressive replacement of the gland by fibrous tissue, destruction of acinar tissue, and eventual destruction of islet tissue. Multiple strictures form in the pancreatic duct, impair drainage and cause further inflammation in the obstructed gland. Protein plugs form in the ducts and later calcify, leading to speckled calcification on plain abdominal X-ray. The exact mechanism whereby alcohol damages the pancreas is uncertain but protein hypersecretion with plug formation may be a factor.

Clinical features

Weight loss is usual. It may be associated with frank malabsorption and steatorrhoea, the bowel motion being pale, bulky, offensive, floating on water, and difficult to flush. Pain is a prominent feature in almost all cases due to alcohol but may be less marked in those with a non-alcoholic basis for their disease. The pain may be precipitated by eating and so contribute to weight loss. It is characteristically epigastric with spread to the back and is often eased by bending forward. Delay in diagnosis may lead to drug addiction in some patients.

Obstructive jaundice may be present if the head of pancreas is inflamed. Jaundice is usually transient or intermittent.

Diabetes mellitus develops in about one-third of patients. It may take several years to become obvious.

Carcinoma of the pancreas appears to be slightly more common in patients with chronic pancreatitis. This may merely reflect the difficulty in distinguishing between the two conditions, and the likelihood that cancer blocks the duct system and predisposes to inflammation.

Investigation and diagnosis

The aims of investigation are to define (1) the degree of exocrine and endocrine functional impairment and (2) the extent of structural damage to the duct system.

Function tests. Exocrine function can be assessed by duodenal intubation and collection of pancreatic juice after stimulation by secretin and CCK. Pancreatic insufficiency may not be evident clinically until 90% of the functional parenchyma is destroyed, but 80–90% of patients with chronic pancreatitis have abnormal function tests with a low secretory volume, low bicarbonate concentration and low enzyme output. Function tests do not discriminate clearly between chronic pancreatitis and other pancreatic diseases.

Steatorrhoea is assessed by measuring faecal fat excretion over 3–5 days while fat intake is controlled at 100 g/day. Normal individuals excrete less than 5 g/day. Alternatively, fat absorption can be measured by isotopic labelling of dietary fat.

Endocrine function is assessed by measurement of fasting glucose concentrations, supplemented if necessary by a glucose tolerance test.

Radiology. Abdominal plain films may reveal speckled calcification in patients with chronic pancreatitis. Ultrasound and CT scanning may detect pancreatic enlargement. Endoscopic retrograde choledochopancreatography (ERCP) is of great value and must always be performed if operation is contemplated. The architecture of the pancreatic duct is revealed and it may also prove possible to outline the biliary tract and so avoid further biliary radiology. Pure pancreatic juice can be obtained for cytological examination to exclude neoplasia.

Management

The principles of medical management are (1) to remove the aetiological agent (e.g. alcohol); (2) to deal with functional insufficiency; and (3) to relieve pain.

The management of functional deficiency includes control of diabetes and replacement of deficient exocrine secretion. A number of commercial enzyme preparations are available (e.g. Cotazym B, Nutrizym) but all are subject to enzymic degradation by gastric acid-pepsin, and steatorrhoea may prove difficult to eradicate. The addition of an H_2 antagonist may prove helpful if steatorrhoea remains troublesome.

For the relief of pain opiates are avoided for as

long as possible, as addiction may result. After removal of the precipitating cause, simple analgesics only should be required. Coeliac plexus block may be successful in providing short-term pain relief but it seldom contributes to long-term management.

Surgical treatment. Operation is indicated if pain persists, if gallstones are present, when inflammation is complicated by pseudocyst or abscess formation, if neighbouring structures such as the bile duct, duodenum or portal vein are being compressed, and when pancreatic carcinoma cannot be excluded. Persisting severe pain is the most common indication for operation.

The object of surgery is to preserve functioning pancreatic tissue by providing adequate drainage or, if this is not possible, to resect the involved portion of the gland. Demonstration of ductal anatomy is essential in selecting the most appropriate operation, and operative pancreatography is mandatory if ERCP has not been successful.

The method of draining the duct system depends on the extent of obstruction. There is rarely a single area of narrowing close to the sphincter of Oddi so that sphincteroplasty (Fig. 37.5) rarely suffices. More frequently there are multiple strictures throughout the length of the duct, which must be slit open by 'filleting' the gland and anastomosing a Roux loop of jejunum to the whole length of the pancreatic duct

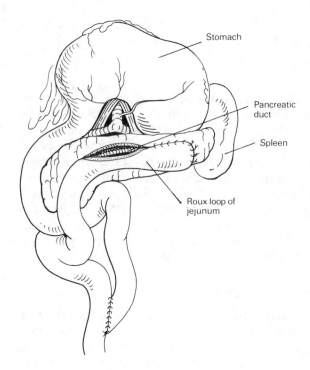

Fig. 37.6 Pancreatic duct decompression

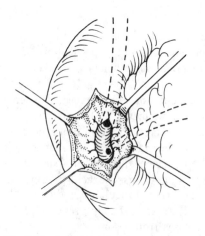

Fig. 37.5 Sphincteroplasty

(Fig. 37.6). Provided the patient ceases to drink alcohol, pain is likely to be relieved following a drainage procedure and pancreatic insufficiency may not worsen.

If drainage is not feasible, part or all of the pancreas may have to be resected. This is a more dangerous undertaking and may compound pre-existing endocrine and/or exocrine insufficiency. This disease is usually most severe in the head of the pancreas so that a Whipple procedure (pancreaticoduodenectomy; see Fig. 37.8) may be indicated. Occasionally, the disease is limited to the distal part of the gland so that distal pancreatectomy is appropriate. In some patients the entire gland may have to be removed (total pancreatectomy), with consequent permanent diabetes and exocrine insufficiency. Careful patient selection is vital, as considerable problems are often encountered in the management of diabetes.

Unfortunately, many patients continue to drink alcohol and the results of surgery are then disappointing.

NEOPLASMS OF THE PANCREAS

Neoplasms of the pancreas arise from ductal or acinar (exocrine) tissue, and in the islets of Langerhans (endocrine). Endocrine neoplasms are rare but are of considerable interest because of the specific clinical syndromes which are produced by excessive hormone secretion.

TUMOURS OF THE EXOCRINE PANCREAS

Benign pancreatic neoplasms are rare and often remain asymptomatic, unless they attain sufficient size to cause pressure on surrounding structures. Such tumours are usually cystadenomas; if small, they may be enucleated but larger tumours require formal resection.

Adenocarcinoma is by far the commonest *malignant* lesion of the exocrine pancreas. Cystadenocarcinoma and sarcoma are extremely rare.

Adenocarcinoma of the pancreas

Aetiology

The cause of pancreatic cancer is unknown. It is increasing in frequency and is now the fourth commonest cause of cancer death in males, and the sixth commonest in females in many Western countries. It accounts for about 10% of all cancers of the alimentary system.

Men are more commonly affected than women, and the peak incidence lies between 55 and 70 years of age. Factors thought to increase the risk of pancreatic cancer include tobacco smoking and a high-fat, high-protein diet. Excessive drinking of coffee was thought to be a risk factor although this is now controversial.

Pathology

The great majority of adenocarcinomas arise from ductal rather than acinar tissue. The head of the gland is more often affected than the body or tail. The cancer spreads locally and disseminates to lymph nodes around the gland. Regardless of the site of origin, spread outwith the reach of surgical resection is the rule by the time the disease is diag-nosed. Survival for more than 5 years from diagnosis is exceptional.

Cancer arising in the periampullary region, duodenum or distal common bile duct has a much more favourable outlook than pancreatic cancer. Biliary obstruction occurs early, leading to discovery of the tumour at a time when resection offers a much better prospect of cure.

Clinical features

Weight loss is invariable and may be the first symptom. Cancer of the head of the pancreas was said to cause painless obstructive jaundice but this is not true. Ill-defined upper abdominal pain is present in most patients and may reflect ductal obstruction with pancreatitis. Neoplastic infiltration can also cause severe pain in the back.

Obstructive jaundice is the best-known feature of cancer of the head of the pancreas. It is usually progressive, unlike the fluctuant jaundice common in calculous obstruction. When cancer originates in the body or tail of the pancreas, jaundice may be due to liver metastases or extension of the cancer into the porta hepatis. In keeping with Courvoisier's law (see Ch. 36), the gallbladder is palpable in some (but not all) patients with obstructive jaundice due to cancer of the pancreas. A distended gallbladder is felt more laterally than expected from the usual surface marking.

Signs and symptoms of pancreatic insufficiency are common. Diabetes mellitus or impaired glucose tolerance is found in 30% of patients with pancreatic cancer and may be the presenting feature. Steatorrhoea due to impaired digestion and absorption of fat may be associated with weight loss.

Thrombophlebitis migrans is a late manifestation in some patients but is not specific for this form of cancer.

Investigation and diagnosis

In patients with jaundice, its obstructive nature is confirmed by examination of the urine, stool and blood (see Ch. 36). Ultrasound scanning wil! detect obstruction and dilatation of the biliary tree, and exclude gallstones. If biliary tract obstruction is demonstrated, percutaneous transhepatic cholangiography or ERCP can be used to define the site of obstruction.

If the diagnosis remains in doubt or if pancreatic cancer is suspected in a patient who is not jaundiced, endoscopic retrograde cholangio-pancreatography is an invaluable investigation. It allows inspection of the stomach and proximal duodenum, and both biliary and pancreatic systems can be defined. Lesions within the gastroduodenal lumen can be biopsied and pancreatic juice sampled for cytological examination.

Pancreatic function tests are of little value. CT scanning may show the pancreatic lesion and any metastases. Angiography to display the vascular anatomy is used only in those few patients in whom pancreatic resection is contemplated.

Every effort should be made to obtain radiological and either cytological or histological confirmation of the diagnosis prior to surgery. Pancreatic tissue can now be obtained for cytology by percutaneous fine needle aspiration, the needle being guided into the target area under ultrasonic or CT scan guidance.

Management

Curative treatment. Surgical resection offers the only prospect of cure. Cancers of the pancreas are usually too advanced to justify resection but in a few selected cases resection may be justifiable when cancer arises in the head of the gland.

The standard operation of radical pancreaticoduodenectomy (Whipple procedure) entails block resection of the head of the pancreas, duodenum, distal half of stomach and common bile duct, with reconstruction of biliary-intestinal, pancreatico-intestinal and gastrointestinal continuity (Fig. 37.7). The operation aims to eradicate the cancer but retain enough pancreatic tissue to sustain adequate endocrine and exocrine function. The operative mortality rate in the past was prohibitively high (10–25%) but is now less than 5% in specialist centres. Although resection offers the only prospect of cure, overall survival rates seldom differ significantly from those achieved by palliative bypass surgery.

Leakage from the pancreaticojejunal anastomosis is the major source of morbidity. Total pancreatectomy avoids this risk but has not proved to be superior in terms of operative mortality or long-term survival. It also confers permanent diabetes and exocrine insufficiency.

The prospects for patients with cancer of the periampullary region, duodenum or distal common bile duct are less gloomy. Radical pancreatico-duodenectomy is associated with a more acceptable

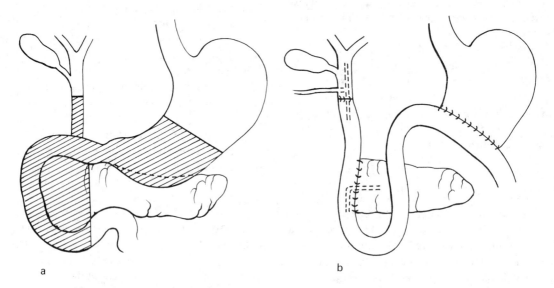

a   b

Fig. 37.7 Whipple procedure showing (a) the area resected and (b) the anstomoses performed. (The gallbladder is usually removed)

operative mortality (less than 5%) and a reasonable 5-year survival rate (30%).

Palliative treatment. Relief of obstructive jaundice and duodenal obstruction are all that can be offered to the majority of patients with pancreatic cancer. Jaundice is usually relieved by cholecystojejunostomy (or choledochojejunostomy), and duodenal obstruction is treated or prevented by gastrojejunostomy. The advent of ERCP now allows relief of jaundice by insertion of a prosthetic stent after endoscopic papillotomy. Encouraging early results suggest that this technique may avoid surgery in these elderly ill patients.

Survival following palliative surgery is usually short and seldom exceeds 12 months. Survival for longer periods should raise doubt regarding the original diagnosis. Cancer and chronic pancreatitis are easily confused at operation so that a biopsy should always be obtained in patients thought to have pancreatic cancer.

Attempts to improve the results of pancreatic surgery by adjuvant chemotherapy or radiotherapy have proved disappointing but continued trials are justified by the poor results of surgery. Pain relief is a vital part of the management of advanced disease, and coeliac plexus block should be considered if pain cannot be controlled by appropriate analgesic therapy.

ENDOCRINE TUMOURS OF THE PANCREAS

Tumours arising in the pancreatic islets are uncommon but may be functional and show endocrine activity. The commonest islet cell tumour is the insulinoma. It arises from B cells and results in oversecretion of insulin producing episodes of hypoglycaemia. Gastrinomas arise from G cells and secrete gastrin to give rise to the Zollinger-Ellison syndrome (see Ch. 30). Tumours of the A cells secrete glucagon.

A number of non-B cell tumours secreting a variety of amines or polypeptide hormones are also described. For example, excess secretion of serotonin causes the carcinoid syndrome (see Ch. 31), and vasoactive intestinal peptide (VIP) secretion produces pancreatic cholera (see later). Such tumours may secrete more than one hormone and a proportion of patients also have tumours or

hyperplasia of endocrine cells at other sites (multiple endocrine neoplasia).

The cell types which give rise to these tumours belong to the APUD series, and have in common the capacity of amine precursor uptake and decarboxylation (see Ch. 23). Rarely, hyperplasia of islet tissue rather than a tumour causes similar endocrine syndromes.

Insulinoma

This is a functioning endocrine tumour arising from the B cells of the islands of Langerhans. Such tumours are generally small (less than 3 cm) and single, and may be situated in any part of the gland. Multiple insulinomas do occur, usually as part of a multiple endocrine neoplasia syndrome (see Ch. 23). The great majority of insulinomas are benign; less than 10% are malignant.

Clinical features

The clinical features of an insulinoma result from inappropriate circulating levels of insulin. Unlike normal islet cells, which secrete in response to changing glucose concentrations in the blood which perfuses them, an insulinoma secretes autonomously. As a result the glucose pool is lowered and the central nervous system starved of glucose. Hypoglycaemic symptoms are usually mild, but over the years there may be intellectual and motor impairment with insidious personality changes.

More severe attacks of hypoglycaemia may occur and give rise to a wide variety of transient psychoneurological symptoms such as bizarre behaviour, sweating, palpitations, and tremulousness. Because of memory lapses, the patient may not recall these events and the diagnosis may be suspected only when the patient is found in hypoglycaemic coma.

Typically, attacks of hypoglycaemia are precipitated by fasting and relieved by taking glucose. Many patients become obese because of the associated hunger. Some patients are regarded as suffering from a psychiatric illness, while others may be diagnosed as epileptics or as suffering from a brain tumour. The diagnosis is difficult and is made within one year of the first symptom in only one-third of patients.

Diagnosis

The diagnosis of insulinoma depends on (1) the demonstration of hypoglycaemia (a fasting blood sugar of less than 2.2 mmol/l) after an overnight (12–14 hour) fast, and (2) the confirmation that the hypoglycaemia is due to excess insulin secretion. Insulin cannot normally be detected when glucose levels are subnormal, but in a patient with an insulinoma, serial plasma insulin assays during a 12–14 hour fast will show persisting insulin levels in the face of falling glucose levels.

Factitious hypoglycaemia caused by insulin injection is a rare problem which is sometimes encountered in medical and nursing staff. It can be excluded by measuring C-peptide levels at the same time as insulin determination. One molecule of C-peptide is produced for every molecule of endogenous insulin produced by the pancreas. If exogenous insulin is being administered, there is no corresponding C-peptide production.

An exaggerated response of insulin secretion to tolbutamide and glucagon has also been described in insulinoma patients but such provocative tests are potentially dangerous and thus no longer used.

Detection of the tumour. Methods of localizing the insulinoma before surgery include ultrasonography, CT scanning and selective angiography but, because of the small size of the tumour, these are successful in only 40% of cases. Selective venous sampling from a catheter inserted into the splenic and portal veins through the liver allows plotting of the concentration of insulin at various sites and may define the point at which excess secretion is entering the venous system.

Treatment

Surgical removal of the tumour is the treatment of choice. Patients may be treated with diazoxide (1 g daily by mouth) until their symptoms and biochemical parameters are fully controlled. The abdomen is then explored and the pancreas mobilized and carefully palpated. If the adenoma is found it is removed. Enucleation is normally

possible but resection of part of the pancreas may be required in some patients.

In the absence of a palpable tumour surgeons used to recommend that the body and tail of the pancreas should be removed in the hope that it contained the impalpable lesion. However, as only about half of such occult tumours are situated in this region, it is better to leave the gland intact. Hypoglycaemia can be controlled with diazoxide, and selective venous sampling used to localize the lesion for removal at reoperation.

If a malignant tumour is found, chemotherapy can be employed using an agent such as streptozotocin. Symptoms of hyperinsulinism can be controlled by diazoxide although nausea, cardiac arrhythmias, leucopenia, hypertrichosis and postural hypotension may be troublesome. Somatostatin analogues may also prove useful.

Glucagonoma

Tumours secreting excessive amounts of glucagon occasionally arise from A cells of the pancreatic islets and produce an unusual clinical syndrome. The most prominent feature is a necrotizing migratory dermatitis which is associated with painful glossitis, stomatitis, bowel upset, weight loss, diabetes mellitus and anaemia. Plasma levels of glucagon are raised and the tumour may be defined by CT scanning or angiography.

Resection of the tumour (which is sometimes benign) reverses the effects described above. Streptozotocin may be beneficial in patients with non-resectable tumours.

Vipoma

Tumours arising in non-B cells of the pancreatic islets can secrete a variety of polypeptides, of which vasoactive intestinal peptide is the most active. Such tumours may be solitary and benign, but half are malignant.

Clinical features

Vipoma causes the syndrome of watery diarrhoea, hypokalaemia and achlorhydria (WDHA syndrome) or 'pancreatic cholera'. There is profuse watery diarrhoea with the passage of 5 litres or more of fluid resembling weak tea and rich in potassium (50–60 mmol/l). The daily loss of potassium may be as much as 300 mmol, causing severe hypokalaemia and metabolic alkalosis. The patient may be confused, and ileus and abdominal distension may lead to a suspicion of intestinal obstruction. Tetany may occur due to hypomagnesaemia.

These symptoms can be intermittent and diagnosis may be delayed for some years. For this reason, malignant tumours have usually metastasized by the time they discovered.

Diagnosis depends on the demonstration of hypokalaemia, achlorhydria and increased levels of VIP in the circulating blood. These tumours are often large and can be demonstrated by CT scanning or angiography.

Treatment

Adequate fluid and electrolyte replacement before surgery is essential. The aim of surgery is to remove the tumour, and in the case of a solitary tumour this may be curative. Subtotal or total pancreatectomy is often required.

In unresectable cases or when metastases are present, streptozotocin or embolization of feeding vessels through arterial catheters may relieve symptoms. Treatment with the recently introduced analogues of somatostatin may also allow useful palliation.

38. The spleen

Anatomy

The spleen is a friable blood-filled organ lying in the left upper quadrant of the abdomen, protected by the ninth, tenth and eleventh ribs. It weighs about 150 g, is ellipsoid or 'coffee bean' in shape and lies with its long axis along the line of the tenth rib.

Its convex outer surface lies against the diaphragm above and its lower pole tests on the splenic flexure of the colon below. Its concave inner surface is related to the fundus of the stomach, the tail of the pancreas and the upper pole of the right kidney. It is surrounded by a fibrous capsule and, except at its hilus, is covered by peritoneum which is reflected as ligaments running to adjacent organs. These are the lienorenal, lienogastric (or gastrosplenic) and lienocolic ligaments. The phrenicocolic ligament, which runs between the splenic flexure of the colon and the undersurface of the diaphragm, provides additional support.

The splenic artery is a branch of the coeliac axis, which carries 40% of the splanchnic blood flow into the spleen and thence into the portal venous system by the splenic vein (Fig. 38.1). The splenic vessels are closely related to the pancreas and run within the lienorenal ligament to reach the splenic hilus, the only part of the spleen without a peritoneal covering. These vessels then continue as the short gastric vessels running within the lienogastric ligament to supply the uppermost part of the greater curvature of the stomach. Both the lienogastric and lienorenal ligament and their contained vessels must be divided during splenectomy.

The spleen is composed of white and red pulp.

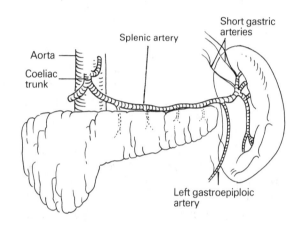

Fig. 38.1 Arterial blood supply of the spleen

Some 25% of the lymphoid tissue of the body is contained within the spleen and forms the *white pulp*, which consists of lymphoid follicles (Malpighian bodies) and lymphatic tissue, containing lymphocytes, macrophages and plasma cells. These cells migrate to the spleen from the bone marrow, and 30–50% of them are thymus-dependent. The *red pulp* is a loose honeycomb of reticular tissue which contains the splenic sinusoids. The blood vessels are carried into the pulp along fibrous trabeculae formed from the capsule. The arterioles first traverse white pulp, where they are surrounded by lymphoid tissue, and then flow into the red pulp and sinusoids (Fig. 38.2). It is controversial whether blood flows through the pulp spaces on its way to the sinusoids or enters the sinusoids directly and then meanders slowly backwards and forwards through the pulp. Erythrocytes move in and out of the pulp tissue so that 1% of the body red cells and 20–30% of the platelets are sequestrated at any given moment.

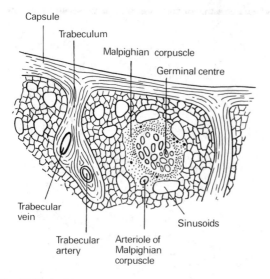

Capsule

Trabeculum

Malpighian corpuscle

Germinal centre

Trabecular vein

Sinusoids

Trabecular artery

Arteriole of Malpighian corpuscle

Fig. 38.2 Architecture of the splenic pulp

Normally the spleen is impalpable and cannot be percussed. When enlarged, it extends downwards and medially below the costal margin. It is then best palpated bimanually, with the patient lying on his right and the left side turned slightly forwards when the distinctive notch on its antero-inferior border will be felt. On percussion an enlarged spleen causes dullness over the ninth rib in the midaxillary line. Splenic enlargement can also be detected by soft tissue X-ray, a splenic scintiscan (using ^{99m}Tc-labelled sulphur colloid which is taken up rapidly by the reticulo-endothelial cells), and by ultrasonic or CT scan.

Function

Haemopoiesis. The spleen is a source of red blood cells and granulocytes in fetal life. Thereafter extramedullary haemopoiesis occurs only in the myeloproliferative syndromes.

Filtration of blood cells. Normal blood cells pass through the spleen unchanged. Abnormal and ageing cells are trapped. Following splenectomy there is an increased number of misshapen red cells in the peripheral blood, some containing nuclear remnants (Howell-Jolly bodies) and others containing clumps of iron (siderocytes). It has been estimated that 20 ml of red cells are phagocytosed daily. White cells and platelets, par-

ticularly when coated with antibodies, also are removed.

Immunological function. The spleen is an important site for effecting both cell-mediated and humoral immunity. Particulate antigens are filtered off and immunoglobulins (particularly IgM) and phagocytosis-promoting peptides (tuftsin) are produced. Following splenectomy immunological responses are impaired.

Storage function. In dogs the spleen acts as a reservoir for blood and in states of shock empties by contraction of its muscular capsule to provide an 'autotransfusion'. This is not a function of the spleen in man.

Endocrine effects. There is some evidence that the spleen exerts a humoral effect on the bone marrow, stimulating erythropoiesis and depressing white cell and platelet counts.

INDICATIONS FOR SPLENECTOMY

While the recommendation to remove the spleen electively usually emanates from the haematologist, the surgeon must be aware of the indications for splenectomy and the criteria which should be fulfilled before accepting a patient for operation. The common indications are outlined below.

Trauma

Injury to the spleen is an indication for splenectomy if the organ cannot be conserved. Spleens involved by pathological conditions such as portal hypertension, polycythaemia and infective mononucleosis are prone to rupture on slight trauma. It must also be appreciated that, following rupture, temporary improvement in the clinical state may precede sudden deterioration. Awareness and careful observation are critical, particularly in patients with a suspected subcapsular haematoma, which can lead to 'delayed rupture'. Splenic injuries are considered in more detail in Chapter 14.

Haemolytic anaemias

Hereditary spherocytosis

This congenital disease is transmitted as an autosomal dominant trait and affects the red blood cells, which are spherical rather than biconcave, unduly fragile and less able to withstand the effects of passing through the splenic pulp. Excess haemolysis results in anaemia, jaundice and splenic enlargement. It is a disease of remissions and relapses with 'haemolytic crises' requiring transfusion. Gallstones occur in 30–60% of cases.

Splenectomy is indicated in all cases when health is impaired. However, it should not be performed before the age of 3–4 years. If gallstones are present, cholecystectomy should be carried out simultaneously.

Acquired haemolytic anaemias

Excess haemolysis may occur secondary to exposure to agencies such as chemicals, drugs, infection, or extensive burns, or it may be an autoimmune phenomenon. In the latter case the red cells are coated with an autoantibody which can be detected by agglutination when antihuman globulin is added to a suspension of the patient's red cells (positive Coomb's test).

Autoimmune haemolytic anaemia affects predominantly middle-aged women and causes severe haemolytic crises superimposed on a background of mild anaemia. Treatment consists of steroids, but if this fails to control the disease and excess sequestration of red cells has been demonstrated, splenectomy may be required.

The purpuras

Idiopathic thrombocytopenic purpura (ITP)

This disease of unknown aetiology is characterized by a low platelet count and short platelet life-span despite plentiful megakaryocytes in the bone marrow. Cyclical episodes of bleeding occur from the gastrointestinal tract and other sites which are associated with petechiae and ecchymoses. Platelet counts are below $50 \times 10^9/1$, bleeding time is prolonged, clotting time is normal and capillary fragility is increased. The spleen is palpably enlarged in only 2–3% of patients and dense adhesions may form around it.

Clinical course. The disease may be chronic or acute. In the *acute* form there is usually a short history of a preceding illness. Spontaneous remission is common and the response to steroids

or splenectomy is excellent. The *chronic* form is characterized by a course of remissions and relapses which may last several years. Its response to steroids is poor and the outcome after splenectomy less satisfactory.

Choice of treatment. The acute form of the disease is treated initially with steroids. A rapid increase in the platelet count is associated with a good prospect of complete and lasting remission when therapy is stopped. If steroid therapy does not result in rapid remission, splenectomy is advised. Splenectomy is the treatment of choice for patients with the chronic form of the disease; steroids are of use only to provide temporary improvement before surgery.

Because of the high incidence of spontaneous remission, splenectomy is not advised for acute ITP in children.

Secondary thrombocytopenia

Splenectomy is contraindicated in secondary haemorrhagic purpuras, although it may be advised if hypersplenism is associated with secondary thrombocytopenia.

Hypersplenism

This syndrome consists of splenomegaly and pancytopenia in the presence of an apparently normal bone marrow and the absence of an autoimmune disorder. There is sequestration and destruction of blood cells in the spleen affecting predominantly white cells and platelets.

Hypersplenism may complicate a number of inflammatory conditions (e.g. rheumatoid arthritis), infections (e.g. malaria), and myeloproliferative and lymphoproliferative disorders. In portal hypertension, splenic congestion frequently leads to splenomegaly and hypersplenism.

The effects of hypersplenism include expansion of the total blood volume to fill the increased vascular spaces of the enlarged spleen and splanchnic bed. There is increased pooling of cells within the enlarged spleen and excess destruction, possibly induced by metabolic damage due to the cells being packed together in the enlarged spleen. In the peripheral blood there is anaemia, leucopenia and thrombocytopenia, but marrow turnover is

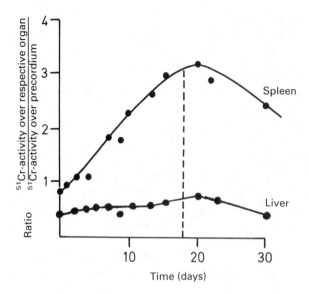

Fig. 38.3 Measurement of the rate of red cell destruction in the liver and spleen using ^{51}Cr-labelled autologous erythrocytes. Radioactivity is measured over the spleen and liver, and in each case compared to that over the precordium. The relative role of the spleen in red cell destruction is determined by the spleen-to-liver ratio, which in this case is 3.2:0.8 = 4.0:1.0

increased, with resultant reticulocytosis and leucoerythroblastosis. Increased amounts of urobilinogen are present in the urine.

Removal of a grossly enlarged spleen carries appreciable morbidity and mortality and by eradicating a large mass of lymphoid tissue puts the patient at risk from serious bacterial infection. It must not be undertaken lightly and the haematologist will take into account the degree of cytopenia, the extent of splenic enlargement, the amount of discomfort caused and the incidence of recurrent infections from leucopenia. Isotopic studies to measure the rate of sequestration of red cells in the liver and spleen are usually performed and operation is advised only if the spleen-to-liver ratio exceeds 2:1 (Fig. 38.3). This is calculated from the 'half-life' of ^{51}Cr-labelled autologous red cells as measured by radioactivity over the spleen and liver compared to that over the precordium.

Proliferative disorders

Myelofibrosis

This condition was once believed to be due to obliteration of the blood-forming elements in the bone marrow by fibrosis. The resulting gross enlargement of the spleen was thought to be a secondary phenomenon to provide a site for extramedullary haemopoiesis. Splenectomy was contraindicated.

It is now recognized that the condition is due to an abnormal proliferation of mesenchymal elements in the bone marrow, spleen, liver and lymph nodes, and that extramedullary haemopoiesis occurs at many sites. Contrary to previous belief, splenectomy does not lead to a lethal aplastic anaemia but decreases transfusion requirements. By relieving the discomfort of a grossly enlarged spleen, it also improves symptoms. However, careful haematological studies are indicated before it is advised.

Lymphomas

The role of splenectomy in the staging and treatment of Hodgkin's disease is considered in Chapter 22. In non-Hodgkin's lymphoma, splenectomy is only rarely indicated, as when a primary neoplasm is confined to the spleen. However, in both myelo- and lymphoproliferative conditions splenectomy may be indicated to reduce transfusion requirements when hypersplenism is a problem.

Other tumours

Apart from lymphomas and leukaemias, tumours of the spleen are rare. Haemangiomas (capillary or cavernous) may reach sufficient size to cause splenic enlargement with a consumptive coagulopathy and haemorrhagic tendency. Most haemangiomas are recognized at operation, when the spleen should be removed.

Miscellaneous conditions

Cysts of the spleen

Cysts of the spleen are rare. They are usually single but occasionally multiple (polycystic disease). Single cysts may be congenital, degenerative or parasitic.

Congenital cysts are due to an embryonic defect and result in a dermoid-like lesion. They are lined by flattened epithelium and contain thin blood-stained fluid or thick creamy material, sometimes with hair and teeth.

Degenerative cysts result from liquefaction of an infarct or haematoma. The wall is fibrous and often calcified and the cyst is filled with brownish fluid or paste-like material.

Parasitic cysts are usually acquired through contact with dogs and are due to infection with *Echinococcus granulosus* (hydatid disease).

Splenic cysts normally cause no symptoms and are often discovered fortuitously by detecting splenic enlargement on clinical examination or abnormal calcification on abdominal X-ray. The diagnosis can be confirmed by ultrasound. Treatment consists of splenectomy. As the cyst may be parasitic, transabdominal needle aspiration is not advised.

Abscess of the spleen

A splenic abscess is rare. It should be suspected when progressive splenic enlargement is associated with bacteraemia and abscess formation at other sites. Splenectomy, although desirable, may not prove feasible. Drainage of the abscess may be the only possible method of treatment.

Splenic artery aneurysm

This is a relatively common complication of atherosclerosis in elderly patients. The calcified wall of the aneurysm is visible on X-ray and there is normally obvious calcification of the tortuous splenic artery. The presence of an uncomplicated atherosclerotic aneurysm is not an indication for surgical treatment. Bleeding can, however, occur and operation is then mandatory.

Rarely, a congenital aneurysm affects the splenic artery. Such aneurysms are more common in women and may rupture during pregnancy. An asymptomatic congenital aneurysm may be discovered on abdominal X-ray as a thin calcified ring shadow. Because of the risk of rupture, it should be treated electively.

As most congenital aneurysms lie close to the splenic hilus, splenectomy is usually required. At other sites excision may be possible.

SPLENECTOMY

Preoperative preparation

As the stomach is handled during splenectomy, a nasogastric tube should always be inserted.

Routine preoperative preparation is as for any abdominal operation, but particular attention must be paid to the full blood count, and coagulation status. In the presence of any bleeding tendency, transfusions of blood or platelets may be required. For thrombocytopenia, platelets should be available to cover the operation and the postoperative phase.

The degree of splenic enlargement should be known before the operation. If in doubt, the surgeon should request a CT scan. A massively enlarged spleen, particularly if due to tropical disease, may give a spurious impression of mobility despite gross adhesion formation. This results from movement of the attenuated diaphragm.

Technique

A normal-sized non-adherent spleen is removed after first mobilizing it medially by division of its lateral peritoneal attachments. The splenic artery and vein are then doubly ligated and divided. Finally, the lienogastric ligament with its contained vessels is divided between ligatures.

When the spleen is enlarged or adherent, preliminary mobilization may not be possible, and the vascular pedicle is dissected first. The lienogastric ligament is first divided between ligatures. The splenic artery is then identified at the upper border of the pancreas and doubly ligated and divided. Alternatively, it may first be ligated in continuity so that the spleen shrinks in size, allowing it to be mobilized and vessels to be ligated close to the splenic hilus.

If there are any adhesions between the spleen and the diaphragm, it is advisable to ligate and divide its vascular supply before interfering with them.

Occasionally a thoracoabdominal incision is necessary to remove a large spleen, but in most cases a long vertical or subcostal abdominal incision is adequate.

Postoperative course and complications

Drainage of the abdomen is not normally required after removal of a normal-sized spleen. After removal of an enlarged organ, bleeding from the pedicle should not occur provided the splenic vessels have been doubly ligated, but oozing from multiple adhesions is common and drainage is therefore advised. Any bleeding tendency, e.g. in a patient with ITP, increases the likelihood of this complication. Hypotension and circulatory collapse within 48 hours of surgery indicate the need to re-explore the abdomen.

Pancreatitis occasionally follows splenectomy. This is due to handling and bruising of the tail of the pancreas during mobilization of the spleen.

Accessory spleens occur around the splenic hilus, in its pedicle or in the omentum, and may account for relapse of the condition for which the splenectomy was performed. Scintiscanning after administration of ^{51}Cr-labelled red cells may be used to detect functioning accessory splenic tissue so that it can be removed at the time of primary surgery.

Local complications of splenectomy include lower lobe collapse and an abscess in the splenic bed.

Following splenectomy there is a transient increase in the platelet and white cell count. This predisposes to a risk of venous thrombosis. Low-dose heparin is therefore advised in all patients undergoing splenectomy.

Loss of lymphoid tissue reduces immune activity and impairs the response to bacteraemia. There is a deficiency in the production of phagocytosis-promoting peptides and immunoglobulin. While the risk of serious infection is greatest when splenectomy is performed in childhood, a slightly increased incidence of death from pneumonia, complicated by disseminated intravascular coagulation and adrenal failure, has been reported in adults. As most infections occur within 3 years of splenectomy, some surgeons advise prophylactic penicillin for this period. This is mandatory in young children. Polyvalent anti-pneumococcal vaccine may also be given before splenectomy.

Splenectomy should be avoided if at all possible in all young children. Lacerations should be sutured and, even when the spleen is ruptured, a partial splenectomy is preferable to total splenectomy if this is feasible.

39. Urological surgery

INVESTIGATION

History

The majority of patients who present in a urological clinic have either a sign or a symptom which suggests an abnormality in the urinary tract. Thus, any patient with blood in the urine (haematuria), *irrespective of other symptoms*, requires a full urological investigation.

There are also patients who present in other clinics complaining of symptoms which may be due to urological problems, e.g. backache from metastatic prostatic carcinoma, fever of unknown origin from renal carcinoma, lethargy and anaemia due to obstructive renal failure or headaches from hypertension of renal origin. Since common things occur commonly, an elderly male complaining of difficulty in passing urine *probably* has outflow tract obstruction due to benign enlargement of the prostate (benign prostatic hyperplasia; BPH). But he may also recently have been prescribed a diuretic, so causing the change in his urinary habits.

Environmental factors must not be ignored. In some parts of the world, bilharziasis is a common cause of haematuria. In the industrialized world, the patient may have been exposed to certain carcinogenic agents which, years later, cause bladder cancer.

Urinary tract symptoms

The site of *pain* must be accurately defined. Pain in the 'side' could originate from the chest, loin or spinal column. Renal pain occurs in the renal angle, i.e. that angle between the 12th rib and the sacrospinalis muscles. Ureteric pain (or colic) may start in the renal angle but typically radiates forwards and downwards into the groin and to either the testes or labia. When the bladder is obstructed acutely, there is characteristic severe central lower abdominal pain. Chronic bladder obstruction may produce only a vague lower abdominal ache even though the bladder is grossly distended. Bladder abnormalities and prostatic diseases may also cause ill-defined perineal or penile pains. A prostate which is grossly enlarged can encroach into the rectum and cause rectal symptoms, including *tenesmus*. The recognition of penile and testicular pain is usually easy.

Urinary symptoms have a character of their own. *Frequency of micturition* is recorded numerically. Thus D/N = 6/3 indicates that the frequency by day is six times and that by night three times. A *poor stream* and *dribbling* are characteristic of a mechanical obstruction in the outflow tract. *Urgency* describes the sudden uncontrollable urge to empty the bladder. This may be associated with incontinence (*urge incontinence*). *Stress incontinence* indicates an involuntary loss of urine due to stress such as straining to lift, running or even laughter. *Dysuria* is painful micturition which is often described as being of a burning or scalding nature.

The patient may use a wide range of phrases to describe alterations in urinary habits. The interrogation must aim to reveal whether the patient is describing obstruction (e.g. poor stream), detrusor contraction (e.g. urgency), infection (e.g. frequency, dysuria) or a more sinister sign of malignancy (e.g. dark, discoloured or brown urine).

Examination

Examination should be full and not confined to the

urinary system. Thus, cardiological, neurological and gynaecological problems may be associated with urinary signs and symptoms. Since many urological patients are elderly, they must be assessed as to their fitness for further investigations and operative treatment. For example, the cardiovascular state of a patient may be relevant to subsequent investigations (e.g. those requiring an anaesthetic) or treatment (e.g. the administration of oestrogens for carcinoma of the prostate).

Physical examination of the *kidneys* is difficult. The patient must be able to relax the abdominal muscles so that the kidney can be lifted with one hand behind the loin and palpated by the other hand pressing downwards (Fig. 39.1). The *ureter* cannot be palpated even though it does pass close to the posterior fornix of the vagina. The *bladder*, if enlarged, is central and rises up out of the pelvis; it is dull to percussion, and in a patient with chronic retention who is lying flat and relaxed it is visible. Abnormalities of adjacent abdominal organs must be sought. For example, a mass in the iliac fossa could be ovarian in origin.

In the male, examination must include the groins, hernia sites, cords, testes and epididymes, which are examined both with the patient standing up and lying down. The penis should always be examined. If it is uncircumcised, it must be confirmed that the foreskin retracts and that the glans and meatus are normal.

In the female, the vulva, urethra and vagina must be examined; a speculum examination should be carried out if there is any suspicion of a vaginal or cervical abnormality. (A full pelvic bimanual examination, whether in males or females, is best

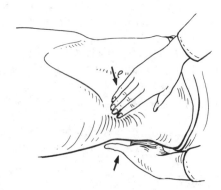

Fig. 39.1 Bimanual palpation of the kidney

carried out under general anaesthesia with a muscle relaxant.)

A rectal examination is mandatory not only to examine the prostate but also to detect abnormalities of the anal margin (e.g. haemorrhoids, fissures) and lower rectum (e.g. carcinoma).

Routine investigations

Urine

Routine 'side-room' examination of the urine consists of testing for protein and sugar with proprietary test-papers. Testing for protein is used as a simple guide to glomerular function. Provided that there is no urinary tract infection, normal urine is almost protein-free. A protein leak of more than 150 mg/24 h requires further investigation of the kidneys. The detection of sugar in the urine may point to a diagnosis of diabetes, and urinary symptoms may be related to this.

In surgical practice, routine *microscopic examination* of a fresh specimen of urine is of limited value. However, the presence of red cells or pus cells may support a diagnosis of stone, tumour or infection. Other abnormalities in the urinary sediment, such as casts or an increase in tubular epithelial cells, are more likely to be associated with renal parenchymal disease. Crystals are often present in patients with renal calculi.

For *microbiological examination* of the urine, a fresh sample must be collected in a sterile container. In order to avoid contamination by normal urethral flora, the patient is asked to pass some urine into the toilet, then, without interrupting the flow, the next part into a special container, and the remainder into the toilet — hence the term *midstream specimen* of urine (MSU). If it is necessary to store the specimen, it should be kept at 4°C. In order to rule out possible contamination during the collection of midstream specimens, fine needle aspiration of a full bladder suprapubically may be required in difficult cases. In the microbiological laboratory, the specimen will usually be examined microscopically for pus cells only. A more detailed microscopic examination of the urine, e.g. for crystals, casts or ova, will need to be carried out on a fresh specimen in the side room of a ward or clinic. To detect organisms the microbiologist will culture the urine in a suitable medium. He will also determine the sensitivity of any organism to antimicrobial agents.

Blood

A guide to overall renal function is provided by measuring blood urea or creatinine. Urea is the major end-product of protein metabolism but its blood level may be influenced by diet and urine flow rate. As the blood urea concentration does not start to rise unless the glomerular filtration rate is reduced to 50% of normal, considerable renal damage can exist in the presence of a normal blood urea. Measurement of serum creatinine is preferred since it is stable, independent of urine flow and little influenced by diet. Measurement of creatinine clearance using the classic formula of UV/P, where U is the creatinine concentration in the urine, V the volume of urine (in ml) over a timed period, and P the creatinine concentration in blood, is required only in patients whose kidneys are failing so that the clinician can estimate when more active treatment of renal failure might be needed.

The blood chemistry may also be examined to exclude a metabolic disorder. The haemoglobin should be checked and will be low in a patient with chronic renal disease. The erythrocyte sedimentation rate (ESR) can be markedly raised in idiopathic retroperitoneal fibrosis, a cause of ureteric obstruction.

A search for tumour secretory products (*tumour markers*) in the blood may help to diagnose and monitor malignant disease. In tumours of the testis, human chorionic gonadotropin and alpha-fetoprotein are valuable tumour markers. Serum acid phosphatase is a useful marker for carcinoma of the prostate.

Intravenous urography

The basic radiological investigation of the urinary tract is *intravenous urography* (IVU). A plain X-ray of the abdomen and pelvis is obtained first to show the areas of the kidneys, ureters and bladder. In addition to the lumbar spine and pelvis, opacities such as stones in the region of the urinary tract will be shown. An iodine-containing contrast material is then injected intravenously and serial X-rays are taken as the contrast is excreted.

The concentration of contrast is influenced by the urine flow, which in turn depends on the hydration of the patient. Routine preparation for an IVU should include fluid restriction for 12 hours. As faeces within the large bowel will diminish the radiographic outline of the urinary tract, an aperient may be given on the day before the X-ray.

An IVU demonstrates the renal pelvis and calyces and the rate of emptying from the kidneys. The calibre of the ureters is seen as contrast passes down to the bladder. Once the bladder has filled with contrast, the patient empties the bladder and a 'post-micturition' X-ray is taken to show the efficiency of bladder emptying and to indicate the amount of residual urine.

Delayed excretion of the contrast is a sign of obstruction somewhere along the urinary tract. Delayed X-rays, taken up to 24 hours after the contrast injection, may then give added detail of the affected kidney and ureter.

Special investigations

Other radiological studies

To define the ureter, pelvis and calyces more clearly, a *retrograde ureteropyelogram* may be necessary. This involves retrograde injection of contrast material through a ureteric catheter placed in the lower ureter (Fig. 39.2). With improved techniques of intravenous urography, retrograde injection is now less commonly used.

The renal vessels can be demonstrated by *renal angiography*. A catheter is passed into the aorta via a femoral artery up to the level of the renal arteries, where contrast medium is injected and serial films are taken. If better definition is required, the renal vessels may be selectively catheterized. Renal angiography is used primarily for the detection of stenosis of the main renal artery, for assessment of the vascularity of a renal mass, or as a preliminary to embolization to infarct a kidney.

To define the bladder, detect ureterovesical reflux or examine the bladder neck and urethra, a

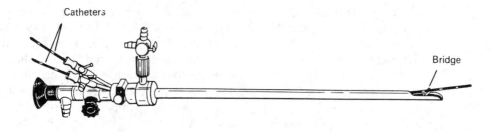

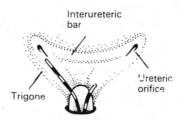

Fig. 39.2 Cystoscope and ureteric catheterization

micturating cystourethrogram (MCU) is required. The bladder is filled with contrast material (via a catheter) and emptying is then studied by X-ray screening. An *ascending urethrogram*, in which contrast medium is injected into the urethra and X-rays are then taken, can be used to define strictures, but is less useful than an MCU.

Ultrasound

The main use of ultrasound in the urinary tract is to distinguish between solid tumours and cysts of the kidney. Other uses include the detection of perirenal collections of fluid which may occur around a transplanted kidney, and the characterization of masses in the pelvis. Ultrasound is of limited value in determining the size or spread of tumours.

Nuclear imaging

Methods using radiolabelled substances are used for two main purposes.

1. *Detection of metastases in bones.* Technetium-99m (^{99m}Tc)-labelled methylene diphosphonate (MDP) is the most reliable marker for detecting metastases in carcinoma of the prostate.

2. *Measurement of renal function.* ^{99m}Tc-labelled

chelates, DTPA (diethylenetetramine penta-acetic acid) and DMSA (dimercaptosuccinic acid) are used for this purpose. DTPA is rapidly excreted through the glomerulus and can be used to provide a measure of the glomerular filtration rate from each kidney. DMSA is concentrated in the renal tubule. As only 5% is excreted, static imaging can be carried out some 2–3 hours after injection. Parenchymal defects such as tumours, haematoma, lacerations or ischaemia may be demonstrated. Differential renal function can be quantified from the DMSA concentration in each kidney.

Urodynamic studies

In their simplest form, urodynamic studies are used to measure maximum urinary flow rate during micturition by a flow meter. The flow meter records the volume of urine passed in a recorded time and converts this into a flow rate expressed as ml/s. The normal flow rate in males is 15–30 ml/s and that in females 20–40 ml/s. It is important to measure the flow rate when the bladder has a capacity of more than 150 ml, otherwise the values may be misleading and reflect bladder dysfunction rather than an outflow obstruction. A flow rate of less than 6 ml/s for a voided volume of 150 ml or more is abnormal. The urinary stream may be so poor that no such quantification is necessary, but in a proportion of patients with equivocal urinary symptoms, the flow rate can be of help in determining the degree of obstruction.

For additional information on the dynamic activity of the urinary tract, measurements of flow rate are combined with *cystometry*. This provides a measure of the residual urine, the capacity of the bladder, the capacity at which a desire to void occurs and the detrusor pressures when the bladder is full and at maximum flow rate. Detrusor muscle pressure is recorded continuously, and any spontaneous contractions during the filling of the bladder may indicate an unstable bladder (a cause of urgency and urge incontinence). The pressures along the length of the urethra may also be measured (urethral pressure profile).

These measurements are of particular value in distinguishing between bladder and urethral abnormalities in an incontinent patient. They also assist in distinguishing between neurological, pharmacological and mechanical causes of outflow tract symptoms.

Semen analysis

Microscopic examination of the semen is a basic investigation in an infertile male. The specimen is collected 3 days after the last ejaculation and examined within 2 hours. Normal semen has a volume of 2–6 ml and a sperm concentration of $20–120 \times 10^6$/ml. More than 60% of the sperms are motile at 2 hours.

The morphology, biochemistry and viability of the sperm may also be studied. In selected cases, immunological tests may help to determine the cause of infertility.

Biochemical screening for stones

The main metabolic causes of urinary tract stones are hyperparathyroidism, idiopathic hypercalciuria, hyperoxaluria and cystinuria. All patients with urinary tract calculi should be screened for such an underlying metabolic abnormality. Serum calcium, phosphate, oxalate and uric acid are measured. More detailed investigation requires 24-hour collection of urine for determination of calcium, phosphate, oxalate and uric acid excretion. The composition of passed or removed stones should be analysed to determine their metabolic type.

URINARY TRACT OBSTRUCTION: OUTFLOW TRACT

The outflow tract is that part of the urinary tract which extends from the bladder neck through the urethra to the external urinary meatus. In older males it is most commonly obstructed by benign hyperplasia of the prostate; in younger males the obstruction may be due to a stricture. Carcinoma of the prostate is a less frequent cause of obstructive symptoms.

Benign prostatic hyperplasia

Pathology

From about the age of 40 years the prostate undergoes progressive change in size and consistency. Enlargement results from hyperplasia of periurethral glandular tissue forming adenomas in the central zone of the prostate. These characteristically form lateral 'lobes', and often a 'middle lobe'. The normal prostatic tissue is gradually compressed to form a shell or capsule around these adenomas. There is considerable variation in the growth rates of the adenomas and in the proportion of stromal and epithelial tissue. A prostate that has been previously infected or has a preponderance of stromal tissue is firm and fibrous on rectal examination. Adenomas with epithelial preponderance can grow to large discrete masses with a total weight of more than 100 g and on examination have a characteristic rubbery consistency. These changes are generally referred to as benign prostatic hyperplasia. The pathological effects of prostatic hyperplasia are summarized in Figure 39.3.

The enlarging adenomas lengthen and obstruct the prostatic urethra, interfere with the sphincter mechanisms of the internal meatus and lead to the signs and symptoms of prostatic obstruction. In order to overcome increasing outflow resistance, the bladder detrusor muscle hypertrophies. The muscle bands form trabeculae between which saccules may form diverticula. Occasionally a diverticulum may become quite large, even larger

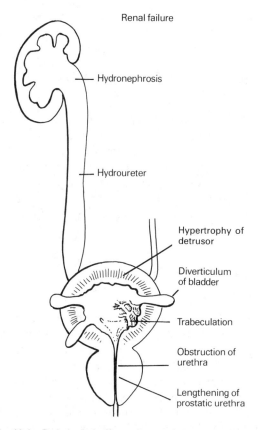

Renal failure

Hydronephrosis

Hydroureter

Hypertrophy of detrusor

Diverticulum of bladder

Trabeculation

Obstruction of urethra

Lengthening of prostatic urethra

Fig. 39.3 Pathological effects of prostatic hyperplasia

than the bladder. Bladder diverticula empty poorly and are liable to the three main complications of urinary stasis: infection, stones and tumour.

With progressive inability to empty the bladder completely (chronic retention), the risk of urinary infection and stone formation increases. Bladder stones have become rare in Western countries but are often seen in areas of poor nutrition and especially in children. The stones are typically of the infective type, mixed calcium oxalate and phosphate. Eventually the residual urine volume may exceed 1 litre, leading to progressive obstruction and dilatation of the ureters (hydro-ureter) and pelvicaliceal system (hydronephrosis) with ultimately obstructive renal failure.

Clinical features

The pathological changes at the bladder neck produce variable signs and symptoms which correlate poorly with the size of the prostate. Frequency, urgency and dysuria are common. Nocturia may become increasingly troublesome. The force of the stream will be noticeably weaker and, with straining in an attempt to empty the bladder, bleeding may occur from vessels at the bladder neck. These clinical features may be separated into two main groups: those that are due to obstruction, i.e. slow stream and hesitancy, and those that are due to an unstable detrusor muscle, i.e. urgency and urge incontinence. These latter irritative symptoms alone are not an indication for prostatectomy.

Increasing frequency may deceive the patient into thinking that he is passing an adequate amount of urine whereas the bladder may be full though painless. The frequency may progress to dribbling incontinence. Such patients are liable to develop the signs and symptoms of obstructive uraemia, including drowsiness, anorexia and personality changes.

Some patients may suddenly stop passing urine (acute retention). This may be precipitated by a urinary infection, cold weather or excessive alcohol, each of which can cause sufficient congestion of the bladder neck to tip the balance from difficult micturition to acute painful retention. If the obstruction has already led to chronic retention of urine (the patient being unable to empty his bladder completely), acute-on-chronic obstruction may occur. If the patient has a bladder stone, he may have obstructive symptoms during micturition and there may also be bladder pain at the end of micturition.

Examination of a patient with symptoms of prostatism will reveal little except enlargement of the gland on rectal examination. The enlargement is symmetrical and smooth, with a median groove between the two lateral 'lobes'. The consistency of an adenoma is described as rubbery. Asymmetry or a hard consistency should raise the suspicion of malignancy.

In a patient with acute painful retention of urine, the size of the prostate is more difficult to determine. This is partly due to the pelvic discomfort but also to the fullness of the bladder, which changes the normal relationship of the prostate to the lower rectum so that the gland appears to be larger than it is. In patients with chronic retention, the painless, enlarged bladder rises up out of the pelvis, almost to the umbilicus. Even if its shape is not visible, the area over it will be dull on percussion. In addition, the patient with chronic retention may be ill from obstructive uraemia.

Investigation

All patients must have a basic assessment of renal function, and haemoglobin and serum electrolytes are estimated routinely. As symptoms of dysuria and frequency may be related principally to a urinary infection (which will have to be treated), the urine must be cultured in all cases. The serum acid phosphatase is measured if the consistency of the gland raises the suspicion of a neoplasm. Intravenous urography is necessary to detect the extent of any of the secondary effects of obstruction on the bladder (e.g. diverticula, stones) and upper urinary tract, and especially to assess the volume of residual urine after micturition. If the patient is uraemic, urography with a high dose of contrast and delayed X-rays will be required.

In some patients, and especially in the elderly, neurological or pharmacological causes of the changes in micturition must be considered. A urodynamic assessment may be necessary.

Treatment

The main clinical decision is whether the patient requires an operation on the prostate. There is no acceptable alternative treatment which will reduce the size of the gland. Patients can be divided into three clinical groups, each requiring a different approach to management.

1. *Symptomatic only.* The patient's assessment of the severity of symptoms is influenced by his age, the social inconvenience caused and by their frequency and progression. Thus, a young man may be greatly inconvenienced by symptoms that are quite acceptable to one who is elderly. If the exact role of the prostate in causing these symptoms is difficult to determine, urodynamic measurements may be helpful, especially if the symptoms appear to be irritative rather than obstructive.

Once it is established that the prostate is the principal problem, prostatectomy is recommended. Very few patients are unfit for this and only if there is a history of a myocardial infarction within the last 3 months should operation be deferred.

2. *Acute retention.* This is an emergency requiring admission to hospital. If there is a history of prostatism, conservative measures to encourage micturition (e.g. sedation, a warm bath) only delay inevitable catheterization.

A self-retaining (Foley) catheter (size 16 Fr) is passed using strict asepsis and connected to a closed bladder drainage system. If it is not possible to pass a urethral catheter, the bladder should be entered directly by puncture with a trocar/cannula device (suprapubic cystostomy). A specimen of urine is cultured and antibiotics are given only if there is microbiological evidence of an infection.

Only if the history of prostatism is short should the urethral catheter be removed after 12 hours, when normal voiding may occur. However, such patients should be advised to have a prostatectomy. Otherwise routine preoperative investigations are performed, followed by operation on the next available operating day.

3. *Chronic retention.* It is essential to determine whether the patient has developed any of the complications of obstruction, especially renal damage. Though the upper urinary tracts may be dilated, renal function is not necessarily impaired.

If the patient is well, with no haematological or biochemical disturbance, there is no indication for preliminary bladder drainage, and prostatectomy may be planned in the usual way.

If the patient is uraemic, with associated biochemical abnormalities, his general fitness for operation must be assessed. Uraemia alone is not a contraindication but hyperkalaemia, dehydration or other evidence of fluid and electrolyte disturbance must be corrected by intravenous fluids. The bladder is catheterized and prostatectomy is carried out as soon as the patient is judged to be fit. It is not necessary to wait unduly long for the blood urea to return to normal, as the risk of infection from prolonged catheterization may be a more serious hazard.

Relief of chronic obstruction is almost always followed by a diuresis due partly to an osmotic (urea) diuresis and partly to renal tubular changes resulting from back pressure. These losses can be detected by keeping accurate intake/output fluid charts. The blood pressure should be monitored and intravenous fluid replacement may be necessary.

Only exceptionally is a patient considered unfit for prostatectomy. He will then need a permanent self-retaining catheter.

Prostatectomy may be performed by open or closed (endoscopic) techniques.

Open prostatectomy. Earlier open procedures were by a transvesical approach in which the bladder was opened and the adenomatous obstruction enucleated from the capsule. Later, a retropubic approach was used in which the adenoma was enucleated through a transverse incision in the prostatic capsule (Fig. 39.4).

These open procedures are now reserved for very large adenomas or when another procedure, e.g. removal of a bladder diverticulum, is required. Apart from the length of hospitalization (10–14 days) and the presence of an abdominal wound, enucleation of some of the smaller adenomas may damage the external sphincter mechanism and cause incontinence. This is a particular problem with more fibrous glands and those that contain a focus of cancer.

Closed (endoscopic) prostatectomy (transurethral resection, TUR). The prostate gland is removed piecemeal by electroresection using an instrument called a resectoscope (Fig. 39.5).

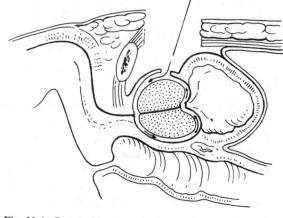

Plane of dissection around prostatic adenoma

Fig. 39.4 Retropubic prostatectomy

The disadvantage of the lengthy apprenticeship needed to acquire the skill to perform this procedure is greatly outweighed by the advantages of patient acceptance, short hospitalization (5–7 days) and the precision of removal of the obstructing tissue. It is now universally accepted as the method of choice. Great damage can be inflicted on the prostatic urethra and even the bladder by inexpert use of a resectoscope, and experience in the technique is essential.

If the patient has a bladder stone, this may be crushed with a lithotrite or removed by suprapubic lithotomy. If there is a diverticulum with a narrow

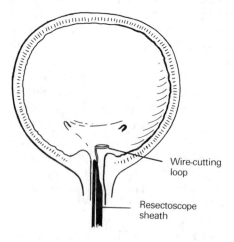

Wire-cutting loop

Resectoscope sheath

Fig. 39.5 Transurethral resection of the prostate

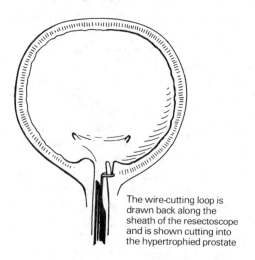

The wire-cutting loop is drawn back along the sheath of the resectoscope and is shown cutting into the hypertrophied prostate

neck, this should be removed through a suprapubic transvesical approach. If the diverticulum is shallow with a wide neck, then only the prostatectomy need be done.

Postoperative care

After either form of prostatectomy, the bladder must be drained by a urethral catheter to allow free drainage while the prostatic bed begins to heal and bleeding stops. After a transurethral resection, the catheter is normally removed on the 3rd postoperative day; after an open procedure, because of the bladder or prostate incision, it is usually left until the 7th postoperative day.

The main postoperative hazard is bleeding. In an open procedure, blood vessels at the bladder neck are sutured, but bleeding within the capsule is less easy to control. In a TUR, coagulation of the blood vessels is more precise but not always complete. If postoperative bleeding is excessive, a clot may form and lead to obstruction (clot retention). Various techniques are used to minimize this hazard; a good flow of urine can be induced by diuretics or by continuous irrigation established through a three-way urethral catheter.

The results from all forms of prostatectomy have continued to improve but transurethral resection is now recognized as the procedure of choice. It has the lowest morbidity and mortality (1%) and requires a shorter hospital stay (50% less) than other procedures.

Obstruction due to prostatic carcinoma

Carcinoma of the prostate is discussed in detail later in this chapter.

Bladder neck obstruction

Occasionally the obstruction to the outflow tract appears to be at the bladder neck. The prostate is often quite small, giving rise to the expression 'prostatism without a prostate'. The cause may be an infective condition such as prostatitis or schistosomiasis, or a neurological disorder, e.g. due to diabetes or a prolapsed intervertebral disc. More commonly, the obstruction is due to dyssynergia, which is the failure of the bladder neck to open when the detrusor contracts.

Characteristically, bladder neck dyssynergia is found in younger middle-aged men, i.e. at an age too young to expect benign prostatic hyperplasia. The urinary stream is poor, though the patient may have thought it normal for him, and there may be frequency and urgency.

The muscular dysfunction that causes dyssynergia may be improved by alpha-adrenergic blocking drugs. However, endoscopic incision or excision of the bladder neck is preferable to long-term drug treatment, but surgery is contraindicated if the risk of retrograde ejaculation and therefore infertility is of concern to the patient.

Urethral obstruction

Lesions of the urethra may be congenital, traumatic, infective or malignant. Each may result in outflow tract obstruction. The common sites of obstruction are shown in Figure 39.6. Foreign bodies, including urinary stones, may also cause obstruction. Any of these causes may be complicated by infection, with periurethral abscess, fistulas and stones occurring as late complications.

Pathology

Congenital lesions. Congenital valves in the posterior urethra occur only in boys. These lie at the level of the verumontanum and may cause gross obstructive changes in the bladder and upper urinary tracts at birth. The diagnosis is confirmed by micturating cystourethrography and treatment consists of endoscopic incision of the valves.

Diverticula of the urethra are rare causes of obstruction. More commonly, diverticula of the urethra occur as a secondary effect of obstruction in women.

Urethral trauma. An important late sequel of urethral trauma is a stricture whose severity is related to both the site and the extent of injury. Thus, a posterior urethral stricture that follows major trauma to the pelvis may be surrounded by dense fibrous tissue, whereas a stricture of the bulb of the urethra may be surrounded by healthy tissues. The former requires major reconstructive

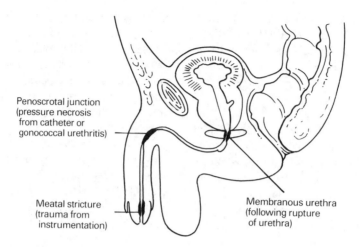

Penoscrotal junction
(pressure necrosis
from catheter or
gonococcal urethritis)

Meatal stricture
(trauma from
instrumentation)

Membranous urethra
(following rupture
of urethra)

Fig. 39.6 Common sites and causes of urethral stricture

surgery, but the latter can be readily managed by urethral dilatation or incision.

It must be remembered that rough inexpert use of any instrument (including a catheter) in the urethra can be followed by stricture formation.

Infective lesions. In the male, the principal organism responsible for inflammatory change, scarring and stricture of the urethra is *Neisseria gonorrhoeae*. The periurethral glands of the bulb of the urethra are the main site of the infection and when treatment is inadequate, stricture formation in this area is likely.

Long-term use of a self-retaining catheter, although not necessarily associated with infection, can also cause an inflammatory reaction in the urethra. This may result in a stricture, most commonly at the external meatus.

The foreskin may cause problems due to infection (balanitis) or narrowing of the orifice (phimosis), or by becoming retracted and stuck (paraphimosis). These are discussed on page 629.

In the female the paraurethral glands, sometimes called the 'female prostate', may become the site of chronic inflammatory change. The urethra becomes narrow, and these women experience recurring infective symptoms or obstructive symptoms without infection, the so-called *urethral syndrome*. Urethral stenosis and incomplete bladder emptying are but part of this difficult clinical problem. In some women symptomatic relief may follow urethral dilatation or urethrotomy.

Tumours of the urethra. Transitional cell tumours, which often occur in association with bladder tumours, and squamous carcinoma of the distal urethra are uncommon tumours which may cause obstructive symptoms.

Clinical features

The change in micturition which is due to urethral narrowing may be indistinguishable from that which occurs with benign prostatic hyperplasia. However, a stricture should be considered if there is a previous history of urethral infection, instrumentation or trauma.

The external meatus must always be examined and, if present, the foreskin retracted for full inspection. The urethra is palpated. It is possible for a stone to be lodged in the urethra yet the patient still pass urine, though with difficulty. In women, the urethra is best examined during cystourethroscopy under general anaesthesia: the urethra can then be palpated against the shaft of the cystoscope.

Investigation

An intravenous urogram may show only incomplete bladder emptying while an ascending urethrogram may not show the posterior urethra adequately because of spasm. A micturating cystourethrogram, in which the behaviour of the urethra during micturition is studied on the X-ray screen, is preferred. Urodynamic assessment of the *urethra and bladder* may be indicated for more complex problems, especially when neurological and mechanical problems coexist.

The final investigation to assess a urethral lesion is urethroscopy. This procedure should be considered as a cystourethroscopy since both urethra and bladder are always examined as a routine. The site and character of the lesion is determined and the degree of narrowing is measured.

Treatment

The precise site and extent of a stricture will have been established by the above investigations. Many simple strictures are treated easily by repeated dilatation with plastic or metal bougies, or may be incised under direct vision using a urethrotome. Most simple short strictures in the region of the bulb respond well to this type of treatment but there is a risk of recurrence which may require some form of operative reconstruction (a urethroplasty). In this procedure a strip of full-thickness skin is used to restore the normal calibre of the urethra.

A long persistent stricture of the anterior urethra will require a two-stage plastic reconstruction. A tight fibrous post-traumatic stricture of the membranous urethra may require transpubic excision of the scar tissue and urethral reconstruction. Stenosis of the meatus is treated by meatoplasty.

If the foreskin cannot be retracted normally (phimosis), and especially if infections are troublesome, circumcision is recommended.

If paraphimosis is present without gross oedema, it may be possible to reduce it manually, compression of the glans allowing the constricting band to be drawn forwards. Otherwise it is necessary to incise the constricting band. Circumcision may be carried out at a later date (see p. 629).

URINARY TRACT OBSTRUCTION: UPPER TRACT

The upper urinary tract includes the renal pelvicalyceal system and the ureters. As with any tubular structure, obstruction may be due to extrinsic, intrinsic or intraluminal causes.

In the kidney, stones within the pelvicalyceal system and congenital abnormality of the pelviureteric junction (PUJ) are the main causes of obstruction; both cause hydronephrosis. In the ureter, the common causes of obstruction are:

1. *Extrinsic*
   Retroperitoneal fibrosis
   External pressure (e.g. carcinoma of the cervix)
2. *Intrinsic*
   Transitional cell tumours
   Tuberculosis/bilharziasis
   Ureterocele
   Ectopic ureter
   Vesicoureteric reflux
   Megaureter
3. *Intraluminal*
   Calculi

More rarely, a sloughed renal papilla or blood clot (from a tumour) may obstruct either kidney or ureter.

During pregnancy there is a physiological dilatation of the ureters due to progesterone, which reduces smooth muscle tone.

Renal and ureteric calculi

Pathology

Stones which form in the kidney are of two main types: infective and metabolic.

An *infective* stone is whitish and chalky and crumbles or breaks easily. It is composed mainly of calcium, ammonia and magnesium phosphates. Such stones develop wherever drainage in the urinary tract is impaired and are usually associated with an anatomical abnormality such as a diverticulum or with long-term recumbency or paraplegia. Their formation indicates an established infection which cannot be eradicated by antibiotics alone. As the stone enlarges, drainage is further impaired and there is progressive damage to the kidney.

A *metabolic* stone, commonly of calcium oxalate, is usually hard and dark with an irregular sharp surface. It develops as a result of an abnormality of the composition of the urine. There may be an abnormal concentration of normal constituents (e.g. due to dehydration), excess excretion of normal constituents (e.g. calcium, as in hyperparathyroidism, or uric acid, as in gout) or the urine may contain abnormal constituents (as in the metabolic disorder of cystinuria). It is likely that several aetiological factors must occur together or in sequence for a stone to form in the urinary tract. As indicated above, all patients with urinary calculi should be screened for metabolic abnormalities.

Up to 80% of the stones seen in the UK are mixed calcium oxalate/phosphate stones. Approximately 10% are magnesium ammonium phosphate stones with a variable proportion of calcium. The remainder are uric acid (95%), cystine (1–4%) and, rarely, xanthine stones.

Clinical features

Renal pain, renal colic or ureteric colic are characteristically unilateral. Renal pain is dull and aching while ureteric colic is acute and severe and occurs in waves which pass down along the line of the ureter. A stone may cause bleeding or there may be symptoms of urinary tract infection. However, a stone in the kidney may remain silent, even one large enough to fill the pelvis and calyces (a 'staghorn' calculus).

Investigation

An intravenous urogram will usually provide all the necessary information on the anatomical position of the stone(s). Routine haematological and biochemical tests are needed to assess overall renal function and to exclude metabolic causes of stones. A urine sample is cultured to determine if there is infection. If an obstruction is acute, relief of the obstruction is the prime clinical need; if it is chronic and has caused renal damage, the surgical approach depends on the function of the affected kidney. This is best determined by radioisotope methods.

Treatment

Symptomatic treatment should be instituted as soon as the diagnosis is confirmed. Large doses of pethidine may be required to relieve pain. The addition of antispasmodics may assist the passage of the stone. The likelihood of spontaneous passage depends both on the size of the stone and on the smoothness of its surface. A stone of less than 0.5 cm in diameter should pass down the ureter. If it becomes fixed, causing increasing hydroureter and hydronephrosis, or if the urine is infected or the patient has increasing pain and fever, the stone must be removed.

A stone in the lower ureter, below the pelvic brim, may be coaxed out endoscopically using a stone basket. The instrument must be used with great care, as otherwise serious damage to the ureter may result. Other stones require methods of treatment that depend on the available expertise or facilities and on the type and size of the stone. Some stones are suitable for extracorporeal shock wave lithotripsy (ESWL), others can be treated by endoscopic ultrasonic disintegration, and yet others may require a direct surgical approach (ureterolithotomy).

Surgical techniques for the removal of fixed stones within the kidney have improved in recent years. Provided the affected kidney contributes more than 10% of the total renal function, attempts to save the kidney should always be made. Removal of a stone from the renal pelvis (pyelolithotomy) should be straightforward.

The surgical approach to stones in the kidney has undergone a major change in the past decade. A stone that is too large to pass down the ureter (usually more than 0.5 cm) can be treated by either percutaneous nephrolithotomy (PCNL) or extracorporeal shock wave lithotripsy. Larger stones in the renal pelvis (up to 2.5 cm in diameter) can be treated by ESWL alone, but still larger stones are best managed by a combination of these techniques. Some stones that extend into the calyces or occupy most of the calyceal system can now be dealt with by these techniques, but others are best removed through an incision in the renal pelvis (pyelolithotomy) which may have to be combined with an incision in the renal cortex (nephrolithotomy). Clamping of the renal vessels gives a bloodless field for operation. If this is to be prolonged for more than 30 min, cooling of the kidney (to 15°C) is recommended. The inside of a calyx may be examined with a nephroscope and small stones removed with forceps or by trapping in a fibrin coagulum. If stones in the lower calyces have damaged the lower part of the kidney, a partial nephrectomy may be necessary.

Pelviureteric junction obstruction (Idiopathic hydronephrosis)

Pathology

Narrowing at the junction between the renal pelvis and the ureter is a common cause of hydronephrosis. As the cause of the narrowing remains obscure, the term 'idiopathic' hydronephrosis is appropriate. Electron microscopy of the narrow area shows normal muscle cells with normal innervation, but the muscle bundles are separated by an excess of collagen fibres which may prevent relaxation of the segment. This abnormality of the PUJ is likely to be congenital. It is often bilateral and is seen in very young children. Gross hydronephrosis may, however, present at any age.

Clinical features

Idiopathic hydronephrosis may be the cause of a large painless mass in the loin; in its grossest form the volume of urine in the hydronephrotic sac may simulate free fluid in the peritoneal cavity. The more usual moderate hydronephrosis causes ill-defined renal pain or ache which may be exacerbated by drinking large volumes of liquid (e.g. tea or beer); the patient may regard these symptoms as 'indigestion'. Rarely, there may be no symptoms and a non-functioning hydronephrotic sac may be found incidentally.

Investigation

An intravenous urogram, with or without delayed films, will provide sufficient information in most cases. The calibre of the ureter in a PUJ obstruction is normal. There are a few patients in whom there is doubt as to whether the dilatation of the pelvis and calyces is truly obstructive in nature. Methods to resolve this include urography and renography during an induced diuresis, and antegrade pressure/flow measurements.

Treatment

Operations on the pelviureteric junction to relieve an obstruction (pyeloplasty) are designed to

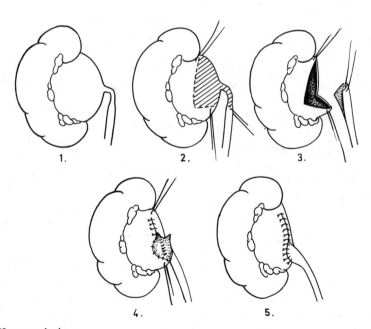

Fig. 39.7 Anderson-Hynes pyeloplasty

remove the obstructing tissue and to refashion the PUJ so that the lower part of the renal pelvis drains freely into the ureter (Fig. 39.7). Occasionally, an aberrant vessel to the lower pole of the kidney crosses the PUJ and gives the appearance of having caused the obstruction (though this is unlikely); in this situation, the PUJ is reconstructed in front of these vessels.

It is not possible to predict the degree of recovery of function (if any) of a kidney after relief of the obstruction. A grossly hydronephrotic kidney should be removed; but if the contralateral kidney is also impaired, even a poorly functioning kidney should be preserved.

Retroperitoneal fibrosis

Pathology

Fibrosis of the retroperitoneal connective tissues may encircle and compress the ureter(s), causing hydroureter and hydronephrosis. Fibrosis occurs in three groups of conditions.

Idiopathic. In this, the largest group, the fibrosis extends across the pelvic brim to involve the ureters and vena cava. The aetiology is unknown though it may be associated with methysergide or analgesic abuse. Mediastinal fibrosis or palmar fascial fibrosis (Dupuytren's contracture) may coexist.

Malignant infiltration. In this group the fibrosis contains malignant cells and represents a metastatic process from primary sites as various as breast, stomach, pancreas and colon; any part of the ureter may be affected.

Reactive fibrosis. Radiotherapy to pelvic organs, resolving blood clot after major vascular or other surgical procedures, or extravasation of sclerosants (e.g. phenol for a nerve block) can lead to fibrotic change in the retroperitoneum.

Since the gross appearance of all three groups of fibrosis may be similar, biopsy of the tissue is essential for diagnosis.

Clinical features

Obstruction due to pelviureteric fibrosis may cause symptoms similar to idiopathic hydronephrosis, i.e. ill-defined renal pain or ache. Some patients complain of low backache.

Investigation

An intravenous urogram will show hydronephrosis and usually hydroureter down to the level of the obstruction. The anatomy of the ureter is often hard to define and a retrograde ureteropyelogram under X-ray screening may be required. It is rarely necessary to pass a ureteric catheter up to the kidney (although it is characteristic of retroperitoneal fibrosis that a ureteric catheter will pass easily through what appears to be a severe obstruction).

A markedly raised erythrocyte sedimentation rate (ESR) is found in more than half of all patients with idiopathic retroperitoneal fibrosis.

Treatment

The relief of obstruction may be difficult. The ureter is dissected out of the fibrous sheet of tissue (ureterolysis) and wrapped in omentum to prevent further involvement in the fibrous process. Although obstruction due to idiopathic retroperitoneal fibrosis may regress with steroid treatment, ureterolysis and biopsy should be the primary treatment and steroids reserved for any recurrence of obstruction.

Transitional cell tumours (see also Urothelial tumours p. 617)

Though most commonly arising in the bladder, transitional cell tumours may occur in any part of the urothelium. During endoscopy, a tumour of the lower ureter may be seen protruding through the ureteric orifice. Tumours higher up in the ureter may not be detected until late; a change in the intravenous urogram may not be obvious until there is a significant degree of obstruction. The tumour may bleed and the clot may cause colic and obstruction.

Although a transitional cell tumour in the upper urinary tract may appear suitable for local excision, radical excision (nephroureterectomy) is recommended because of the difficulties in follow-up examination of this area. Conservative surgery may be considered in the elderly and *will* be necessary in those with bilateral upper tract tumours.

Miscellaneous conditions

A variety of congenital and acquired abnormalities of the ureter and ureteric orifice may result in obstruction.

Congenital abnormalities

A *ureterocele* develops behind a pin-hole ureteric orifice; the intramural part of the ureter dilates, bulges into the bladder and can become very large. Incision of the pin-hole opening will relieve the obstruction.

An *ectopic ureter* occurs with congenital duplication of one or both kidneys (duplex kidneys). Developmentally, the ureter has two main branches and, if this arrangement persists, the two ureters of the duplex kidneys may drain separately into the bladder (Fig. 39.8). One of the ureters enters normally on the trigone, while the ectopic ureter (from the upper renal moiety) may enter

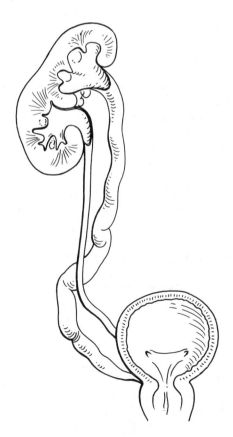

Fig. 39.8 Duplex kidney

either the bladder or, more rarely, the vagina or seminal vesicle.

A ureter that is ectopic within the bladder is liable to have an ineffective valve mechanism so that urine passes *up* the ureter on voiding (vesicoureteric reflux). Reflux can occur in normally sited ureters if the normal intramural ureter fails to act as a valve. The pressure of refluxing urine behaves as an intermittent obstruction which in children may lead to serious renal damage. Vesicoureteric reflux is treated by reimplantation of the ureter with the formation of an effective valve.

In primary obstructive *megaureter* there is dilatation of the ureter in all but its terminal segment without obvious cause and without vesicoureteric reflux. Although this condition has been compared to Hirschsprung's disease, there are normally no ganglionic cells in the ureter so that the megaureter cannot be due to neuromuscular incoordination. Radiographic and pressure/flow studies may be needed to determine whether there is a functional obstruction to the flow of urine. Narrowing of the ureter and reimplantation may be necessary.

Infections

Tuberculosis of the urinary tract may involve the ureter. Progression of the disease leads to strictures and even complete obstruction. This process may be silent and a so-called 'autonephrectomy' may be detected at a later date. This is now rare.

Bilharziasis affecting the urinary tract is common in parts of Africa and in the Middle East. Ureteric fibrosis and obstruction are part of the process that can affect the whole of the urinary tract if untreated. Many patients present in such an advanced state of the disease that surgical treatment is not feasible.

Both these infections require specific drug treatment. When the ureters are involved and obstructed, a variety of reconstructive surgical procedures may have to be considered to conserve renal function and to correct obstruction and/or reflux.

RENAL CYSTS

Simple cysts of the kidney are usually single. They

are almost always asymptomatic and of interest only because they are often found incidentally on intravenous urography. The differential diagnosis between a cyst and a renal carcinoma must then be made. Ideally, a cyst should be diagnosed and treated at the same session in the radiology department (Fig. 39.9). Fluid from the cyst is examined cytologically; if there is any suspicion of tumour cells, then the cyst must be explored. Malignant change in a cyst can occur but is very rare.

Polycystic kidney disease is a congenital anomaly (dominant) that affects both kidneys and often leads to chronic renal failure in middle life. Despite their very large size the cystic kidneys cause few symptoms. Infection or bleeding into a cyst can occur and may require exploration to relieve the symptoms. This condition may be a cause of haematuria.

TUMOURS OF THE URINARY SYSTEM

Benign adenomas are small and usually incidental findings. Haemangiomas are rare but may cause dramatic haematuria.

Primary malignant tumours are nephroblastoma (or Wilms' tumour) in children and renal carcinoma in adults. Metastases from other tumour sites may occasionally be found in the kidney.

Nephroblastomas

These tumours usually occur in children under 4 years of age. They account for 10% of all childhood malignancies.

Pathology

The tumour is probably derived from embryonic mesodermal tissue and microscopically has a mixed appearance of spindle cells, epithelial cells and muscle fibres. The growth is rapid and there is early local spread, including invasion of the renal vein. Invasion of the renal pelvis occurs late, so that haematuria is not common. Tumours presenting in the first year of life have a better prognosis than those diagnosed later. Distant metastases most commonly appear in the lungs, liver and bones.

Clinical features

The cardinal sign is a large abdominal mass which is often first noted when the baby is bathed. Some of the unusual clinical features associated with a renal carcinoma in adults, e.g. fever or hypertension, may also be present.

Investigation

An intravenous urogram is essential. The main differential diagnosis is from a neuroblastoma affecting the adrenal (see p. 353), but other causes of a large kidney, such as hydronephrosis and cystic disease, must also be considered. The tumour is bilateral in 5–10% of cases.

The chest is X-rayed in all cases.

Treatment

A transabdominal nephrectomy with wide excision of the mass is carried out after preliminary ligation of the renal pedicle. This is followed by radiotherapy and chemotherapy using a combination of actinomycin D and vincristine. As a result of this treatment, the prognosis of this

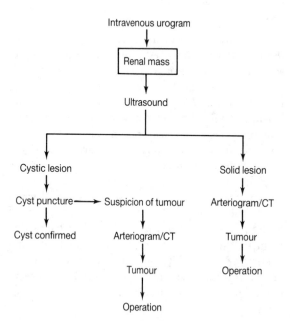

Fig. 39.9 Differential diagnosis of a renal mass. More precise tumour staging is possible with computed tomography (CT). An arteriogram will provide more information about renal vessels and tumour vascularity

tumour has improved greatly. Five-year survival rates (previously 10%) are now 80%.

Renal carcinoma

This is the commonest malignant tumour of the kidney. The incidence in males is three times greater than in females, and most patients are over 40 years of age.

Pathology

The tumour arises from renal tubules. Haemorrhage and necrosis within the tumour gives a characteristic mixed golden yellow and red appearance to the cut surface. Microscopically there are clear and granular cell types; the former are more common. There is early spread of the tumour into the renal pelvis, causing haematuria. Invasion of the renal vein, often extending into the inferior vena cava, also occurs early. Direct spread into perinephric tissues is common, so that the whole fascial envelope and kidney should be removed 'en bloc'. Lymphatic spread occurs to para-aortic nodes, while blood-borne metastases (which may be solitary) may develop almost anywhere in the body.

Clinical features

The triad of pain, haematuria and a mass is an important but late feature. A remarkable range of systemic effects may occur early. These include fever, a raised ESR, polycythaemia, disorders of coagulation, and abnormalities of plasma proteins and liver function tests. The patient may present with pyrexia of unknown origin (PUO) or, rarely, with a neuromyopathy.

Systemic effects may also be due to secretion by the tumour of products such as renin, erythropoietin, parathormone and gonadotropins. These abnormalities disappear when the tumour is removed but may reappear when metastases develop, i.e. they can be used as markers of tumour activity.

Investigation

The investigation of a renal carcinoma is as for any space-occupying lesion or mass in the renal parenchyma. The main differential diagnosis is from a simple renal cyst. The sequence of investigations used is that which gives the maximum information with the least number of tests and which facilitates the diagnosis and treatment of simple renal cysts. The tests most commonly used are ultrasonography, needle aspiration, CT scanning and arteriography (see Fig. 39.9).

Additional information about the extent to which a tumour has spread into the renal vein is obtained from an inferior vena cavagram. A chest X-ray (including tomograms) and an isotope bone scan are necessary to detect metastases.

Treatment

A radical nephrectomy that includes the perirenal fascial envelope and ipsilateral para-aortic lymph nodes is performed whenever possible. Preoperative radiotherapy is of no benefit but postoperative radiotherapy may be given if the surgical excision is incomplete. Infarction of the kidney by renal artery embolization at the time of arteriography can be used to reduce the vascularity of the tumour mass and to facilitate removal of larger tumours. There is no effective chemotherapy for these tumours, although some are believed to be hormonally sensitive.

Because of the unusual features associated with renal carcinomas, a nephrectomy should always be considered. Not only may systemic effects disappear, but there may even be regression of a solitary metastasis. Solitary metastases tend to remain single for long periods of time and excision or radiotherapy is often worthwhile.

Urothelial tumours

The urothelium is the transitional cell lining of the urinary tract that extends from the renal papilla to the external urinary meatus. Approximately 8000 new cases of tumours arise from this source each year in the UK. The incidence of these tumours is increasing, possibly due to environmental carcinogens.

There is a high incidence of urothelial cancer in workers in certain chemical, dyestuff and rubber-moulding industries. This has led to the identification of carcinogens (naphthylamines and benzidine) which are now banned from industrial use. Carcinogens associated with hairdressing and leather work have also been suspected. Smoking and analgesic abuse are associated with a higher incidence of urothelial cancer.

The vast majority of urothelial tumours occur in the bladder.

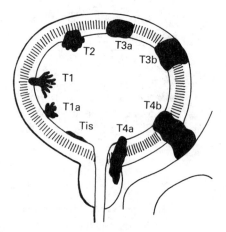

Fig. 39.10 T-categories of bladder tumour. Tis = carcinoma-in-situ

Pathology

Almost all tumours are transitional cell carcinomas. A squamous carcinoma may occur in urothelium that has undergone metaplasia, usually due to chronic inflammation or irritation following a stone or bilharziasis. An adenocarcinoma is a rarity and usually occurs in a urachal remnant in the dome of the bladder.

The appearance of a transitional cell tumour ranges from a delicate papillary structure to a solid ulcerating mass. The appearance correlates well with subsequent behaviour, i.e. papillary tumours are relatively benign while those which ulcerate are mostly malignant.

A *biopsy* is essential for three reasons: (1) to confirm the diagnosis; (2) to determine the degree of cell differentiation (i.e. the *grade*); and (3) to determine the depth to which the tumour has penetrated the bladder wall (i.e. the *stage*).

The TNM system of tumour classification is also applicable to bladder tumours (Fig. 39.10).

Assessment of the *primary tumour* (T) is of prime clinical importance and requires bimanual examination under anaesthesia to judge the degree of penetration through the bladder wall. This is especially important for T2 and T3 tumours (see Fig. 39.10).

Involvement of *regional and juxtaregional lymph nodes* (N) is assessed by both clinical examination and radiography, including lymphography and urography.

Assessment of *distant metastases* (M) requires both clinical examination and radiography.

Histopathological examination allows much more accurate assessment of the tumour and is of great help when deciding the best form of treatment. Biopsy tissue can give accurate information on superficial tumours but invasive tumours cannot be assessed precisely without examining the full thickness of the bladder wall.

Clinical features

More than 80% of patients will have noted haematuria, which is usually painless. It should be assumed that such bleeding is from a tumour until proved otherwise. In women, symptoms of cystitis are so common that occasional bleeding may be thought to be part of an infective problem. In men, symptoms of prostatism are common and may include bleeding.

Bleeding at the end of micturition, and especially if the colour is pink/red, suggests that the site of bleeding is in the bladder; uniformly dark-coloured urine suggests that the source is in the upper tract.

A tumour at the lower end of a ureter or a bladder tumour involving the ureteric orifice may cause obstructive symptoms, but usually there are few other complaints apart from discoloration of the urine. Examination is usually unhelpful. Rectal examination will detect only far-advanced tumours.

Investigation

The urine may contain obvious blood. Cytological examination of the urine is not helpful in the initial assessment but can be used in the follow-up of certain patients, e.g. those exposed to industrial carcinogens. Microbiological testing for mutagens in the urine is a new development.

Because upper tract tumours are much less common than bladder tumours, they may be overlooked in the presence of an obvious bladder tumour. Both may occur together and the whole of the urothelium must be examined on the excretion urogram. If there is any suspicious defect in the ureter, a ureteropyelogram is necessary.

Cystourethroscopy and examination under anaesthesia are the basic investigative procedures for all suspected bladder tumours. With the patient under relaxation anaesthesia, the bladder and tumour are examined bimanually to determine the depth of spread. The physical features of the tumour(s) are noted, the normal bladder mucosa is inspected and biopsies are taken from the tumour and any suspicious area. For some tumours the definitive treatment may then be carried out.

Treatment

Upper tract tumours. The management of these tumours is discussed on page 616.

Superficial bladder tumours. Small superficial tumours (T0 and T1) are treated by endoscopic diathermy or, if larger than 2–3 mm, by transurethral resection. Indeed, most superficial tumours can be treated by transurethral resection and even multiple extensive tumours can be managed in this way. Occasionally a tumour in the upper half of the bladder is best treated by open operation, provided that at least 2 cm of healthy bladder wall can be included (partial cystectomy); in that site transurethral resection is awkward and even unsafe.

Histological examination may show that an apparently superficial tumour has invaded superficial bladder muscle (T2). Provided the resection has been complete and the tumour is well or moderately well differentiated, no further treatment is indicated. If, however, the tumour is poorly differentiated and the exact depth of invasion cannot be determined, treatment should be as for an invasive tumour (see below).

Intravesical chemotherapy (using ethoglucid,

thiotepa or mitomycin) is useful to treat multiple low-grade transitional cell carcinoma and to reduce the recurrence rate of low-grade superficial tumours. The drug is instilled weekly for 3 months and the bladder is then re-examined. If there has been a response, regular treatment is recommended. If there are further new tumours, they will require to be treated by extensive diathermy or even cystectomy.

Carcinoma-in-situ (Tis) may occur either in association with a proliferative tumour, often in an apparently normal mucosa, or as a separate entity, when there may be only a generalized redness (*malignant cystitis*). The behaviour of carcinoma-in-situ is unpredictable and some progress rapidly to invasive bladder cancer. The tumour responds well to intravesical BCG treatment but if there is any doubt about the response, and especially if there is any pathological evidence of progression, more aggressive treatment is needed (see Invasive bladder tumours below).

Invasive bladder tumours. The management of invasive (T3) tumours is much debated. The combination of a short preoperative course of radiotherapy followed by total cystectomy is recommended for younger patients (under 65 years of age). The morbidity and mortality associated with such a radical procedure increases with age and some surgeons believe that a radical course of radiotherapy is a better option. Unfortunately this may not always cure the tumour and a 'salvage' cystectomy may then be needed for tumour recurrence or for symptoms such as intractable bleeding.

A cystectomy always necessitates diversion of the urine. In an ileal conduit (or ureteroileostomy) the ureters are implanted into a short segment of ileum which then opens onto the abdominal wall as an ileostomy (Fig. 39.11). Alternatively, the ureters may be implanted into the sigmoid colon (ureterosigmoidostomy), but complications such as renal infection and metabolic disturbances make this procedure less popular (Fig. 39.12).

An invasive T4 tumour, fixed to the pelvis or surrounding organs, is inoperable and only symptomatic palliative primary treatment can be given.

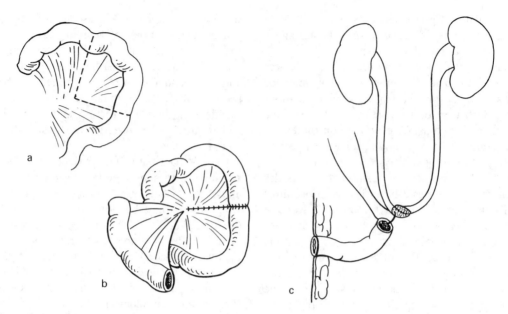

Fig. 39.11   Ileal conduit urinary diversion. (a&b) Isolation of segment of ileum. (c) Uretero-ileal anastomosis

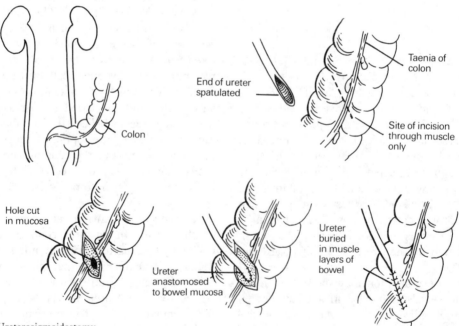

Fig. 39.12   Ureterosigmoidostomy

The place of chemotherapy in combination with any of these treatments is not yet established. Both cisplatin and methotrexate have an effect on transitional cell cancer but the response rates in the treatment of metastatic disease are only modest (about 20%).

The prognosis of bladder tumours depends on the stage and grade of the tumour. The 5-year survival rate varies from 20–30% in those with deep muscle invasion to 50–60% in those with mucosal tumours. Overall the 5-year survival rate is about 35%.

Invasive tumours may sometimes develop in the posterior (prostatic) urethra. These tend to be aggressive in behaviour and require aggressive combination treatment.

Carcinoma of the prostate

In the UK this is the sixth most common malignancy in males, arising in 6000 new patients each year and increasing in frequency. The tumour is common in northern Europe and the US (particularly in negroes) but rare in China and Japan. It rarely occurs before the age of 50 and is uncommon before the age of 60. The mean age at presentation is approximately 70 years. The aetiology is unknown but hormonal and possibly viral factors are implicated.

Pathology

Almost all malignant tumours of the prostate are carcinomas. Microscopically, carcinoma of the prostate is not always easy to diagnose. This is especially true of small foci. If a prostate is examined by serial sections a small malignant focus will be detected in almost all men over the age of 80 years.

Three degrees of biological malignancy can be recognized:

1. *Clinical*: the prostate is believed to be malignant on palpation and this diagnosis is confirmed by histology.

2. *Latent*: the tumour is found incidentally, usually in a prostatectomy specimen.

3. *Occult*: the tumour presents with metastases.

The TNM system is used for classification of carcinoma of the prostate. T0 denotes a latent, incidentally diagnosed tumour, while categories T1–T4 indicate progressive degrees of involvement of the gland. These are shown in Figure 39.13.

Metastatic spread to pelvic lymph nodes occurs early. One-third of clinically localized tumours have in fact spread to regional nodes. Metastases to bone, mainly the lumbar spine and pelvis, are common; more than half of all new cases have such metastases.

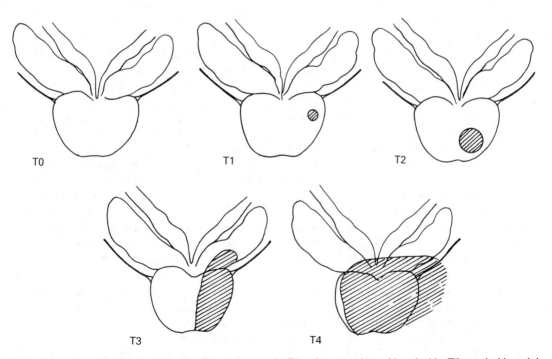

Fig. 39.13 T-categories of prostatic carcinoma. T0 = microscopic; T1 = intracapsular and impalpable; T2 = palpable nodule within gland; T3 = extending beyond capsule; T4 = fixed

Clinical features

The majority of patients present with 'prostatic' symptoms of frequency, urgency and dysuria. One-quarter present with acute retention of urine. Occasionally the tumour extends posteriorly around the rectum and causes an alteration in bowel habit.

Symptoms and signs due to metastases are much less common and include back pain, weight loss, anaemia and obstruction of the lower ends of the ureters.

On rectal examination the prostate feels nodular and stony hard. The diagnosis must never be made on clinical grounds alone; many irregular prostates, even with nodules, are not malignant. Conversely, 10–15% of malignant prostates are not palpably abnormal on rectal examination.

Investigation

Since most patients present with outflow tract obstruction, an intravenous urogram and serum creatinine determination are used to assess the urinary tract. An X-ray of the pelvis or lumbar spine (to investigate backache) may show osteosclerotic metastases as the first evidence of a prostatic malignancy.

Whenever possible, the diagnosis should be confirmed by needle biopsy (either transperineal or transrectal) of a suspicious part of the prostate or by histological examination of tissue removed by endoscopic resection should this be necessary to relieve outflow tract obstruction.

The patient is assessed for distant metastases (M) by measuring the serum acid phosphatase and by a skeletal survey by X-ray or radioisotope bone scan. Serum acid phosphatase is a useful marker of tumour metastases although normal values do not rule out spread of the tumour. Its main use is as a monitor of response to treatment and progress of the disease. A bone scan is more sensitive in detecting metastases than X-rays or acid phosphatase and repeat scans are useful to monitor the progress of the disease.

Lymphography is practised by some but is inaccurate and therefore unnecessary. Staging pelvic lymph node dissection is also unnecessary because the usual treatment recommended in the UK would not be influenced by the information gained.

Treatment

Prostatic cancer, like that of the breast, is sensitive to endocrine influences. In 1941 Charles Huggins, Professor of Urology in the University of Chicago, concluded from a series of experimental studies that since the growth of all types of prostatic cells could be inhibited by oestrogens or castration and stimulated by androgens, the malignant prostate might also respond to endocrine manipulation. This concept led to the first successful treatment of this tumour.

The management is best considered in four clinical groups:

1. *Incidental or focal cancer.* Such patients will have had a prostatectomy, the diagnosis having been made incidentally on histological examination of the prostatic tissue. A patient with a focus of well-differentiated carcinoma who has no evidence of bone metastases has a normal life expectancy. Since these men have no other symptoms and no other evidence of tumour, they need only be watched. If the focus contains undifferentiated cells, treatment by radiotherapy should be considered. Such tumours can recur and progress to a more advanced stage of clinical cancer.

2. *Localized prostatic cancer; no evidence of bone metastases.* Radiotherapy is recommended. Endocrine treatment should be kept in reserve until there is evidence of progression of the tumour. Radical excision of the prostate is practised in some parts of the world but not in the UK.

3. *Metastatic prostatic cancer.* Most patients fall into this category. They should be treated either by androgen depletion (orchidectomy) or by androgen suppression (e.g. stilboestrol 1 mg three times a day). Oestrogens should not be given to patients with cardiovascular disease since salt retention may precipitate further cardiovascular problems, including hypertension and cerebrovascular bleeding. Gonadotropin-releasing hormone analogues are now under trial.

4. *Secondary treatment.* A small proportion of

patients fail to respond to endocrine treatment. A larger number of patients respond for a year or two, but then the disease progresses. Other oestrogens, or progesterones, are of limited value but chemotherapy with 5-fluorouracil, cyclophosphamide or nitrogen mustard may be effective. Radiotherapy will relieve localized bone pain. For severe generalized bone pain, hypophysectomy can be effective palliative treatment.

Prognosis

The life-expectancy of a patient with an incidental finding of focal carcinoma of the prostate is that of the normal population. With tumours localized to the prostate, a 10-year survival rate of 40–50% can be expected but if metastases are present this falls to 10%. Only 50% of patients will survive 3 years. The overall 5-year survival rate of all patients with carcinoma of the prostate is approximately 25%.

Testicular tumours

Tumours of the testis, although uncommon, occur mainly in younger men between the age of 20 and 40 years. In the UK there are about 500 new cases per year. A particular feature of these tumours is that they secrete 'tumour markers' which provide good indices for both diagnosis and prognosis.

The prognosis in the non-seminomatous tumours has been dramatically improved by recent advances in chemotherapy.

Pathology

There are two main tumour types: seminoma and teratoma. Together, these account for 85% of all tumours of the testis. Malignant lymphoma, yolk-sac tumours, interstitial cell tumours and Sertoli cell/mesenchyme tumours make up the remainder.

Seminoma. This tumour arises from seminiferous tubules and is of relatively low grade malignancy. The cut surface has a uniformly grey appearance. Microscopically, the cell type varies from well-differentiated spermatocytes to undifferentiated round cells. Metastases occur mainly via the lymphatics and may spread to the lungs.

Teratoma (non-seminomatous tumours). This tumour arises from primitive germinal cells. The tumour may contain cartilage, bone, muscle, fat and a variety of other tissues and is classified according to the degree of differentiation. Well-differentiated tumours are the least aggressive. A trophoblastic teratoma represents the other extreme and is highly malignant. Most teratomas have an in-between pattern. Occasionally, both teratoma and seminoma occur in the same testis.

Clinical features

The history is often vague. The patient may blame an injury or there may be pain and swelling suggestive of inflammation. In this event the patient may wrongly have received treatment for 'acute epididymitis'. Very rarely, a patient may complain of gynaecomastia (usually associated with a teratoma).

Irrespective of the history, any new painless testicular lump in a young man (20–40 years) must be regarded with suspicion. A hydrocele in a young man demands early exploration. A testicular tumour may be accompanied by a blood-stained effusion in the tunica vaginalis.

The peak age for a teratoma is 20–30 years and for a seminoma 30–40 years. However, either may occur at any time from childhood to old age.

Investigation

As soon as a tumour is suspected, and before orchidectomy, blood should be examined for alphafetoprotein (AFP) and the beta-subunit of human chorionic gonadotropin (HCG). The levels of these classic 'tumour markers' are increased in extensive disease.

Accurate staging of the tumour requires detailed investigations, including lymphography and intravenous urography, CT scans of lungs, liver and retroperitoneal area, and an assessment of renal and pulmonary function.

Tumours are staged according to the following (Royal Marsden Hospital) classification.

I   Lymphogram negative, no evidence of metastases

II Lymphogram positive, metastases confined to abdominal nodes

III Involvement of supra- and infradiaphragmatic lymph nodes, no extralymphatic involvement

IV Extralymphatic involvement

Treatment

Through an inguinal incision the cord is ligated and divided at the internal ring and the testis is removed. Subsequent treatment depends on the histological report. Radiotherapy remains the treatment of choice for a seminoma since this tumour is very radiosensitive.

The management of a teratoma is more debatable because of the wide histological variations. Traditionally radiotherapy was advised but the use of combination chemotherapy (vincristine, actinomycin D, bleomycin plus cisplatin) has greatly improved the prognosis so that the exact place of radiotherapy and also of retroperitoneal lymph node dissection as part of management will have to be re-evaluated.

The tumour markers AFP and beta-HCG are most valuable in monitoring the response to treatment and in detecting recurrent disease. Both markers should be measured at regular intervals in all patients with testicular tumours for at least 2 years after they are considered to be tumour-free.

Computerized tomography, in addition to being useful for staging the tumour, can be used to follow the response of enlarged lymph nodes to treatment.

Prognosis

The 5-year survival rate for seminoma is 90–95%. That for teratomas is more variable and depends on tumour type, stage and volume. With more favourable tumours the 5-year survival rate may be as high as 95% but in more advanced cases 60–70% is more usual.

Carcinoma of the penis

This unusual tumour is generally attributed to poor hygiene associated with a non-retractable foreskin; it is very rare in circumcised men. It occurs only in the elderly.

Pathology

The tumour may be either a papillary or an ulcerating squamous cell carcinoma. Local spread is early and the tumour may ulcerate and fungate. Lymphatic spread to inguinal lymph nodes is common but infection of the tumour may also lead to inguinal node enlargement.

Clinical features

The patient may present with either a purulent or a blood-stained discharge. Unfortunately, many patients do not seek help until the lesion is advanced and ulcerating, and some present only when much of the penis is already destroyed and the inguinal lymph nodes are involved.

Investigation

The diagnosis must be confirmed by biopsy.

Treatment

Early tumours respond dramatically to bleomycin. An initial circumcision is required to keep the tumour area clean and treat any infection. Advanced tumours require partial amputation and bilateral block dissection of the inguinal lymph nodes. Inoperable tumours are treated by palliative radiotherapy.

TRAUMA

Kidney and renal pedicle

Aetiology and pathology

Open injuries. The kidney and renal pedicle may be injured by a gunshot or stab wound. Inadvertent damage during percutaneous needle biopsy of the renal parenchyma can cause severe bleeding and rarely an arteriovenous fistula. Open lacerations of the parenchyma, collecting system or pedicle are usually associated with other injuries within the abdomen.

Closed injuries. These are of two main types.

1. *Direct blunt injury* may be caused by a fall against the edge of the bath (or similar hard object) or by a blow or kick in the loin. These injuries are commonly associated with fractured ribs and, if on the right side, with injury to the liver.

2. *Major renal trauma* may occur as a result of rapid deceleration, as occurs for example in aircraft or road accidents. The pedicle is injured rather than the kidney. Deceleration injuries to the pedicle may cause intimal tears, spasm or thrombosis of the vessels.

The late effects of renal trauma include perirenal collection of urine (urinoma), scarring of the kidney, or renal artery stenosis (hypertension). Hydronephrosis may be an early or late complication.

Clinical features

While a gunshot wound is obvious, a penetrating wound from a knife may appear trivial even if it involves several important deep structures.

Commonly, a child or young person presents with a history of injury (sometimes trivial) to the loin followed by haematuria. Usually, the worse the haematuria, the worse the renal damage. Thus, a bruise or contusion of the kidney causes mild haematuria, a laceration moderate haematuria, while a fragmented kidney causes gross haematuria. A mass in the loin which is increasing in size is characteristic of severe injuries.

In severe injuries there will also be signs of shock (tachycardia, low blood pressure, pallor and sweating). These patients may have injuries to other organs.

Damage to the renal pedicle may cause few signs or the patient may be severely shocked.

Investigation

Urgent excretion urography is indicated to determine the extent of renal damage. A shocked patient must be resuscitated but urographic information about the other kidney must always precede emergency surgery.

With mild contusion the urogram may be normal. With increasing damage there is distortion of the renal outline and calyces and extravasation of contrast. Non-visualization of the kidney implies serious damage, especially to the pedicle, and is an indication for angiography.

Angiography is also helpful in assessing parenchymal/vascular damage in patients in whom surgical exploration is considered likely to be required; it is not necessary in those who need urgent exploration.

A renal scan using technetium-labelled dimercaptosuccinic acid and ultrasound are of more help in the follow-up of an injured kidney than in its immediate care.

Treatment

A contusion of the kidney is managed conservatively by bed rest and observation.

Lacerations which are part of an open injury are explored to determine the overall extent of the damage. Those from a closed injury may be treated conservatively at first, but should be explored if the haematuria persists or the loin swelling increases. Severe lacerations with fragmentation of the kidney must be explored.

The extent of the operation depends on the severity of the laceration. Whenever possible, a partial rather than total nephrectomy should be carried out.

Ureter

Aetiology and pathology

Open injuries. Rarely, a ureter may be damaged by a knife or a bullet. This is always associated with other injuries.

The principal cause of injury to a ureter is inadvertent damage during an operation involving the colon, rectum, bladder, major abdominal blood vessels and, most commonly of all, the uterus. The anatomical relationship of the ureter to these organs makes it inevitable that it is frequently affected by direct spread of a variety of pathological conditions. Surgical damage may lead to complete or partial obstruction with subsequent hydronephrosis, or to a urinary fistula. A fistula may occur either immediately (if damage to continuity is not recognized at operation) or later (if the injury to the ureter is one which causes later necrosis). The urine may leak to the skin (cutaneous fistula), form a 'urinoma' or, after a gynaecological operation, leak through the vagina (ureterovaginal fistula).

Closed injuries. The ureter is occasionally damaged in major accidents, e.g. where the victim is 'run over'.

Clinical features

The patient may complain of renal pain after an operation. However, even a completely obstructed kidney may cause few symptoms. If there is infection in the obstructed kidney, the patient may be extremely ill with pain, fever and rigors.

Any excessive 'watery' discharge from a wound is suspicious. A urinary fistula may cause little or no symptomatic upset but if infection is added the patient may become extremely ill.

Investigation

A rapid way to determine whether a watery discharge is urine or serum is to measure the concentration of urea in the fluid. Alternatively, intravenous methylene blue will quickly appear in a urinary leak. An intravenous urogram will show the side of the damage. Whether the ureter is cut or injured, there is always some hold-up in the contrast on the affected side. This differs from the urogram in a patient with a *vesicovaginal* fistula, where the upper tract is usually normal.

If there is still uncertainty as to whether a vaginal leak is from the ureter or bladder, discoloration of a vaginal swab after intravesical instillation of methylene blue will confirm that the leak is from the bladder.

Occasionally, cystoscopy and ureteric catheterization are indicated.

Treatment

Early exploration of the wound is advised to avoid the risks of infection. Provided it is of sufficient length, a damaged lower ureter can be reimplanted directly into the bladder. If the ureter is short, then the gap may be bridged by a tube of bladder (Boari flap) (Fig. 39.14) or simply by drawing up the bladder and fixing it to the psoas muscle (psoas hitch).

If the ureter is too short for these procedures, it may be joined to the other ureter (ureteroureterostomy). However, if there is infection, or the patient has a poor prognosis because of the underlying disease, it may be best to remove the kidney or embolize the renal artery.

Bladder

Aetiology and pathology

Open injuries. The bladder may rupture as a result of a penetrating injury to the lower abdomen. In this case the bladder, urethra and

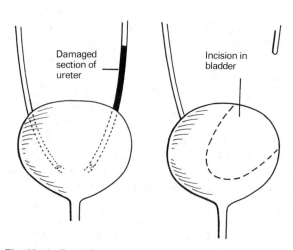
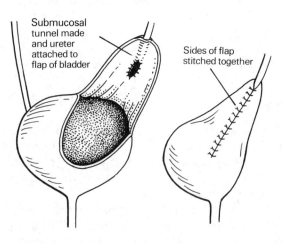

Fig. 39.14   Boari flap

rectum are all likely to be damaged. The bladder may also be injured in the course of extensive cancer operations in the pelvis. Occasionally, a large inguinal or femoral hernia may include bladder in the medial wall of the sac, and this may be damaged during repair of the hernia. Unrecognized damage during surgical procedures may lead to a wound fistula, a vesicovaginal fistula or a vesicocolic fistula.

Fistulas may also occur as a result of inflammatory or neoplastic bowel disease.

Closed injuries. Two types of closed bladder injury may occur. Two different mechanisms are involved.

1. *Intraperitoneal.* Typically, the patient has been drinking alcohol, has a full bladder and is assaulted and kicked in the abdomen. The dome of the bladder ruptures and urine extravasates into the peritoneum (Fig. 39.15a), causing intestinal ileus and abdominal distension.

2. *Extraperitoneal.* Extraperitoneal rupture is usually due to a major road traffic accident in which the pelvis has also been fractured (Fig. 39.15b).

An extraperitoneal leak in the bladder may also occur in the course of resecting the prostate or a bladder tumour. The extravasated urine then causes a local inflammatory reaction so that the small bowel may become adherent to the pelvic peritoneum. This is dangerous should the patient later require pelvic irradiation.

Clinical features

The ileus and distension that occur with intraperitoneal rupture of the bladder are often detected late because of the circumstances surrounding the injury. However, the patient will soon note that he is anuric and seek advice.

Extraperitoneal extravasation of urine, if part of a major accident, will only add to what already are severe pelvic symptoms. When the leak occurs during an endoscopic procedure, the patient will later complain of suprapubic pain with varying degrees of lower abdominal tenderness.

Investigation

Generally, the circumstances of the bladder injury will establish the diagnosis. If confirmation of a bladder injury is required, a water-soluble contrast material is injected via a urethral catheter and the bladder examined on the X-ray screen.

Treatment

Intraperitoneal rupture of the bladder demands laparotomy. The bladder rupture is oversewn, the abdominal viscera are examined for other injuries and drainage by a urethral catheter is established. An extraperitoneal rupture of the bladder requires surgical exploration to remove blood and serum, to correct bony injuries, to close the tear in the bladder and to establish bladder drainage.

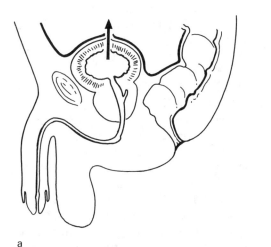
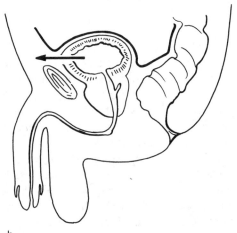

a   b

Fig. 39.15 Rupture of the bladder. (a) Intraperitoneal. (b) Extraperitoneal

If urine has extravasated during any pelvic operation, a urethral catheter to keep the bladder empty is usually all that is needed. Very rarely a suprapubic drain may be required.

Urethra

Aetiology and pathology

Open injuries. Penetrating injuries resulting in damage to the anterior or posterior urethra are rare.

Closed injuries

Anterior urethra. Damage to this part of the urethra is typically due to falling astride a hard object, although a well-aimed boot can cause a similar injury. This may be either a contusion or a laceration. A laceration may be partial or complete.

Posterior urethra. The mechanism of injury to this part of the urethra is similar to that causing extraperitoneal rupture of the bladder, e.g. a road traffic accident. For such an injury to damage the urethra, a fracture of the pubis or fracture-dislocation of the pelvis must occur. Both posterior urethra and bladder are damaged in 10% of cases. The urethral rupture may be partial or complete.

An injury to the posterior urethra may also be iatrogenic. Inexpert instrumentation of the urethra can tear the mucosa and cause a false passage and subsequent stricture formation.

Clinical features

Anterior urethral injuries are usually located at the bulb of the urethra so that the patient presents with a haematoma of the perineum. Should this haematoma become infected, there may be sloughing of the skin, urethra and even scrotal tissues.

Because of the mechanism of injury, patients with posterior urethral tears are usually shocked and require resuscitation before a detailed assessment of the pelvic injuries can be made. If the patient has passed clear urine, the bladder and urethra are probably intact. If there is blood at the external meatus a urethral injury must be suspected. A distended bladder can occur either

because of spasm of the urethral sphincter or because of a torn posterior urethra.

Investigation

If the physical signs suggest an anterior urethral injury and the patient has passed clear urine, no further steps need be taken. If there is blood at the external meatus or the urine is blood-stained, a urethrogram using a water-soluble contrast material may demonstrate the extravasation.

There is a strongly held view that any investigative procedure of the posterior urethra is dangerous and may worsen the urethral injury. A catheter should never be passed in the emergency room 'just to see'.

If the patient passes clear urine, then nothing further should be done. If, however, the urine is blood-stained, retrograde urethrography may be carried out. The radiological distinction between an extraperitoneal bladder rupture and a rupture of the membranous urethra may be difficult. Catheterization for these injuries is best carried out at the time of other surgical procedures with full aseptic precautions.

Treatment

Any patient with an injury to the bulb of the urethra will have a perineal haematoma. This will resolve if the urethral injury is only a contusion. As there is always the risk of infection, prophylactic antibiotics are indicated.

A large haematoma may need to be drained. If this is necessary, the urethra is likely to be lacerated. The extent of injury should be defined and the urethra repaired if possible. The bladder is drained either by a urethral or by suprapubic catheter.

The treatment of a posterior urethral injury depends on the expertise available. It is quite acceptable to perform a suprapubic cystostomy and deal with the injury to the urethra at a later date. If, however, a laparotomy is necessary for other reasons, this may also give an opportunity to pass a catheter. If the rupture is incomplete, the catheter will act as a splint. If the rupture is complete, the ends of the urethra can be approximated and splinted by the catheter.

The late complication of these injuries is stricture.

EXTERNAL GENITALIA

Penis

Circumcision

The foreskin is normally non-retractile in the first few months of life. By the end of the first year, 50% will retract; but it may be 3–4 years before all will do so. Provided that the parents are reassured of these facts, there is no reason, *apart from religious grounds*, to remove the foreskin within the first few years of life.

In some children the foreskin remains non-retractile beyond this age and this should be treated by division of preputial adhesions or by circumcision. Otherwise, secretions may collect under the foreskin, leading to infection (balanitis) and narrowing of the orifice (phimosis). In those whose foreskin can retract, but not easily, pain during intercourse may be a problem in later years. If there are difficulties in keeping the glans and coronal sulcus clean, accumulated secretions may predispose to carcinoma of the penis.

Urologists are familiar with the problem of a non-retractile foreskin in patients who later need a cystoscopy or urethral catheterization.

If a poorly retracting foreskin remains retracted, it can act as a tight band and cause engorgement and oedema of the glans (paraphimosis). This demands urgent treatment. It may be possible to compress the glans and draw the foreskin forwards, but, if this fails, the tight band must be incised under general anaesthesia. Later elective circumcision is advocated.

Congenital abnormalities

Hypospadias. Failure of fusion of embryonic folds results in abnormal placing of the external urinary meatus along the ventral surface of the penis. The opening may be coronal, penile, scrotal or even perineal. With these latter sites the corpus spongiosum is scarred and fibrosed, leading to a ventral curvature or *chordee* of the penis.

The aim of treatment is to correct the chordee by excising the fibrosis and then to perform one of several available plastic surgical techniques to make a new urethral opening in the normal position on the glans. These procedures should be completed before the boy goes to school.

Epispadias. In this condition, the external urinary meatus opens on the dorsal surface of the penis. The extent of the malformation varies from a penile abnormality to a gross failure in development of the bladder and urethra. Severe deformity is due to extension of the cloacal membrane onto the lower abdominal wall preventing the two halves of the wall from closing over the developing bladder. As a result, the mucosa of the whole bladder and the ureteric orifices are exposed and form the infraumbilical part of the abdominal wall (exstrophy). The urethra lies opened out and the testes are undescended; additional abnormalities include separation of the symphysis pubis and rectal prolapse.

Reconstruction of these deformities is not always successful and urinary incontinence may remain a major problem and require treatment by urinary diversion.

Disorders of erection

Priapism. In this uncommon condition there is a maintained erection, unassociated with sexual desire. It occurs in association with leukaemia, disorders of coagulation, renal dialysis and sickle-cell trait and is believed to be due to sludging of venous blood in the sinuses of the corpora cavernosa. Thus the painful erection affects the corpora cavernosa but not the corpus spongiosum or glans.

A variety of non-operative methods to relieve the congestion, e.g. spinal anaesthesia or heparinization, have been tried but without success. Aspiration of the thickened blood is also ineffective.

Operative treatment by insertion of a venous shunt (e.g. saphenous vein to corpus cavernosum or corpora cavernosa to corpus spongiosum), when carried out within 6–12 hours, gives satisfactory results and the patient can achieve normal erections subsequently.

If treatment is delayed or incomplete, the erectile tissue is damaged and the patient will be impotent.

Peyronie's disease. This is the occurrence of a

hard fibrous plaque (or plaques) in the wall of a corpus cavernosum causing a lateral curvature of the penis. The cause is obscure but is possibly related to trauma leading to the formation of hard scar tissue in a corpus cavernosum. In addition to the deformity, the patient complains of pain during intercourse.

Various treatments including cortisone injections, vitamins and radiotherapy have been tried for this condition, but without much success. Excision of the plaque with replacement by a dermal patch graft, or excision of a wedge of tissue on the convex (opposite) border of the penis may prove effective. It is suggested that the condition will eventually improve without treatment but reliable data are scarce.

Impotence

Impotence may be psychogenic, organic or drug-induced. Although *loss of libido* may be due to a generalized illness or endocrine disease, the majority of patients who complain of *impotence* have a psychosexual disturbance which may require psychosexual therapy.

Psychogenic causes can be established from a careful history that includes details of sexual habits. However, it is always important to exclude organic causes so that the correct advice may be given to the patient.

Organic impotence may occur with diabetes mellitus or neurogenic disorders, after major pelvic injury or operations (e.g. total cystectomy), or with vascular disease of the pelvic vessels (e.g. Leriche syndrome), priapism and Peyronie's disease. Most of these conditions cause irreversible impotence, but angiography may help to define a treatable abnormality of the arterial supply to the penis.

There is no drug treatment, and the only treatment in selected cases is to implant a pair of silicone rods into the corpora cavernosa to allow successful intercourse.

Drug-induced impotence occurs in patients receiving oestrogen treatment for prostatic cancer. In addition, a range of antihypertensive drugs may cause loss of erection or inability to ejaculate. Drugs such as barbiturates, benzodiazepams, corticosteroids, phenothiazines and spironolactone may all affect libido.

Scrotum

Examination of the scrotal contents should follow a simple routine. With the patient supine, the configuration of the scrotum and the scrotal wall is first observed. The contents of the scrotum are then palpated between the thumb and index and middle fingers. In sequence the testes, head, body and tail of the epididymis, the cord and the external inguinal ring are checked. With the patient standing and the doctor seated, examination of the contents is repeated, specifically excluding an inguinal hernia and a varicocele (see below).

Undescended testes (cryptorchidism)

Normally both testes should be in the scrotum within 6 months of birth. However, the testes may be excessively mobile and readily retract towards the external inguinal ring or into the inguinal canal, especially when the patient is examined in a cold room. Such *retractile* testes may easily be misdiagnosed as being incompletely descended. Care must be taken to examine the baby in a warm room or after a bath.

Undescended testes are of two types: incompletely descended and ectopic.

Incomplete descent of the testis. Such a testis is arrested in its normal pathway to the scrotum. Usually this is within the inguinal canal, more rarely within the abdomen. The testis is smaller than normal and cannot be palpated. Its ability to produce sperm is doubtful.

As the spermatic cord is short, such testes are difficult to bring down into the scrotum by operation (orchiopexy). If this can be carried out before the age of 6 years, the testis may be of some use; otherwise it should be removed.

Occasionally, an incompletely descended testis is situated just inside the external inguinal ring through which it can be coaxed (*emergent testis*). If the child is approaching puberty when this diagnosis is made, a 5-day course of human chorionic gonadotropin may encourage enlargement and descent.

Testes that remain incompletely descended have a 1 in 40 chance of becoming malignant; the risk is doubled if the testis is retained in the abdomen.

Ectopic testis. It is important to distinguish an ectopic from an incompletely descended testis. An ectopic testis has developed normally but after passing through the external inguinal ring its further descent is impeded. It either remains in the superficial inguinal pouch (common) or is transposed to perineal, femoral or prepubic sites (rare).

Because an ectopic testis is normal in size, it is palpable and its cord is normal. Operative placement in the scrotum (*orchiopexy*) is achieved without difficulty. Provided this is done at an early age, preferably before the age of 6 years, spermatogenesis is believed to occur normally.

However, even if the diagnosis is not made until later (frequently this is just before puberty), orchidopexy should still be performed. The use of gonadotropins to treat ectopic testes is illogical.

The operation of orchiopexy consists of mobilizing the testis and its cord and placing the testis in the scrotum. Various methods are used to stop the testis from retracting back towards the inguinal canal. The simplest is to place the testis in a pouch between the dartos muscle and scrotal skin (Fig. 39.16).

As indicated above, mobilization of an ectopic testis and placement in a dartos pouch is easy. Because of the shorter cord, an incompletely descended testis can be brought into the scrotum only with difficulty and various manoeuvres may be necessary to gain length.

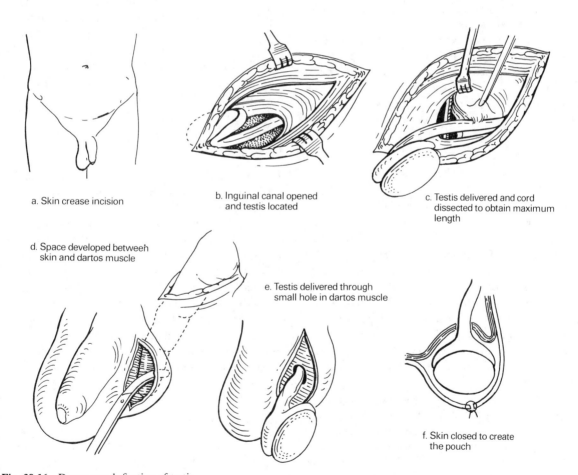

a. Skin crease incision

b. Inguinal canal opened and testis located

c. Testis delivered and cord dissected to obtain maximum length

d. Space developed between skin and dartos muscle

e. Testis delivered through small hole in dartos muscle

f. Skin closed to create the pouch

Fig. 39.16 Dartos pouch fixation of testis

Torsion of the testis

Torsion of the testis is due to an abnormality of the visceral layer of the tunica vaginalis which completely covers the testis so that it is suspended within the parietal layer and can twist the cord. Torsion is a surgical emergency. Delay in diagnosis or treatment may lead to loss of the testis.

Characteristically the patient, usually a teenager, presents with an acutely tender, swollen testis of sudden onset. There may be a history of minor trauma or of previous episodes of pain in the testis due to partial torsion. On examination there is a red, swollen hemiscrotum which is usually too tender to palpate. Misdiagnosis of the swelling as an epididymo-orchitis, which is rare in teenagers, is a serious error.

The scrotum must be explored as soon as possible so that the twist can be reversed and the blood supply restored. If this is not done within 12–18 hours, the testis infarcts and must be excised. If the testis is viable, it is fixed, e.g. by creating a dartos pouch. Since the underlying abnormality of the tunica is bilateral, the other testis must be fixed to its parietal tunica vaginalis *at the same time*. Otherwise, torsion may occur later on that side. This could be disastrous for the fertility of the patient.

Hydrocele

This is a common condition, especially in older men, in which fluid collects in the tunica vaginalis, resulting in an enlarged but painless scrotum. The inconvenience of its size usually leads the patient to seek advice.

The cause of most hydroceles is unknown (idiopathic). The fluid is straw-coloured and rich in protein. In some patients it develops as a reaction to epididymo-orchitis. Rarely, and this is more sinister, it may develop with a malignant testis (secondary hydrocele). The fluid may then be blood-stained.

On examination of the scrotum there is a smooth oval swelling above which a normal spermatic cord can be palpated. The fluid around the testis transilluminates when a torch is held against the scrotum, but in long-standing hydroceles this may be difficult to elicit owing to fibrosis and thickening of its wall. It is important always to seek this physical sign and also to examine the neck of the scrotum carefully to exclude an inguinal hernia as the cause of the swelling.

It may be possible to palpate the testis and confirm that it is normal, but this is unusual as it lies behind and is enveloped by the hydrocele. If there is doubt about an associated pathology, the fluid should be aspirated by needle and syringe and the testis re-examined. If there is still doubt, immediate exploration is indicated to exclude a testicular tumour.

Injury to the scrotum may result in a swelling that resembles a hydrocele but does not transilluminate because the tunica has filled with blood (*haematocele*).

Aspiration alone does not cure an idiopathic hydrocele and the tunica soon refills with fluid. It is possible to obliterate the sac by injecting a sclerosant after aspiration, but preferably it should be excised or everted so that recurrence is prevented.

If the hydrocele fluid becomes infected, incision and drainage of the pus are necessary. Similarly, a haematocele may require treatment by incision and drainage.

Varicocele

The veins of the pampiniform plexus are dilated and tortuous, producing a swelling in the line of the spermatic cord which assembles a 'bag of worms'. It is more common on the left side because of the right-angled drainage of the testicular vein into the renal vein, which renders it more liable to stasis. In some men, varicocele is associated with infertility. A dragging sensation in the scrotum may cause concern.

Treatment by scrotal support is no longer advised. The spermatic vein can be ligated at the internal inguinal ring or embolized through a venous cannula inserted by femoral or jugular routes.

Cyst of the epididymis

Cysts in the epididymis arise from diverticula of the vasa efferentia. The distinction between a cyst of the epididymis and a hydrocele is easy. Epididymal cysts are almost always multiple and therefore nodular on palpation; they are located above and behind the testis, which is palpably separate from the cysts, and always transilluminate brightly.

A solitary epididymal cyst may even resemble a testis, so giving rise to fables of three testes.

Sometimes the fluid within an epididymal cyst is opalescent and contains sperms (it is then called a *spermatocele*). Usually the fluid is clear.

It is best to leave these cysts alone unless increasing size warrants excision. This operation requires careful dissection to remove the cyst completely. Often several other little cysts are present which, if not removed, will eventually increase in size and produce a so-called recurrence. If all the cysts are removed, the pathway for sperms will almost certainly be damaged. A bilateral operation could result in sterility.

Epididymo-orchitis

Acute epididymo-orchitis is the preferred term to describe either acute orchitis or acute epididymitis, for both testis and epididymis are involved in the acute inflammatory reaction. Further, the spermatic cord is often thickened (funiculitis). After the infection has subsided, the epididymis alone may remain thickened and irregular, so that chronic epididymitis may be diagnosed. Thus a late effect of tuberculosis is an irregularly hard (craggy) epididymis.

Apparent involvement of the testis alone may be a feature of viral infections such as mumps orchitis. Late syphilis results in a gumma of the testis, but this is now seen only in museum specimens.

The usual cause of epididymo-orchitis is bacterial spread, either from infected urine or from gonococcal urethritis. The affected side of the scrotum is swollen, inflamed and very tender. In all cases the urine or urethral discharge must be cultured. Sometimes there is no evidence of a bacterial cause and a viral aetiology is then likely.

Treatment consists of antibiotics, bed rest and a scrotal support. The choice of antibiotic depends on the results of culture and sensitivity determination of the organism responsible. If there is any doubt about the diagnosis, the testis should be explored.

Abscess formation is now rare, but if signs of localization or fluctuation develop, the pus should be drained. An important late complication of epididymo-orchitis is infertility.

Infertility

The investigation and management of infertily requires the assessment of both partners, but only aspects of male infertility will be discussed here. While more patients are now being referred for investigation, the management of infertility is still very limited in its success. Often it consists only of clarifying the diagnosis and appropriate counselling.

A detailed history is essential, particularly with regard to factors that may contribute to an abnormal sperm count. These include previous operations (e.g. for hernia), illnesses such as mumps and tuberculosis, bacterial infections, (e.g. gonococcal), and certain drugs (nitrofurazone, cyclophosphamides and possibly some tranquillisers). Excessive smoking, alcohol intake, obesity and working in a hot environment may all suppress spermatogenesis. The patient should also be asked about any psychosexual problems, including impotence or premature ejaculation.

Physical examination may be entirely normal. Body build and hair distribution are noted. Testicular size is a crude but useful guide to spermatogenic potential. For example, a tall male with female hair distribution and pea-sized testes almost certainly has Klinefelter's syndrome. Examination of the scrotum may reveal dilated spermatic veins (varicocele).

The principal investigation in the male is analysis of the seminal fluid. The values given as 'normal' are only a guide, for undoubtedly pregnancy can occur with low sperm concentrations (oligozoospermia). However, the lower the concentration of sperms, the less the chance of pregnancy.

If a patient has no sperm (azoospermia), it is necessary to distinguish between obstruction and primary spermatogenic failure. This may be possible by measuring plasma gonadotropins (FSH). A normal value indicates obstruction which is usually in the epididymis. In these patients the testes are also normal in size. More detailed tests such as immunological compatibility and chromosome analysis may be necessary but these require special facilities.

Management

There is no treatment for a patient with azoospermia due to primary spermatogenic failure. A testicular biopsy to confirm the diagnosis is all that can be done.

Azoospermia due to obstruction may be treated by a bypass anastomosis (epididymovasostomy). This may be successful if the obstruction is in the tail of the epididymis, but if it is elsewhere in the epididymis or in the vasa efferentia, the results are very poor.

Patients with oligozoospermia are initially advised to reduce their weight, improve dietary and smoking habits, and (if possible) adjust their occupation or working environment. It is always helpful to ensure that the patient has an understanding of the basis of reproductive biology and especially the timing of intercourse in relation to the menstrual cycle. These measures alone often lead to a successful pregnancy.

The role of a varicocele as a cause of infertility is debatable. There is evidence that some varicoceles affect testicular temperature, and therefore spermatogenesis, and ligation of these veins is widely practised to avoid this effect. Most series have shown overall improvement in semen analysis following the ligation, but none of these studies are controlled.

Drug treatment for oligozoospermia is disappointing; clinical trials are in progress but no one treatment can at present be recommended. As a result various worthless drugs continue to be prescribed.

Vasectomy and vasectomy reversal

Bilateral ligation of the vasa deferentia, in the neck of the scrotum, is now widely practised as a form of permanent contraception. This is usually done as an outpatient procedure under local anaesthesia. Each vas is divided and ligated, and the ends are separated in order to avoid recanalization.

It is essential to repeat the semen analysis 6–8 weeks postoperatively to confirm azoospermia. Three negative tests are required for assurance that fertilization cannot occur.

Reversal of a vasectomy may be requested, usually because of remarriage. Reported pregnancy rates vary from 50% to 80% following this microsurgical technique.

DISORDERS OF CONTROL OF MICTURITION

Anatomy of the outflow tract

The *fundus* of the bladder consists of interlacing bundles of smooth muscle, the detrusor, which do not lie in defined layers. They are attached to the deep muscle layer of the trigone. During the storage phase of micturition the detrusor stretches to accommodate the increased volume of urine but without an increase in intravesical pressure (compliance).

The *trigone* forms the base of the bladder and includes both ureteric orifices and the internal urethral orifice. It has two muscle layers: (1) the superficial trigonal muscle which merges with the ureteric muscle and extends down into the proximal urethra and (2) the deep trigonal muscle to which is attached the detrusor muscle.

The *proximal urethral sphincter mechanism* (internal meatus) in the male consists of specially adapted fibres of detrusor muscle, arranged in a circular fashion in the region of the bladder neck, together with the proximal urethral extension of superficial trigonal smooth muscle. The detrusor muscle fibres at the bladder neck form the pre-prostatic sphincter which is richly supplied with sympathetic nerves and closes tightly with ejaculation.

The *distal urethral sphincter mechanism* (external sphincter) consists of intrinsic urethral (striated) muscle which surrounds the urethra distal to the verumontanum and forms the external urethral sphincter. This mechanism is innervated from the sacral cord segments S2–4 by motor fibres which reach the sphincter by the pelvic plexus, unlike the periurethral striated muscle of the pelvic floor and rectum which are innervated by the pudendal nerves.

In the female the external urethral sphincter extends over the whole length of the urethra but is most prominent in the middle third of the urethra, which it surrounds.

Neurological control of micturition

The *parasympathetic* fibres arise from S2, 3 and 4 as preganglionic axons, relay through the pelvic ganglia and, as postganglionic nerves, supply the detrusor muscle. These (cholinergic) nerves stimulate detrusor contraction.

The *sympathetic* fibres arise from T11–L1 and relay in the pelvic ganglia. The exact role of the sympathetic nerves in the control of micturition has not been fully clarified. It is, however, known that alpha-adrenergic receptors at their nerve terminals are found mainly in the smooth muscle of the bladder neck and proximal urethra, whereas beta-receptors are in the fundus of the bladder. The alpha-receptors respond to noradrenaline by stimulating contraction, while the beta-receptors relax the smooth muscle. It is possible that the sympathetic neurones play a role in both urethral closure and detrusor relaxation during the filling phase of the micturition cycle.

The somatic motor innervation of the (striated) external urethral sphincter and pelvic floor is derived from the same cord segments (S2–4) but by different neural pathways to those already outlined. Afferent nerves are carried in both the parasympathetic and pudendal pathways and transmit sensory impulses from the bladder, urethra and pelvic floor. These sensory impulses not only pass to the cerebral cortex and the micturition centre but also to the cord as part of the spinal cord reflexes. Thus bladder filling stimulates afferent impulses which then stimulate pelvic floor contraction, so adding to urethral compression.

Cortical control is a basic part of the micturition cycle described below. The higher centres suppress detrusor contractions and their main function is to inhibit micturition until such times that it is appropriate to micturate. Afferent impulses pass to the brain via the posterior columns and lateral spinothalamic tracts. Thus bladder sensation is transmitted bilaterally and is lost only when both tracts are divided. The higher centres are situated in the pons, anteromedial aspect of the frontal lobe, the cingulate gyrus and the paracentral lobule.

The micturition cycle

The series of events that occur continuously within the bladder are known as the micturition cycle, which has three phases.

1. *Storage (or filling) phase.* Because of the high compliance of the detrusor muscle the bladder fills steadily without either bladder sensation or change in intravesical pressure. Eventually the volume is sufficient to induce the desire to void, which marks the end of this phase.

2. *Postponement (or inhibitory) phase.* Voluntary control is now exerted over the desire to void, which then disappears temporarily. Compliance of the detrusor allows a further increase in capacity until the next desire to void. Just how often this desire need be inhibited depends on many factors, not the least of which is finding a suitable place in which to void.

3. *Emptying (or micturition) phase.* The act of micturition is initiated first by voluntary and then by reflex relaxation of the pelvic floor, followed by reflex detrusor contraction. Intravesical pressure remains greater than urethral pressure until the bladder is empty.

The normal control of micturition requires coordinated reflex activity of autonomic and somatic nerves, as described above. These responses depend on normal anatomical structures and normal innervation. There are thus two main types of disorders of micturition: (1) structural and (2) neurogenic. Examples are extensive carcinoma of the prostate that has damaged the sphincter mechanism (structural) and a spinal cord injury that has damaged the innervation (neurogenic).

Structural disorders

Investigation

Abnormalities of function of the lower urinary tract are notoriously difficult to assess because of the frequently dual underlying pathology. For example, incontinence in an elderly man may be due to cortical deficiency resulting from cerebral degeneration but could also be due to chronic outflow tract obstruction resulting from prostatic hypertrophy.

The history is important but may be deceptive, mainly because different abnormalities can produce similar symptoms. The exact character of the urinary abnormality must be determined so that, if possible, structural causes can be separated from neurological causes. Details of drug treatment are noted. Diuretics and drugs with anticholinergic side effects may tip the balance when there is already dysfunction. Urine is tested for glycosuria and infection.

In addition to intravenous urography there are now a range of more specific methods for assessing micturition but not all are required for a diagnosis. Their value lies in resolving specific clinical questions relating to management. These methods include radiology (cystourethrography), urodynamic studies (uroflowmetry, cystometrography and urethral pressure measurement) and direct inspection (cystourethroscopy and pelvic examination under anaesthesia).

In summary, a full clinical history and physical examination, with cystourethroscopy and bimanual examination of the pelvic contents, remain the basic initial methods for investigation of structural disorders.

Structural causes of incontinence in the male

Operation. Removal of the prostate gland is a common cause of disorders of control of micturition in males. In this operation the internal urethral mechanism is deliberately excised posteriorly but the distal mechanism is left strictly alone; any damage to this sphincter will affect continence. Episodes of incontinence commonly follow removal of the urethral catheter but usually stop within several days. More persistent incontinence can be classified as follows.

Dribbling incontinence. This is an uncommon complication which is due to structural damage to the external urethral mechanism. Recovery is unlikely. It may be treated either by an appliance or by an operative procedure (with or without an artificial sphincter) that narrows the urethra.

Stress incontinence. This occurs with any sudden increase in abdominal pressure, as with coughing. Since the damage to the sphincter is mild, it usually responds to physiotherapy.

Urge incontinence. This is not due to sphincter weakness but to involuntary bladder contractions in an uninhibited or unstable bladder. Removal of the prostatic obstruction alone is usually sufficient to correct the symptoms of urgency and urge incontinence, but antispasmodic drug treatment may be necessary.

Bed-wetting that occurs after prostatectomy may be due to urge incontinence or poor tone in the pelvic floor, or to both. Physiotherapy and drug treatment may help.

Other operative procedures on the urethra, such as repeated dilatations for urethral stricture or urethroplasty, may be followed by incontinence as classified above.

Disease. *Carcinoma of the prostate* may grow locally to involve adjacent urethral structures. Repeated transurethral resections for recurring obstruction may be necessary. The net effect of these is to change the posterior urethra into a rigid tube so that dribbling incontinence occurs, i.e. leakage of urine during the storage phase. An indwelling catheter or condom incontinence appliance may be necessary.

Benign prostatic enlargement may induce urgency of micturition alone or with other obstructive symptoms. An early sign of benign enlargement, a 'post-micturition dribble', is probably due to a small amount of urine that is trapped between the proximal and distal mechanisms. A similar complaint may occur with prostatitis and early outflow changes of bilharziasis. (The development of chronic retention with overflow or dribbling incontinence is referred to on page 605.)

Chronic illness and debility, especially in an elderly patient, may lead to incontinence because of poor tone in the periurethral striated muscle of the pelvic floor; this may be worsened by some loss of the cortical inhibition of micturition.

Structural causes of incontinence in the female

Incontinence of urine is more prevalent than generally suspected. As many as 50% of nulliparous young women may have some degree of stress incontinence and in approximately 20% this may be a daily occurrence. Overall, approximately

10% of women aged 15–64 years are incontinent twice or more per month. This figure rises rapidly in older patients and in geriatric units. Only a fraction of the younger women seek advice, either because of embarrassment or because of stoical acceptance of some incontinence as a normal event.

Childbirth and operations. Multiparous women commonly lose some of the tone in the muscles of the pelvic floor with each pregnancy. Symptoms may range from occasional stress incontinence to dribbling incontinence. Examination shows weakening of the pelvic floor muscles and anterior vaginal wall (cystocele). It is important to distinguish stress incontinence from urge incontinence, for the former responds to surgical procedures designed to support the bladder neck and strengthen the anterior vaginal wall, while the latter should be treated by drug therapy. Stress incontinence is characterized by an involuntary loss of urine during coughing, laughing, sneezing or any other activity that raises the intra-abdominal pressure suddenly. A cough, however, may stimulate involuntary detrusor contractions, which cause motor urge incontinence. This differential diagnosis can be made only by urodynamic assessment. Urge incontinence may thus be motor, due to unstable detrusor contractions, or sensory, in which infection or stones produce excessive sensory stimulation.

In parts of the world where obstetric services are poor, prolonged labour may lead to a *vesicovaginal fistula*, which presents as continuous dribbling incontinence. The association with delivery is usually clear, but a small fistula may be missed. Investigation of dribbling incontinence must distinguish between urethral damage and a fistula. Treatment of a fistula consists of closing the fistula either through the vagina or through a suprapubic approach.

Hysterectomy may also be followed by urinary incontinence, suggesting damage to the ureter(s) at the time of operation. Again, the association of an operation with incontinence should indicate a diagnosis of *ureterovaginal fistula*. Investigations are directed to establishing which ureter has been damaged. Treatment consists of reimplanting the ureter into the bladder.

Disease. Cystitis is a common condition in women which, in addition to the symptoms of frequency, urgency and dysuria, sometimes causes sensory urge incontinence. Treatment of both the infection and bladder spasm is required.

Chronic interstitial cystitis (Hunner's ulcer) is a chronic inflammatory condition which, in addition to causing frequency and dysuria, may also cause urgency and urge incontinence. Treatment is often unsatisfactory. Hydrostatic dilatation may be effective or the patient may respond to treatment with steroids.

The *urethral syndrome* is characterized by symptoms of cystitis but there is no infection. There may be some incontinence. These patients often have a degree of urethral stenosis and treatment by urethral dilatation or incision may be successful. However, the urethral syndrome usually responds to treatment by regulating micturition habits and by careful perineal hygiene.

Dribbling incontinence in a child should raise the suspicion of an *ectopic ureter* in which the lower of the two ureters from a kidney opens outside the control of the urethral mechanism. The abnormal ureter must be relocated in the bladder.

Carcinoma of the cervix or its treatment by radiotherapy may cause vesicovaginal fistula and hence incontinence.

Neurogenic disorders

Investigation

As with the investigation of structural disorders a full history, including an interview with relatives, is required. Examination must include the plantar reflexes and the sensation and tone of the anal canal. Once again, glycosuria and urinary infection should be sought.

Urodynamic, radiological and electromyographic studies may all be required to determine the appropriate management.

Aetiology of abnormal micturition

Impaired cortical control. Diseases affecting the frontal lobe can alter the pattern of micturition by increasing or decreasing the frequency or affecting the social awareness of incontinence. Lesions such as cerebral thrombosis or cerebral degeneration may produce incontinence by failing to inhibit the postponement phase of micturition. The paracentral lobule controls the activity of skeletal muscle, so that lesions in this area may cause sustained pelvic and perineal muscular contraction. It must be remembered that a disorder of micturition may be accentuated by or even be due to the physical inability to prepare for micturition.

Emotional states may affect the postponement of micturition, giving rise to 'giggle' incontinence and possibly to enuresis in some patients. Incontinence with epilepsy is also due to a loss of inhibitory control. Hysteria can lead to acute retention in women. Excessive *sensory stimuli*, as with the pain of cystourethritis in women, may cause 'sensory urge incontinence'.

Drugs, including alcohol, may alter the cortical control of micturition. Sedatives can affect the postponement phase and precipitate incontinence, especially at night. The intoxicated patient may lack the mental alertness to maintain continence or may continually suppress the desire to void, leading to prostatic congestion and retention.

Damage to the spinal cord. Two aspects of disease or injury to the spinal cord will influence the nature and prognosis of disordered micturition: the level of the disease and the completeness or incompleteness of the damage.

Injury at or below the spinal reflex centre (S2, 3, 4). The injury may be a fracture of the spine at the level of T12 and L1 which damages the conus medullaris or a central prolapsed intervertebral disc leading to cauda equina injury or spinal stenosis. The bladder distends without sensation and the external sphincter is flaccid. Thus the cystometrogram is flat. The patient develops retention with overflow, but emptying is possible with abdominal straining or hand pressure.

Injury above the sacral segments (upper motor neurone lesions). Trauma such as fractures of the cervical spine, whiplash injuries or gunshot wounds is the commonest cause of injury to the spinal cord. Tumours such as angiomas may compress the cord or the cord may be injured during surgical removal of the tumour. Diseases affecting the spinal cord include multiple sclerosis, transverse myelitis at this level and cervical cord stenosis.

If the central connections are disrupted, the patient develops a reflex bladder with impaired or absent cortical control. The bladder fails to empty completely and, because of the uncoordinated action of the detrusor and sphincter, develops a thick, trabeculated wall. Usually the central connections are not completely disrupted and there may be some sensation and some cortical inhibition.

Damage to pelvic nerves. Operative procedures may interrupt the autonomic pathways, especially when the dissection involves the side walls of the pelvis, as in radical dissection of the rectum or the uterus. Similarly, a lumbar sympathectomy or surgery for aortic aneurysm may disrupt the neural pathways in the pelvis.

Diseases affecting the autonomic system, principally diabetes mellitus, also affect the control of micturition.

With the loss of sensation and contraction, the bladder becomes an atonic sac, prone to the main complication of stasis infection. The external sphincter remains closed by uninhibited tonic contractions, but the internal sphincter is partly open since it partly depends on detrusor activity.

Causes within the bladder. Primary failure of the detrusor has been described but usually it is a sequel of chronic overdistension.

Atonic myogenic bladder is caused by prolonged outlet obstruction and is found in the late stages of bladder decompensation. The commonest cause is silent prostatic obstruction, where progressive loss of the desire to void results in overflow incontinence. In women, conscious prolonging of the postponement phase can lead to a large, atonic bladder.

Principles of management of disorders of micturition

1. The diagnosis must be as complete as possible. More than one mechanism may account for the disordered micturition. When, after full clinical examination, the diagnosis is still in doubt a full urodynamic assessment must be undertaken. A urodynamic assessment is mandatory in all patients with a suspected or proven neuropathic bladder.

2. Infection is the single most sinister complication and every effort must be made to prevent it.

3. Renal damage (from vesicoureteric reflux) and chronic infection are the most serious complications of bladder and urethral dysfunction, and prevention of these complications takes priority in subsequent treatment.

4. Early management of a spinal injury consists of continuous bladder drainage with a fine urethral catheter. Infection must be avoided.

5. If there is evidence that the spinal reflex is intact, reflex activity may return to the bladder.

6. Reflex activity leads to uncoordinated micturition. The bladder becomes thick-walled and sacculated and there is vesicoureteric reflux.

7. In the absence of reflex activity, a large atonic bladder must be expressed manually.

8. If this is unsatisfactory, the distal urethral mechanism should be incised. Resection of the proximal urethral mechanism may also be needed.

9. For severe reflux and recurrent urinary infections, urinary diversion is indicated.

10. Carefully selected cases may be treated by an artificial sphincter whose opening and closing is under the patient's control. If the patient is not suitable for such a device, and especially in women in whom incontinence is otherwise difficult to control, a urinary diversion may need to be done early.

40. Neurosurgery

Although there is evidence that so-called primitive man trepanned skulls and that in medieval times crude attempts were made at trepannation, tumour removal and nerve section, surgical neurology is a relatively new specialty. Conditions affecting the central nervous system which may require surgical intervention may be classified as follows.

1. Congenital disorders
2. Degenerative disorders
3. Vascular disorders
4. Infection
5. Neoplasia
6. Trauma (see Ch. 14)
7. Miscellaneous disorders

These disorders may affect the central nervous tissue itself, the coverings of the nervous tissue such as the meninges, or the bony compartments containing the nervous system. The signs and symptoms produced may be *generalized* (e.g. headache, vomiting, alterations in conscious level) due to increase in intracranial pressure, or *localized* (e.g. paralysis, sensory defect), resulting from damage in a specific area from trauma, local pressure, ischaemia or haemorrhage.

Increased intracranial pressure

The central nervous system is enclosed in a rigid bony framework, and increases in mass content produced by tumour, haemorrhage, oedema or failure to reabsorb cerebrospinal fluid result in an increase in pressure within the framework, particularly within the cranium. In children, the ununited cranium permits expansion of intracranial contents with smaller increases in intracranial pressure than in adults, although in certain situations hydrocephalus results (see p. 649).

Intracranial pressure normally fluctuates throughout the day and may increase during coughing, defaecation or any circumstances producing an increase in intrathoracic pressure. Such transient rises do no harm; only sustained increases produce disorders.

Increases in intracranial pressure lower perfusion pressure (i.e. intracerebral arterial pressure minus intracranial pressure), but initially autoregulatory processes maintain an effective perfusion pressure of above 40 mmHg. Intracranial vessels dilate as extracranial pressure increases, resulting in increased cerebral flow. If raised intracranial pressure is unrelieved, bradycardia, hypertension and respiratory abnormalities (e.g. apnoea) develop with eventual progression to irreversible oedema, vasoparalysis and death.

Pressure may not increase uniformly throughout the intracranial and spinal cavities, producing distortion of vessels and local ischaemia. Marked displacement of intracranial structures may occur and lead to three major types of herniation.

Transfalcine herniation. The cingulate gyrus herniates beneath the free edge of the falx. The anterior cerebral artery may be compressed sufficiently to produce medial hemisphere infarction, but otherwise there are no obvious clinical signs except deterioration in conscious level.

Transtentorial herniation. The medial part of the temporal lobe is pushed downwards through the tentorial notch to become wedged between the tentorial edge and the midbrain (Fig. 40.1). The opposite cerebral peduncle is pushed against the sharp tentorial edge, and the midbrain and uncus become wedged at the tentorium. The

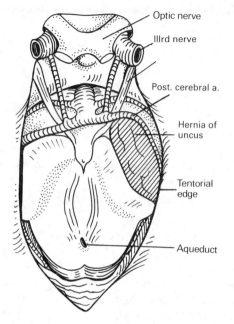

Fig. 40.1 Transtentorial herniation

aqueduct is compressed, obstructing flow of cerebrospinal fluid, and venous obstruction produces midbrain haemorrhage. The condition of the patient rapidly deteriorates. Epidural haematomas, or tumours or contusions of the temporal lobe are the usual causes.

Upward herniation is less common, but sometimes occurs with posterior fossa tumours. The pons and superior cerebellum become impacted at the tentorium.

Foraminal herniation. The cerebellar tonsils and medulla are displaced downwards through the foramen magnum, and cerebellar impaction occurs (Fig. 40.2). This may follow lumbar puncture and removal of cerebrospinal fluid in patients with raised intracranial pressure. Deterioration with loss of consciousness and decerebration is rapid. Thus, lumbar puncture should *not* be performed in patients suspected of having increased intracranial pressure.

Signs and symptoms of increased intracranial pressure

The principal symptoms are headache, vomiting and visual disturbance (Hippocratic triad), and papilloedema may be detected. Clinical suspicion should be aroused by any one of these signs or symptoms.

Headache is common in patients with tumour, but may be absent. It is usually generalized, dull and aching, exacerbated by straining, coughing or defaecation, and classically worse in the morning, when it may be accompanied by vomiting.

Nausea or vomiting is more common in posterior

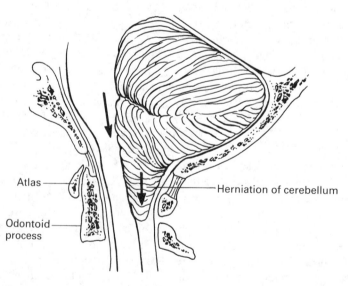

Fig. 40.2 Foraminal herniation

fossa tumours than supratentorial lesions and may be due more to medullary displacement than to generalized increase in pressure.

Visual disturbance in the form of transient *amblyopia* or blurred vision may occur in one or both eyes, particularly during straining or stooping. In the early stages of *papilloedema*, the retinal veins appear full and there is blurring of the nasal margin of the optic disc. Later, the disc becomes reddened and congested, with haemorrhagic streaks radiating from its edges, and filmy exudates form. Papilloedema is often present or more marked in one eye, but this is usually of no localizing significance.

Weight loss and anorexia may be present and usually indicate the presence of a tumour.

Bradycardia and *mild hypertension* are common in the later stages. *Intellectual deterioration* and *disorders of consciousness* occur as intracranial pressure rises progressively.

Assessment of consciousness level

Swelling, ischaemia or displacement of brainstem structures result in dysfunction of the reticular activating system in the brainstem which is concerned with consciousness. Continuing brainstem compression leads to deterioration of consciousness, coma and death.

Table 40.1 Glasgow coma scale

Eyes open	spontaneously	4
	to verbal command	3
	to pain	2
	no response	1
Best motor response		
to verbal command	obeys verbal command	6
	localizes pain	5
	flexion withdrawal	4
to painful stimulus	abnormal flexion (decorticate rigidity)	3
	extension (decerebrate rigidity)	2
	no response	1
Best verbal response	orientated and converses	5
	disorientated and converses	4
	inappropriate words	3
	incomprehensible sounds	2
	no response	1
Total number of points (minimum 3, maximum 15)		—

Assessment of consciousness level is invaluable in the observation of patients with a variety of neurological disorders, where even minor changes in consciousness level may indicate the need for urgent treatment. The following classification of disordered consciousness has found general acceptance.

Grade 1 *Alert and orientated* (AO). Patient responds readily and accurately to question and command, and is orientated in time, place and person.

Grade 2 *Disorientated* or *confused* (D). The patient is disorientated in time, place and person.

Grade 3 *Drowsy — vocal response to stimuli* (VRS). The patient can be roused briefly by strong stimuli to respond vocally.

Grade 4 *Stuporous — purposeful response to stimuli* (PRS). The patient can be roused briefly by strong stimuli to respond purposefully but not vocally.

Grade 5 *Coma — absent or abnormal response to pain* (ARP). The patient does not respond vocally or purposefully. There is a diminished or absent corneal reflex, depressed or absent cough or swallowing reflexes, sluggish or fixed pupils. Superficial reflexes are absent. Deep reflexes are diminished and the response to painful stimulation, particularly midline sternal pressure, is decorticate or decerebrate.

Several coma classifications have been proposed, the most useful of which is the Glasgow coma scale (Table 40.1). This records the patient's responses to stimulation in terms of vocal response, motor response and pupillary reaction.

Focal signs of intracranial lesions

Compression or destruction of different parts of the brain often produces subtle signs and symptoms long before there is evidence of increased intracranial pressure. The following signs are general pointers to the site of the pathology but are not specific. Displacement and resulting ischaemia frequently produce symptoms from parts of the brain distant to the causative lesion.

Frontal lobe. Lesions of the frontal lobe are associated with intellectual and emotional changes, and may cause expressive dysphasia (dominant lobe lesion) and focal epilepsy. Contralateral faciobrachial weakness in convexity lesions, and contralateral lower limb weakness in medial lesions. Lateral gaze paralysis with the eyes deviated to the side suggests a destructive lesion on that side, while lateral gaze fixation with the eyes deviated to the side is more likely to be due to an irritating lesion on the opposite side. Urinary and faecal incontinence and anosmia may develop as the disease progresses.

Parietal lobe. Convexity lesions cause contralateral faciobrachial sensory loss, while medial lesions are associated with sensory loss in the lower limb. Astereognosis and sensory epilepsy also point to parietal lobe damage. Dominant lobe lesions produce receptive and global aphasia.

Occipital lobe. Patients with occipital lobe lesions may develop dyslexia (dominant lobe) and hemianopia.

Temporal lobe. Lesions in the temporal lobe may produce emotional changes, temporal lobe epilepsy, memory loss or receptive auditory disorder.

Cerebellum. Ipsilateral weakness, hypotonia, ataxia, dysmetria, and nystagmus may all suggest a cerebellar lesion.

Brainstem. Lesions of the brainstem are commonly associated with cranial nerve palsies, and long-tract motor and sensory signs.

Cerebellopontine angle. Functional disturbance may develop in all or some of the 5th–12th cranial nerves. Weakness of the contralateral arm and/or leg and ipsilateral ataxia may also occur.

Basal tumours. Anosmia (unilateral or bilateral), optic nerve atrophy and paresis of eye movement may suggest a basal tumour.

Pituitary or *parapituitary tumours.* Patients with such tumours may show early signs of visual disturbance and endocrine abnormalities.

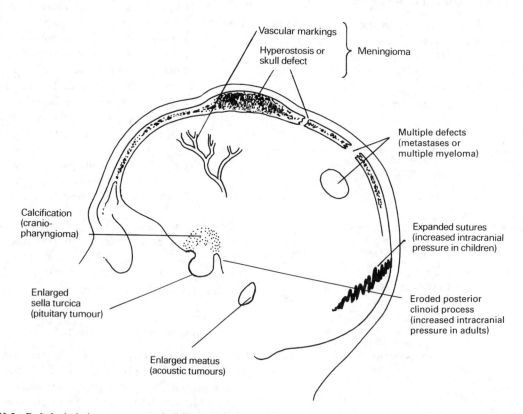

Fig. 40.3 Pathological changes seen on skull X-ray and some of their causes

Reaction of central nervous system to injury or infection

The reaction of the central nervous system to injury is similar to that of other tissues. Oedema is, however, more prominent due to damage to the blood-brain barrier allowing albumin, sodium ions and water to pass into the extracellular fluid. Oedema may be exacerbated by a number of factors, including a rise in Pa_{CO_2}. The injured area becomes surrounded by increased numbers of glial cells which act as phagocytes to remove dead neurones and other material, and which tend to localize infection. Fibrosis (gliosis) or scarring is the final outcome.

Oedema may result in loss of function of involved neural cells, with recovery of function as the oedema resolves. Irritation of cells may also result from oedema, or from their involvement in the scar process, leading to epilepsy, or pain if pain fibres are involved. Replacement of destroyed neurones by regeneration is not possible in the central nervous system.

Investigation of neurological disorders

Although many sophisticated investigations are available, a detailed history and careful examination are essential if they are to be used rationally.

A *full blood count* is needed in all patients. Severe anaemia should arouse the suspicion of metastatic disease, while polycythaemia in a patient with posterior fossa symptoms suggests cerebellar haemangioblastoma. A raised white count suggests infection.

Lumbar puncture and *CSF examination* may assist in or confirm the diagnosis of meningitis, subarachnoid haemorrhage, or neoplasm. The investigation should not be carried out in patients with suspected raised intracranial pressure because of the risk of foraminal herniation and cerebellar coning.

Plain radiography

X-rays of the *skull or spine* should be obtained routinely. Metastatic disease of the spine or skull is often clearly seen. A narrowed intervertebral disc space confirms a provisional diagnosis of prolapsed intervertebral disc. Congenital disorders may be revealed by the abnormal shape of the skull. Raised intracranial pressure in children produces expansion of the sutures, while in adults the posterior clinoid processes are thinned. Enlargement of the sella turcica or internal auditory meatus may occur in patients with pituitary or acoustic tumours respectively, while the vascular markings of the skull may be enlarged in the region of a vascular tumour such as a meningioma. Bony erosion or overgrowth (hyperostosis) are other features of meningioma. Calcification of the pineal gland or choroid plexus may reveal displacement of these structures, while abnormal calcification may develop within certain cysts or tumours (Fig. 40.3).

A *chest X-ray* should always be obtained. About 25% of cerebral tumours are secondary deposits from lung cancer. The chest X-ray may also reveal metastases from other primary sites.

Contrast radiology

Dye may be injected to outline the spinal cord and nerve roots (*myelography* or *radiculography*; Fig. 40.4) or the cerebral ventricles (*ventriculography*; Fig. 40.5). The ventricles and basal systems may also be filled with air injected via lumbar puncture (*pneumo-encephalography*). This technique is contraindicated if raised intracranial pressure is suspected. *Angiography* may reveal lesions such as aneurysms and arteriovenous malformations, and display the relationship of important arteries to tumours. Angiography and ventriculography have been largely superseded by computerized axial tomography but still hold an important place in investigation.

Other imaging techniques

Computerized axial tomography (CT) is a non-invasive, accurate diagnostic technique which can be performed without risk. Ventricular enlargement and displacement, and the extent of tumours and abscesses with their associated oedema can be clearly shown. Haemorrhages and clots show up as dense areas, and the presence of even small

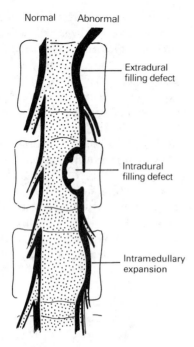

Fig. 40.4 Myelographic appearances of normal and abnormal spinal canal

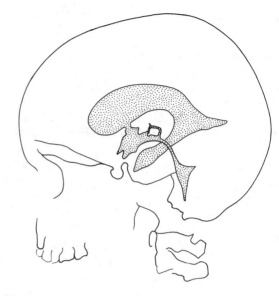

Fig. 40.5 Contrast radiology: normal ventriculogram

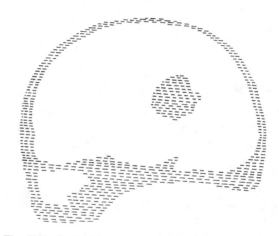

Fig. 40.6 Cerebral isotope scan showing increased uptake of isotope by tumour

haemorrhages and associated oedema may indicate subarachnoid haemorrhage. Intravenous contrast injection may 'enhance' the density of some lesions such as tumours.

Cerebral isotope scanning. Technetium-99 is usually used as a marker. Vascular tumours such as meningiomas, metastases and some gliomas are readily revealed (Fig. 40.6), while the vascularity of the neck muscles tends to obscure posterior fossa tumours. Although isotope scanning does not provide as good anatomical detail as computerized axial tomography, it is a valuable method of assessing tumour vascularity following radiotherapy or chemotherapy, and may also be used to study cerebral blood flow and cerebrospinal fluid flow.

Magnetic resonance imaging (MRI) and *positron emission tomography* (PET scanning) are new developments not generally available. Both provide information on certain brain lesions which cannot be provided by CT or isotope scanning.

Electrophysiological measurements

Electroencephalography is less used than formerly, (except in epilepsy) because of the availability of

other techniques. *Intracranial pressure monitoring* is of some value in assessing the response to treatment of raised intracranial pressure.

CONGENITAL LESIONS

Congenital malformations of the central nervous system are relatively common. Although genetic counselling and advances in intrauterine diagnosis are reducing the number of babies born with severe defects, minor defects undoubtedly continue to occur. The causative role of viral infection and ingestion of certain drugs and toxic substances during pregnancy is well established, and therapeutic abortion may have to be considered in some cases. Children with mild defects who are likely to live independent lives should be offered immediate surgical treatment. Those with major defects are often denied surgery because this is thought unlikely to allow them to live independent lives. Unfortunately a proportion of such children survive with much greater defects than if surgery had been undertaken. Currently, therefore, at least simple corrective surgery is offered to all, except those with severe defects associated with bladder abnormalities.

Spinal defects

These are common. *Dysrhaphism* is due to defective closure of the neural tube, and includes conditions such as spina bifida occulta, simple meningocele and meningomyelocele. Closure of the neural tube begins in the mid-dorsal region and extends cranially and caudally. Thus, thoracic defects are rare and cervical defects uncommon, while lumbar and lumbosacral defects are common.

Spina bifida occulta

This common condition is not usually associated with neurological defect. The overlying skin may be hairy or dimpled, or have an associated fat pad. Occasionally a fibrous band tethers the cord, producing increasing symptoms as the vertebral column grows and the spinal cord 'ascends' the vertebral canal. The onset of paraesthesia or sphincter disorders is usually due to an associated lesion such as a cord lipoma, or to *diastemyelia* where the cord is split by a projection from the posterior surface of a vertebral body. A sinus may connect the skin and spinal canal in a few cases and is a rare cause of meningitis in children. Plain X-rays may reveal an abnormality of the lamina or failure of fusion of the laminar arches.

Patients with neurological disorders require surgical treatment. Paraesthesia, backache and sphincter disorder due to tethering by a fibrous band may be dramatically relieved by division of the band. Splitting of the cord by a bony spur can be dealt with by careful removal of the spur. Intraspinal lipomas are often diffuse. Although removal has been facilitated by the introduction of microscopic techniques, severe neurological disturbances may result.

Simple meningocele

The defect is usually lumbar and results from failure of fusion of laminae (Fig. 40.7). The subarachnoid space is distended and protrudes through the defect. The arachnoid fuses with the skin, forming a membrane to which nerve roots may be adherent. The cord, however, is nor-

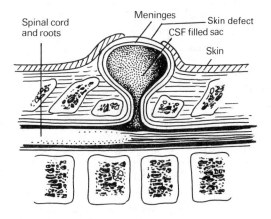

Fig. 40.7 Simple meningocele

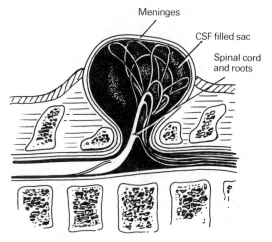

Fig. 40.8 Meningomyelocele

mal and usually there are no neurological abnormalities.

Meningomyelocele

The condition occurs most commonly in the lumbar region. Spinal nerve roots and the cord adhere to the membrane because of distension of the central canal and may be exposed on the surface (Fig. 40.8). Craniocerebral malformations such as hydrocephalus are commonly associated.

There is usually serious motor and sensory loss affecting the lower limbs and sphincters due to involvement of the cauda equina. Bladder paralysis is of the lower motor neurone type with paralysis of the detrusor muscle and pelvic floor musculature.

These patients often require complex and lengthy corrective procedures, and urinary continence is difficult to achieve.

Syringomyelia and syringobulbia

Distension of the central canal of the cord or paraventricular extension of the fourth ventricle results in syringomyelia or syringobulbia respectively. Although the genesis of the condition is debated, most believe it to result from failure of closure of the connection between the fourth ventricle and the central canal, coupled with failure of development of exit foramina in the membrane around the cerebellar tonsils.

Symptoms, which are steadily progressive, appear in the third decade and affect men more commonly than women. In the cord, distension of the central canal gradually compresses and destroys the decussating pain and temperature pathways, producing 'dissociated sensory loss' (loss of pain and temperature sensation but not of touch) over the upper part of the body, most often in the fingers. Pain, however, is a common presenting symptom. Trophic lesions develop on the hands and arms due to loss of pain sensation. The small muscles of the hand are often involved early, with resultant deformity and wasting. Ultimately the long tracts become involved, producing paresis and sensory changes below the level of the lesion. Denervation arthritis (Charcot's joints) may occur.

The condition is treated by creating an opening in the membrane around the cerebellar tonsils to allow drainage of cerebrospinal fluid. Occasionally a persisting communication with the central canal may be plugged. A posterior fossa approach is used. Isolated cysts of the cord can be drained by direct puncture either via a laminectomy or percutaneously. Orthopaedic deformities may require correction, e.g. arthrodesis of unstable joints.

Malformations of the skull

These are less common than spinal defects.

Meningocele and encephalocele

Protrusion of the meninges (meningocele) or of the meninges together with brain (encephalocele) through a skull defect occurs most commonly in the occipital region and is usually associated with other abnormalities such as hydrocephalus and mental retardation.

Craniostenosis

Premature fusion (before 4 years of age) of one or more skull sutures results in restriction of the growing brain and an increase in intracranial pressure. The shape of the skull is determined by which sutures fuse. Associated ophthalmic disorders such as exophthalmus are common. Severe cases are treated by excision of the fused sutures. The edges are then lined with dura or plastic material to retard re-union and allow the brain to expand.

Orbital hypertelorism

This group of malformations is produced by overgrowth of anterior fossa structures resulting in widening of the intercanthal distance and persistence of clefts and fusion lines. The disorder is relatively common in a mild form, but in its most advanced form produces gross malformation requiring treatment by excision of the central sutures and transposition of the lateral masses.

Epidermoid cysts

These contain cheesy debris and arise from skin which has been engulfed by bone. They expand the bone and erode the skull, producing a characteristic scalloped lytic area.

Miscellaneous malformations

Malformations associated with autosomal abnormalities (e.g. Down's syndrome, microencephaly, macroencephaly, porencephaly) are not correctable. Tuberous sclerosis is a form of neuroectodermal dysplasia associated with mental retardation and epilepsy in which astrocytes form pale firm 'tubers' in the cortex and subependyma which occasionally become malignant. Angiomatous malformations of the skin (usually in the distribution of the ophthalmic branch of the trigeminal nerve), or of the retina and meninges (Sturge-Weber syndrome) may be associated with epilepsy and mental retardation. The vessels rarely rupture and symptoms are related to the epilepsy.

Hydrocephalus

Cerebrospinal fluid is produced by the intraventricular choroid plexus. It passes from the lateral ventricles via the narrow foramen of Munro into the slit-like third ventricle and then through the aqueduct of the upper brainstem into the widening fourth ventricle. From here the fluid passes via 'exit foramina' in the lower part of the fourth ventricle into the cisterna magna, afterwards flowing over the surface of the brain and spinal cord to be absorbed by cerebral veins and arachnoid granulations. Hydrocephalus results when the rate of production of cerebrospinal fluid exceeds that of absorption and is usually associated with increased intracranial pressure. Though a choroid plexus papilloma may produce hydrocephalus by oversecretion of CSF, much the commonest cause of hydrocephalus is obstruction to flow with failure of CSF to reach sites of absorption (Fig. 40.9).

Obstruction may be congenital, due to failure of communications between ventricles (as in aqueduct stenosis), or acquired as a result of tumour or fibrosis (gliosis) following infection or

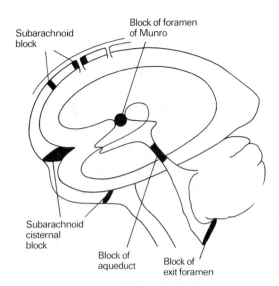

Fig. 40.9 Hydrocephalus: sites of CSF blockage

haemorrhage. For the sake of simplicity, the acquired types of hydrocephalus are also considered in this section. Obstruction within the ventricular system leads to so-called *non-communicating* or *internal hydrocephalus*, while in *communicating* or *external hydrocephalus* the ventricular system is patent, but absorption by the arachnoid granulations is prevented by blood or fibrosis, or occasionally by their failure to develop.

Hydrocephalus usually presents at birth or in early infancy with characteristic enlargement of the head. Presentation in later childhood or in adult life is associated with the signs and symptoms of raised intracranial pressure.

If the cause of hydrocephalus can be removed (e.g. cysts, thin membranes, certain tumours), this should be done after preliminary drainage of the ventricles via a right frontal burr hole. Lumbar puncture should be avoided because of the risk of medullary 'coning'. If the cause cannot be removed, a ventricular shunt may be inserted (Fig. 40.10). A catheter is introduced into a lateral ventricle and tunnelled subcutaneously into the neck, where it is inserted into the internal jugular vein and passed into the superior vena cava or right atrium (ventriculo-atrial shunt). Alternatively, the catheter can be tunnelled to the peritoneal cavity (ventriculo-peritoneal shunt). The catheter has a one-way valve to prevent reflux

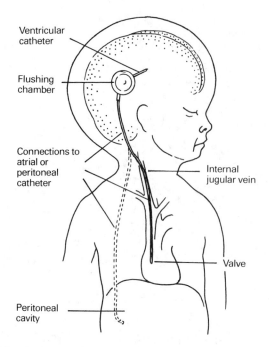

Fig. 40.10 Ventriculo-atrial shunt (continuous line) and ventriculo-peritoneal shunt (interrupted line) to relieve hydrocephalus

of blood, and a chamber which may be compressed to prevent clotting and encourage flow. Despite this, blockage is frequent, especially in children, necessitating revision or replacement of the catheter.

Cerebral palsy

Cerebral palsy may result from agenesis, birth injury or infection. There is often a history of neonatal distress, cyanosis and feeding difficulties. Although many patients have normal intelligence, mental subnormality is common and signs of retarded development become apparent as the child grows. Spasticity and athetoid movements become marked, and the abnormal movements may be so violent that the patient cannot sit up. Joint contractures may develop. In milder cases, the patient has a characteristic 'scissor' gait with adduction of the legs and equinus varus posture.

Treatment consists of physiotherapy and special education in mild cases, but major disability often progresses so that the patient becomes helpless and unable to dress or feed himself. Joint deformities

may be relieved by tendon transposition or neurectomy. Stereotactic destruction of thalamic or cerebellar nuclei is successful in relieving lower limb spasticity, and to a lesser degree spasticity of the upper limbs.

DEGENERATIVE DISEASES OF THE VERTEBRAL COLUMN

Degenerative changes in the intervertebral discs are common at all levels. Intervertebral discs consist of three parts: the *cartilage end plates* which adhere to the cancellous bone of adjacent vertebral bodies; the central semifluid *nucleus pulposus* which is relatively incompressible and inelastic, and the slightly elastic *annulus fibrosus* which surrounds it and retains it and which regulates and restricts movement of the spine. The disc is subject to severe and repeated compression, and degenerative changes may allow protrusion of the nucleus pulposus. This can occur through the cartilage end plate or horizontally through the annulus fibrosus. Horizontal protrusion usually occurs in a posterolateral direction and is of considerable clinical importance if the cord or nerve roots are subjected to direct pressure.

Herniation of the nucleus pulposus is usually a gradual and intermittent process so that symptoms tend to remit between exacerbations. Acute herniation may, however, occur, usually in response to severe trauma with flexion injury. The annulus fibrosus ruptures, allowing posterior (central) protrusion of the nucleus with sudden severe neurological deficit.

If the nucleus pulposus has lost substance by protrusion or desiccation (as occurs in advancing age), the relaxed fibres of the annulus fibrosus bulge outwards and the 'disc space' narrows. Strain on the apophyseal joints then results in osteophyte formation and narrowing of the intervertebral foramina. Osteophyte formation occurs around the disc margin. This condition is known as *spondylosis* (Fig. 40.11). With continuing degeneration, osteophytes may protrude on the cord or nerve roots.

Spinal *osteoarthritis* is a disorder affecting the posterior apophyseal joints and producing back pain without distant radiation. It should be distinguished from spondylosis (which depends on

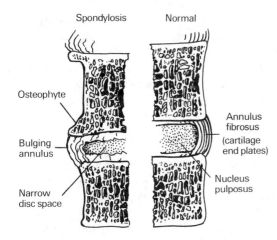

Fig. 40.11 Intervertebral disc of normal spine and in spondylosis

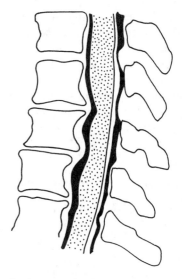

Fig. 40.12 Cord compression by cervical spondylosis

disc degeneration) although the two frequently coexist in older patients.

Cervical spine

Cervical spondylosis

Degenerative changes in the cervical spine are common and may start as early as adolescence. Compression of a nerve root in an intervertebral foramen produces pain, usually in the neck but often radiating to the shoulder or arm, which is exacerbated by rotation of the neck. The most commonly affected level is C5–6.

Plain X-ray of the spine shows narrowing of one or more disc spaces and foramina with osteophyte formation. Myelography may demonstrate nerve compression, and in severe cases compression of the cord (Fig. 40.12).

Treatment is initially conservative and comprises physiotherapy, neck traction and prescription of a supporting cervical collar. For more severe compression, as evidenced by weakness and paraesthesia, conservative therapy is not effective and decompression is required. Through an anterior approach a central core of disc and related vertebra is removed and the lateral portion of the disc is curetted away. A dowel of bone taken from the iliac crest is then hammered into the central core to stabilize the two vertebrae (Fig. 40.13).

Acute cervical disc prolapse

Acute prolapse is uncommon and fortunately most protrusions are small. The patient experience sudden acute neck pain radiating down the arm in the area of the involved root or roots. Symptoms usually resolve following conservative management

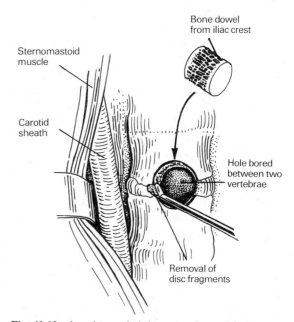

Fig. 40.13 Anterior cervical decompression and fusion

with analgesics, neck traction and use of a cervical collar. Persistence of symptoms is an indication for surgery, and patients with major prolapse and long-tract signs (which may include quadriparesis) require urgent operation.

The disc fragments may be removed through a posterior approach or, less commonly, by anterior decompression; this is usually accompanied by vertebral fusion.

Thoracic spine

Thoracic disc degeneration with formation of osteophytes and foraminal narrowing is relatively common, although surgical treatment is seldom required.

Acute disc prolapse is uncommon. It requires urgent surgery because the narrow calibre of the vertebral canal in the thoracic region favours cord compression. Acute pain in the distribution of the segmental nerves may be accompanied by paraparesis or paraplegia depending on the degree of prolapse.

An anterolateral or posterolateral approach is used to avoid injuring the acutely compressed spinal cord.

Lumbar spine

Disorders of the lumbar spine are extremely common. Low backache (*lumbago*), with pain radiating down one or both legs (*sciatica*) may be caused by a variety of conditions. Metastases from lung, breast or prostatic cancer should always be considered, but degenerative disease of the vertebrae and discs accounts for the majority of cases.

Lumbar spondylosis

As a result of bulging of the annulus fibrosus, osteophytes form at the disc margins. Posterior osteophyte formation reduces the diameter of the vertebral canal, while additional stress on the posterior joints results in hypertrophy of the joint bone and ligaments, reducing the canal laterally. There is thickening of the laminar arch, and the ligamentum flavum degenerates, losing its elasticity and tending to buckle on extension. All lumbar vertebrae may be affected, but the severe

changes described here usually occur only at the lower lumbar level. Radiculography confirms the diagnosis.

Most patients can be managed conservatively with exercise and support, but those with severe symptoms require decompression by laminectomy.

Acute lumbar disc prolapse

Acute disc prolapse is most common in the fourth and fifth decades of life and occurs more frequently in men. It is often associated with degenerative spinal disease elsewhere. Trauma which subjects the disc to torsional stress (e.g. twisting while carrying heavy weights) may precipitate rupture of the annulus fibrosus, allowing protrusion of the nucleus pulposus.

Rupture through the central portion of the annulus may compress the roots of the entire cauda equina, causing severe back pain (without a predominant root involvement), urinary retention and weakness below the knees. This *cauda equina syndrome* requires urgent surgical relief.

More commonly the prolapse occurs posterolaterally and compresses and angulates the nerve emerging at that level. The commonest sites for prolapse are at the L4–5 and L5–S1 level, the roots affected being L5 and S1 respectively. Prolapse above L4–5 becomes less common as one ascends. The majority of patients recover on conservative management, but those with symptoms persisting for more than 6 weeks should be offered surgical treatment.

Signs and symptoms. Pain is the predominant symptom, and is exacerbated by coughing and sneezing. Tendon jerks and muscle power are diminished according to the site of the lesion. Straight leg raising stretches the sciatic nerve and pulls on nerve roots, resulting in pain if the roots are stretched over a disc protrusion. Straight leg raising is measured in degrees and reflects the amount of root compression. The limit of straight leg raising is normally 80–90°, but it may be reduced on the affected side to less than 30°. Dorsiflexion of the foot at the limit of straight leg raising often exacerbates the pain. Examination of the back usually reveals flattening of the lumbar spinal curve and mild lumbar scoliosis, concave to the side of the lesion. This scoliosis is exaggerated when the patient is asked to bend forward.

L5–S1 prolapse compresses the root S1 and produces pain which radiates down the back of the thigh and lateral aspect of the leg onto the lateral border of the foot and the lateral three toes. Sensory changes may be detected in this distribution. The ankle jerk is diminished or absent, and plantar flexion of the foot is weak, so that the patient has difficulty in standing on his toes.

L4–L5 prolapse compresses the root of L5, causes pain which radiates from the back down the back of the thigh and then passes medially from the lateral aspect of the leg to the dorsum of the foot and into the great toe. Sensory changes may also be detected in this distribution. The ankle jerk is normal, but dorsiflexion of the foot is weak.

L3–L4 prolapse compresses the root of L4 and produces pain and sensory disturbance down the front of the thigh and medial aspect of the leg on to the medial malleolus. The knee jerk is diminished or absent, and there is quadriceps weakness.

Investigation. Full examination of the abdomen (including rectal examination) is imperative as retroperitoneal or pelvic pathology may also produce severe back pain with radiation if nerves become involved.

The diagnosis is often apparent from the history and physical examination, although some difficulty may arise when an adjacent root is involved in addition to the root at the level of the prolapse. Posteroanterior and lateral X-rays of the lumbar spine are essential and often show narrowing of the involved disc space. Radiculography is indicated if the diagnosis remains in doubt.

Treatment. Immediate strict bed rest is mandatory. The patient should lie flat and should not sit up for meals, although he may be allowed up for toilet purposes. Most patients improve within 2–3 weeks and are allowed up after 4 weeks.

Patients with major protrusions are unlikely to respond satisfactorily and should be offered early surgery. Any patient who has not progressed satisfactorily after six weeks' bed rest also requires operation. The prolapsed material is removed through a posterior approach. The results of operation are good for those with acute prolapse, though pain may recur if there is generalized spinal disease.

Spondylolisthesis

Spondylolisthesis is caused by a bilateral defect in the pars interarticularis of the neural arch of the fifth lumbar vertebra (spondylolysis) which allows the anterior part of the vertebra (comprising body, pedicles, transverse processes and superior articular facets) to slide forward upon the sacrum.

Spondylolysis is probably not a congenital defect although there is an inherited tendency in some patients, and signs and symptoms may appear in childhood, most often between 10 and 15 years of age. Vertical stresses on a weakened neural arch may be responsible for the slipping, while in adults it may follow stress fracture in mature bone or result from facet deficiency due to degenerative joint disease.

In children, the condition is usually painless, though a prominent lumbar lordosis may be detected. The normal presenting symptom in adolescents or adults is backache exacerbated by exercise. Sciatica may develop as a result of S1 root pressure. The diagnosis is confirmed radiologically.

Symptomatic younger patients are treated by lumbosacral fusion, but, as this is a major undertaking, older and less fit patients are usually managed with a spinal brace.

Spinal stenosis

This is a congenital condition in which there is generalized narrowing of the vertebral canal. Symptoms do not occur until middle life, and are associated with other degenerative changes, such as spondylosis, which are more likely to produce symptoms as a result of the narrow canal. Several nerve roots are often affected.

Treatment is similar to that for spondylosis although decompression by laminectomy (with or without fusion) is more frequently necessary.

VASCULAR DISORDERS

The metabolic demand of the brain is greater than that of any other organ and requires a considerable blood supply. The cerebral blood flow of 800 ml/min (16% of cardiac output) is provided by two systems: the carotid arteries, which supply the forebrain, and the vertebral arteries, which supply

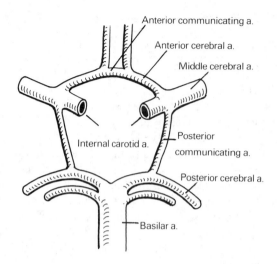

Fig. 40.14 Circle of Willis

the hindbrain. The two systems communicate freely in the circle of Willis (Fig. 40.14), and occlusion of a major artery may be complicated by anastomotic flow.

The common carotid artery divides into the external carotid artery, which supplies the soft tissues of the head and the dura, and the internal carotid artery, which enters the skull to supply the brain. After passing through the carotid sinus, the internal carotid artery divides into the anterior cerebral artery and the middle cerebral artery. The two vertebral arteries join within the skull to form the basilar artery, which supplies the cerebellum and brainstem and then divides into the posterior cerebral arteries, which pass through the tentorium to supply the occipital lobe and the posterior two-thirds of the medial aspect of the hemisphere.

Disorders of the central nervous system resulting from vascular disease are due mainly to occlusion or haemorrhage.

Occlusive vascular disease (see also Ch. 21)

Symptoms most often result from occlusive disease of *extracranial* vessels. The lumen of the carotid or vertebral vessels may be narrowed or occluded by arteriosclerotic changes in the aortic arch, in the neck (particularly at the carotid bifurcation) or at the level of entry into the skull. While arteriosclerotic disease may be widespread in the cerebral vessels, *intracranial occlusion* is usually embolic.

Transient ischaemic attacks (TIA)

Small thrombi and platelet aggregates attached to atheromatous plaques, and occasionally small portions of the plaques themselves, may embolize and become lodged in small intracranial vessels, and so produce sudden and alarming symptoms which are often transient. Sudden occlusion of the carotid artery commonly causes unilateral blindness and contralateral weakness, with associated speech disorder if the dominant hemisphere is affected. Auscultation over the carotid bifurcation will reveal a bruit in 70% of patients, and ophthalmodynamometry may show lower pressure on the affected side. The extent of the lesion can be revealed by angiography, although this is not without risk.

About 50% of patients with TIA will have a major stroke within 5 years if the primary lesion is not treated. Stenotic lesions in the neck arteries are relatively easy to remove; those arising in the aortic arch are more difficult. Gentle handling of the carotid artery is essential to avoid dislodging thrombi. If the pressure in the distal carotid artery is less than 50 mmHg, a bypass procedure is used to lessen the risk of postoperative stroke. The value of carotid endarterectomy is debated, many opponents contending that aspirin therapy is equally effective.

Unfortunately many of these patients suffer from generalized arteriosclerotic disease and a high proportion die from myocardial infarction within a few years of surgery.

Cerebral thrombosis

Stenotic lesions may progress to complete occlusion, with thrombus formation extending up the carotid tree. If the collateral circulation via the circle of Willis is defective, cerebral infarction occurs. In the past, extracranial-intracranial anastomosis was commonly advocated to improve the precarious circulation. However, it is now believed that this is of no value for prophylaxis of arteriosclerotic lesions but useful in aneurysm surgery.

Haemorrhage

Intracranial haemorrhage may be intracerebral, subarachnoid, subdural or extradural. Extradural and subdural haemorrhage usually result from trauma and are considered separately in Chapter 14.

Intracerebral haemorrhage

Intracerebral haemorrhage is relatively common in the middle-aged and elderly. The risk is particularly high in patients with hypertension and diabetes, and justifies the prophylactic treatment of hypertension. In hypertension the perforating arteries of the middle cerebral arteries develop micro-aneurysms which rupture and tear open the internal capsule. Intracerebral haemorrhage may also occur from rupture of 'berry' aneurysms located deep within the brain, from arteriovenous malformations, or from trauma producing brain lacerations.

The onset is abrupt and the majority of patients become comatose with stertorous respiration and flaccid hemiparesis. About 30% of patients die within 3 days, but some survive with partial recovery of function.

Emergency procedures to remove acute intracerebral haematomas are rarely successful since bleeding continues. If patients survive the initial haemorrhage, evacuation of the clot through a burr hole may result in marked improvement.

Subarachnoid haemorrhage

In more than 50% of patients the haemorrhage is due to rupture of an aneurysm, while in 15% arteriosclerotic disease is the cause. Arteriovenous malformations, trauma, and haemorrhage in association with tumour or infection account for the remainder.

Intimal proliferation with degeneration of the internal elastic lamina produces weakness of arterial walls, particularly at sites of congenital weakness in the circle of Willis. Failure of the media to develop allows the intima to bulge and form an aneurysm. The majority of aneurysms occur in the anterior portion of the circle of Willis; only 15% are sited in the posterior portion.

Although 10% of patients present with symptoms due to local pressure effects of the aneurysm (e.g. 3rd cranial nerve palsy in posterior communicating artery aneurysm) or with signs suggesting tumour, the majority have no symptoms until the aneurysm ruptures. Sometimes the patient has pre-ictal symptoms of vague headache or neck pain, while the first haemorrhage (ictus) may be relatively mild and pass unrecognized.

Rupture of the aneurysm into the subarachnoid space produces sudden severe headache, neck stiffness and photophobia. Kernig's sign indicates meningism. The patients' consciousness level is affected in varying degrees, ranging from mildest disorientation to deep coma, and sudden death may occur. These symptoms, apart from meningism, are mostly due to vasospasm. The focal signs depend on the vessels affected, but are commonly related to the aneurysm's parent vessel. For example, rupture of a middle cerebral artery aneurysm commonly produces faciobrachial paresis. Associated rupture into brain substance is more serious than subarachnoid haemorrhage, and is the usual cause of sudden death.

Diagnosis and assessment. The diagnosis is confirmed by lumbar puncture. The fluid is evenly blood-stained, in contrast to a 'traumatic tap', which progressively clears. Oxyhaemoglobin

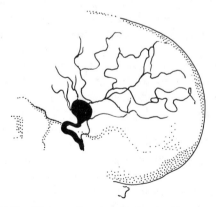

Fig. 40.15 Diagram of angiogram showing internal carotid aneurysm

appears within a few hours of haemorrhage, giving an orange colour to the supernatant fluid. By 3 days bilirubin (due to red cell breakdown) is present and gives the supernatant fluid a characteristic yellow colour (xanthochromia).

A special grading system (Botterell) is used to assess the patient:

Group A
Grade 1 Conscious, with or without signs of subarachnoid blood.
Grade 2 Drowsy, without significant neurological deficit.

Group B
Grade 3 Drowsy and confused or with mild neurological deficit.
Grade 4 Major neurological deficit and generally deteriorating, possibly the result of intracerebral clot.
Grade 5 Moribund or nearly so, with vegetative disturbance and extensor rigidity.

In practice, group A patients are fit for angiography, group B patients are not. Patients in group A have a much better prognosis and are fit for definitive surgery directed at the aneurysm. Patients in group B may sometimes be improved by removing intracerebral clot.

Skull X-rays usually show no abnormality, although a giant aneurysm may erode a clinoid process or have a calcified wall. A CT scan may reveal a large aneurysm but is more useful in detecting oedema or intracerebral haemorrhage. Angiography should be deferred until the patient is in group A and has no evidence of vasospasm. Although the clinical picture may suggest the site of the aneurysm, it is important to have a complete picture of the cerebral circulation, as aneurysms are commonly multiple (Fig. 40.15).

Management and prognosis. Mortality is high in the first week but falls steadily after the second week. Without operation, 60% of patients die within 2 months, and of those who survive the first haemorrhage 50% die within 5 years if not treated. Thus, surgical treatment should always be considered after the first haemorrhage. It has been suggested that the best time to operate is during the second week following the first haemorrhage,

provided the patient is in group A. Others believe that operation should be performed immediately after diagnosis.

While awaiting surgery the patient is confined to bed rest and given oxygen. Sedation may be required. If neurological signs are present, dexamethasone (10 mg initially and 4 mg 6-hourly thereafter) is given. Hypertension is treated by hypotensive drugs, with the aim to reduce blood pressure by 10%. Antifibrinolytic therapy may slightly reduce the risk of rebleeding but only at the expense of increased morbidity from other complications.

Most aneurysms are now treated by a direct approach. Using the operating microscope, the neck of the aneurysm is exposed and a special clip applied (Fig. 40.16). The wall of the aneurysm can be strengthened by coating it with plastic material or by wrapping it in gauze to cause a fibrous reaction. The mortality rate of operation (less than 5%) is substantially less than with non-operative treatment, but despite meticulous technique vasospasm may occur and result in brain oedema requiring energetic treatment with steroids and other anti-oedema agents.

Common carotid artery ligation is the procedure of choice for aneurysms within the cavernous sinus or for giant aneurysms of the carotid system, provided angiography has revealed a satisfactory

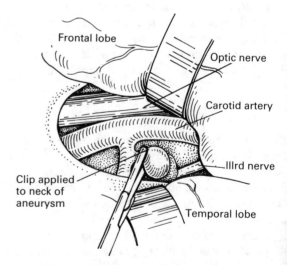

Fig. 40.16 Treatment of internal carotid aneurysm by clipping the neck of the aneurysm

cross-circulation. The procedure is normally done under local anaesthesia so that the patient's speech, behaviour, sensation and motor function can be monitored after clamping of the common carotid artery. If these remain satisfactory for 5 minutes, the vessel is ligated and the clamp removed.

Arteriovenous malformations

These congenital malformations may occur close to ventricular walls, in the substance of the brain or on the cerebral cortex. Composed of a complex mass of abnormal arteriovenous connections, they vary in size from small lesions undetectable by conventional angiography to large masses occupying major portions of brain. The lesions frequently bleed and are the commonest source of subarachnoid haemorrhage in younger patients. They may also cause epilepsy. Once bleeding has occurred, the risk of re-bleeding is high. Within 10 years 20% of patients die and a further 30% suffer severe disability from recurrent haemorrhage. The prognosis improves with increasing age at the first bleed.

Arteriovenous malformations are best demonstrated by angiography, although CT scans enhanced by contrast media will reveal moderate-sized to large lesions. Calcification may occur and will be shown on plain X-rays. Occasionally a bruit may be heard.

The lesion may be locally excised or removed by block resection (lobectomy). Preoperative embolization of contributing vessels with small plastic spheres may facilitate resection, and small anomalies may be sealed completely by selective catheterization or embolization. Stereotactic radiotherapy is an alternative to resection.

Spinal arteriovenous malformations

These lie over the posterior surface of the cord and form loops of vessels which may involve cord substance. Thrombosis frequently occurs, producing cord ischaemia. Symptoms are often progressive, and include pain, weakness and ultimately paraplegia. Excision using the operating microscope is the only available treatment, but its long-term value is uncertain.

INFECTION

Infection of the central nervous system and its coverings acquires surgical importance if it produces a mass (abscess or oedema), hydrocephalus or osteomyelitis, or if it occurs as a result of a breach in or absence of the coverings of the brain (Fig. 40.17).

Intracranial infection

Osteomyelitis of the skull

Bone may become infected by penetrating wounds, during surgery, by local extension from sinuses, the middle ear or mastoid, or by blood-borne infection. Pus may track into the subgaleal space or involve the overlying scalp to produce 'Pott's puffy tumour', and there is often an associated small extradural abscess. The infection is difficult to eradicate and may require removal of large areas of calvarium, which may subsequently be replaced with an acrylic plate.

Extradural abscess

Extradural abscess is usually secondary to osteomyelitis and most often occurs close to the middle ear, the mastoid air cells or the paranasal

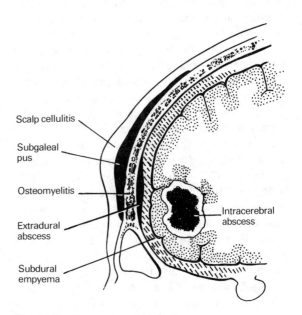

Fig. 40.17 Types of cranial infection

sinuses. Trauma is another cause. Pus may infiltrate the pericranium to produce Pott's puffy tumour and frequently breaks through the dura to produce meningitis, subdural empyema or cerebral abscess.

Systemic upset is usually severe. There is local tenderness, and focal neurological signs may result from thrombophlebitis of superficial cortical veins. Facial nerve paralysis is frequent when mastoiditis is the source.

Treatment involves administration of large doses of antibiotics, drainage, excision of any infected bone and drainage of infected sinuses or mastoid air cells as appropriate.

Subdural empyema

Subdural empyema (pus within the subdural space) is commoner than cerebral abscess in the western world. It may follow penetrating wounds or surgery, but is most commonly associated with paranasal or ear infection, which may spread to the subdural space along emissary veins or via dural sinuses.

Pus may spread over the whole hemisphere, beneath the falx, to involve the opposite hemisphere, or beneath the tentorium. It may accumulate in multiple sites, making treatment difficult. Although accumulation of pus exerts pressure on the brain, symptoms are largely due to venous thrombosis. Patients may present with disordered consciousness, paresis and epilepsy, or with signs of meningitis. Spread of infection is revealed by altering localizing signs. Deterioration of consciousness in patients with a history of frontal sinusitis or ear infection should arouse suspicion of subdural empyema.

Plain X-ray of the skull may reveal opaque air sinuses, but the diagnosis is confirmed by angiography or CT scan. Immediate treatment is indicated. Multiple burr holes are made to drain the pus, and catheters are inserted through which antibiotics are instilled 4-hourly in addition to systemic administration. The common infecting organisms are staphylococci and streptococci, which determines the choice of antibiotic until bacteriological reports are available. Occasionally, a large area of skull may have to be removed to achieve adequate decompression. Anticonvulsant treatment is continued indefinitely. Despite these measures, the mortality is 20–35%, and residual paresis and epilepsy are common.

Cerebral abscess

Although the brain is relatively resistant to infection, abscess formation may occur, particularly if there has been previous damage due to haemorrhage, trauma or anoxia. Initially there is a cerebritis (encephalitis) following which the brain tissue necroses to form pus surrounded by a tough glial capsule resistant to passage of antibiotics.

Abscesses may occur, in descending order of frequency, as a result of:
1. direct extension from the paranasal sinuses, mastoid or middle ear;
2. haematogenous spread, most commonly in patients with bronchiectasis or lung abscess, or in patients with cyanotic heart disease with a right-to-left shunt; or
3. direct penetrating trauma.

The presentation is often acute, with high fever, progressive disturbance of consciousness and evidence of increasing intracranial pressure. If the abscess is chronic and walled off, systemic signs of infection may be minimal and the patient may present with signs of a slowly expanding localized mass.

Diagnosis requires a high degree of suspicion and is now confirmed by CT scanning. Electroencephalography may show large delta waves.

Treatment. Urgent treatment is essential. In the acute stage of encephalitis, systemic antibiotics in high doses and anti-oedema agents are administered in an effort to localize the infection. Once localization has occurred, the abscess is drained through burr holes and a catheter is inserted into the cavity so that antibiotics can be instilled regularly. Alternatively, the abscess is tapped every few days with a brain cannula. Systemic antibiotics are continued for 10 days while the size of the cavity is monitored by CT scanning. If the patient does not become rapidly more alert following drainage of an abscess, excision is indicated. Encapsulated abscesses and cerebellar abscesses are excised.

Nearly 50% of patients with cerebral abscess develop epilepsy, and anticonvulsant therapy should be continued indefinitely. With early diagnosis, the mortality is low. The overall mortality rate of 30–50% reflects failure to make an early diagnosis.

Infections of the spine

Tuberculosis

Tuberculosis of the spine is still relatively common in Third World countries. The bovine bacillus, from infected milk, is the usual agent and most commonly affects the thoracic spine.

Infection initially affects the anterior border of one or more vertebral bodies where it causes caseous necrosis. It then spreads through the disc space to affect the adjacent vertebrae. The disc space narrows because of loss of fluid. A paraspinal abscess develops which may compress the cord and nerve roots, and the disc may sequestrate into the abscess. The anterior part of the vertebral body may collapse if there is sufficient damage, producing angulation (kyphosis) of the spine and, in severe forms, a gibbus. In 10% of patients angulation is severe enough to produce cord compression and paraplegia.

The patient presents with back pain, limitation of spinal movement and systemic signs of infection. Cord compression produces neurological deficits. Spinal X-rays show narrowing and irregularity of the disc space with erosion of the vertebral body, and a paravertebral abscess may be seen as a soft tissue mass. Angulation is seen with more advanced disease.

Early treatment carries a good prognosis, and even if cord compression has occurred from an epidural abscess, the chances of recovery are usually good. The late form of Pott's paraplegia is due to ischaemic changes in the cord and carries a poor prognosis for recovery. If tuberculosis is suspected, chemotherapy is instituted and the patient is nursed in bed in a plaster cast. Once adequate chemotherapy has been given, the diagnosis is confirmed by biopsy, infected material is removed and, if necessary, the spine is stabilized by bone grafting.

The presence of pus or signs of compression are indications for urgent drainage. All necrotic material is removed and bone grafts (from resected rib or iliac crest) are inserted to stabilize the spine.

Osteomyelitis of the spine

The usual infecting organism is *Staphylococcus aureus*. The infection most often arises as a result of haematogenous spread from boils, dental root infections, tonsillitis or otitis media, but may follow local trauma or operation.

The infection is most common in adolescence and early adulthood, and is much more common in males. In contrast to spinal tuberculosis, the lumbar region is most frequently infected, the illness is usually more acute and severe, and large paravertebral abscess and vertebral collapse are rare. Radiological signs are absent in the first 10–14 days, after which signs of bone erosion and regeneration and loss of disc space begin to appear.

Treatment consists of immobilization in a plaster cast and administration of large doses of the appropriate antibiotic, as determined by culture of material from the primary site or by blood culture. Any associated abscess should be drained via an anterolateral approach and the area debrided. If the resultant defect is large, bone grafting may be required.

Epidural abscess

Epidural abscess may arise from haematogenous spread (e.g. from an infected skin lesion or the urinary tract) or from local spread of a vertebral infection.

The patient develops severe pain and signs of cord compression, with retention of urine. Plain X-rays are usually normal in the absence of an established bone infection, but myelography confirms the compression.

Antibiotics and urgent evacuation of the pus are indicated. In the absence of local bone infection, a laminectomy approach is used, but an anterolateral approach can be used if the abscess is secondary to vertebral infection.

NEOPLASMS

Intracranial tumours

Primary intracranial tumours show a bimodal age incidence, with a small peak at 6–7 years of age, a decline until puberty, and thereafter a progressive rise in incidence, with a maximum in the fifth decade. Both sexes are equally affected. Apart from certain tumours such as cholesteatomas and craniopharyngiomas, which arise from cell remnants, their cause is unknown. They rarely metastasize, and death usually results from the consequences of continued growth within the confined space of the skull.

About 50% of intracranial tumours are metastatic, the most frequent primary sources being lung and breast. Intracranial tumours may present with general or localized effects. Diagnosis is easy when tumours are large, but early diagnosis while the tumour is still small facilitates treatment and improves prognosis.

CT scanning and angiography (Fig. 40.18) are essential investigations in the diagnosis and localization of intracranial tumours. Histological verification is mandatory and a tumour biopsy should be obtained if at all possible. Cell culture is important for immunological investigation and determination of sensitivity to treatment.

Tumours arising from the skull

Osteoma

This relatively common benign tumour is usually solitary. It usually arises in a paranasal sinus or in the orbit. Osteomas usually grow outwards to produce a palpable hard mass but may grow inwards to compress the underlying brain and meninges. Osteomas growing within a sinus may produce obstruction and sinusitis, while those in the orbit may cause proptosis and diplopia.

Symptomatic osteomas should be excised.

Chordoma

These rare malignant neoplasms are thought to arise from remnants of the notochord. They occur in the spheno-occipital region of the skull or the sacrococcygeal region of the spine. They are highly vascular, firm grey tumours which erode bone and, in the skull, invade the optic chiasma, the sella and cavernous sinus. They also displace the pons. Although malignant, they are relatively slow-growing. Complete surgical removal is rarely possible, but radiotherapy may slow the growth rate and prolong life for a few years.

Glomus jugulare tumours

These tumours arise in the middle ear and invade the posterior fossa. They often present with bleeding from the ear and examination reveals a soft fleshy red mass protruding through the drum. Invasion of the internal jugular vein is common. Invasion of the middle ear produces tinnitus, deafness and facial paresis, while intracranial growth produces signs and symptoms of a cerebellar pontine angle tumour.

Radical excision of the petrous and occipital bones followed by irradiation is indicated.

Histiocytosis

This group of disorders is characterized by tumours which contain histiocytes and which erode bone.

Eosinophilic granuloma normally presents between the ages of 8 and 15 years as a solitary lesion in the skull or spine. It causes pain, swelling, tenderness and systemic disturbance. The prognosis is good: some lesions resolve spontaneously, others heal after curettage and/or radiotherapy.

Hand-Schuller-Christian disease becomes manifest in earlier childhood. The tumour usually

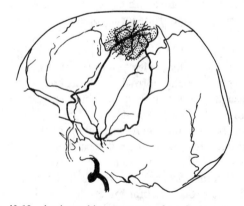

Fig. 40.18 Angiographic appearance of meningioma

involves the base of the skull to produce proptosis and diabetes insipidus, and occasionally other pituitary dysfunction. Its progress, though steady, is usually slow and relatively benign, but in 25% the prognosis remains poor despite radiotherapy.

Letterer-Siwe disease may be regarded as an acute form of Hand-Schuller-Christian disease, with onset in infancy. In addition to the skull, many other organs are involved. Progression is rapid, leading to death within weeks.

Multiple myeloma

Myeloma usually occurs after the age of 50 years and affects males twice as often as females. The tumour is multicentric and, in addition to the skull, vertebrae and other bones are involved. The condition may be confused with metastases from a primary solid tumour. Systemic cytotoxic chemotherapy is indicated.

Paget's disease (osteitis deformans)

This condition of unknown aetiology produces thickening, softening and deformity of bone which later densely scleroses. Both sexes are equally affected and the condition usually begins between the fourth and sixth decades. The skull is most frequently affected and is enlarged and thickened. When the base of the skull is involved, encroachment on the optic or auditory foramina may produce visual or auditory disturbance. Sarcomatous change occurs in 10% of patients.

There is no known treatment and management is usually confined to pain relief. Entrapped nerves may require surgical decompression, while radiotherapy is effective in the management of localized pain. Calcitonin is used increasingly in systemic management.

Metastatic tumour

The skull is a common site for metastases from cancers of the lung, breast, prostate, thyroid and kidney. The lesions are usually osteolytic, although metastases from breast and prostate may be osteoblastic. Local radiotherapy may be indicated for a rapidly enlarging metastatic tumour.

Tumours arising from the meninges

Meningiomas

These account for 20% of all brain tumours. They arise from arachnoidal cells and are therefore most commonly found close to the intracranial sinuses. About 90% occur in the supratentorial region. They are slow-growing and often highly vascular, deriving most of their blood supply from meningeal vessels. They are usually rounded or bossellated and embedded in the brain, but tumour cells may invade bone or spread widely over the dura (meningioma en plaque). The overlying skull may be rarefied or thickened (due to hyperostosis) with production of a palpable mass.

The signs caused by meningiomas depend on their location. The parasagittal region is the commonest site for supratentorial meningiomas, and their proximity to the motor cortex results in focal seizures, particularly in the leg. They frequently invade the sagittal sinus.

Meningiomas are treated by surgical excision. If the sagittal sinus is involved, it should be resected and replaced with a vein graft to reduce the risk of recurrence.

Pituitary and parapituitary tumours

Pituitary tumours (see also Ch. 23) account for 15% of all intracranial tumours. They produce effects due partly to endocrine change and partly to local pressure (Fig. 40.19)

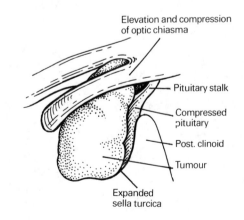

Elevation and compression of optic chiasma

Pituitary stalk

Compressed pituitary

Post. clinoid

Tumour

Expanded sella turcica

Fig. 40.19 Pituitary tumour

Chromophobe adenoma

This, the commonest of the pituitary tumours, is occasionally cystic due to haemorrhage. Gradual tumour growth compresses the remaining pituitary tissue, producing hypopituitarism, and expands and erodes the sella turcica. Penetration of the roof of the sella causes pressure on the optic chiasma and nerves, giving rise to the characteristic visual field defect of bitemporal hemianopia.

The tumour is removed via a craniotomy or by the transphenoidal route (Fig. 40.20). Residual tumour is treated by postoperative radiotherapy.

Eosinophilic adenoma

The tumour is usually small (a microadenoma) and its effects are due to oversecretion of growth hormone. In children the tumour causes gigantism, but it usually occurs in middle life, causing acromegaly. The eosinophilic adenoma is not infrequently part of a chromophobe adenoma, and is then associated with the features of local expansion described above.

The tumour is usually removed by a transphenoidal approach, leaving the rest of the pituitary intact (see Fig. 40.20). Pituitary irradiation has the disadvantage that normal pituitary tissue is also destroyed. Recently, bromocriptine (in a dose increasing up to 20 mg daily) has been used successfully but treatment must be continued indefinitely. Dizziness, postural hypotension and confusional states may be troublesome side effects.

Prolactinomas

These tumours cause galactorrhea and amenorrhea. They are frequently microadenomas but may enlarge, particularly during pregnancy, when they may cause visual defects. Bromocriptine is useful in reducing tumour bulk prior to surgery.

Basophilic adenoma

These rare microadenomas secrete ACTH and occur more commonly in women. Oversecretion of ACTH results in Cushing's disease (see Ch. 23).

The preferred treatment is transphenoidal removal of the tumour.

Craniopharyngioma

These tumours develop in remnants of Rathke's pouch and present either in childhood or in later life. Most are multicystic and they may reach a large size. The majority lie anterior to the pituitary stalk, although some may occur within the sella.

Visual field defects occur early and are due to compression. Progressive growth results in hypopituitarism due to hypothalamic involvement, and eventually causes signs and symptoms of raised intracranial pressure.

Complete surgical removal is the treatment of choice for small solid tumours. If the tumour is large, and particularly if it is cystic, puncture and aspiration of the cyst contents followed by radiotherapy is safer and more effective.

Cholesteatoma

These tumours are characteristically pearly-white and glistening, and are composed of layers of large finely granular cells. They may arise in the suprasellar region but are most commonly found in the posterior fossa at the cerebellopontine angle or within the fourth ventricle or cerebellum.

Complete removal is not often possible, but partial removal often prolongs survival.

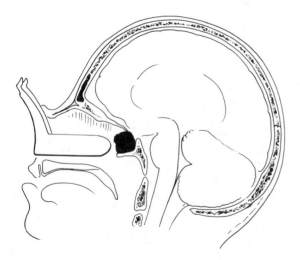

Fig. 40.20 Transphenoidal approach to pituitary tumour

(This condition should not be confused with cholesteatoma of the middle ear.)

Neurinomas

Neurinomas of the cranial nerves account for about 5% of primary intracranial tumours and affect almost exclusively the acoustic nerve. Bilateral tumours may occur in generalized neurofibromatosis but are rare.

The tumour develops within the internal auditory meatus, which it erodes and expands. The 8th and 7th cranial nerves become stretched over the tumour as it grows into the cerebellopontine angle (Fig. 40.21). Early symptoms are due to 8th nerve involvement and include progressive nerve deafness, tinnitus and vertigo. Further tumour growth results in 7th nerve compression and facial weakness, while upward extension may damage the trigeminal nerve and lead to diminution in facial sensation. Large tumours may eventually compress the pons and cerebellum and cause ataxia and nystagmus, while gradual displacement of the brainstem angulates the aqueduct and fourth ventricle to produce internal hydrocephalus. The neurinoma may reach a large size before the patient is first seen by the surgeon. Patients with early symptoms are frequently misdiagnosed as having Menière's disease.

Plain X-rays show enlargement of the internal

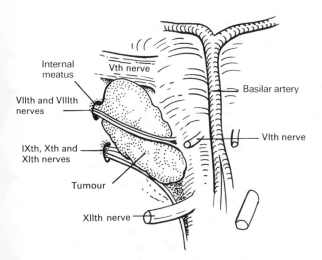

Fig. 40.21 Right acoustic tumour in the cerebellopontine angle seen from the front

auditory meatus, while the tumour itself is usually clearly demonstrated by CT scanning.

Treatment consists of surgical removal via a posterior fossa approach. It is usually possible to preserve the facial nerve if the operating microscope is used and the effects of nerve stimulation are carefully observed.

Intracerebral tumours

Metastatic tumours

Metastatic tumours account for almost 50% of intracerebral neoplasms, the common primary sites being lung and breast. They are found in about 20% of autopsies in patients with cancer. They are multiple in about 50% and because of the breakdown in the blood-brain barrier are usually associated with considerable oedema. About 80% of patients have papilloedema.

Multiple metastases are inoperable and are best treated by cytotoxic therapy or hormonal manipulation, if appropriate (e.g. breast). Whole-brain radiotherapy may produce some improvement, while gross oedema can be reduced by steroids such as dexamethasone. If a metastasis is single and accessible, the patient is otherwise well and there is no evidence of wide extension of the primary tumour, surgical removal of the metastasis may be considered. The surgical mortality is less than 10% and survival ranges from 3 to 12 months. although in patients without a demonstrable primary tumour the median survival is about 2 years.

Gliomas

Gliomas arising from the supporting cells of the brain (the glia) are much the commonest primary brain tumour and account for 25% of all intracranial tumours. They are classified histologically as astrocytomas and oligodendrogliomas. Astrocytomas are often initially slow-growing, but may be rapidly invasive (glioblastoma multiforma). The less common oligodendrogliomas are slow-growing, sometimes become calcified and have less tendency to infiltrate the brain.

Complete removal of gliomas is difficult and is often prevented by infiltration of the tumour. The cerebellar astrocytoma of childhood is an exception in that removal is usually feasible and curative. Gliomas confined to a single lobe may be removed by lobectomy, but more usually resection is incomplete. Recurrence is common despite postoperative radiotherapy, but may take several years before becoming manifest. Unfortunately, many gliomas occupy vital cerebral areas, for example the speech area, so that radical removal would produce unacceptable brain damage, in this case aphasia and hemiplegia. A humane surgeon will therefore not subject these patients to radical surgery. Judicious use of radiotherapy, steroids, chemotherapy and immunotherapy are preferable in such cases and will prolong useful independent life for many months. Hydrocephalus may be treated by appropriate shunts, while aspiration of unresectable cystic tumours usually results in considerable improvement in the patient's condition.

Some gliomas present as emergencies with rapid onset of coma and decerebration. Prompt administration of anti-oedema agents, and ventricular drainage to relieve hydrocephalus may improve the patient's condition and allow adequate investigation and appropriate definitive treatment.

Ependymomas

Ependymomas arise from ependyma in the walls of the ventricles, and from ependymal remnants in the central canal (see later). They are most common in the fourth ventricle and produce hydrocephalus. They may emerge from the fourth ventricle into the cisterna and spread over the brainstem, producing multiple cranial nerve palsies.

With the help of the operating microscope many of these tumours can now be safely and completely removed.

Medulloblastomas

These malignant tumours of childhood arise from the roof of the fourth ventricle and, like ependymomas, tend to seed through the cerebrospinal fluid pathways, so that in some patients the presenting symptoms may be due to lumbar or sacral root lesions. Treatment consists of partial

removal followed by radiotherapy to the entire central nervous system.

Tumour biopsy

The importance of histological verification of tumour type cannot be overemphasized if appropriate treatment is to be instituted. Stereotactic biopsy has now replaced other methods of tumour sampling.

Spinal tumours

Primary spinal tumours are about one-sixth as common as intracranial tumours. Almost 60% are benign, and many of the remainder are radiosensitive to varying degrees and thus have a better prognosis than intracranial lesions. Metastatic tumours are as common as primary tumours.

The majority of spinal tumours arise in relation to the coverings. The commonest early symptoms are pain due to root displacement and associated mild spastic paraparesis, more marked in one leg, which may drag during walking. Bladder function is usually impaired. Intrinsic tumours of the cord (intramedullary tumours) account for only 5% of spinal tumours and, in contrast to extramedullary tumours, usually present with sensory symptoms and signs due to involvement of the decussating spinothalamic pain and temperature fibres.

Clinical differentiation between intra- and extramedullary tumours is not always easy. Plain radiology plus myelography are needed to make the distinction.

Epidural tumours

Epidural tumours account for more than half (55%) of all spinal tumours. About 90% are malignant and 75% are due to metastatic spread from a primary site elsewhere.

Lymphoma is the commonest non-metastatic tumour, but leukaemic infiltration and myeloma may also involve the epidural space and produce cord compression. Metastatic deposits in the vertebrae may be the first manifestation of the disease, and tumour cells may enter the epidural space. These lesions most commonly affect the thoracic spine, and symptoms progress rapidly.

Treatment consists of decompression, laminectomy and removal of the epidural tumour, followed by local radiotherapy and systemic treatment appropriate to the primary disease.

Intradural tumours

Intradural tumours account for 45% of all spinal tumours. The great majority are extramedullary rather than intramedullary. Nearly all intradural tumours are primary tumours and more than half are benign. Progression tends to be slow, in contrast to epidural lesions.

Extramedullary tumours. Meningiomas and schwannomas are the common lesions. Meningiomas are ten times as common in females as in males. They are firm hemispherical tumours occurring most commonly in the thoracic region. They usually present after the age of 40 years and compress the cord and nerve roots. Surgical removal is followed by an excellent prognosis.

Schwannomas affect the sensory roots more commonly than the motor roots. They tend to grow out through the intervertebral foramen and expand, producing a 'dumb-bell' tumour. They are as common as meningiomas. The much less common neurofibroma occurs as part of generalized neurofibromatosis. The prognosis is excellent following removal of the tumour, although the attached nerve root may have to be resected.

Intramedullary tumours. Ependymomas are the commonest intramedullary lesion and usually affect the conus and filum terminale. They arise at the centre of the cord and expand slowly rather than invade. Complete removal is often possible and is followed by a good prognosis.

Gliomas, usually astrogliomas, are most often found in the thoracic region. They infiltrate the cord to produce a fusiform swelling. They can usually not be removed completely but with microscopic techniques incomplete removal followed by radiotherapy may allow survival for 5 years or longer.

MISCELLANEOUS CONDITIONS

Disorders of movement

Parkinson's disease

Parkinson's disease affects 0.1% of the population overall, with an incidence of 1% in those over 50 years of age. The characteristic histological features are depigmentation of the substantia nigra and the presence of inclusion bodies in many neurones of the brainstem nuclei and spinal cord grey matter. The cause is unknown in 80% of cases (idiopathic parkinsonism). Postencephalic parkinsonism has an earlier onset than the idiopathic form. It usually becomes manifest 10–20 years after an attack of encephalitis. Blepharospasm and oculogyric crises are particularly common in this form of the disease.

Arteriosclerotic parkinsonism occurs in older patients and is often of sudden onset. Rigidity and akinesia are more common than tremor. Psychotropic drug-induced parkinsonism may follow administration of drugs such as the phenothiazines. The condition regresses in two-thirds of patients following withdrawal of the drug.

The onset of tremor, akinesia or bradykinesia, and rigidity may be sudden or insidious. Common early complaints include a painful limb, clumsiness or weakness. The tremor is often unilateral and affects distal muscles. The fully developed clinical picture is unmistakeable with the mask-like face, flexed posture, festinating gait and tremor. Swallowing becomes difficult, leading to drooling and aspiration, and weight loss is common. Idiopathic parkinsonism is progressive, leading to death or severe disability in 15–20 years.

The majority of patients are treated medically, surgery being reserved for patients with severe tremor. Stereotactic radiofrequency lesions are made in the *nucleus ventralis lateralis* of the thalamus, which is an important relay centre of the motor system. Results are good.

Chorea

Chorea causes rapid and purposeless involuntary contractions of facial or limb muscles at rest which also interfere with voluntary movement. Chorea may follow thrombosis of brainstem vessels. *Huntington's chorea* is an autosomal dominant disorder associated with progressive dementia, which becomes evident in adult life. There is widespread neuronal loss in the cortex, caudate and putamen. Although stereotactic thalamotomy will relieve chorea it is rarely undertaken.

Choreoathetosis

Choreoathetosis with spasticity is common in young patients with cerebral palsy. Stereotactic dentatotomy converts the spastic paresis into a flaccid one, improves speech and feeding, and allows the limbs to attain greater facility.

Torsion dystonia

This disease is characterized by sustained muscle contractions, which may be spasmodic or continuous. It usually results from birth injury or cerebral anoxia, but is occasionally inherited. Partial forms are relatively common in adults (e.g. orofacial dyskinesia and dystonia or torticollis). A good response is often obtained by stereotactic thalamotomy or dentatotomy.

Epilepsy

Onset of epilepsy at any age requires investigation to determine its cause. This is particularly important in *late-onset epilepsy*, which is often due to a tumour or vascular lesions which may be relieved by surgery. Epilepsy may continue after removal of the cause, but is then usually easier to control by long-term anticonvulsant therapy.

Idiopathic epilepsy can usually be managed satisfactorily by drug therapy, but if satisfactory control cannot be achieved, surgery is considered after accurate localization of the focus of discharge. A cortical lesion may be carefully excised, using electrocorticography to ensure that the whole of the epileptic focus is removed.

Temporal lobe epilepsy is not infrequently associated with definite, though small, cortical or subcortical haematomas. If the focus is well-localized, temporal lobectomy gives excellent results.

Intractable grand mal seizures sometimes respond to stereotactic thalamotomy.

Psychiatric disorders amenable to surgery

Surgical treatment of mental disorder has been discredited by the indiscriminate use of gross frontal leucotomy in the past and is only now regaining reputable status. Full cooperation with the referring psychiatrist is essential, and surgery is only recommended after frank discussion with the patient and his or her relatives. In the UK the provisions of the Mental Health Act (1983) must be considered.

Intractable anxiety states which do not respond to medical treatment may be improved by a discrete stereotactic leucotomy which interrupts white matter pathways from various parts of the limbic lobe, such as the orbital frontal gyri.

Aggressive disorders, particularly those associated with temporal lobe epilepsy, may respond to stereotactic amygdalotomy.

Hyperactivity of severe grade is difficult to manage, but stereotactic hypothalotomy is sometimes useful.

INTRACTABLE PAIN

Intractable pain (i.e. pain not responding to conservative measures) requires careful assessment before recommending procedures which themselves may be extensive or hazardous. A detailed history and clinical examination are essential, and factors which exacerbate the pain should be noted. It is also important to determine whether the pain is in any way related to anxiety or drug dependence or whether it is a means of seeking attention. Many hospitals now operate special 'pain clinics' where patients are examined and their problems are discussed by a team of physicians, surgeons, anaesthetists and psychiatrists before management is initiated.

Intractable pain may be iatrogenic. Careful attention to surgical technique and adequate reassurance and information both before and after the operation reduces this risk. Adequate pain relief should always be provided during the painful early postoperative period, but powerful analgesics (which carry a high risk of addiction) are rarely required for more than 48 hours.

Some patients seeking pain relief merely require reassurance while others may need a change in their drug regimen. A third group, however, merit specific treatment of an underlying cause. Surgical procedures to relieve pain should not incapacitate the patient and should aim to secure complete and long-lasting relief. Patients with incurable malignant disease in whom survival is likely to be short

Table 40.2 Surgical treatment of intractable pain

Peripheral procedures	Central procedures
Neurectomy	*Spinal cord*
Surgical posterior	Spinothalamic tractotomy
rhizotomy	(cordotomy)
Intrathecal chemical	Myelotomy
rhizotomy	
Epidural techniques	*Brainstem*
	Spinothalamic tractotomy
	Thalamus
	Thalamotomy

are not usually considered for surgical procedures, provided their pain can be controlled by drugs without severe side effects. Patients with a longer expectation of life and those in whom life-expectancy is shortened by analgesic drugs should be offered surgery. The success rate is high in patients with malignant disease, possibly because they die from the disease before the pain recurs. In patients with pain from benign disease the success rate is lower (except in those with clear-cut conditions such as trigeminal neuralgia).

The procedures available for surgical pain relief are summarized in Table 40.2.

Peripheral procedures

Peripheral neurectomy

Most nerves are mixed nerves so that peripheral neurectomy produces not only anaesthesia but also paresis and loss of other normal sensation. Facial pain is an exception, as neurectomy can be limited to purely sensory fibres. Splanchnicectomy, now usually performed chemically by local injection of alcohol, is sometimes helpful in the management of intractable upper abdominal pain such as that due to pancreatic cancer.

Posterior rhizotomy

Posterior rhizotomy (division of nerve roots) is a satisfactory procedure for pain syndromes due to direct nerve involvement, but because of the extensive overlap of dermatomes (especially on the trunk) several nerve roots have to be divided to

obtain a relatively small area of anaesthesia. Surgical rhizotomy requires extensive laminectomy and is now often replaced by *percutaneous rhizotomy*. Electrodes are introduced percutaneously into the appropriate intervertebral foramina, and the roots are destroyed by electro- or radio-frequency coagulation. The procedure may be repeated, and is suitable for patients in poor general condition. Percutaneous rhizotomy carries a greater risk of motor root injury than surgical rhizotomy.

Intrathecal chemical rhizotomy

This is suitable for patients with pain involving a large area or multiple sites. Injection of alcohol is effective but carries a high risk of paresis so that its use is restricted to those already paralysed. Phenol produces fewer unwanted side effects and may control pain for many months. Hypertonic saline is the safest of all, but pain relief rarely lasts for more than 3 months. It is therefore most suitable for patients with a short life expectancy.

Intrathecal steroids

Local intrathecal injection of steroids is sometimes effective in the management of chronic back pain (particularly chronic lumbar pain from arthritis) and severe continuous pain following laminectomy. The effect is quite unpredictable, but some patients obtain relief of pain for a few weeks. The effect is presumed to be due to a local anti-inflammatory action but there may be a strong placebo component.

Epidural anaesthesia

Epidural anaesthesia has become increasingly popular in recent years and has the advantage that an epidural catheter can be left in situ postoperatively so that the level of analgesia may be topped up if necessary, thus avoiding the need for systemic opiates. When used for intractable pain, epidural anaesthesia has the disadvantage of providing only temporary relief.

Epidural morphine. Recent work demonstrating the presence of morphine receptors within the cord has stimulated the use of epidural morphine in the management of postoperative and chronic pain. The results are still uncertain.

Central procedures

Spinothalamic tractotomy (cordotomy)

Spinothalamic tractotomy (Fig. 40.22) is an excellent operation for pain relief in patients with malignant disease when life expectancy exceeds 6 months. It is less satisfactory for those with pain due to benign causes. Cordotomy removes pain and temperature sensation but preserves touch. It is usually performed at the cervical level, but section at C1 is required to obtain analgesia of arm and shoulder.

The procedure is usually performed percutaneously, using either rough aiming or a stereotactic technique. Local anaesthesia is used to allow the patient to be assessed during the operation and thus reduce the risk of damage to motor tracts and to bladder and respiratory fibres.

Myelotomy

Bilateral cordotomy carries a high risk of respiratory or bladder dysfunction and is very rarely indicated. However, bilateral analgesia can be produced by cutting the cord longitudinally in the midline and thus dividing the decussating fibres (see Fig. 40.22). This is done as an open procedure in the lumbar region and is useful for

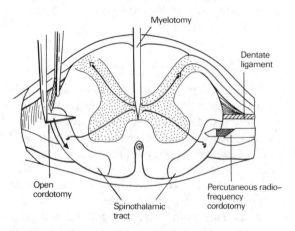

Fig. 40.22 Spinal cord tractotomy and myelotomy for intractable pain

intractable pain following abdominoperineal excision of the rectum. Cervical myelotomy for pain arising at higher levels is usually carried out by a percutaneous stereotactic technique.

Brainstem tractotomy

The spinothalamic tract can be divided at the medullary level to relieve widespread cervical and facial pain. The risk of operative damage to neighbouring structures is reduced if a stereotactic technique is employed.

Thalamotomy

Stereotactic thalamotomy is useful in patients with long-standing pain or pain which seems to be of central (affective) origin, and in those in whom a more peripheral procedure has failed. Alternatively, stimulating electrodes can be placed in thalamic nuclei which can be activated by the patient using a battery-operated coil placed subcutaneously.

Additional techniques

Cingulotomy

Severe pain is often accompanied by emotional distress, especially in terminal malignancy, so that a technically successful pain-relieving procedure may not provide the expected relief. Addition of a simple tranquillizer may be effective, but in some patients with this so-called 'psychic' pain, stereotactic cingulotomy to interrupt circuits in the limbic system may be required.

Sympathectomy

The use of splanchnicectomy in the management of intractable abdominal pain, e.g. from chronic pancreatitis, has been mentioned. Sympathectomy is also effective in relief of *causalgia*, the burning pain and autonomic dysfunction that results from partial injury to major nerve trunks.

Electroanalgesia

Newer techniques using nerve fibre stimulation rather than destruction have been introduced following the demonstration that stimulation of a peripheral nerve trunk reduces pain sensation over the distribution of the nerve. Activation of A fibres may interfere with the perception of a painful stimulus, possibly at spinal cord level, or there may be a release of enkephalins.

Electrodes are implanted close to the nerve trunk in question, or at higher levels in the nervous system such as the high epidural spine, which can be activated by the patient using a small power pack when he feels the need for more analgesia. Early results are encouraging but require fuller assessment.

Hormonal ablation

Hypophysectomy for the relief of pain due to metastases from hormone-dependent tumours, particularly those arising from the breast or prostate, is no longer popular, and has been largely superseded by antihormone drug therapy.

Trigeminal neuralgia

The standard treatment of trigeminal neuralgia used to be long-term administration of the drug carbamazepine. However, adverse drug reactions such as rash, drowsiness and ataxia are frequent, and pain recurrence after months or years is not uncommon. Consequently, radiofrequency trigeminal rhizotomy is now recommended for initial treatment. It produces analgesia without loss of ordinary sensation in the face and the corneal reflex is preserved.

Pain relief in advanced oropharyngeal cancer

Extensive analgesia is required. This may be achieved by dividing, through a posterior fossa approach, the 5th nerve, nervus intermedius, 9th and 10th cranial nerves and the upper three cervical nerves on the appropriate side. This is a major procedure in debilitated patients and better results are obtained by stereotactic tractotomy of the trigeminal tract of the upper cervical cord under local anaesthesia.

SPECIAL NEUROSURGICAL TECHNIQUES

Access

While the general principles of all surgical operative techniques apply in neurosurgery, there are certain specific requirements of access to the nervous system.

Burr holes

Burr holes are simple skull perforations made to remove fluid, pus or blood from the cranium, or to enable instruments to be passed into the brain. The standard burr holes are made in the frontal, parietal and occipitoparietal regions along the pupillary plane (Fig. 40.23). Temporal burr holes may be made immediately above the zygoma to allow access to the middle meningeal artery in extradural haematoma, or directly above the root of the ear to drain a temporal lobe abscess.

After shaving the head, local anaesthetic sol-

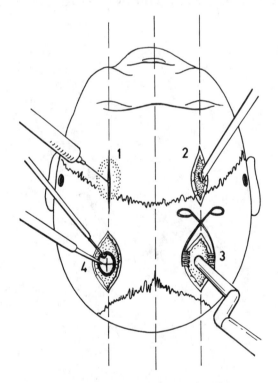

Fig. 40.23 Sites of standard burr holes. Technique: (1) infiltration and incision; (2) scraping away the pericranium; (3) drilling of cranium; (4) incision of dura

ution with adrenaline is injected into the skin of the scalp. If the procedure is being done under general anaesthesia, 1:200 000 adrenaline solution is used to assist haemostasis. An incision is made down to bone and the pericranium scraped away. A small self-retaining retractor is placed in the wound and the skull is perforated using a brace and bit. A burr is then used to enlarge and smooth out the hole. Modern power tools combine these functions. The dura is now exposed. It is picked up with a sharp hook and opened using a cruciate incision (see Fig. 40.23).

For temporal and occipital burr holes the overlying muscle must first be incised and retracted to expose the skull.

Craniotomy

A flap of skin and skull is formed which is replaced over the defect at the end of the procedure.

The line of incision is marked out and infiltrated with a solution of local anaesthetic and adrenaline

in saline. The scalp incision is made with the assistant compressing the scalp against the skull to reduce bleeding. Artery forceps or clamps are then applied to the scalp edges to prevent further bleeding. The scalp flap is elevated, and the lines of incision in the skull are marked by diathermy. The pericranium is incised and scraped away from the lines of incision.

Burr holes are now made. Using a guide, a Gigli saw is passed under the skull between two burr holes and the skull is divided between these two points. This process is repeated until the bone has been completely separated from the skull. A small muscle attachment is usually left to carry the blood supply to the skull flap (Fig. 40.24).

This classical technique is being replaced with the quicker and easier method of using a straight incision and skin retraction. Only two temporal burr holes are needed and the bone flap is cut using a craniotome.

Bleeding from the exposed dura is controlled by diathermy or gelatin packs, or by dural traction. This is achieved by suturing the periphery of the dura to the pericranium around the defect (Fig. 40.25). Raised intracranial pressure, as evidenced by a tight dura, may be reduced by mannitol or ventricular puncture.

The dura is then opened after elevation on a

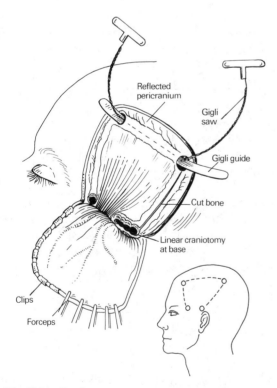

Fig. 40.24 Craniotomy

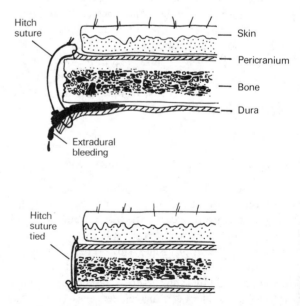

Fig. 40.25 Control of dural bleeding with 'hitch' sutures

small hook, and the incision is extended with scissors while the brain is protected by a small swab.

Craniectomy

In urgent situations, e.g. when immediate access is required for removal of an intracranial haematoma, there may not be time to 'turn a flap'. A single burr hole is then made and extended by piecemeal excision of the skull with bone forceps, making a defect referred to as a craniectomy. The defect may have to be corrected at a later date by insertion of a plastic or metal mould (cranioplasty).

Craniectomy is always used for posterior fossa exploration, as the thick posterior neck muscles will cover the area without leaving an unsightly defect.

Laminectomy

Exposure of the spinal cord and nerves is achieved by partial or complete laminectomy. The skin and underlying muscles are infiltrated down to the laminae with a solution of local anaesthetic and adrenaline and an incision is made down to the spinous processes. The wound is held open with a self-retaining retractor. The paraspinal muscles are then separated from the processes and lamina, and retracted with a larger self-retaining retractor (Fig. 40.26).

The spinal processes over the desired length of spine are removed at their bases, and the lamina is removed with bone rongeurs, taking care to protect the underlying spinal dura. The dura is incised longitudinally and its cut edges are sutured to the muscles.

In partial laminectomies or (hemilaminectomies) the spinal processes are preserved while the lamina is removed on one side. In *fenestration* procedures for the removal of a prolapsed intervertebral disc, the disc and nerve root are exposed by opening the ligamentum flavum at the appropriate level and, if necessary, removing a small piece of adjoining lamina.

Stereotactic surgery

First used in experimental animals in 1906, and

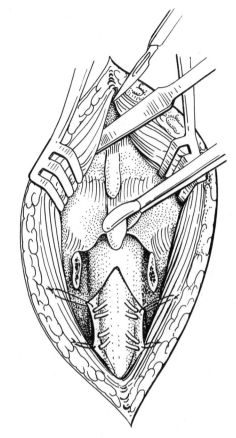

Fig. 40.26 Laminectomy

introduced into clinical practice in 1947, stereotactic surgery is being increasingly used in neurosurgery.

Although the apparatus needed for stereotactic operations may seem complex, the underlying principles are simple, enabling the operator to determine the position of a point in space relative to a known reference point or points. Most stereotactic frames employ the Cartesian coordinate system with three fixed intersecting planes at right angles — coronal, sagittal and horizontal (Fig. 40.27). The position of a point in space can be defined in all three planes, and a probe moved precisely to that point.

The instrument is securely fastened to the skull (or spine) and, using specially prepared brain or spinal stereotactic atlases, the coordinates of the target area are determined. Accuracy may be improved by injection of radio-opaque material to

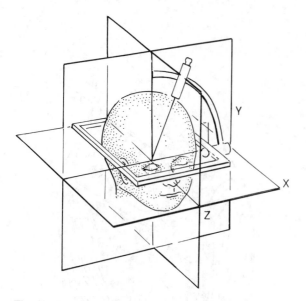

Fig. 40.27   Principles of stereotactic apparatus used to locate (and treat) the target area

outline the ventricles or by obtaining electrical recordings from known areas. Under fluoroscopy, on which a measuring grid also appears, the tip of the probe is advanced to the target area. A lesion is then made by either cutting (using a leucotome), freezing (using a cryoprobe), heating (by radiofrequency electrode) or irradiation (using isotopes). Alternatively, stimulating electrodes may be introduced and left in situ if required. Recent renewed interest in the technique has centred mainly on its use for accurate tumour biopsy or excision and for interstitial radiation (by introducing radioactive isotopes).

41. Practical procedures

PROCEDURES ON BLOOD VESSELS

Venepuncture

The antecubital fossa is the most convenient site for venepuncture. Here the median cubital vein, median vein of forearm and the cephalic vein are easily accessible, but the median nerve and the brachial artery must be avoided. A 21-gauge needle is used for adults and a 23-gauge needle for children. A venous tourniquet is placed around the upper arm. Small veins become more engorged if the fist is clenched several times or if the veins are tapped briskly. The skin is cleaned with isopropyl alcohol and the elbow is fully extended. The needle is inserted obliquely through the skin overlying the vein in a 'two-step' fashion: first through the skin, then through the vein wall. A distinct reduction of resistance to the passage of the needle is appreciated as the lumen of the vein is entered. The needle is advanced 2 or 3 mm within the vein and then stabilized with the left thumb (Fig. 41.1). The plunger of the syringe is *gently* withdrawn until the volume of blood required is obtained (too rapid withdrawal may cause haemolysis which can invalidate some results, e.g. potassium). The tour-

niquet is released and the needle is withdrawn. Pressure over the puncture site for one minute prevents haematoma formation. The needle is removed from the syringe and the blood is gently injected into appropriate tubes. Tubes which contain anticoagulants must be gently inverted several times to allow sufficient mixing to prevent clot formation. The tubes are now labelled with the patient's name and hospital number, and the time and date of sampling. Preliminary or delayed labelling introduces an unacceptable risk of error.

Venepuncture for blood culture

This requires more careful preparation than routine venepuncture. The hands are washed and dried on a sterile towel. An assistant applies the venous tourniquet. The patient's skin is prepared with isopropyl alcohol applied with a sterile cotton wool ball carried on sterile forceps. Venepuncture is performed with strict 'no-touch' technique and blood is withdrawn. The needle is then withdrawn from the vein and removed from the syringe and a second needle is substituted to inject 5 ml aliquots of blood into paired blood culture bottles (two aerobic, two anaerobic). All bottles are immediately sent to the laboratory and/or placed in an incubator at 37°C.

Peripheral venous cannulation

Most intravenous infusions are given into the cephalic vein in the forearm or into a vein on the flexor or extensor aspect of the forearm. In these situations the cannula does not cross joints, making splints unnecessary and allowing the patient to use the arm freely. Cannula units com-

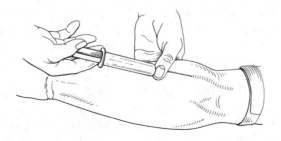

Fig. 41.1 Venepuncture

673

prise an outer polythene or Teflon sheath, the cannula proper, and an inner metal needle. A large variety are commercially available and 'Venflon', 'Intraflon', 'Abbocath', 'Quick-Cath' and 'Medicut' are all easy to use. A 16- or 18-gauge cannula is used for most purposes in adults but a 14-gauge cannula is required for rapid blood transfusion. The preliminary preparation for venepuncture is repeated. A small bleb of local anaesthetic is raised intradermally at the proposed site of skin puncture. The vein is steadied by the left thumb which applies gentle pressure and traction distally. Venepuncture is made with the cannula unit and is confirmed by 'flashback' of blood into the observation chamber. The cannula unit is then advanced up the vein while the right hand withdraws the inner metal needle. The venous tourniquet is released, the infusion tubing set (previously primed with isotonic saline solution) is connected to the cannula and the infusion started. The cannula is fixed securely to the skin with adhesive tape and the infusion tubing folded in a U-loop and secured with adhesive tape (Fig. 41.2).

Peripheral intravenous cannulation requires no more than clean hands, antiseptic skin preparation and a strict 'no-touch' technique for the part of the cannula which lodges within the vein. Cannula sites are inspected daily and the cannula is removed at the first sign of swelling, erythema or tenderness over the vein.

Central venous cannulation

Central venous cannulation allows measurement of central venous pressure and can be used for parenteral nutrition. Long cannulas (60 cm) are inserted via the basilic vein at the elbow, while short cannulas (20–30 cm) are inserted directly into the subclavian or internal jugular veins. Cannula units vary considerably but a 16-gauge cannula is generally used. Systems in which a Teflon cannula is introduced through and retained by a shorter outer cannula (e.g. Surcath, Intramedicut) are preferred. This avoids the risk of accidental division of the cannula and possible embolization inherent in systems in which the cannula is introduced through and retained by a metal needle (e.g. Bardicath, Drum-Cartridge). Silastic cannulas specially designed for long-term intravenous nutrition are also available (e.g. Nutricath and Leadercath).

Central venous cannulas are always inserted under sterile conditions, ideally in the operating theatre. The operator scrubs up and wears a gown, mask and gloves. The patient's skin is prepared with antiseptic solution and draped with sterile towels. The precise method for insertion of each cannula unit is clearly described in the manufacturer's instructions, which must always be consulted.

Local anaesthetic is injected intradermally. Cannulation of the basilic vein is performed above the elbow skin crease to permit free use of the arm. In other respects the procedure is similar to peripheral venous cannulation. Cannulation of the internal jugular vein and subclavian vein is performed with the patient tipped 20° head-down to achieve adequate venous congestion. Preliminary test venepuncture with a 21- or 19-gauge needle identifies the vein with least risk of trauma to adjacent structures.

The *internal jugular vein* is best entered in the triangle between the sternal and clavicular heads of the sternocleidomastoid muscle (Fig. 41.3). The operator stands behind the patient's head, which is rotated a few degrees towards the opposite side. The cannula is introduced at the apex of the triangle at an angle of 45° to the skin. It is directed downwards parallel to the sagittal plane or up to 15° medially.

The *subclavian vein* is best entered by the infra-clavicular approach. The infraclavicular pulsation of the subclavian artery is defined with the left index finger. The cannula is introduced 5 mm medial to this point, just below the clavicle, and directed upwards at an angle of 45° to the

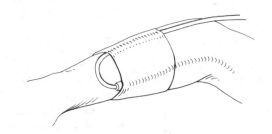

Fig. 41.2   Cannula and infusion tubing secured

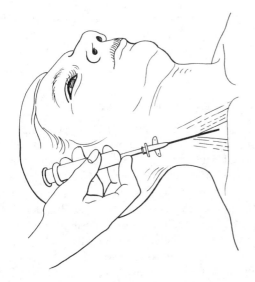

Fig. 41.3 Cannulation of the internal jugular vein. Note the triangle between the sternal and clavicular heads of the sternocleidomastoid muscle

sagittal plane, passing immediately below the clavicle and in front of the first rib to enter the subclavian vein at a depth of some 4–5 cm (Fig. 41.4).

Other approaches to the internal jugular vein and the subclavian vein are also possible. All approaches have the potential hazard of entering the pleural cavity. It is therefore essential to check the correct placement of the cannula in the venous system by a 'flowback' test. The infusion tubing set (previously primed with isotonic saline solution) is connected to the cannula. The infusion fluid bag is then lowered below the level of the patient and the infusion commenced. Blood flows retrogradely up the tubing. If this does not occur, the cannula is not in the venous system. The head-down position is now changed to horizontal and the fluid bag is raised above the patient. Free flow now occurs into the superior vena cava. A chest X-ray is taken to exclude pneumothorax and to visualize the tip of the cannula. It may need to be advanced or withdrawn. When a satisfactory position is obtained in the superior vena cava, the cannula is sutured to the skin to prevent accidental dislodgement. The skin puncture site is dabbed with antiseptic solution and covered with a sterile dressing.

Cannulas inserted for intravenous nutrition are tunnelled in the subcutaneous tissue to emerge on the chest wall at a distance from the site of entry into the vein (Fig. 41.5). This minimizes the risk of sepsis spreading down the tract direct into the vein.

Central venous pressure (CVP) manometry

To measure the central venous pressure, a three-way tap is placed in the infusion line so that a vertical limb of tubing can be used as a manometer reflecting the pressure within the great veins draining into the right atrium (Fig. 41.6).

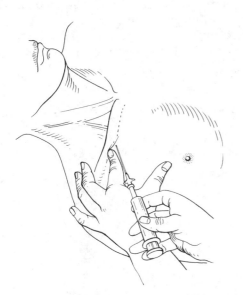

Fig. 41.4 Cannulation of the subclavian vein

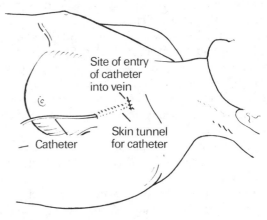

Site of entry
of catheter
into vein

Catheter

Skin tunnel
for catheter

Fig. 41.5 Skin tunnel for central venous catheter

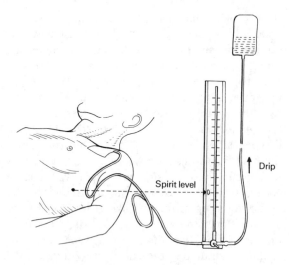

Fig. 41.6 Measurement of central venous pressure. Note the midthoracic point (marked by a black dot) which is used as the zero reference point

The patient is placed horizontal. The midthoracic point (the point at which the midaxillary line is intersected by a vertical plane from the sternal angle) is then defined and a spirit level is used to define the zero point on the manometer (see Fig. 41.6). Alternatively, the sternal angle itself can be used as a reference point; with the patient lying horizontal, the level of the sternal angle then corresponds to a reading of +5 cmH$_2$O on the manometer.

The three-way tap is turned first to allow fluid from the infusion set to fill the manometer to about 20–25 cmH$_2$O; it is then turned to allow fluid from the manometer to drain into the central venous cannula. The level of fluid in the vertical limb drops rapidly before stabilizing at a level which fluctuates by some 0.5–1.0 cmH$_2$O with inspiration and expiration. The lowest point of the meniscus on inspiration indicates the central venous pressure in centimetres of water above the midthoracic point. The normal range is 5–12 cmH$_2$O. As soon as the measurement is made, the three-way tap is turned to restore flow from the infusion set through the cannula. Sequential measurements must be made with the patient lying horizontal.

Low central venous pressure is corrected by rapid infusion of crystalloid, colloid or blood as appropriate and in sufficient volumes to restore the central venous pressure to the normal range. High central venous pressure indicates fluid overload and further intravenous infusions are strictly limited.

Venous cutdown cannulation

This procedure is rarely required. Even when it is impossible to cannulate a peripheral vein, it is seldom difficult for an experienced operator to cannulate the internal jugular vein or the subclavian vein. Only in shocked or very obese patients may this prove impossible. In such cases cutdown cannulation of the basilic vein at the elbow, the cephalic vein in the deltopectoral groove, or the long saphenous vein at the ankle or groin may be life-saving. Cutdown of the long saphenous vein at the groin or ankle should be regarded only as a temporary expedient in a grave emergency, as it is associated with the risk of deep venous thrombosis. Cephalic vein cutdown is gaining in popularity for the insertion of catheters for parenteral nutrition. It avoids the risk of pneumothorax.

Venous cutdown cannulation is performed under local anaesthesia and in sterile conditions. The skin is incised transversely over the chosen vein. The subcutaneous fat is opened with the points of dissection scissors. The vein is exposed and cleared all round over a length of 1 cm. The distal end of this segment is ligated with an absorbable ligature. The proximal end is elevated on a second absorbable ligature to prevent venous

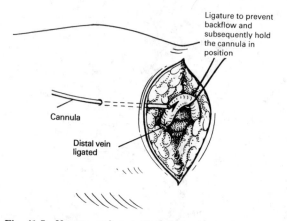

Fig. 41.7 Venous cutdown cannulation

backflow, and a transverse venotomy is made with a scalpel. The largest cannula that will fit the vein is introduced through the skin 2 cm below the incision and passed up the vein (Fig. 41.7). The proximal ligature is tied securely but without undue compression of the cannula. The infusion set is then connected to the cannula and the infusion commenced rapidly. The skin is closed with non-absorbable sutures and the cannula is sutured to the skin to prevent accidental dislodgement. Finally the wound and the skin puncture site are dabbed with antiseptic solution and covered with a sterile dressing.

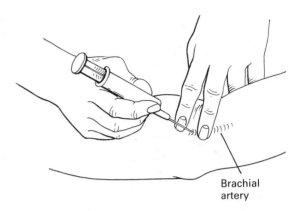

Brachial artery

Fig. 41.8 Brachial artery puncture

Arterial puncture

Arterial puncture is performed to measure the P_{aCO_2}, P_{aO_2}, pH and bicarbonate concentration or to monitor arterial pressure. The brachial artery at the elbow or the radial artery at the wrist are the sites of choice for arterial puncture. A 21-gauge needle and a pre-heparinized syringe containing a metal agitator are used. If the syringe is not pre-heparinized, 5000 units of heparin in 1 ml solution are drawn into the syringe. The plunger of the syringe is fully withdrawn and the air in the barrel and excess heparin are expelled. The residual heparin not only anticoagulates the blood but also lubricates the syringe.

The course of the artery is defined by palpation of its pulse between two fingers placed longitudinally 1 cm apart. The skin is cleaned with isopropyl alcohol. The needle is inserted at an angle of 45° to the skin, bevel upwards, and advanced directly into the artery (Fig. 41.8). Blood pulsates into the syringe under its own pressure; 4–5 ml is sufficient. The needle is withdrawn and an assistant applies firm pressure over the puncture site for 3 minutes to prevent haematoma formation. The needle is removed from the syringe and any small air bubbles are expelled through the nozzle before and a cap is applied. The syringe is gently inverted several times to heparinize the blood. The sample is sent immediately for analysis. If any delay is anticipated the syringe must be placed in ice.

To monitor arterial pressure, an indwelling cannula is inserted and connected to a manometer.

All used needles and cannulas must be placed, immediately after use, directly into a labelled receptacle, ideally one designed specifically for this purpose. The possibility of human immunodeficiency virus (HIV) infection from accidental needle stabs and of hepatitis B from small volumes of blood demands rigorous precautions.

INTUBATION, CATHETERIZATION AND ASPIRATION

Nasogastric intubation

The patient is asked to sit up for this procedure. If he or she is particularly apprehensive, the nostril may be anaesthetized with local anaesthetic spray. A size 14 Fr or 16 Fr radio-opaque tube is suitable for most adults but a size 18 Fr or 20 Fr tube is preferred for patients with intestinal obstruction. The tube is thoroughly lubricated with KY jelly and then passed into the nostril parallel to the hard palate and not in the direction of the external contour of the nose (Fig. 41.9). The patient breathes through the mouth and is encouraged to swallow as soon as the tube is felt at the back of the throat. The tube is gently advanced with each swallow and is readily passed into the stomach. Sips from a glass of water help those who find it difficult to swallow spontaneously.

The presence of the tube in the stomach is confirmed by blowing 20 ml air rapidly down it while auscultating over the stomach; a bubbling noise should be heard. Gastric contents are now aspirated with a syringe. The ideal length of tube

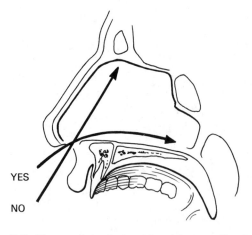

Fig. 41.9 Nasogastric intubation. Note the correct direction for inserting the tube

in the stomach is about 10–15 cm. The tube is therefore advanced to midway between the 50 and 60 cm marks and then secured firmly to the nose and cheek with adhesive tape.

Oesophageal tamponade

The Sengstaken tube is a gastric aspiration tube with inflatable gastric and oesophageal balloons, distension of which compresses the overlying oesophageal and high gastric veins. It is used for emergency treatment of bleeding oesophageal varices.

A modification, the Minnesota tube (Fig. 41.10), has an additional channel to allow the aspiration of saliva from the oesophagus above the level of the oesophageal balloon.

Before passing the tube, the oesophageal and gastric balloons are checked. It is also important that efficient suction apparatus is available. The nose is anaesthetized with local anaesthetic spray and the tube is thoroughly lubricated with local anaesthetic jelly. The tube is passed through the nose or mouth and into the back of the throat. As with routine nasogastric intubation, the patient is encouraged to swallow and the tube is gently advanced with each swallow. The procedure is, however, much more uncomfortable and few patients with bleeding varices are able to cooperate well with the operator. Coughing and spluttering is usually a sign that the tube is in the larynx and it must be withdrawn before further attempts are made to advance it.

The tube is passed so that the junction between the oesophageal and gastric balloon is 50 cm from the incisor teeth, and the gastric balloon is inflated

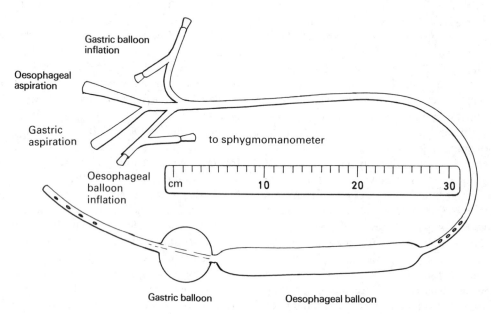

Fig. 41.10 Minnesota tube

with 30 ml Gastrografin. An X-ray is taken to confirm that the balloon is inflated in the stomach. The balloon is now filled with water to a total volume of 150 ml and then drawn back to impact at the cardia. An assistant holds the tube in this position with slight tension. The oesophageal balloon is inflated with air to a pressure between 30 and 40 mmHg, checked by attachment to a sphygmomanometer. A 5 cm cube of sponge rubber is secured around the tube as close to the nose as possible. The assistant now releases the tube and the sponge pulls back snugly against the nose. This ensures continuous 'fixed traction' on the tube with reliable compression of varices in the gastric fundus in addition to those in the oesophagus.

The stomach is aspirated regularly through the main lumen of the tube. The oesophagus cannot be aspirated with the Sengstaken tube and saliva starts to pool as soon as the oesophageal balloon is inflated. The patient is therefore nursed in a semi-prone position so that saliva can be spat out of the mouth. With the Minnesota tube these secretions can be aspirated.

It is essential to deflate the oesophageal balloon for 5–10 minutes every 6 hours to avoid the risk of ischaemic necrosis of the oesophageal mucosa. If possible, the pressure in the oesophageal balloon should be reduced to 25 mmHg after 12 hours. Normally the tube is not kept in position for more than 24 hours.

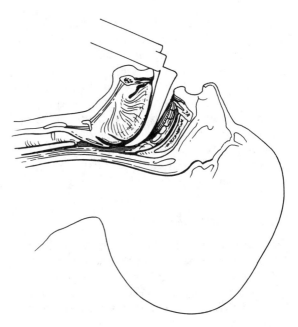

Fig. 41.11 Laryngoscope in position

Endotracheal intubation

The operator stands behind the patient's head. The patient's cervical spine is extended. Dentures are removed. Secretions or vomit are cleared from the mouth and pharynx by suction. An assistant presses on the cricoid cartilage to prevent reflux of oesophageal contents into the pharynx.

The Mackintosh laryngoscope is held in the left hand. The curved blade is passed down the right side of the tongue to engage its tip in the vallecula anterior to the epiglottis (Fig. 41.11). The assistant hooks a finger in the right angle of the mouth to improve the view while the laryngoscope is lifted vertically and the blade pulls the tongue and epiglottis forwards to expose the vocal cords (Fig. 41.12).

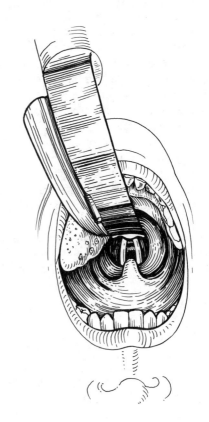

Fig. 41.12 Vocal cords displayed

A lubricated, cuffed endotracheal tube is passed under direct vision between the vocal cords and into the trachea. The average external diameter of suitable tubes is 9 mm for adult males and 8 mm for adult females. The cuff of the tube is inflated until an airtight seal is formed. The assistant discontinues cricoid pressure and the laryngoscope is removed. The endotracheal tube is connected to a re-breathing bag or a self-inflating 'Ambu-bag' and ventilation is started. The chest is observed and auscultated to confirm inflation of both lungs.

Urethral catheterization

Urethral catheters are inserted under sterile conditions. The operator scrubs up and wears a gown and gloves. The patient's skin is prepared with antiseptic solution and draped with sterile towels. All items that will be required are laid out on the sterile catheter tray.

For *males* a 14 or 16 Fr self-retaining Foley balloon catheter is used (Fig. 41.13). If the operator is right-handed, the penis is grasped with the left hand. Traction is applied down the shaft to retract the prepuce. All further manoeuvres are performed with the right hand. The glans and the inner aspect of the prepuce are prepared with antiseptic solution applied by a swab carried in forceps. The catheter is lubricated by drawing it across a large drop of sterile KY jelly on a gauze swab. The catheter is then placed in a sterile tray which is transferred to rest over the patient's thighs close to the penis. The penis is held vertically and the catheter is introduced using forceps (Fig. 41.14). When the catheter is in the bulbar urethra, the penis is directed towards the feet while traction is maintained, and the remainder of the catheter is inserted. Urine flows into the sterile tray. The left hand is released from the penis and

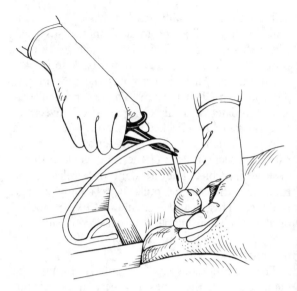

Fig. 41.14 Catheterization

used to steady the inflation limb for the catheter balloon while 10–20 ml water is injected. The catheter is gently withdrawn until the balloon engages at the bladder neck. The prepuce is drawn down over the glans to prevent paraphimosis.

The sterile drainage tube is fitted to the catheter and secured to the pyjama trousers to avoid traction directly on the catheter.

For *females* an 18 or 20 Fr self-retaining Foley balloon catheter is used. The labia minora are separated with the thumb and fingers of the left hand to expose the urethral meatus immediately anterior to the vagina. The pudenda is now swabbed with antiseptic solution. Two swabs are used, each being swept once across the pudenda from anterior to posterior and then discarded. The remainder of the procedure is performed in a similar fashion to catheterization in the male, although the catheter need only be inserted to half its length before the drainage tube is connected and the balloon is inflated.

Suprapubic catheterization

Suprapubic catheterization is indicated when urethral catheterization cannot be performed or is contraindicated. The bladder must be distended to at least midway between the pubic symphysis and the umbilicus. A 16 Fr Ingram trocar catheter

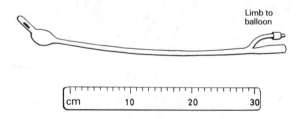

Limb to balloon

Fig. 41.13 Foley balloon catheter

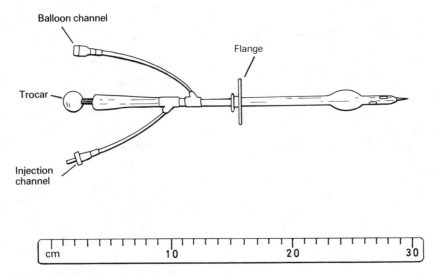

Fig. 41.15 Ingram trocar catheter

(Fig. 41.15) of the Foley type is used and the procedure is carried out under sterile conditions.

The operator scrubs up and wears a gown and gloves. The patient's skin is prepared with antiseptic solution and draped with sterile towels. Local anaesthetic is infiltrated at an angle of 70° through all layers of the midline of the abdominal wall two fingerbreadths above the pubic symphysis. The depth at which the bladder lumen is entered is then determined by aspiration with the syringe.

A small stab incision is then made in the skin with a scalpel. The shaft of the catheter is held firmly between left thumb and index finger some

4–5 cm higher than the estimated depth of the bladder lumen. This prevents 'overshoot' as the right hand thrusts the trocar and catheter through the abdominal wall (Fig. 41.16). The catheter is advanced fully with the left hand while the trocar is withdrawn simultaneously with the right hand. An assistant attaches the sterile drainage tube to the catheter. The catheter balloon is inflated with 5 ml water. The length of catheter within the bladder is adjusted so that the balloon is 2–3 cm away from the bladder wall. The snug-fitting flange is slid down the catheter to make contact with the skin and then sutured to it to prevent accidental displacement of the catheter.

Abdominal paracentesis

Abdominal paracentesis is performed to relieve the discomfort caused by abdominal distension with ascitic fluid or to obtain a specimen of ascitic fluid for cytological examination. The bladder must be emptied, if necessary by preliminary catheterization. A 'Trocath' peritoneal dialysis catheter (Fig. 41.17) with multiple side perforations over a length of 8 cm is used and inserted under sterile conditions. The operator scrubs up and wears a gown and gloves. Local anaesthetic is infiltrated at an angle of 70° through all layers of the abdominal wall. This can be done either in the midline one-

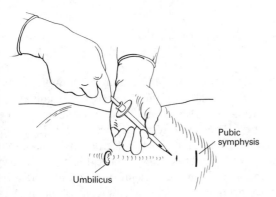

Fig. 41.16 Suprapubic catheterization

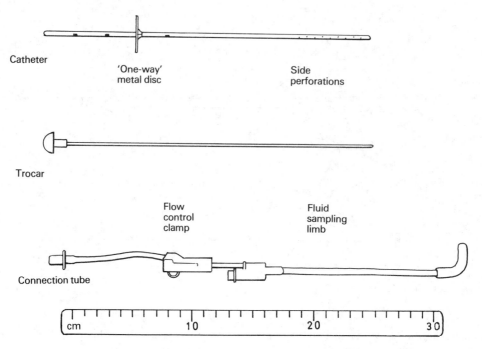

Fig. 41.17 'Trocath' peritoneal dialysis catheter

third of the way between the umbilicus and the pubic symphysis, or in the right or left iliac fossa at the junction of the outer to middle-third of a line from the anterior superior spine to the umbilicus. The depth at which the peritoneum is entered is then determined by aspiration with the syringe. The vicinity of scars should be avoided, as adhesions between scar and bowel increase the risk of puncture of the bowel.

A 3 mm stab incision is made in the skin with a scalpel. The trocar is introduced into the catheter and the shaft of the catheter is held firmly between left thumb and index finger some 4–5 cm higher than the estimated depth of the peritoneum. This prevents 'overshoot' as the right hand thrusts the trocar and catheter through the abdominal wall into the peritoneum (Fig. 41.18).

The catheter is now advanced further with the left hand while the trocar is withdrawn with the right hand. If any resistance is noted, the catheter is withdrawn 2–3 cm, rotated 180° and then advanced again. The minimum final length of catheter within the peritoneal cavity must be 10 cm. If this position is not obtained, the side

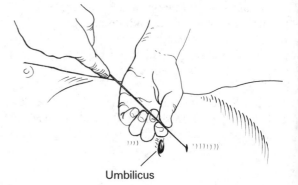

Umbilicus

Fig. 41.18 Insertion of peritoneal dialysis catheter

perforations of the catheter may come to lie within the abdominal wall and allow troublesome extravasation of ascitic fluid in the subcutaneous tissues. The one-way metal disc is slid down the catheter to make contact with the skin and secured to it with adhesive tape. The catheter is divided some 4 cm above the metal disc and attached via a connection tube with a flow control clamp to a sterile drainage bag.

Pleural aspiration

Pleural aspiration is performed to drain large pleural effusions. The procedure is carried out with the patient in the upright position, resting his elbows and forearms on a table. The seventh or eight intercostal space is identified and marked in the plane of the inferior angle of the scapula. Lower spaces are not suitable, as the diaphragm lies too close to the chest wall. The procedure is performed under sterile conditions. The operator scrubs up and wears a gown and gloves. The patient's skin is prepared with antiseptic solution and draped with sterile towels. Local anaesthetic is infiltrated through all layers of the chest wall at an angle of 70° downwards. The depth at which the pleural space is entered is determined by aspiration with the syringe. A 2 mm stab incision is made in the skin with a scalpel and a wide-bore needle with a central stilette is inserted at an oblique downward angle so that its tip comes to lie 0.5–1.0 cm within the pleural cavity. The needle is stabilized in this position by artery forceps, a needle guard or by the left thumb and index finger resting firmly against the skin. The patient is told to hold his breath for a few moments while the stilette is removed and the needle is connected to a 50 ml syringe with a three-way tap closing off the limb to a drainage tube (Fig. 41.19). The

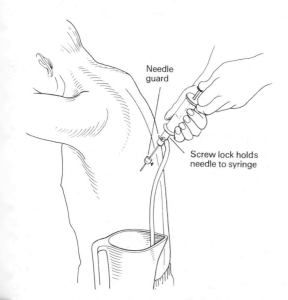

Fig. 41.19 Pleural aspiration. Note screw-lock on needle to maintain position

Needle guard

Screw lock holds needle to syringe

syringe is aspirated until full, the three-way tap is turned to close the limb to the aspiration needle, and the contents of the syringe are ejected via the drainage tube into a jug. The three-way tap is then turned to close the limb to the drainage tube and the cycle of aspiration and ejection is repeated. The procedure is stopped when the patient starts to cough (this is often the case after 1.0–1.5 litres has been removed) or when the aspiration is complete. The patient is told to hold his breath again for a few moments while the needle is withdrawn and the skin puncture site is covered with a sterile dressing.

An alternative, and to some a preferable method, is to insert a small drainage tube which is connected to an underwater sealed drainage system to which gentle suction is applied.

More accurate placement of the drain is possible by using ultrasound to guide the drain tube to the most dependent part of the pleural cavity, taking care to avoid the diaphragm.

Intercostal tube drainage

Intercostal intubation is performed to drain a large pneumothorax, haemothorax or pleural effusion. The second intercostal space in the midclavicular line is most suitable for a pneumothorax, while the ninth intercostal space in the posterior axillary line is preferred for drainage of a haemothorax. The procedure is carried out under sterile conditions using a 'Trocath' catheter. Sizes 20–26 Fr are suitable for adults, the larger sizes being essential for adequate drainage of blood. The operator scrubs up and wears a gown and gloves. Local anaesthetic is infiltrated widely at the chosen site. If a rib is encountered by the needle tip, the tip is 'walked' up the rib to enter the pleura above the rib edge. The depth at which the pleural space is entered is determined by aspiration with the syringe. A stab incision is made in the skin with a scalpel. The shaft of the catheter is held firmly between the left thumb and index finger some 3 cm higher than the estimated depth of the pleura. This prevents 'overshoot' as the right hand thrusts the trocar and catheter through the chest wall in the chosen interspace into the pleural cavity (Fig. 41.20).

The point of the trocar is directed towards the

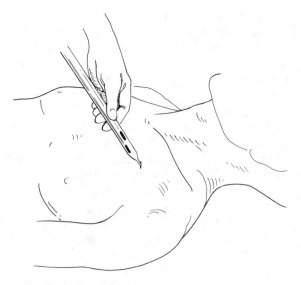

Fig. 41.20   Intercostal intubation with 'Trocath' catheter

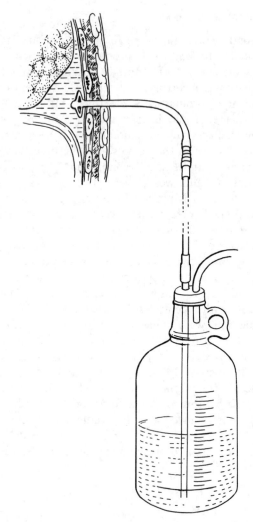

Fig. 41.21   Waterseal drainage bottle attached to Malecot catheter

apex of the pleural cavity. The catheter is then advanced with the left hand while the trocar is withdrawn with the right hand. The catheter is clamped with a heavy artery forceps and then sutured to the skin with a heavy suture to prevent accidental dislodgement. A 'Z' suture is placed loosely in the skin around the emerging catheter. The catheter is connected to a sterile drainage tube which emerges under a waterseal in a drainage bottle (Fig. 41.21). The artery forceps is removed from the catheter and the patient is asked to cough gently to expel much of the air or blood within the chest. The drainage bottle may then be connected to a suction apparatus to maintain a negative pressure of up to 30–40 mmHg and prevent loculation of air or fluid.

The catheter may be removed 12–24 hours after drainage has ceased and when chest X-ray confirms a well expanded lung. The patient is told to hold his breath for a few moments. An assistant presses the margins of the skin wound against the catheter. The 'Z' suture is held taut, the catheter is removed and the suture is tied firmly. A sterile dressing pad is applied over the sutured wound. A repeat chest X-ray is obtained to confirm that air has not entered the pleural cavity during removal of the catheter.

Lumbar puncture

Lumbar puncture is performed to obtain samples of cerebrospinal fluid or to insert therapeutic substances. The patient is asked to lie on the left side on a firm couch with the spine flexed and the knees drawn up to the abdomen. This position opens up the interspinous spaces. The right shoulder and right hip must lie vertically above the left shoulder and left hip. Lumbar puncture is performed under sterile conditions. The operator scrubs up and wears a gown and gloves.

The patient's skin is prepared with antiseptic solution and draped with sterile towels. The space between the spinous processes of the third and fourth lumbar vertebrae is identified at the point where the vertical line joining the highest points of the iliac crests crosses the spine. Local anaesthetic is injected as an intradermal 'bleb' and then infiltrated in this space to a depth of 2–3 cm. A lumbar puncture needle with a central stilette is inserted in the midline and aimed towards the umbilicus. At a depth of 3–4 cm the dura is pierced. A distinct drop in resistance to further passage of the needle confirms that it is in the subarachnoid space. The stilette is removed and cerebrospinal fluid drips out of the needle.

The needle is removed when the procedure is completed and the puncture site is covered with a sterile dressing. The patient must lie flat in bed for the next 24 hours. Severe headache is an indication that cerebrospinal fluid is leaking through the dura into the epidural space. This is managed by an epidural 'blood patch', a procedure best performed by an anaesthetist familiar with epidural anaesthetic techniques.

WOUND CLOSURE

The operator should practise the techniques of surgical knot tying first with heavy cord and then on patients undergoing elective surgery under general anaesthesia. Thereafter he may consider suturing minor superficial incised lacerations and only later progress to deeper or ragged lacerations. All wounds are thoroughly cleaned with antiseptic solution, and a generous volume of local anaesthetic is then infiltrated into the surrounding tissues. Lignocaine 1% is commonly used. The maximum dose for adults is 200 mg, so the volume is limited to 20 ml. If larger volumes are required, a more dilute solution may be used. Lignocaine with adrenaline may be preferred but must never be used on fingers, toes or penis, as vasoconstriction may cause ischaemic necrosis.

Wounds are sutured under as near sterile conditions as possible, although in busy casualty departments it is accepted that gowns are unnecessarily cumbersome and gloves alone will generally suffice. Once the local anaesthetic has become effective, the entire wound is inspected. Incised lacerations present few problems. The layers are usually easily defined and foreign body fragments are uncommon. Ragged lacerations are more difficult. The layers are sometimes difficult to define and foreign body fragments including grit, glass, clothing and hair are common. These are removed and the wound is irrigated with antiseptic solution or with hydrogen peroxide. The irregular margins of all damaged tissue layers are excised, leaving healthy regular tissue defects to be sutured. In the face, excision must be restricted to an absolute minimum.

In suturing any wound, the following principles must be observed.

1. Tissues should be handled gently. Rubbing wounds with swabs to remove blood should be avoided; swabs should be *pressed* on to the wound and blood allowed to soak into the swab, which is then removed.

2. Meticulous attention to haemostasis is essential.

3. Foreign material or devitalized tissue should be removed. Heavily contaminated wounds are best not sutured primarily but treated by delayed primary or secondary suture.

4. 'Dead' spaces in the wound should be closed with absorbable sutures (catgut or Dexon). If this is not possible, a drain or drains should be led from the dead space prior to closing more superficial layers. Alternatively, the wound may be left open and subsequently treated by secondary suture or by skin grafting.

5. Sutures should be tied just tight enough to approximate tissues without tension. Excessively tight sutures or the use of tension to approximate skin or deeper tissues causes ischaemia of the wound edges with delay in healing and an increased risk of wound infection.

Suturing the skin

Non-absorbable sutures (see below) are generally preferred for skin and require subsequent removal. Interrupted sutures are preferred and have the advantage over continuous sutures that, should the wound become infected, removal of one or two appropriately sited stitches may allow adequate drainage of the wound.

The sutures should be placed equidistant from one another, taking equal 'bites' on either side of the wound. A sufficient number of sutures should be inserted to maintain apposition of the skin edges without any gaping between sutures. More than this is unnecessary. The size of bite is determined by the amount of subcutaneous fat and by whether or not the subcutaneous fat has been separately sutured. In the abdomen the bite is approximately 5 mm on either side of the wound, whereas on the face a 1–2 mm bite is preferred. The wound edge is picked up with toothed dissecting forceps, and the needle is introduced through the skin at an angle as close to vertical as possible and brought out on the other side at a similar angle.

Similar principles apply when using a continuous suture.

A subcuticular stitch, inserted as a continuous suture, is preferred by some surgeons and has the advantage of avoiding the small pinpoint scars at the site of entry and exit of the traditional suture, or the ugly cross-hatching that results if sutures are tied too tightly or left in too long.

The following times are normally recommended for removal of sutures:

face and neck	4 days
scalp	7 days
abdomen and chest	7–10 days
limbs	7 days
feet	10–14 days

However, cosmetic results as good as those achieved by subcuticular suturing can be obtained by removing sutures in half the above times and replacing them by adhesive strips (e.g. Steristrip, Clearol).

Suture materials

Non-absorbable sutures

Non-absorbable sutures fall into three basic categories.

1. *Natural braided* (e.g. silk). This has good 'handling' qualities and knots easily and securely. It has the disadvantage of causing significant tissue reaction and is possibly associated with a higher rate of wound infection than synthetic materials.

2. *Synthetic monofilaments* (e.g. nylon, prolene). These sutures pass easily through tissues and cause little tissue reaction. They are, however, more difficult to handle than silk, and the knot is rather insecure so that multiple 'threads' are required to ensure security.

3. *Braided synthetics* (e.g. Mersiline, Ethibond, braided nylon). These sutures attempt to combine the virtues of both the above types while avoiding their disadvantages, and are now the preferred materials for skin closure, except for facial wounds, for which a monofilament suture is the material of choice.

Absorbable sutures

Absorbable sutures such as catgut (plain or chronic), Dexon, Vicryl and PDS are rarely used for skin closure except in circumcision, where removal of sutures may be uncomfortable for both patient and nurse. Absorbable sutures are also widely used for subcuticular skin closure.

Choice of suture gauge

Very fine sutures (4/0 or 5/0) are recommended for the face, neck, hands and digits. Elsewhere, sutures of 3/0 or 2/0 gauge are used. Sutures thicker than 2/0 are not necessary for skin.

Needles

Needles used in skin suture are cutting needles. Near the point they are triangular in cross-section, with one side of the triangle being longer than the other two. When inserting the needle, this longer side should be parallel to the wound edge.

The needles may be hand-held or used with a needle holder. Hand-held needles may be straight or curved, while those designed to be used with a needle holder (which are generally smaller) are always curved to varying degrees.

Other techniques of skin closure

Adhesive strips

Provided that the skin surface around the wound is flat, adhesive strips (Steristrips, Clearol) may be used instead of sutures. The cosmetic results are good. Such strips may be used to replace sutures after early removal.

Metal clips or staples

Metal clips (e.g. Michel clips) or staples are used by some surgeons, particularly on thyroid incisions, and are favoured by many gynaecologists. They give a good cosmetic result but have the disadvantage that they can catch easily on clothing, producing discomfort.

42. Medico-legal problems

Surgeons more than any other medical practitioners are confronted in everyday practice by potential medico-legal problems.

Consent to treatment

A doctor may not force recommendations on a patient. Treatment performed without consent may amount to assault and result in litigation. In every instance, the patient should be given as much information about proposed treatment as the doctor considers to be in his or her best interest. For minor procedures such as venepuncture verbal consent is adequate, but for operative procedures written consent must be obtained. The nature and purpose of the proposed operation are explained to the patient by a doctor. The patient is then asked to sign a consent form which the doctor countersigns. For patients under the age of 16 years, written informed consent of the parent or guardian is obtained.

If immediate treatment is necessary to save the patient's life, verbal consent is acceptable. When the patient's condition does not allow even this, the proposed treatment should be discussed with a near relative. If none is readily available, the patient should be given such treatment as the doctor considers necessary to preserve life and health.

In the UK, if a patient is compulsorily detained under the Mental Health Act, treatment immediately necessary to preserve life and health may be given without consent. For all other procedures, the informed written consent of the patient should be obtained before an operation is performed. If the patient is unable or unwilling to give his consent to a non-urgent operation, it should not be performed. If this prohibition jeopardizes the patient's health, the surgeon and psychiatrist should act in good faith and in the best interests of the patient.

Patients with mental illness who are not compulsorily detained under the Mental Health Act have exactly the same rights as ordinary patients.

Jehovah's Witnesses who consent to operation but refuse to consent to transfusion of blood or blood products place the surgeon in a dilemma. If the surgeon agrees to the limitations set by the patient, a conditional consent form prepared by one of the medical defence societies should be signed by the patient and countersigned by the surgeon and a witness.

The operation

Preoperative examination

Every patient about to have an operation under general anaesthesia must be examined preoperatively. The responsibility for this may rest with either the surgical staff or the anaesthetic staff. The declared policy of the individual surgical unit should be known to all staff working in it. The history should include a list of previous operations and previous anaesthetics (noting any untoward reactions to either), past history and a systematic enquiry including current drugs and known allergies. In addition to a full physical examination, urinalysis must always be performed. A full blood count and electrolyte estimation, chest X-ray and ECG are prudent for all but the shortest examinations under anaesthetic. The decision as to whether a patient is fit for anaesthesia and the proposed operation rests with the anaesthetist and the surgeon in consultation.

Premedication

Ideally, the premedication should be ordered directly by the anaesthetist. In many instances, however, local policy dictates that the surgical staff prescribe the premedication. The anaesthetist should be consulted if there is any doubt about the drug or the dose to be given.

Safeguards against wrong operations

Performing a wrong operation or operating on the wrong patient is both avoidable and indefensible. A series of safeguards to prevent these disasters has been recommended by the medical defence societies. These care summarized below.

1. All patients should wear identity bracelets including forenames, surname and hospital number. This is checked when the patient is sent to theatre. In paediatric wards the identity bracelet is of the type which cannot be removed by the child.

2. The operation list shows the patient's full name and hospital number. The nature of the operation is written in full, never abbreviated.

3. Patients are sent for by name and number by the senior nurse in the operating theatre.

4. The anaesthetist checks that the correct patient has been brought to the anaesthetic room.

5. The surgeon sees the patient and reviews the case notes before anaesthesia is commenced.

The following safeguards are recommended to prevent an operation on the wrong side, limb or digit.

1. The side to be operated on is marked by the surgeon with indelible ink before the patient comes to theatre.

2. The words 'right' and 'left' are written in full in the patient's notes and on the operation list.

3. To avoid ambiguity in describing digits, the fingers are described as thumb, index, middle, ring and little finger and the toes are described as great, second, third, fourth and little toe.

Discharge against medical advice

When a patient decides to discharge himself from hospital and the doctor feels that discharge is not in the best interest of the patient, the reasons for this advice are clearly explained. The patient is asked to sign a form which indicates that he is voluntarily taking his own discharge from hospital against the advice of his doctor. His signature on this form is witnessed by two persons. The general practitioner is informed about the patient's discharge from hospital, his condition and any further treatment which is considered advisable.

When the patient has a mental illness, the doctor may feel that there are grounds for compulsory detention under the Mental Health Act. The mental welfare officer is then contacted. If he agrees that detention under the Act is in the best interest of the patient or society, he will make application to the Court for formal admission to a mental hospital and compulsory detention.

Confirmation of death

It is the statutory duty of the doctor who has attended the deceased during his last illness to supply a death certificate to the Registrar of Deaths. Although a certificate may be issued if the body has not been seen after death, it is desirable that identification and examination are performed. The pupils are tested for reaction to light. The precordium is auscultated for heart sounds and the optic fundus is inspected with an ophthalmoscope for fragmentation of blood in the retinal vessels.

There are circumstances in which a death certificate should not be issued until the death has been reported to the coroner in England and Wales or the procurator-fiscal in Scotland. These include sudden death when the doctor has not seen the patient before or (in England and Wales) when a doctor has not attended the deceased within 14 days of death; death after trauma or neglect or in suspicious, unnatural or violent circumstances; death during an operation or before recovery from an anaesthetic; death within 24 hours of admission to hospital; and deaths about which complaints or litigation may be expected.

If the doctor is in any doubt about issuing a death certificate, he should discuss the matter first with the coroner or procurator-fiscal.

Cremation

Before a cremation may take place, two medical

certificates are required: Forms B and C. Form B is completed by the usual medical attendant of the deceased or the doctor signing the death certificate. Form C is completed by a medical practitioner of at least five years' standing who is neither a relative of the deceased nor a partner of the doctor completing Form B. A fee is payable for each certificate.

Removal of tissues for transplantation

Under the Human Tissues Act of 1961, a registered doctor who is satisfied that life is extinct may remove the required organ for transplantation provided either the deceased has requested in writing or orally in front of two witnesses that his body be used for therapeutic purposes, medical education or research, or the person in possession of the body is satisfied that the deceased expressed no objection and the next of kin have no objection to removal of tissues for transplantation.

The increasing use of life-support systems to maintain respiratory function in patients with severe head injury or spontaneous intracerebral catastrophe has resulted in the definition of stringent criteria of 'brain death'. When these criteria have been confirmed independently by two senior doctors, withdrawal of the life-support system may be considered after discussion with the patient's next of kin. Members of transplant teams should not be involved in these decisions. If the relatives are favourably disposed towards tissue transplantation, organs may be removed before the life-support system is disconnected.

Clinical research

Clinical research presents moral and ethical problems rather than legal ones. Proposed research projects should be presented in detail to the Hospital Ethical Committee. Approval may be expected when the research project has a direct bearing on the illness for which the patient is being treated and does not involve additional invasive or painful investigations. Ethical criteria are stricter when the research project may contribute to the advancement of knowledge but is of no immediate benefit to the patient. Nevertheless, approval is usually given provided there is no unnecessary

pain and no risk to the patient's health or well-being. If ethical doubt persists, the matter is referred to a medical defence society.

Informed verbal consent is always obtained from the patient and obtaining written consent is prudent in all but the simplest projects.

Laboratory requests and reports

Great care must be taken in labelling and completing all laboratory request forms and in labelling specimen containers. Inappropriate advice may result from incorrect information on the request forms, incorrect or insufficient samples, or by sending the request form for one patient with the specimen from another. The greatest potential hazard is in blood transfusion, where labelling errors may result in a fatal incompatible blood transfusion. Before blood transfusion is commenced, the patient's name, hospital number, date of birth, blood group and serial number on each unit of blood are checked, at the patient's bedside, on both the laboratory form and the blood bag label to ensure that they correspond. This is confirmed by a second observer.

Laboratory reports must be scrutinized and acted upon without undue delay, and individual surgical units must define policies to ensure that important information is not overlooked. Important outstanding reports may be available by telephone from laboratories at certain times and so permit earlier treatment of critically ill patients than would be possible by awaiting the 'routine' arrival of the written report. Such communications should be made directly to the ward doctor or written in a book specially kept for this purpose.

Confidentiality

The professional relationship between a doctor and his patient is based on the understanding that information which is given to the doctor in his professional capacity is confidential. There are, however, instances in which a breach of professional secrecy is justified. In Court, a doctor may be directed to divulge information. He may request that this information is disclosed in writing but, if this is overruled, failure to comply risks prosecution for contempt of court. Professional secrecy may also be breached when a doctor feels he has a duty to protect the patient or an innocent third party from avoidable harm. There are three common situations in which this problem arises.

1. *Fitness to drive a motor. vehicle.* If, for example, a patient is subject to fainting or fits or to a lack of motor coordination which will impair his ability to drive safely, efforts should be made to persuade him to notify the licensing authority. The introduction of the driving licence valid until the 70th birthday has placed a great burden of responsibility on the driver to report any disability and an equal burden of responsibility on the doctor to persuade him to do so. If the patient does not agree to divulge the information himself, it is considered ethical for the doctor to disclose it to the licensing authority.

2. *Non-accidental injury to children.* When a doctor suspects he is dealing with non-accidental injury to a child, it is considered ethical to disclose confidential information. Health authorities should be able to investigate actual or possible cases of non-accidental injury to children. If this service is not available, the children's officer of the local authority, or the officers of the National Society for the Prevention of Cruelty to Children, are appropriate persons to inform. The doctor should advise the parents that it is in the interests of the child to disclose clinical information to the appropriate authority and that it is preferable to do so with their agreement.

3. *Police investigation of a crime.* A doctor may be asked to divulge information given in confidence. Only if it clearly appears to be in the interests of public safety to do so, should the information be given. In doubtful cases, the prudent doctor will consult his Defence Society.

In all other circumstances, requests for confidential information should be denied unless the patient has given informed written consent.

Notifiable diseases

All doctors must remember that certain diseases are by statute notifiable to health authorities. Those which may be encountered in surgical wards include anthrax, dysentery, erysipilas, tuberculosis and infective enteritis.

All cases of diarrhoea of undetermined cause, of gas gangrene and clostridial wound infections, and of suspected serum hepatitis should be reported to the hospital infection officer without delay, as should any unusual 'runs' of wound or other infections in the ward.

At present, testing for HIV (human immunodeficiency virus) antibody can only be performed if the patient gives his informed consent.

The police

There are frequent occasions in surgical practice when the doctor comes into contact with the police. Even when the police are acting in the interests of the patient, information should only be disclosed with the consent of the patient. As has been stated previously, the doctor may be faced with difficult decisions when the police are investigating a crime allegedly committed by the patient. The duty of the doctor in possession of information which might assist the police in their pursuit of a criminal is not clear in law and must be left to individual conscience and judgement. In most circumstances the doctor will seek guidance from his defence society before divulging to the police any information received in professional confidence. However, when the nature of the crime is extreme or the potential dangers to society are great, the doctor may feel that these factors take precedence over the rules of professional secrecy.

When an inpatient is in police custody, it is usual for a police officer to remain with him during his stay in hospital. When there is no accompanying police officer, the police may request information about the time of discharge of the patient from hospital and this should be given. When a patient is brought to hospital after a road traffic accident, the question of driving under the influence of alcohol frequently arises. The police may request a blood sample for blood alcohol analysis. The doctor in charge should satisfy himself that neither the request for the sample nor the actual taking of it will be prejudicial to the patient's condition. The sample should not be taken by the hospital staff but by a police surgeon. Blood taken by a hospital doctor from an unconscious patient as part of the routine admission investigations should not be made available to the police. If requested, it may be preserved in the hospital and released later if the patient or his legal representative consent.

Court appearance

Most doctors will at some time be required to appear in court. For the junior doctor this will usually be as a witness to fact if he has been involved in the care of the patient in the case. For the senior doctor it will usually be as an expert witness whose specialized knowledge is such that he is called solely to express his opinion.

Legible and comprehensive notes (see below) must be made when treating any patient, not just those whose case is likely to result in legal proceedings. They must be referred to before appearance so that a clear knowledge of the facts is available.

Divulgence of professional confidence in Court is discussed on p. 691.

Clinical records

The importance of accurate and legible clinical records in hospital practice cannot be overemphasized. Complaints against hospital doctors frequently allege that clinical examinations have been omitted or have been cursory. Claims that inappropriate treatment has been given are less common. Oral evidence to refute this is more likely to impress the court if it is backed up by a contemporary entry in the clinical notes. It should be remembered that in the event of a complaint against a doctor, a court may require the case records to be examined by the medical advisors of the complainant. Facetious or rude entries should never be made in case notes.

The Data Protection Act (1984) allows any patient access to data about him- or herself. If requested, a copy of the data and an interpretation must be provided. Exemptions to this access exist but have yet to be tested in Court.

Case notes remain the property of the Secretary of State but, as indicated above, there are occasions when a court may order compulsory disclosure of clinical notes. In such instances the applicant issues a summons to the doctor or hospital accompanied by written evidence to justify the application. The doctor or hospital may then request a hearing at which the arguments for and against the production of case notes are heard. If the court orders the production of the case notes, they are disclosed to the applicant's medical advisors only and not to his legal advisors or to the applicant himself. Whenever such applications are made, the doctor should seek advice from his defence society immediately.

Professional negligence

Negligence may be defined as a failure to display the competence and to exercise the care which might reasonably be expected of the doctor and which results in damage to the patient. Two common examples which affect junior hospital doctors are prescribing an antibiotic for a patient who is known to be hypersensitive to it and failing to X-ray a patient in whom there is clinical doubt about bone injury. More obvious examples of negligence are operation on the wrong patient, limb or digit.

When a letter of complaint is received from a patient or his lawyer, the case notes should be carefully perused and a factual report about the case made. Copies are sent first to the doctor's defence society and to the hospital legal advisor. A further copy is retained by the doctor. All correspondence including the letters of complaint, threats of proceedings or claims for compensation are forwarded to the defence society. If the incident involved an instrument, needle, swab or foreign body, this should be retained where possible.

Index